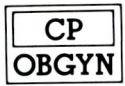 Clinical Perspectives in Obstetrics and Gynecology

Series Editor:

Herbert J. Buchsbaum, M.D.

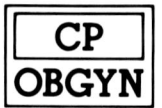 Clinical Perspectives in Obstetrics and Gynecology

perspective *noun:* . . . the capacity to view subjects in their true relations or relative importance.

Each volume in Clinical Perspectives in Obstetrics and Gynecology will cover in depth a major clinical area in the health care of women. The objective is to present to the reader the pathophysiologic and biochemical basis of the condition under discussion, and to provide a scientific basis for clinical management. These volumes are not intended as "how to" books, but as a ready reference by authorities in the field.

Though the obstetrician and gynecologist may be the primary provider of health care for the female, this role is shared with family practitioners, pediatricians, medical and surgical specialists, and geriatricians. It is to all these physicians that the series is addressed.

Series Editor: Herbert J. Buchsbaum, M.D.

Published Volume:
Buchsbaum: *The Menopause*

Forthcoming Volumes:
Futterweit: *Polycystic Ovarian Disease*
Lavery and Sanfilippo: *Pediatric and Adolescent Obstetrics and Gynecology*
Galask: *Infectious Disease in the Female Patient*
Lifshitz: *Strategies in Surgical Gynecology*

Infertility

Diagnosis and Management

Edited by

James Aiman

Associate Professor
Department of Gynecology and Obstetrics
Director, Section of Reproductive Endocrinology
The Medical College of Wisconsin

With 52 halftone and 84 line illustrations.

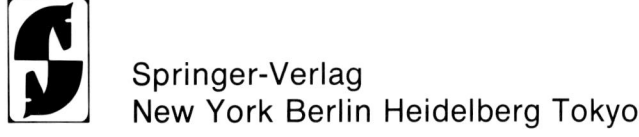

Springer-Verlag
New York Berlin Heidelberg Tokyo

Editor

James Aiman, M.D., Department of Gynecology and Obstetrics, Section of Reproductive Endocrinology, The Medical College of Wisconsin, 8700 West Wisconsin Avenue, Milwaukee, Wisconsin 53226, U.S.A.

Series Editor

Herbert J. Buchsbaum, M.D., Department of Obstetrics and Gynecology, University of Texas Health Science Center at Dallas, 5323 Harry Hines Boulevard, Dallas, Texas 75235, U.S.A.

Library of Congress Cataloging in Publication Data
Main entry under title:

Infertility, diagnosis and management.

(Clinical perspectives in obstetrics and gynecology)
Bibliography: p.
Includes index.
1. Infertility—Addresses, essays, lectures. I. Aiman, James. II. Series. [DNLM: 1. Infertility—Diagnosis. 2. Infertility—Therapy. WP 570 I437]
RC889.I562   1984   616.6'92   83-20395

© 1984 by Springer-Verlag New York Inc.

All rights reserved. No part of this book may be translated or reproduced in any form without written permission from Springer-Verlag, 175 Fifth Avenue, New York, New York 10010, U.S.A.
The use of general descriptive names, trade names, trademarks, etc., in this publication, even if the former are not especially identified, is not to be taken as a sign that such names, as understood by the Trade Marks and Merchandise Marks Act, may accordingly be used freely by anyone.

While the advice and information of this book is believed to be true and accurate at the date of going to press, neither the authors nor the editors nor the publisher can accept any legal responsibility for any errors or omissions that may be made. The publisher makes no warranty, express or implied, with respect to material contained herein.

Media conversion and composition by Bi-Comp, Inc., York, Pennsylvania, U.S.A.
Printed and bound by Halliday Lithograph, West Hanover, Massachusetts, U.S.A.
Printed in the United States of America.

9 8 7 6 5 4 3 2 1

ISBN 0-387-90940-0 Springer-Verlag New York Berlin Heidelberg Tokyo
ISBN 3-540-90940-0 Springer-Verlag Berlin Heidelberg New York Tokyo

To Joannie, Dan, and Pat

Contents

	Preface	ix
	Contributors	xi
1	A History of Human Fertility *James Aiman*	1
2	The Psychology of Infertility *Barbara Eck Menning*	17
3	The Hypothalamus: Physiology and Pathophysiology *G. William Bates*	31
4	The Pituitary: Physiology and Disorders in Infertile Women *Douglas C. Daly, Daniel H. Riddick*	51
5	The Normal Menstrual Cycle *G. Rodney Meeks*	83
6	Anovulation and Ovulation Induction *Mary G. Hammond*	101
7	The Cervix in Reproduction *Gilbert G. Haas Jr., Phillip C. Galle*	123
8	Uterine Function and Abnormalities Causing Infertility *G. William Bates, Winfred L. Wiser*	143
9	The Fallopian Tube: Physiology and Pathology *Carlton A. Eddy*	161
10	Male Reproductive Physiology *Ronald S. Swerdloff, Shalender Bhasin*	177
11	Male Infertility: Diagnosis and Medical Management *Rebecca Z. Sokol, Ronald S. Swerdloff*	185
12	The Surgical Management of Male Infertility *Howard Frey, Jacob Rajfer*	199
13	Extracorporeal Fertilization and Embryo Transfer *Anibal A. Acosta, Jairo E. Garcia*	215

14	Environmental Factors in Infertility	231
	A. F. Haney	
15	Habitual Abortion	247
	Barry E. Schwarz	
16	Endometriosis	255
	Lewis Russell Malinak, James M. Wheeler	
17	Artificial Insemination	277
	James Aiman	
18	Reproductive Performance of Previously Infertile Couples	289
	Richard J. Worley, William R. Keye Jr.	
19	Primary Amenorrhea	303
	James Aiman	
20	Adoption	329
	Mary Reistroffer	
21	The Ethics of Reproductive Intervention	337
	Dennis J. Doherty	
22	Legal Issues in Reproduction	345
	Peggy A. Hardwick	
	Index	359

Preface

The authors of this book have a goal—to describe the management of infertility from the perspective of physiology and anatomy gone awry. To accomplish this goal, the chapters devoted to the causes of infertility begin with a description of the normal structure and function of the organ or system causing the infertility. We believe that understanding the normal will result in rational and effective diagnosis and treatment of infertility. Our intent is that this book be a useful resource for those who care for infertile couples.

For an infertile couple, success is the delivery of a normal and healthy infant. Chapters that describe the causes and treatment of habitual abortion and the reproductive performance of previously infertile couples emphasize the hazards that exist between conception and birth. Our environment is one of these hazards, one that may also affect reproduction before conception. A chapter is devoted to a description of environmental agents that affect reproduction, the mechanisms of their effect, and methods to predict those present and future environmental agents which might also affect reproduction.

We have a second, equally important, goal—to stress that infertility is an intensely personal problem, yet a subject of societal and cultural significance. The importance of this dimension is emphasized in the chapters describing the history of human fertility, the psychology of infertility, adoption, ethics, and the legal issues in reproduction. The myths of reproduction reflect our need to understand the mechanisms of our fertility and the causes of infertility. Symbols of fertility are abundant in art and literature; artists express a concern for human fertility as eloquently as the scientists who define the mechanisms of reproduction and the physicians who care for infertile couples. The response of a couple to their infertility is also symbolic—of their grief for a child that never was. Understanding the psychology of infertility is as important as recognizing the physical cause because the psychologic dimension can affect a couple's response to their medical management.

Whether ethics and legislation concerning reproduction constrain or guide us in the care of infertile couples is irrelevant. Pertinent is the fact that society exerts its will and expresses its dictates by ethical formulations and statutes. Understanding the ethical and legal dimension of reproduction provides an effective framework in which to manage the physical dimension of infertility.

The contributing authors are expert in the care of infertile couples and possess an ability to teach with the written word. All have written lucid descriptions of subjects of their special interest. Others also have helped in the preparation of this book. Dr. Herbert Buchsbaum, the Series Editor of *Clinical Perspectives in Obstetrics and Gynecology*, advised and encouraged me during the planning and implementation of this book. The staff of Springer-Verlag helped to make the preparation of this book a pleasant and rewarding endeavor.

James Aiman

Contributors

Anibal A. Acosta, M.D.
Professor of Obstetrics and Gynecology, Eastern Virginia Medical Center, Norfolk, Virginia, U.S.A.

James Aiman, M.D.
Associate Professor of Gynecology and Obstetrics; Director, Section of Reproductive Endocrinology, Medical College of Wisconsin, Milwaukee, Wisconsin, U.S.A.

G. William Bates, M.D.
Professor, Department of Obstetrics and Gynecology, University of Mississippi Medical Center, Jackson, Mississippi, U.S.A.

Shalender Bhasin, M.D.
Assistant Professor of Medicine, Department of Medicine, University of California, Los Angeles School of Medicine, Harbor-UCLA Medical Center, Torrance, California, U.S.A.

Douglas C. Daly, M.D.
Assistant Professor of Obstetrics and Gynecology; Director, In Vitro Fertilization Unit, University of Massachusetts School of Medicine, Worcester, Massachusetts, U.S.A.

Dennis J. Doherty, PH.D.
Acting Director, Regional Center for the Study of Bioethics, Medical College of Wisconsin; Visiting Professor of Medical Ethics, Department of Neurology, Medical College of Wisconsin; Associate Professor of Christian Ethics, Department of Theology, Marquette University, Milwaukee, Wisconsin, U.S.A.

Carlton A. Eddy, PH.D.
Associate Professor, Department of Obstetrics and Gynecology; Director of Reproductive Research, University of Texas Health Science Center, San Antonio, Texas, U.S.A.

Howard L. Frey, M.D.
Adjunct Assistant Professor of Surgery/Urology, University of California, School of Medicine, Los Angeles, California, U.S.A.

Phillip C. Galle, M.D.
Assistant Professor, Department of Obstetrics and Gynecology, Medical College of Georgia, Augusta, Georgia, U.S.A.

Jairo E. Garcia, M.D.
Assistant Professor, Department of Obstetrics and Gynecology, Eastern Virginia Medical School, Norfolk, Virginia, U.S.A.

Gilbert G. Haas, Jr., M.D.
Associate Professor of Obstetrics and Gynecology; Director, Section of Reproductive Endocrinology and Infertility, University of Oklahoma Health Science Center, Oklahoma City, Oklahoma, U.S.A.

Mary G. Hammond, M.D.
Assistant Professor of Obstetrics and Gynecology, University of North Carolina, School of Medicine, Chapel Hill, North Carolina, U.S.A.

A. F. Haney, M.D.
Associate Professor of Obstetrics and Gynecology; Director, Division of Reproductive Endocrinology and Infertility, Duke University Medical Center, Durham, North Carolina, U.S.A.

Peggy A. Hardwick
University of New Mexico Law School, Albuquerque, New Mexico, U.S.A.

William R. Keye, Jr., M.D.
Assistant Professor of Obstetrics and Gynecology; Head, Division of Reproductive Endocrinology and Infertility, University of Utah, School of Medicine, Salt Lake City, Utah, U.S.A.

Lewis Russell Malinak, M.D.
Professor, Department of Obstetrics and Gynecology, Baylor College of Medicine, Houston, Texas, U.S.A.

Barbara Eck Menning, M.S.N., M.P.H.
Founder and Director of RESOLVE, Inc. from 1973–1982; Continuing Care Coordinator, Sancta Maria Hospital, Cambridge, Massachusetts, U.S.A.

G. Rodney Meeks, M.D.
Assistant Professor of Obstetrics and Gynecology, University of Mississippi Medical Center, Jackson, Mississippi, U.S.A.

Jacob Rajfer, M.D.
Associate Professor, Department of Surgery, Division of Urology, University of California Medical Center, Los Angeles, California, U.S.A.

Mary Reistroffer, M.S.W.
Professor of Social Work, University of Wisconsin-Extension, Milwaukee, Wisconsin, U.S.A.

Daniel H. Riddick, M.D., PH.D.
Professor of Obstetrics and Gynecology, Director of Reproductive Endocrinology and Infertility; Coordinator, Resident Education, University of Connecticut Health Center, Farmington, Connecticut, U.S.A.

Barry E. Schwarz, M.D.
Associate Professor and Vice-Chairman, Department of Obstetrics and Gynecology, The University of Texas Southwestern Medical School at Dallas, Dallas, Texas, U.S.A.

Rebecca Z. Sokol, M.D.
Assistant Professor of Medicine, UCLA School of Medicine; Associate Director, Male Reproductive Research Center, Harbor General Hospital, Torrance, California, U.S.A.

Ronald S. Swerdloff, M.D.
Professor of Medicine, UCLA School of Medicine; Chief, Division of Endocrinology, Harbor-UCLA Medical Center, Torrance, California, U.S.A.

James M. Wheeler, M.D.
Resident, Department of Obstetrics and Gynecology, Baylor College of Medicine, Houston, Texas, U.S.A.

Winfred L. Wiser, M.D.
Professor and Chairman, Department of Obstetrics and Gynecology, University of Mississippi School of Medicine, Jackson, Mississippi, U.S.A.

Richard J. Worley, M.D.
Associate Professor and Vice-Chairman, Department of Obstetrics and Gynecology, University of Utah School of Medicine, Salt Lake City, Utah, U.S.A.

A History of Human Fertility

James Aiman

The Ice Age

Fifty-thousand years ago a man died and was buried in the Shanidar cave in the Zagros mountains of Iraq. His family and fellow tribesmen went into the surrounding fields and gathered flowers to lay at his grave. This documented act of deliberate burial reveals a sense of compassion in a group of nomads who chose to delay their journey long enough to honor a dead companion.

To begin a history of human fertility with a story of death is not unusual since death and birth are each a part of the human experience. It is from the perspective of man's concern for his fertility and mortality exemplified in this ritual burial that a history of human fertility can begin.

In that time our ancestors lived a nomadic existence. They sustained themselves by hunting—a way of life forced on them as the only means of survival in a hostile, Ice Age environment. Out of this hunting existence there developed three important effects: the establishment of a base camp (which set the precedent for future villages), the division of labor, and the need for cooperation. A natural consequence of this spirit of cooperation was the compassion shown this man who died 50,000 years ago.

During the Ice Age, our ancestors were forced to depend on animals for food, clothing, and even weapons. Edible plants were a transitory source of food found only beyond the boundaries of the constantly advancing and receding ice. The rigors of hunting on the edge of ice also changed the strategy of hunting. A lone man could not stalk his prey as well as a group of hunters, so cooperation was necessary to assure survival. Our ancestors learned to follow herds, to anticipate their actions, and, ultimately, to adopt their habits, including their migration. Survival in this time was precarious and few could expect to live to 30 years. Without understanding the biologic process of procreation, Ice Age man must have understood the necessity to nurture their young for the tribe would pass out of existence unless the number of hunters was maintained. So children were protected and women were esteemed as essential members of their tribe—in part for their unique ability to bear children, but also because they performed vital functions in the early division of labor.

The art of man is a reflection of his concerns and early symbols of fertility appear at this time. Even 25,000 years ago the breast and the pelvis of women were associated with fertility and these parts are prominent in the Venus of Willendorf (Fig. 1–1).

The Ice Age ended in 10,000 B.C. Wild grasses became abundant and our ancestors learned to supplement their diet by harvesting these grasses. In 8,000 B.C. a wild form of wheat, which had 14 chromosomes, hybridized with a natural goat grass, which also had 14 chromosomes. The result of this union was a fertile hybrid of 28 chromosomes: Emmer wheat. Its seeds were plumper but they still were sown by scattering in the wind. A second genetic accident then occurred—Emmer wheat combined with another goat grass and

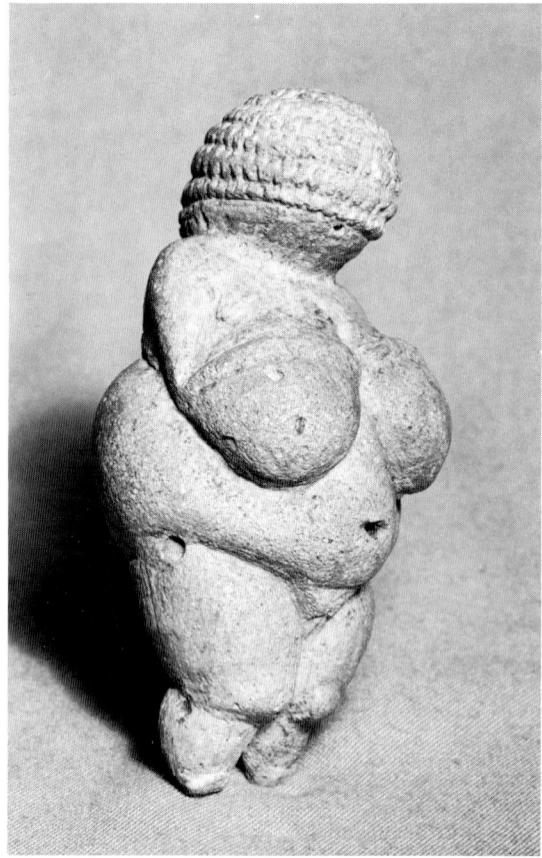

Fig. 1–1. Venus of Willendorf. A 4.5-inch limestone statuette sculpted about 25,000 B.C. (Found in Willendorf, Austria in 1908. Naturhistorisches Museum, Vienna.)

the resulting hybrid, now with 42 chromosomes, became bread wheat, which is fertile because of a specific gene mutation. The ears of bread wheat are heavier and the husks are sturdier. If the husks are broken, the chaff scatters in the wind but the seeds drop to the ground. Now man learned to sow the seeds in the spring and reap the harvest in the fall. This is perhaps the most profound change in human history, for our ancestors' existence changed from the nomadic hunter to the stationary farmer. It is from this time that recorded history begins and we can know more directly our ancestors' beliefs regarding their fertility.

Ancient Riverine Civilizations

The first great civilizations were nurtured in the fertile valleys of four rivers: the Nile in Egypt, the Tigris and Euphrates in Mesopotamia, and the Indus in northern India. In Egypt, wheat and barley became the basis of a pregnancy test.

> Put wheat and barley seeds into separate cloth purses and tell the woman to pass her water on it every day . . . If both sprout she will give birth . . . If they do not sprout she will not give birth at all.
> Egypt
> 3000 B.C.

This ancient obstetrician further suggested that if the wheat sprouted first, the child would be a boy, but if the barley sprouted before the wheat, then the child would be a girl. This concern for sex prediction and sex selection occurs in all times, even in the present. In addition to the diagnosis of pregnancy, ancient Egyptian physicians also suggested a means of evaluating an infertile woman.

> To distinguish her who shall conceive from her who will not conceive, pour thou fresh oil . . . examine her.
> Kahun papyrus
> ca. 2000 B.C.

The Kahun papyrus was one of several devoted to medicine. The Ebers papyrus discussed methods to diagnose amenorrhea, treat threatened abortion, and cure gonorrhea. In the Brugsch or Berlin papyrus, the augmented cardiac output in pregnancy was recognized by the prominent pulse of a gravid woman.

By 1000 B.C., the Egyptian sage Ani was advocating marriage as the most expedient means of bearing and rearing children in an ordered society.

> Marry a wife when you are young, she will bring your son into the world. Let her give birth for you while you are young. It is wise to make children; happy the man whose family is numerous.
> *Maxims of Ani*
> Egypt, 1000 B.C.

While Egyptian civilization was born and nurtured along the banks of the Nile river, another great civilization began in the fertile crescent between the Tigris and Euphrates rivers. Our ancestors in Mesopotamia were also concerned with their fertility and worshipped goddesses to assure their ability to procreate (Fig. 1–2).

Fig. 1–2. Fertility goddess. Clay figurine carved about 6000 B.C. (Oriental Institute, University of Chicago.)

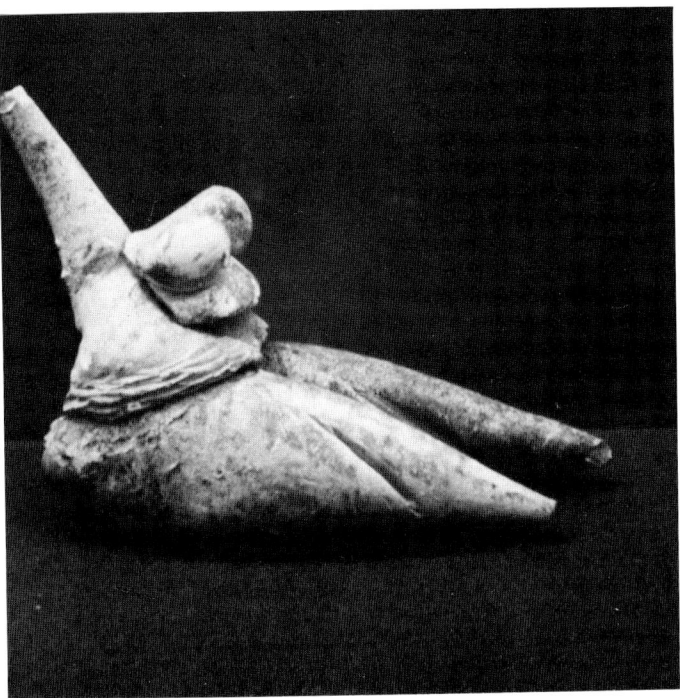

This neolithic goddess of fertility was carved in stone about 6000 B.C. and was found near Kermanshah, Iran. The head, arms, and feet may have been lost over the last 8,000 years, but perhaps this ancient artist never added these parts to emphasize the breasts and pelvis—symbols of fertility.

In this time, Hammurabi constructed a set of 286 laws that defined and legislated human interaction in a growing society. Among his laws, Hammurabi fixed the penalty for causing an abortion.

> If a man has struck a free woman with child, and has caused her to miscarry, he shall pay 10 shekels for her miscarriage. If that woman die, his daughter shall be killed.
> Hammurabi
> 2000 B.C.

The penalty for inflicting testicular damage was equally harsh and severe.

> If a woman has crushed a man's testicle in an affray, one of her fingers shall be cut off. And if, although a physician has bound it up, the second testicle is affected with it and becomes inflamed, both her nipples shall be torn off.
> Hammurabi
> 2000 B.C.

This code contains an implicit recognition of the role of the testis in reproduction. No similar penalty exists for injury to any other part of a man's anatomy. In this law, an immune mechanism causing infertility was also implied. That is, injury to one testis could lead to damage of the second. This particular code of Hammurabi bears a striking resemblance to a Jewish law in the book of Deuteronomy.

> When men fight with one another, and the wife of the one draws near to rescue her husband from the hand of him who is beating him, and puts out her hand and seizes him by the private parts, then you shall cut off her hand.
> Deuteronomy 25:11–12

The ancient Babylonians, like their Egyptian neighbors to the west, had a formula for a pregnancy test.

> To know a woman who will bear from a woman who will not bear: Watermelon pounded and bottled with the milk of a woman who has born a male child; make it into a dose. To be swallowed by the woman. If she vomits, she will bear. If she belches, she will never bear.
> Babylon
> ca. 1200 B.C.

Restriction of the milk for this formula to mothers who bore male children probably indicates this person's bias toward male offspring.

East of the fertile crescent of Mesopotamia, there developed a third great civilization along the Indus river of northern India. In each of these early civilizations there developed a creation myth, a story of a great flood, and epic legends of heroism that contain hints of man's concern for his fertility. In Egyptian legend, Ishtar descends into the underworld because "the maid in the street no man drew near." In the Maha-Bharata, an epic account of a war between the 5 sons of Pandu and their 100 cousins, there appears the following:

> If these rites and sacrifices move thy favor and thy grace
> grant me offspring, prayer-maiden worthy of my noble race.
> Maha-Bharata
> ? 1000 B.C.

Athens and Rome

Early in the millenium before the birth of Christ, the city-state of Athens gave birth to philosophers and physicians whose thoughts influence us today. The physician Asklepios became deified and temples were erected in his name. An early legend attributed to the power of Asklepios is that of Agamede.

> Agamede dremt a snake was lying on her belly and there-upon she had five children.
> Asklepios—temple cult
> 600 B.C.

The snake is an ancient symbol of fertility. In the book of Genesis, a snake tempted Eve and she ate of the tree of forbidden knowledge. In the legend of Agamede and in the book of Genesis, the snake may be a phallic symbol and the knowledge Eve acquired may have been carnal.

During the time of the Persian wars, Hippocrates wrote of a test for fertility.

> If a woman does not conceive, and wishes to ascertain whether she can conceive, having wrapped her in blankets, fumigate below with oil of roses, and if it appear in the nostrils and mouth, know that of herself she is not unfruitful.
> Hippocrates
> 460–377 B.C.

Oil of roses is a volatile and aromatic compound. Being wrapped, the fumes ascend in her genital tract. If her fallopian tubes are patent, then the vapors will enter the abdominal cavity, and will be absorbed into her circulation and tasted—much in the manner of a test of circulation time.

Hippocrates also recognized the relationship between lactation and menstruation. He wrote, "If you wish to stop the flow of menses, apply as large a cupping instrument as possible to the breasts."

Aristotle, teacher of Alexander the Great, proposed a mechanism for conception:

> Here the milk is the body and the fig juice or the rennet [seminal fluid] contains the principle which causes it to set.
> Aristotle
> 300 B.C.

The "milk" represents menstruation. Aristotle differed from his contemporaries by proposing the theory of epigenesis that held that the fetus is not preformed, but comes to exist only after union of man and woman. This theory of epigenesis was contrary to the prevailing opinion and remained so until the eighteenth century. Most believed that the fetus existed in a miniature state within the ovaries of women. Boys came from the right ovary and girls from the left. Others believed that the testes regulated reproduction and boys came from the right testis and girls from the seed of the left testis. Although Aristotle denied this, such myths were prevalent and persist even to the present. In a certain Indian tribe today, it is custom for a woman to squeeze her husband's left testis at the moment of ejaculation. This is intended to favor the birth of male offspring. If she subsequently has a daughter, she is beaten because it is assumed that she did not squeeze either soon or hard enough.

In ancient Greek society all deformed children were allowed to die by exposure. It was also customary to expose many newborn daughters. This custom was adopted by the ancient Romans. The "Laws of Romulus" required Roman families to raise all male children but only the first-born female. Subsequent female children and deformed children were allowed to die by exposure at specific locations set aside for this. The decline of the Roman Empire was, in part, the result of a population insufficient to sustain a large empire.

As early as 700 B.C., Hesiod acknowledged the necessity of marriage and encouraged it despite what he perceived to be some limitations.

> He who evades, by refusing marriage, the miseries that women bring upon us will have no support [children] in the wretchedness of his old age.
>
> Hesiod
> 700 B.C.

Six hundred years later, Gallius also commented on the tribulations of marriage.

> If it were possible to live without wives, gentlemen, we should all save ourselves the trouble. But since Nature has decreed that we can neither live with them in peace, nor without them at all, we should act with future benefits rather than present comforts of mind.
>
> Gallius (Rome)
> 131 B.C.

The Roman philosopher Cicero, when asked if he would remarry, replied that he "could not cope with philosophy and a wife at the same time." However, Cicero forgot that he would have to repay his wife's dowery. Shortly after he divorced Terentia, Cicero remarried.

To combat a declining birth rate, Roman laws were enacted as early as 403 B.C. that prohibited celibacy and required remarriage within 12 to 18 months. Rome also enacted the "Rights of Three Children," which provided a reward for couples having 3 or more children. The value of children is also expressed in Psalm 127.

> Like arrows in the hand of a warrior are the sons of one's youth. Happy is the man who has his quiver full of them.
>
> Psalm 127

In the book of Genesis (30:14) it is written that ". . . Rachel envied her sister Leah and cried out to her husband, Jacob, 'give me children or I shall die.'" Rachel then requested of Leah that she "Give me I pray thee of thy son's mandrakes." Mandrake roots or mandragora are traditionally used as an aphrodisiac. In Ancient Egypt, they were called the "phallus of the fields" and in Arabic civilization "devil's testicles." If mandragora was an aphrodisiac, Juvenal recognized that the testes served an endocrine function.

> There are girls who adore unmanly eunuchs—smooth, so beardless to kiss, and no worry about abortions.
>
> Juvenal
> 100 A.D.

Obviously, he also recognized the role of the testes in reproduction.

The function of menstruation has also been discussed since antiquity. Aristotle considered menstruation to be the matrix for conception. Democritus thought menstruation was a manifestation of some uterine ferment while Pliny believed that it was a method of cleansing the uterus. Galen, an eminent physician who lived between 130 A.D. and 200 A.D., considered menstruation to be a means of disposing of excess blood.

An ancient Chinese physician explored the relationship between menstruation and fertility and concluded that conception was most likely to occur within the first few days after menstruation. It was not until 1839 A.D. that a physician named Augustin Nicholas Gendrin suggested that ovulation controlled menstruation.

In 98 A.D., Soranus, a physician from Ephesus (Asia Minor) came to Rome. He observed that

> When the menses flow freely the milk is checked, but while the milk is flowing, the menses no longer appear.
>
> Soranus
> 98 A.D.

Rufus, also of Ephesus, wrote an early description of the fallopian tubes and described them as "varicose vessels . . . springing from the female testicles."

Galen wrote over 400 medical treatises and for the next 1,200 years his observations were accepted without question. Galen performed anatomic dissections, but only in animals and commonly in sheep. Because of his animal dissections, he concluded that the human uterus was bicornuate. He believed that male children were conceived in the right horn and female children in the left.

The Middle Ages

The invasion of Rome in 410 A.D., the first in 800 years, was one of many events that signalled the end of an empire that held prosperity, power, and scientific achievement as its ideals. The long decline of the Roman Empire, the growth of poverty, and the spread of violence in secular authority necessitated a new ideal to console the human misery in an era now called the Middle Ages. An age of power yielded to an age of faith that came to focus on the principles taught by Christ. The Christian Church became the vehicle that supplied the ideal of faith and grew to be as powerful as any secular authority in the Middle Ages. The Church suppressed doctrines that challenged its secular or religious authority and called these doctrines heresies. Many scientific advances, including those of medicine, were often considered heretical to church doctrine although the teachings of Hippocrates, Galen, and Soranus were accepted. The value of these medical teachings diminished with each successive mistranslation and misinterpretation. In the lands of the eastern Mediterranean the power of the Church was less pervasive and here ancient traditions were kept alive while scientific inquiry was encouraged.

Islam was born in 610 A.D. with Mohammed's vision. The Islamic faith expanded rapidly in the Middle East and into northern Africa and southern Spain. With the spread of Islamic thought came the scientific method developed by Jabir (500 years before Roger Bacon proclaimed that method to Europe), the medical teachings of Avicenna and Rhazes, and translations of Aristotle and Hippocrates.

In western Europe, scientific medicine survived in the Middle Ages chiefly owing to Jewish physicians who practiced a Graeco-Roman form of medicine. Maimonides (1135 to 1204 A.D.) wrote his *Medical Aphorisms* during exile in Egypt and reduced Galen to 1,500 short statements covering all branches of medicine. In 1150 A.D. Saint Hildegarde lamented that "the cause of menstruation is the fall of Eve." Trotula (Dame Trot of nursery rhyme fame), a teacher at the medical school of Salerno, predicted the sex of an unborn child by putting two or three drops of milk (or blood if milk was not yet available) into spring water. If the drops sank, the child would be a boy; if they floated, a girl. In this time massages to relevant parts of the anatomy and ingestion of asses' dung were recommended as effective treatment of infertility.

The spread of Islam and the influence of Jewish physicians were essential in keeping advances in medical knowledge alive in the West. The Crusades of 1095 A.D. to 1291 A.D. failed to halt the advance of the Seljuq Turks, strengthen the Byzantine Empire, improve the commercial and economic conditions of western Europe, or rescue Jerusalem for Christianity. However, the Crusades did succeed in one respect: The secular life of Europe was enriched by contact with Moslem commerce, science, and medicine.

During the Middle Ages, the feudal system became a way of life. The concept of courtly love was developed and epitomized in the legend of King Arthur and his Knights of the Round Table. One byproduct of this concept was a rigid code of moral conduct forced on women—the proverbial pedestal. To assure compliance with this moral code, various instruments were developed to assist medieval women in the male quest to ensure her chastity and fidelity (Fig. 1–3). The origin of such devices is disputed but they may have been brought back from the Crusades, along with other accoutrements of Islamic society including science and medicine. Western Europe was now on the verge of a renaissance of thought.

The Renaissance in England

In 1485, the War of Roses between the Houses of York and Lancaster ended. Henry Tudor became Henry VII, King of England. Henry's oldest son, Arthur, married Katherine of Ara-

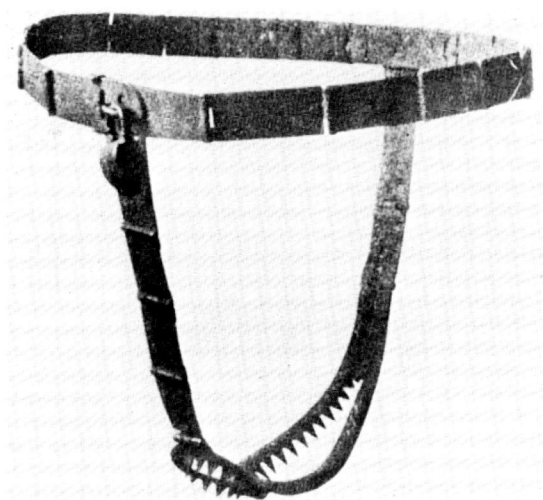

Fig. 1–3. Iron chastity belt. (Found in Wurzburg, Germany in 1885. (From Ploss H and Bartels M: Woman, London, Wm Heinemann, 1927.)

gon. Arthur died within several months of the wedding so Henry VII arranged Katherine's marriage to his second son, also named Henry. Henry VII's third child, a daughter named Margaret, married King James IV, of Scotland. At the death of Henry VII in 1509, his second son became King Henry VIII (Fig. 1–4). Katherine, first wife of Henry VIII, miscarried 5 times, had a daughter, Mary, but bore her husband no sons. Henry had his marriage to Katherine annulled to marry Ann Boleyn, who bore Henry a daughter Elizabeth and may have had an episode of pseudocyesis. Ann was later executed for adultery. Henry then married Jane Seymour, who bore Henry's only male heir, the future Edward VI, who became King of England at age 9 in 1547. Edward reigned only 6 years and died in 1553, possibly of tuberculosis. Henry VIII's daughter by his first wife then ascended the throne as Queen Mary I. During her 5 year reign, she became known as "Bloody Mary" for her efforts to reinstitute the Catholic faith in England. Bloody Mary never conceived although she did suffer with pseudocyesis on one occasion. At Mary's death in 1558, her half-sister Elizabeth, Henry VIII's daughter by his second wife, became Queen and ruled without marrying until her death in 1603. Upon hearing of the birth of a son, James, to her distant cousin Mary, Queen of Scotland, Queen Elizabeth lamented that "the Queen of Scots is mother of a fair son, and I am but a barren stock." Several years after Elizabeth's death, Ben Jonson surmised that

> She had a membrane on her which made her incapable of man, though for her delight she tried many.
>
> Ben Jonson
> 1615 A.D.

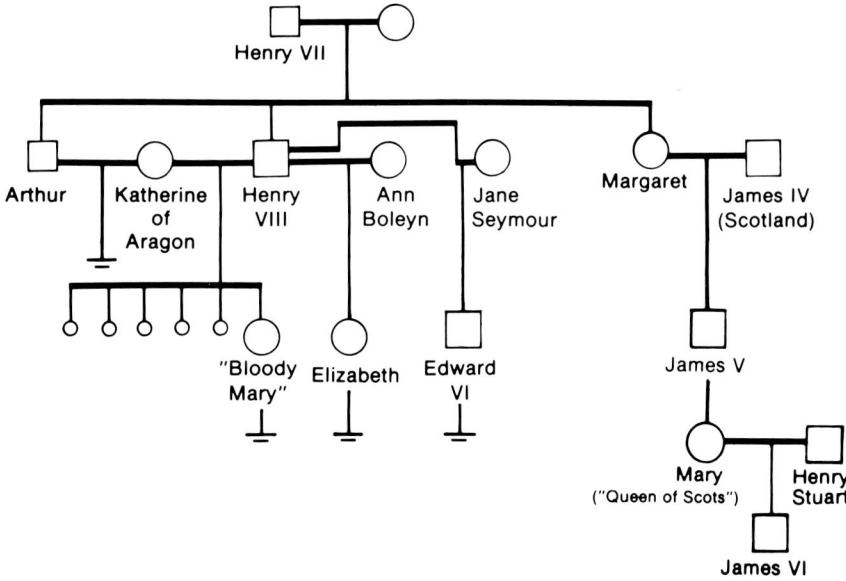

Fig. 1–4. The Tudor family. Each small circle is a spontaneous abortion. This is an incomplete pedigree that illustrates the line of succession.

However, it may be that Elizabeth never married to avoid handing the reins of power to a husband. Since none of Henry VIII's three children had offspring, the English crown passed to James VI of Scotland, whose great-grandmother Margaret was sister to Henry the VIII (Fig. 1–5). Because of infertility, the English crown passed from the Tudor to the Stuart family and James VI of Scotland became James I of England. James I is most famous for introducing the table fork into common usage and commissioning a bible that bears his name. James I was succeeded by his son, Charles I, who was beheaded by Cromwell in 1649. During this time the Renaissance faded and yielded to what history now calls the Age of Enlightenment. In 1660, the son of Charles I became King Charles II and formed a secret pact with Louis XIV of France in which he agreed to restore Catholicism to England. Whereas the ruling family in England had a problem of relative infertility, it was said of the French monarch that

> If Louis XIV was not the father of all his subjects, he was of many.
>
> Anonymous

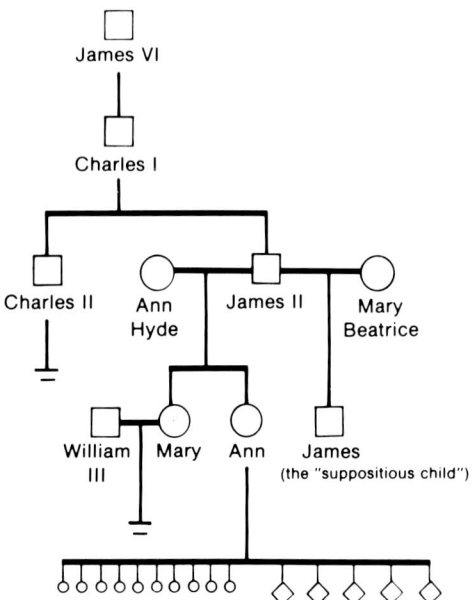

Fig. 1–5. The Stuart family. Mary Stuart ("Queen of Scots") was the granddaughter of Margaret Tudor, the sister of Henry VIII. Mary's second husband was Henry Stuart (Lord Darnley), who was also a grandchild of Margaret Tudor and Margaret's second husband, Archibald Douglas, Earl of Angus. James VI of Scotland became James I of England.

At his death in 1685, Charles II was succeeded by his brother, James II, whose first wife bore him two daughters, Mary and Anne.

After the death of his first wife, James II married Mary Beatrice, a Catholic, who bore him what has become known as the "suppositious child." The birth of this child, a boy named James, was not witnessed and there was suspicion that the midwife had smuggled a newborn male into the queen's chamber. As a result, it became custom for a government minister to witness the birth of all royal offspring, a custom that did not end until the birth of Elizabeth II's first child, Charles, in 1947. For this reason, and because James' second wife was Catholic, they were forced into exile in November 1686. James II's eldest daughter, Mary, and her husband became William III and Mary, rulers of England. She too suffered an episode of pseudocyesis but had no children. The English throne then passed to her sister, Ann, who ultimately had 10 miscarriages and 5 neonatal deaths. The royal obstetrician at this time was Hugh Chamberlen, whose family invented the obstetric forceps. Within 140 years, 5 English monarchs were infertile and 4 separate families ruled England.

During the fifteenth and sixteenth centuries, the Renaissance of art and science was in full flower. Van Eyck portrayed marriage in his *Giovanni Arnolfini and His Bride* (Fig. 1–6). The Flemish bridal chamber has many symbols that reflect the social and economic role of marriage in that society. The rich furnishings and cloth are symbolic of the husband's obligation to provide material goods and protection for his wife. In the background is a high-backed arm chair with a carving of Saint Margaret, patroness of childbirth. Behind the wife is the bridal bed in which the marriage is to be consummated in order to make it legally binding. With her left hand, the bride is lifting her dress to expose her blue underdress, a sign of acquiescence. The terrier-like dog in front of the couple is a symbol of fidelity and the apples by the window are a reminder of Adam and Eve's original sin.

Men's and women's feelings about children are symbolized in the many madonna portraits, in which the bond between mother and child is prominent. (Fig. 1–7). Leonardo da Vinci also portrayed fertility in an anatomic drawing of a gravid uterus, upon which he

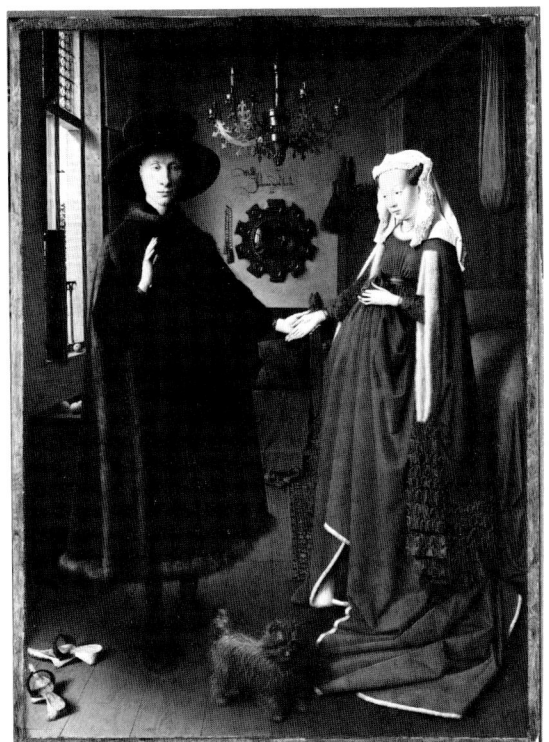

Fig. 1–6. *Giovanni Arnolfini and His Bride,* Jan van Eyck, 1434. Some believe that the bride was already pregnant. On the wall above the mirror is the inscription Johannes de eyck fuit hic ("Jan van Eyck was here"). (Reproduced by courtesy of the Trustees, The National Gallery, London.)

de Humani Corporis Fabrica. Vesalius and others changed anatomy, and all of medicine, into a science of personal observation. Vesalius accurately illustrated the anatomy of the female (Fig. 1–8).

Nine years later Bartolomeo Eustachio, a student of Vesalius, illustrated the uterine vasculature. It was Eustachio who advised a husband to insert his finger into his wife's vagina after they had intercourse to push the semen into the cervix. She conceived and this may be the first recorded instance of artificial insemination.

The Age of Enlightenment

The rebirth of scientific inquiry during the Renaissance stimulated a phenomenal growth in our understanding of anatomy, physiology, and medicine in the seventeenth and eighteenth centuries. William Harvey lived from

wrote ". . . how the great vessels of the mother pass into the uterus."

This period in our history was no less a renaissance in medicine. The 1,200-year teaching of Galen that all gynecologic disorders were due to malpositions of the uterus was no longer accepted. The anatomist Berengarius stated that

> In the fundus of the uterus you will see a certain depression indicating a right and left but I have not found in the uterus any other division.
>
> Berengarius
> 1514 A.D.

Recall that Galen had taught that the uterus was bicornuate. For the first time in more than 1,200 years, tradition in the West gave way to experimentation and personal observation. In 1543, Vesalius published his atlas of anatomy,

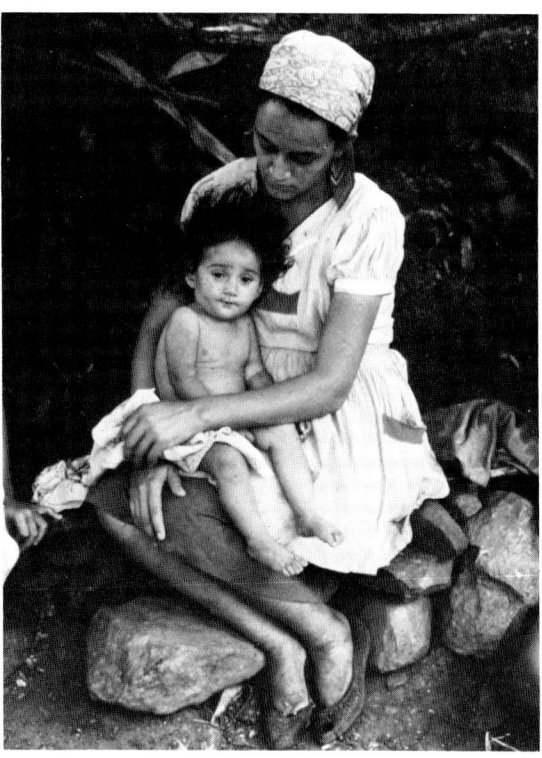

Fig. 1–7. Mother and Child. A Salvadoran refugee enfolding her child. (Photographed by Skeeter Hagler. Reproduced with permission of the *Dallas Times Herald.*)

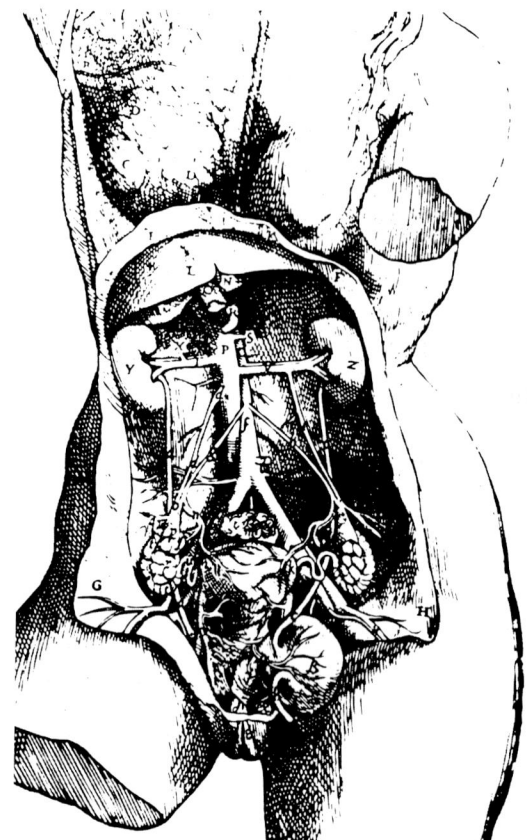

Fig. 1–8. The female pelvic organs. Vesalius (Andreas Wittig). *De Humana Corporis Fabrica*, 1543.

After a dormant period of 1,200 years and within the space of 150 years, Vesalius published an accurate atlas of human anatomy, William Harvey introduced the scientific method to Western medicine and renewed an ancient theory of conception, and Fallopius described the tubes that now bear his name. In 1672, Regner de Graaf described ovarian follicles, although he was only partially accurate since he considered the entire follicle to be the ovum.

Five years later, in 1677, Leeuwenhoek used his invention, the microscope, and first saw sperm, which were illustrated by Niklass Hartsoeker (Fig. 1–9). Although Harvey had renewed the theory of epigenesis, it was still not completely accepted and there were those who still believed that the sperm contained a pre-

1578 to 1657 and was the personal physician of James I. Although he is best known for his work on the circulation of blood, he also wrote *On the Generation of Animals* in 1651. In this work, he resurrected the theory of epigenesis first proposed by Aristotle. Like Aristotle, Harvey contended that the fetus was not preformed, but developed only after the union of a male and female component. Harvey believed that

> . . . women are most prone to conceive either just before or just subsequent to the menstrual flux . . .
> William Harvey
> *De Generatione Animalium*
> 1651 A.D.

Along with Vesalius, Harvey is important to medicine because he relied on personal observation and did not appeal to prior authority.

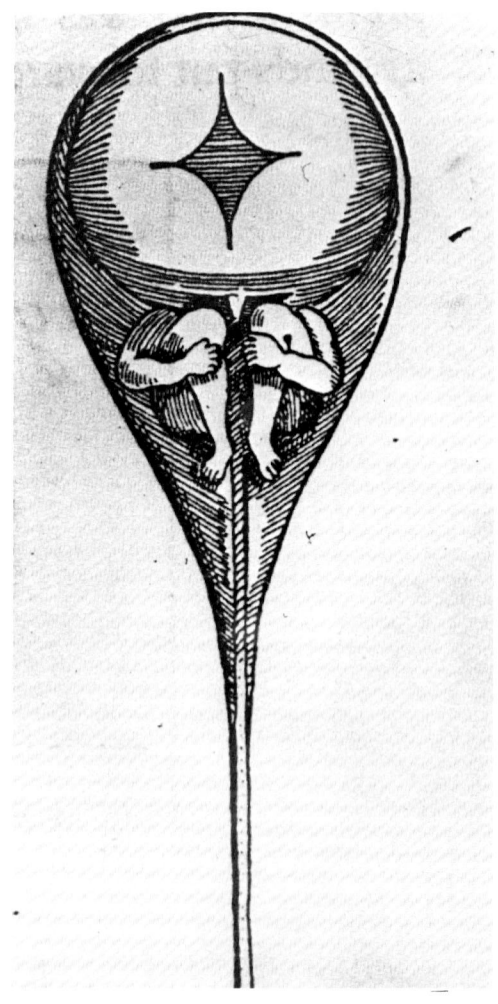

Fig. 1–9. A human spermatozoa. Niklaas Hartsoeker. *Essai de Diotropique*, 1694.

formed embryo. Four years later Malpighi described the endometrium and the corpus luteum in his work *de Utero Epistola*.

Continuing a long tradition of sex prediction, Nicholas Culpepper proposed a means of diagnosing the presence of a male fetus.

> If she have conceived a Male Child the right eye will move swifter and look more clear than the left. The right pap will also rise and swell beyond the left . . .
> Nicholas Culpepper
> *Directory for Midwives*
> 1651 A.D.

Sir Kenelm Digby proposed a medication to procure conception.

> An Excellent Remedy to procure Conception consists of the syrups of Mother-wort and Mugwort, Spirit of Clarey, root of English Snakeweed . . . Stamp all of these into an Electuary. Put it in Gally Pots and keep it for use.
> Sir Kenelm Digby
> *Choice and Experimental Recipes in Physics & Chirurgery*
> 1668 A.D.

Birth, Death, and Population Growth

By the year 1700 the ancient Greek and Roman custom of disposing of unwanted children had been abandoned and the necessity for cooperation between man and woman to procure conception was accepted. The uterus, fallopian tubes, endometrium, ovarian follicle, and corpus luteum had been described with reasonable accuracy. Sperm were seen for the first time, although their true role was not yet appreciated. Until this time, the growth of human population was agonizingly slow (Table 1–1). From 1 million B.C. until 8000 B.C., the human population doubled only every 250,000 years. In the next 10,000 years, until 1750 A.D., the human population doubled only every 1,500 years. Until 1750 A.D., the dominant social pressure was to bear a large number of children because there were significant limits to human fertility (Table 1–2). Even in 1700 A.D. women had a short reproductive life span. Diseases and malnutrition limited women's fer-

TABLE 1–1. Human Population

YEAR	POPULATION
1,000,000 B.C.	500,000
8,000 B.C.	8,000,000
1 A.D.	300,000,000
1750 A.D.	800,000,000
1800 A.D.	1,000,000,000
1850 A.D.	1,300,000,000
1900 A.D.	1,700,000,000
1950 A.D.	2,500,000,000
1974 A.D.	3,900,000,000
(2000 A.D.)	(6,400,000,000)

tility. Long birth intervals reduced the number of children born to any woman. Coitus interruptus existed as a means of contraception. In certain societies, late marriage and delayed fertility were encouraged.

Perhaps above all else, human fertility was limited by human mortality (Table 1–3). In 1750, the estimated maternal mortality was 24 mothers per 1,000 births. This compares to a figure of 0.09 mothers per 1,000 births (or 9/100,000) today. In the last 250 years, fetal, neonatal, and infant mortality have also dropped from levels that represented a threat to population growth. When maternal mortality rates are high and life expectancy is short, the number of children that are needed to maintain a static population is high (Table 1–4). With a life expectancy of 20 years, each woman must bear 6.5 children. By 1800 A.D., the life expectancy of a woman was 50 years and the number of children needed to sustain the population dropped to 2.8. Today, a woman living in a developed country can expect to live 72 years. If she bears more than 2.2 children, the population grows. Until 1700 the annual rate of increase in the population had

TABLE 1–2. Limits to Fecundity

Short reproductive life
Disease (e.g., tuberculosis, parasitic)
Malnutrition
Long birth interval (lactation, social taboos)
High infant mortality
Infanticide
Contraception
Late marriage
Delayed fertility

TABLE 1-3. Human Mortality

DATE	MATERNAL (No./1,000)	FETAL (No./1,000)	NEONATAL (No./1,000)	INFANT (No./1,000)
1750	24	29	58	437
1800	—	—	—	240
1870	—	—	—	153
1930	6	40	40	67
1948	—	23	20	34
1978	0.09	10	10	15

been 0.2% to 0.3% (Fig. 1–10). Beginning in the eighteenth century, we have increased our numbers at an ever increasing rate—a rate that is currently 1.7%. Today, we exist in a condition totally unique in the history of man. A large rate of population growth is operating on the largest population ever to inhabit the planet earth.

Are we in danger of growing faster than our food supply, as proposed by the Reverend T. R. Malthus (1766 to 1834)? Since 1950, there has been a 50% increase in our population. In that same time, there has been a 100% increase in the supply of food (Fig. 1–11). The Malthusian prediction does not appear to be a matter for concern—yet. However, the rate of increase in the production of grain, fish, livestock, and all other foodstuffs has declined since the mid- to late 1970s and in some instances there have been actual declines in the quantity of food sources. At the present rate of population growth, the weight of all earth's inhabitants will exceed the weight of earth herself in 700 years.

We are, indeed, viewing the dynamics of human population from a vantage point totally unique in our history. But, if women who are infertile were not allowed to conceive, there would be no perceptible decline in the growth of our population. Allowing infertile women to remain so is an ineffective and misdirected means of population control.

The Last 250 Years

If the human population has grown at a dizzying pace in the last 250 years, so too has our understanding of conception. Karl Ernst von Baer expanded the work of de Graaf and described the ovum within the Graafian follicle. William Hunter described the seminiferous tubules in 1762. In 1786, nearly 100 years after Leeuwenhoek first saw sperm, Lazzaro Spallanzani proved that sperm were essential for conception. At this time George Washington was commanding the Continental army but could not father children. John Hunter, brother of the man who described the seminiferous tubules, reported the first successful instance of artificial insemination using the husband's sperm. In 1866, J. Marion Sims, known best for his repair of vesicovaginal fistulae, successfully inseminated a woman with sperm from a donor.

Whereas William Hunter described the seminiferous tubules and Lazzaro Spallanzani noted that sperm were essential for conception, it was Albert von Kolliker, in the middle of the nineteenth century, who described sperm coming from the seminiferous tubules. He stated that sperm fertilized the ovum, and suggested that hereditary characteristics were conveyed by the cell nucleus. Martin Berry observed fertilization in a rabbit in 1843 and Oscar Hertwig described the union of the sperm and egg nuclei during the process of fertilization. In addition to reporting a successful case of insemination with sperm from a donor,

TABLE 1-4. Number of Children to Maintain a Static Population

FEMALE LIFE EXPECTANCY (YEARS)	NO. OF CHILDREN
20 (Homo africanus)	6.5
28 (10,000 B.C.)	4.5
32 (1640 A.D.)	4.1
50 (1800 A.D.)	2.8
72 (1980 A.D.)	2.2

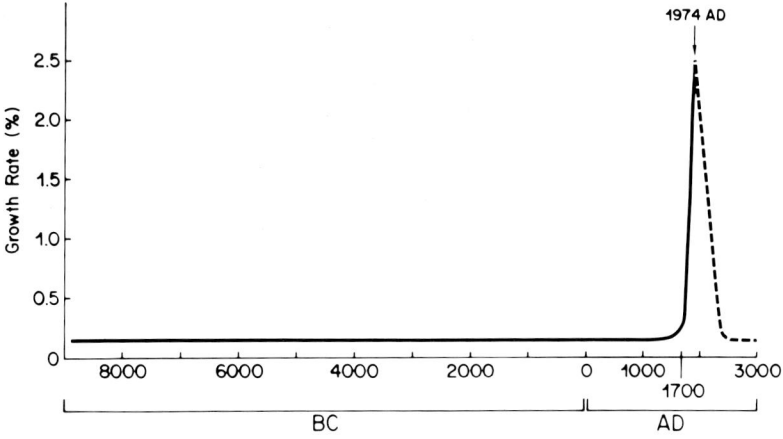

Fig. 1-10. Population growth rate. In 1983 the rate is approximately 1.7%.

Marion Sims was one of the first to time the fertile period of women correctly. In the same year, 1866, James Matthew Duncan wrote *Fecundity, Fertility and Sterility*, the first scientific work in this area of medicine. In 1871, Karl Sigmund suggested that a woman menstruated because she failed to conceive.

Late in the nineteenth century, Jacob Bruno Noeggerath insisted that gonorrhea caused salpingitis and subsequent sterility. Sixty-one years earlier, the emperor Napoleon divorced Josephine because she failed to bear him a child during 15 years of marriage. While married to Josephine, Napoleon contracted a case of what his physicians called "cystitis" shortly after he returned from one of his efforts to expand the French boundaries. Josephine was undoubtedly infertile as a result of tubal disease.

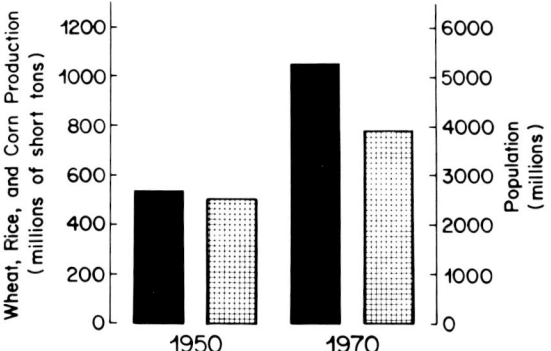

Fig. 1-11. Population and food production in 1950 and 1970. The solid bars are food production and the hatched bars represent world population.

In 1879, Albert Neisser discovered the gonococcus bacteria. Forty years earlier, the city of Vienna reported 6,000 to 7,000 women infected with gonorrhea and 30,000 cases of gonorrhea were treated in 3 hospitals in London during the year 1856. Sixty percent of Parisian prostitutes were found to be infected by gonorrhea in 1860. In 1865, the French government estimated that gonorrhea was responsible for 20,000 days lost in 3 months by members of the Imperial Guard.

At the close of the nineteenth century, Brown-Sequard injected himself with a crude extract of testes and described a rejuvenating effect. At this time, evidence was also accumulating that the ovaries served an endocrine as well as a reproductive function. In 1893, menopausal symptoms were cured by the subcutaneous injection of follicular fluid. Two years later, Dr. R. T. Morris grafted ovarian tissue in oophorectomized women and noted a transient reestablishment of menses. In 1903, J. Whitridge Williams wrote:

> From the evidence before us, we conclude that the two processes [ovulation and menstruation] occur about the same time. . .
> J. Whitridge Williams
> 1903 A.D.

Despite accumulating evidence for the endocrine function of the ovary, Dr. Arthur W. Johnstone concluded that:

> There is not an iota of proof that the ovary has any other function than the manufac-

ture of eggs... The ovary is in no sense a gland.

Arthur W. Johnstone
1900 A.D.

Yet, 22 years later Edward Doisy could recall that

... He [Edgar Allen] had noted in his work on the estrous cycle of the mouse that development of the ovarian follicle just preceeded the appearance of the cornified squamous cells in the vagina—so he injected some follicular fluid which had been aspirated from sows ovaries into ovariectomized mice and found the cornified cells typical of estrus.

Edward Doisy
1922 A.D.

Six years later, in 1928, George Corner and Willard Allen described their experiments leading to the discovery of progesterone.

We have been able to prepare alcoholic extracts of the corpora lutea of swine which produce in spayed rabbits a condition of the uterus identical with normal progestational proliferation.

George Corner & Willard Allen
1928 A.D.

While these men were exploring the endocrine function of the human ovary, Zondek and Ascheim stimulated ovarian function by implanting pituitary tissue in hypophysectomized mice. These early studies culminated in 1958 when Gemzell, Diczfalusy, and Tillinger induced ovulation with gonadotropins.

A great economic depression followed the stock market crash in 1929. In the same year, Ogino in Japan and Knaus in Germany proved that ovulation ordinarily takes place 12 to 16 days before menstruation. The findings of these 2 men are today used as the basis of natural family planning.

A change in basal temperature during the menstrual cycle was first described by Squire in 1868 and Van de Velde suggested in 1905 that the shift in basal temperature may be related to ovulation. But it was not until the 1930s and 1940s that the biphasic basal temperature pattern of ovulating women was correlated with changes in the endometrium, the cervix, and the vagina.

Three hundred and ninety years after Fallopius first described the uterine tubes and 80 years after Noeggerath associated gonorrhea with tubal occlusion, Hellman described the use of polyethylene stints in human tuboplastic operations. In the earlier decades of the 20th century, Isador Rubin described his insufflator to test for tubal patency (Fig. 1–12). He also illustrated the results of his test when the tubes were patent (Fig. 1–13).

The complex interaction of sperm and cervical mucus was described by Max Hühner, who died in 1947. His observations are the origin of the postcoital test, today used extensively to evaluate infertile couples.

Since the beginning of recorded history, our understanding of the physiologic processes of conception has expanded enormously. However, man's concern for his fertility has not been limited to the realm of medicine.

First he becomes the seed of a man, which is light gathered from all limbs of the body. Man nourishes himself within himself as

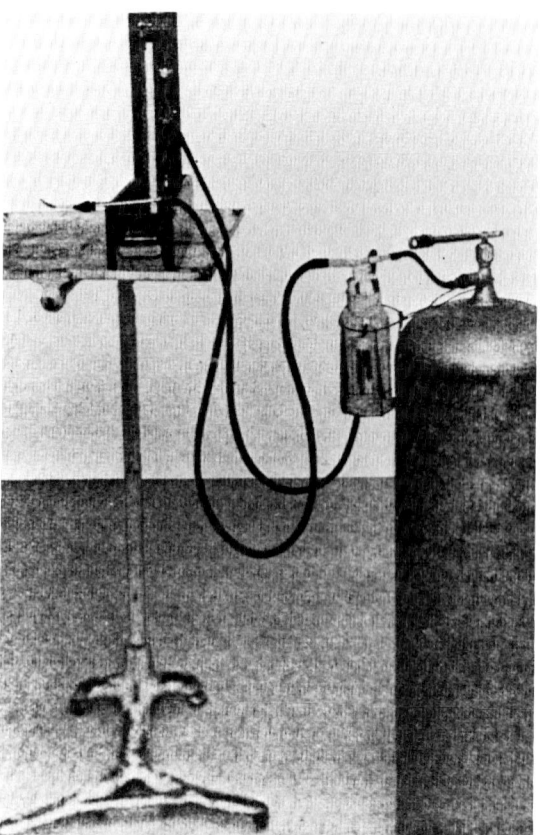

Fig. 1–12. Isador Rubin's original tubal insufflator.

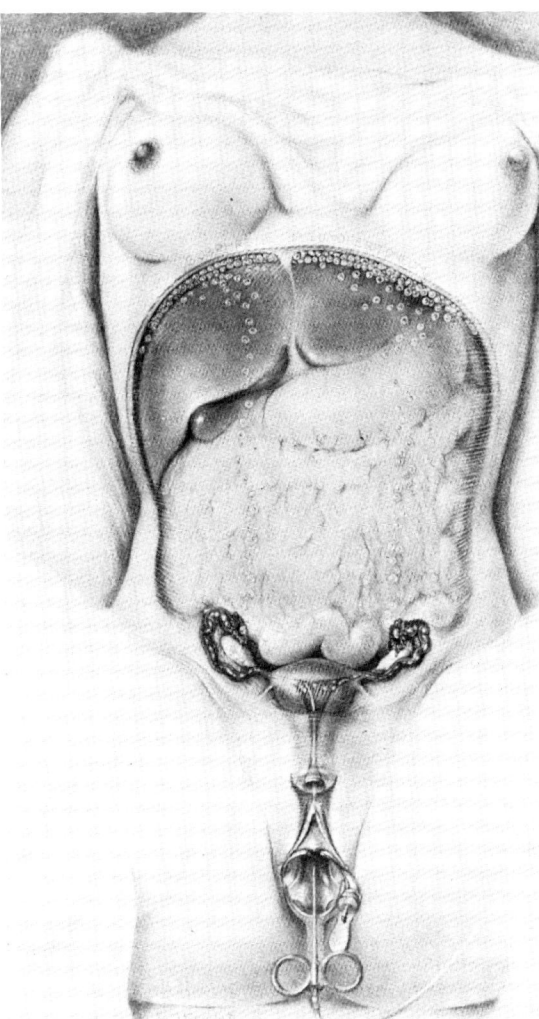

Fig. 1–13. Rubin's illustration of tubal insufflation and the resulting pneumoperitoneum.

seed. When he ejects that seed into a woman, he himself is born. That is his first incarnation.

The seed merges in the woman's body; because it becomes her body, it does not harm her. She nourishes the self of the man within. Protect her for she is protecting the seed. Before and after the birth of the child, man blesses the child, blessing himself. Man lives in his child; that is his second incarnation.

Aitareya Upanishad
ca. 1000 B.C.

"If I had a child" she thought to herself; "if I had him inside me as a child!"—and her limbs turned molten at the thought, and she realised the immense difference between having a child to oneself, and having a child to a man whom one's bowels yearned towards. The former seemed in a sense ordinary; but to have a child to a man whom one adored in one's bowels and one's womb, it made her feel as if she was sinking deep, deep to the center of all womanhood and the sleep of creation.

Lady Chatterley's Lover
D.H. Lawrence
1932 A.D.

BIBLIOGRAPHY

Barraclough G, ed. The Times concise atlas of world history. London: Times Books Limited, 1982.

Behrman SJ, Kistner RW. Progress in infertility. Boston: Little, Brown & Co., 1975.

Bronowski J. The ascent of man. Boston: Little, Brown & Co., 1973.

Barney GO. The global 2000 report to the president: entering the twenty-first century. New York: Penguin Books, 1982.

Brown LR, McGrath PL, Stokes B. Twenty-two dimensions of the population problem. Population Reports, Series J, 1976;11:177–202.

Brown LR. World population trends: signs of hope, signs of stress. Population Reports, Series J, 1977;13:237–251.

Brown LR. Building a sustainable society. New York: WW Norton & Co., 1981.

Carroll HJ, Embree AT, Mellon K, Schrier A, Taylor AM. The development of civilization, vol. 1. Chicago: Scott Foresman & Co., 1961.

Coale AJ. The history of the human population. In: Freedman R, Berelson B, eds. The human population. San Francisco: WH Freeman & Co., 1974.

Coomaraswamy AK. Status of Indian women. In: Needleman J, Bierman AK, Gould JA, eds. Religion for a new generation, 2nd ed. New York: Macmillan Publishing Co., 1977;278–292.

Darwin C. The descent of man and selection in relation to sex. Detroit: Gale Research Co., 1974.

Dewhurst J. Royal pseudocyesis. History of medicine. 1980;May/June:12–17.

Durant W, Durant A. The story of civilization. New York: Simon & Schuster, 1961.

Ebbel B (trans.). The Papyrus Ebers. London: Oxford University Press, 1937.

Editorial. Energy: facing up to the problem, getting down to solutions. National Geographic, 1981; February.

Ellis H. Studies in the psychology of sex. New York: Random House, 1942.

Evans JR, Hall KL, Warford J. Health care in the developing world: problems of scarcity and choice. N Engl J Med 1981;305:1117–1127.

Graham H. Eternal Eve: The history of gynecology and obstetrics. Garden City, New York: Doubleday & Co., 1951.

Greenblatt RB. Love lives of the famous, a physician's reflections. Lancaster, England: MTP Press, 1978.

Greenblatt RB. Search the scriptures. Modern medicine and biblical personages. Philadelphia: JB Lippincott Co., 1978.

Greenblatt RB. Induction of ovulation. Philadelphia: Lea & Febiger, 1979.

Gregory H (trans.). Ovid, the metamorphoses, New York: New American Library (Mentor Classic), 1958.

Henry A, Piotrow PT. Age at marriage and fertility. Population Reports, Series M, 1979;4:105–159.

Himes NE. Medical history of contraception. New York: Schocken Books, 1970.

Jensen NF. Limits to growth in world food production. Science 1978;201:317–320.

Lawrence DH. Lady Chatterley's lover. New York: New American Library (Signet Classic), 1959.

Leaky RE. Origins. New York: EP Dutton, 1977.

Mauldin WP. Population trends and prospects. Science 1980;209:148–164.

Pimental D, Oltenacu PA, Nesheim MC, Krummel J, Allen MS, Chick S. The potential for grass-fed livestock: resource constraints. Science 1980;207:843–848.

Plowden A. The house of Tudor. New York: Stein & Day, 1976.

Ravenholt RT, Chao J. World fertility trends, 1974. Population Reports, Series J, 1974;2:21–39.

Reining P, Tinker I, eds. Population: dynamics, ethics, and policy. Washington, D.C.: American Association for the Advancement of Science, 1975.

Rodwell JM (trans.). The Koran. JM Dent & Sons, Ltd. (Everyman's Library), 1977.

Ross MA, Piotrow PT. Periodic abstinence. Population Reports, Series I, 1974;1:1–19.

Speert H. Iconographia Gyniatrica. Philadelphia: FA Davis Co., 1973.

Speert H. Obstetrics and gynecology in America, a history. Baltimore: Waverly Press, 1980.

Tannahill R. Sex in history. New York: Stein & Day, 1980.

Williams JW. Obstetrics. New York: D Appleton & Co., 1903.

Yeats WB, Purohit S. The ten principal upanishads. New York: Collier Books, 1975.

Zaehner RC (trans.). Hindu scriptures. London: JM Dent & Sons, 1966.

The Psychology of Infertility

Barbara Eck Menning

> When Rachel saw that she bore Jacob no children . . . she said to Jacob
> "Give me children or I die!"
> Genesis 30:1

Introduction

Most American families now plan their fertility as meticulously as they do their education, choice of career, life style, and financial investments—measuring all factors and waiting until the moment when starting a family is just right. For 75% of the 28 million couples of reproductive age in the United States, their meticulously planned fertility proceeds without difficulty or delay. However, fertility cannot be instituted at will for the remaining 7 million couples who are either absolutely infertile (3 million), subfertile (2.8 million), or who experience a long interval before conception (1.2 million). Stated in a different context, there are more than *3 times* as many infertile couples as there are annual deaths (all causes) in the United States. While the diagnosis and therapy of infertility have improved greatly for some causes of infertility, still only 50% of these couples will become fertile with medical care. Not all the couples whose infertility cannot be resolved fail because medical therapy is unsuccessful. Many fail to achieve fertility because they lack the knowledge of available resources and encounter such barriers to care as lack of transportation, limited financial resources, and mistrust of the care they receive. Because of these barriers, many are as yet uncounted in the roll of those who are infertile. I believe there is a silent epidemic of infertility owing to these barriers and to the apparent freedom of sexual mores, with its increased sexual activity at an earlier age and the resultant risks with contraception or genital infection.

Today's cures in infertility are not achieved without cost. A couple may incur tremendous emotional and financial expenses. Years may elapse before the longed-for baby is born to them. But for 4 to 5 million couples in the United States, conception or birth of a living, healthy child will prove impossible. This population represents one of the most silent and neglected groups in our country. They are not physically sick, merely heartsick. They continue to work, to function, to carry out their lives in a state of involuntary childlessness, the thought of which can pervade every waking moment and make decisions for the future next to impossible.

Alternatives for family building have never been more difficult. Adoption of the local, healthy infant of one's own race may be a very lengthy process. While there are as many out-of-wedlock pregnancies as there ever were, more than 90% of single mothers are now choosing to keep their babies instead of surrendering them for adoption. A couple requesting a white infant may wait 3 years or more just to begin a home study with an adoption agency. Increasing numbers of couples are exploring international adoption or reconciling themselves to a life without children.

When male infertility is the problem, couples are turning in record numbers to the choice of donor insemination. These alternatives force the couple to face issues and decisions that may be as difficult as the original problem of infertility.

From 1973 to 1982, I worked as a counselor and advocate for infertile couples. As founder and first director of RESOLVE, Inc., a national, nonprofit organization that offers infertility counseling, referral, and support groups, I became aware of the psychologic and social issues that infertility causes for both women and men. In preparing this chapter, I am drawing more upon my clinical experience in counseling and leading 15 support groups than upon the scant research and literature available to clinicians. Physicians, more than any other health professional, interact with infertile couples at maximum points of crisis and stress. Unfortunately, some physicians feel that management of feelings is not within their province and prefer to work solely with the physical problem of infertility. I write this chapter as an appeal to all health professionals to consider the entire psychosocial context within which the couple presents for management. Only in this way can comprehensive care be given.

Infertility as a Life Crisis

During the infertility investigation and treatment an infertile person commonly experiences a state of *crisis*, a disruption in his or her steady state or a period of disequilibrium. Common in any state of crisis are (1) a stressful event posing a threat that is insoluble in the immediate future; (2) a problem that overtaxes the existing resources of the person(s) involved because it is beyond traditional problem-solving techniques; (3) a perception that the problem is a threat to important life goals of the person(s) involved; and (4) a reawakening of some unsolved key problems from both near and distant past.

A crisis is usually time limited and resolved within 6 weeks or less. With or without help, each person attempts to resolve his or her crisis since our minds and bodies cannot tolerate a state of disequilibrium for an indefinite period of time. There are three possible outcomes: The person may emerge from the crisis state with the same level of functioning; the person may emerge from the crisis with increased strength and emotional insight; or the person may regress to a less stable level of functioning. Since there may be a series of crisis states in a protracted infertility situation, there is a very real risk of maladaptive behavioral changes, just as there is the real opportunity for positive growth and increased insight. How the person is managed by the clinician may mean the difference.

It is naive for a physician who treats infertility to say that emotions are not within his or her province of care. Whether by acts of omission or commission, the physician very much affects the outcome of the crisis state. The person in crisis is extremely vulnerable, and can be gravely hurt by indifference, lay psychiatric advice, or an admonishment to "buck up" or "relax!" Each member of a couple, as if by tacit agreement, rarely develops a crisis at the same time. This may lead the one who is dysfunctional to believe that the other cannot understand what he or she is experiencing. The partners may have little to give each other, forcing them to depend upon outside help. The physician is a person of immense importance at such times. If he or she cannot provide the necessary counseling, at the very least the physician should be an important bridge to therapeutic intervention.

There is a positive side to the disequilibrium and vulnerability of the crisis state. Since existing coping mechanisms have failed, the person is very open to suggestions of growth and change. Old and unsuccessful coping patterns are often discarded at times of crisis; new and more appropriate methods may be learned. The anxiety that most people in crisis experience is a high energy state. If this energy can be focused upon a tangible problem by a skilled counselor, it can be used to resolve the situation. While it is not always possible to resolve the infertility problem itself, counseling may pave the way to better communication between the couple, or between the couple and their significant others. Counseling may help the couple feel more in control of their investigation and treatment. The most fundamental goal of crisis intervention should be *primum non nocere*—above all, do no harm. The optimal goal is to help the couple emerge from the crisis state with increased strength and emotional insight.

The Feelings of the Infertile Couple

Infertility is a complex life crisis that evokes many feelings. Some of these feelings are rational, based on the very real and difficult events of the social and medical situation. Others may be more irrational, based, in part, upon myths and superstitions or on childlike magical thinking. Although feelings vary in order and intensity, most people face a similar syndrome of feelings as they attempt to work through their infertility. The sequence of feelings I have most often observed is described here.

SURPRISE. The first reaction most people have to their infertility is one of total shock and surprise. Most couples in their childbearing years are used to thinking in terms of prevention of pregnancy. They naturally assume that they will have children if and when they desire them. For the couple, it is ironic that they discover their infertility after having used some form of contraception, sometimes for many years. The discovery of an infertility problem is felt most keenly by those who are highly achievement oriented, and who believe themselves capable of surmounting any obstacle if only enough effort and will are exerted.

DENIAL. "This can't happen to me!" Denial is also a common response with infertile couples, especially if the initial tests reveal an absolute and untreatable problem in either partner. Denial serves a purpose. It allows the mind and body to adjust at their own rate to an overwhelming situation. Denial is only dangerous when it becomes a long-term or permanent coping mechanism. I have seen chronically depressed women who staunchly maintain that they never wanted a family. I have also seen men and women who refused to apply the label "infertile" to themselves in spite of 5 to 10 years of involuntary childlessness. People who need this level of defense may require psychotherapy of some duration.

ANGER. When couples enter into infertility investigations and treatment, they surrender much of their control over their bodies. Even in the best doctor-patient relationship, frustration, helplessness, and embarrassment may be present. Anger is a predictable response to loss of control. The anger may be quite rational, as when it is focused on real and correctly perceived insults, social pressure from family and friends to "produce," and the inconvenience of the tests and treatments. The anger may also be irrational, as when it is projected onto such targets as the physician or the marriage partner, or groups such as Pro-Choice abortion advocates or people who "breed like rabbits." This irrational anger is usually a front for a more primary feeling, such as intense loss and grief that the couple is unable to acknowledge. Whatever the source or the type of anger, it is necessary for the person to express it. Anger tends to dissipate in the telling (and retelling) of the indignities producing it. This can be done without detriment to the angry person or to the object of the anger in a milieu such as a peer support group.

ISOLATION. It is common for infertile couples to state that they are the only people they know who cannot achieve a pregnancy. Infertility is a difficult subject for most people to discuss. It is very personal and inherently sexual. Couples may keep their infertility a secret because they do not wish to be objects of pity. Nor do they wish to receive unsolicited advice, such as, "Relax!" or, "Why don't you take a second honeymoon!" Secrecy may have several negative effects. It usually increases the pressure from family and friends on the couple to plan and start a family. More importantly, it isolates the couple from their potential sources of support and comfort in a time of great stress. In extreme instances, infertile couples may be so sensitized to the sight of a pregnant woman or a child that they withdraw from any social situation that might produce such a contact. This may even involve a change of work or living situation.

Isolation may also occur between the members of a couple. The woman may despair over her husband's inability to empathize with her feelings about menstruation, her fixation with her basal temperature chart around ovulation, or her nervous hopes if a menstrual period is overdue. The man may find it impossible to share his anxiety over being "counted and scored" by a semen analysis, or having to perform sex on demand whether or not he feels like it. The result may be a breakdown in communication and a loss of pleasure in the sexual relationship. Marital stress and tension over sexual intercourse are so commonly present in certain phases of infertility that their absence is rare. Since the couple may often have no others to validate their feelings, they may presume that not only are they infertile, but that their marriage and sex life are also in jeopardy. Infertile couples are always relieved to find others who share the same frustrations and concerns. One of the most helpful ways to ease the isolation of infertility is to help such couples find each other and encourage them to join in a support group experience.

GUILT. Another reason for the secrecy that so often surrounds infertility is the presence of guilt. Each of us needs to construct a cause-and-effect relationship for events that have occurred. The infertile couple review their mutual and individual histories and search for a guilty deed for which they are being punished. Premarital sex, use of contraception, a previous abortion, venereal disease, extramarital coitus or interest, masturbation, homosexual thoughts or acts, and even sexual pleasure itself are some of the common events to which these couples assign the cause of their infertility. Once the guilty deed is discovered, the infertile person may go to great lengths to atone and achieve forgiveness. Atoning may take any form, from religious acts, to personal denial, to working in painful areas such as counseling of unwed mothers or teaching other people's children. Guilt and atonement appear to have no relationship to the educational level of the person. Some of the most sophisticated people I have counseled have applied a mystical belief in "God's punishment" to their own infertility, even in the absence of belief in a religion! The teachings of the Old Testament and folklore from early civilization often portray childlessness as a falling from grace, a test, or punishment by a higher power. People who have poor self-esteem seem particularly vulnerable to guilty thoughts about infertility. Believing in their hearts that they really do not deserve a pregnancy and child, they may keep their infertility secret for fear it might be discovered how "bad" they really are.

GRIEF. Without question, the most compelling feeling of conclusive infertility is grief. This state may be preceded by a period of depression, as the final throes of testing or treatment are pursued to no avail. Once all hope for pregnancy and live birth is abandoned, the appropriate and necessary response should be grieving. It is a strange and confusing kind of grief—involving the loss of a potential, not an actual, life. Society has elaborate rituals to comfort the bereaved in death. Infertility is different. There is no funeral, no wake, no grave upon which to lay flowers. Family and friends may never even know. The infertile couple often grieves alone. Stillbirth or miscarriage, while very tragic, are more often perceived as an actual death. Family and friends are more often aware of the loss and offer solace and support.

Infertility represents many losses: of children, of genetic continuity, of fertility and related sexuality, and of the pregnancy experience itself. For each individual, some of these losses are keener than others and grieving is often quite focused and specific. Failure or inability to grieve over infertility is the most common problem I have encountered when dealing with infertile couples. There are some very logical reasons why grief may fail.

Why Grief May Fail

UNRECOGNIZED LOSS. Because infertility represents the loss of a potential, not actual object, the couple may not realize that they are entitled to grieve. This may be unwittingly abetted by suggestions from the doctor at the moment of conclusion ("You can always adopt.") that send the couple immediately in search of an alternative.

UNCERTAINTY OVER THE LOSS. A conclusive diagnosis is never reached in a certain percentage of infertile couples. There *could* be a spontaneous pregnancy in any cycle and the couple *could* seek yet another expert opinion.

The moment for grieving is elusive—the couple holds back their grief until the moment of certainty. This state of uncertainty is like having a loved one "missing in action." Possible loss is not actual loss. For some, a resolution of grief does not occur until the woman completes her menopause.

LACK OF A SOCIAL SUPPORT SYSTEM. Grieving is intense and painful. There may be great reluctance to succumb to the feelings without the reassuring presence of family and friends to give comfort. Thirty percent of the population in America moves every year. We are an increasingly mobile society that is without roots or ties to the extended family. When the need to grieve arises, infertile people may find themselves far away from the loved ones they need for comfort. Those who find themselves isolated often seek the help of a therapist, counselor, or support group.

As painful as the initial grieving may be—accompanied by weeping and sobbing, and physical symptoms such as loss of appetite, exhaustion, choking or tightness in the throat—it does run a predictable course and it does end. It is helpful to point this out to the person who is afraid to give in to the feelings. Assisting a person or couple through griefwork can be a very rewarding experience. As a "grief facilitator," I have often seen the catharsis and restorative powers of grief resolved.

RESOLUTION. The desired goal in any crisis, including infertility, is its successful resolution. The process of resolution requires that each of the feelings described be discovered, worked through, and overcome. Feelings are never resolved permanently. They may be activated by special reminders, such as anniversaries of losses, or by new and different crises. But the feelings are never as difficult or overwhelming as they once were. Reactivation is usually brief and can be accepted by the person rather philosophically. People I have counseled about infertility describe the state of resolution in some of the following ways: There is a return of energy, perhaps even a surge of zest and well-being; a sense of perspective emerges, which puts infertility in its proper place in life; a sense of optimism and faith returns; a sense of humor returns and some of the past absurdities may even become grist for storytelling. The concepts of sexuality, self-image, and self-esteem are reworked to become disconnected from childbearing and become wholesome and complete. Plans that build a life around the obstacle of infertility are begun again. The couple is ready to act with confidence in selecting an alternate life plan (such as adoption). Once resolution is achieved, the couple is ready to get on with their lives.

Some Areas of Special Concern

Commonly, couples expend the most energy on those feelings where they are most vulnerable. For example, the person accustomed to high achievement may need a prolonged period of anger to deal with the loss of power and control; a person of low self-esteem may spend much more time in guilt and atonement feelings. To illustrate how complex infertility and its attendant feelings may be, I have selected five situations that are representative of the most difficult infertility crises. Each of these may help the clinician to understand the unique pain and sorrow of each aspect of infertility, and ways the couple may be comforted and guided toward resolution. The situations described are miscarriage and stillbirth, the "normal infertile" couple, the couple who select donor insemination, secondary infertility, and the woman who faces hysterectomy or loss of ovarian function. References are provided for the reader who wishes to learn more about these subjects.

MISCARRIAGE AND STILLBIRTH. This aspect of infertility is concerned not with the inability of a couple to achieve a pregnancy, but with problems resulting from the loss of a pregnancy. Miscarriage* is a more common occurrence than many people realize. One in six recognized pregnancies ends as a miscarriage and as many as 30% of all conceptions may end before the birth of a living child. Seventy-five percent of all miscarriages occur in the first trimester and most of these are caused

---
* The term *miscarriage* is used instead of the more medically correct term *spontaneous abortion* to avoid confusion with therapeutic abortion.

by unavoidable and untreatable problems. These random errors rarely repeat themselves in the childbearing years of normal couples. Women who have repeated miscarriages must be counted as infertile since they have not borne a live child. Couples who have great difficulty conceiving may have up to a 40% risk of miscarriage—perhaps because of the very problems that made conception difficult, but perhaps also because infertile couples are older than normally fertile couples. A miscarriage may be a potentially dangerous, even life-threatening situation. When emotional aspects are added to the physical trauma, it may be seen as a life event of critical importance.

Miscarriage is almost always totally unexpected and it may be over within a matter of minutes in early pregnancy. The threat of a miscarriage may linger for days or even weeks and, occasionally, medical intervention is successful in preventing loss of the pregnancy. The couple going through such efforts to preserve the pregnancy may experience alternate states of hope and despair as they await their fate. Regrettably, the onset of bleeding and cramping will usually end with expulsion of the gestation.

There are a number of issues unique to the experience of miscarriage. One of the most troublesome is the practice of many hospitals of admitting the patient threatening to miscarry to the obstetric unit. There she may be with laboring and newly delivered women and also near the newborn nursery. Hospitals justify this policy by reasoning that miscarriage is not a routine gynecologic event and is best managed in the cleaner obstetric area where the delivery room is available for surgical intervention. The emotional effect on the couple, however, may be profound. The couple who have experienced a miscarriage should, at the very least, be screened from laboring and newly delivered women. A special indicator should be posted on the door so that hospital staff are aware of the situation. The husband should not be treated as a visitor but be allowed unlimited access to his wife. Privacy from all but the few caring for her will facilitate the couple in expressing their grief.

The need for grieving after a miscarriage is obvious, especially for those couples who have longed for a child. Unfortunately, many hospital personnel are uncomfortable with this basic human emotion. They may look upon grieving as suffering or as a disturbance to the welfare of other patients. It is all too common for doctors to prescribe sedation, tranquilizers, or even mood-elevating drugs so that no one need be "upset." Probably the best management of the grieving couple is the earliest possible discharge, so that both griefwork and recovery can take place unimpeded at home.

The reaction of significant others to news of a miscarriage is usually one of abbreviated support (one person termed it a "mini-death") and assurances of successful pregnancy in the near future. It has been my experience that if well-meaning family and friends say anything at all, it is usually the wrong thing. "It's a blessing. The baby wouldn't have been normal!" "Next year at this time you'll be up to your elbows in diapers!" Such platitudes and assurances are not only medically unsound, but they also invalidate the couple's right to grieve for this particular loss.

Couples who have endured 5 or 6 or more miscarriages before giving up hope come to receive news of a pregnancy with dread and forboding rather than joy. They keep the pregnancy a secret for fear of raising anyone's hopes and practice denial to prevent their own nervous hopes from mounting with each passing week. The emotional toll in such cases is exhausting and some couples may finally choose sterilization in preference to any more attempts at pregnancy.

Stillbirth, the loss of a baby that has reached sufficient gestation to be viable outside the uterus (usually after 28 weeks), is a much less common occurrence and is usually not a recurring event. There are several possible situations, each fraught with its own pain and turmoil. There may be a cessation of fetal life and the woman is admitted to the hospital knowing her baby is dead before delivery. Death is not anticipated when a baby expires during the labor or delivery process, or in the neonatal period as a result of congenital abnormalities. Finally, there may be a physical crisis for both mother and child, such as premature separation of the placenta, where bleeding may be profuse and oxygenation of the baby is impaired. This may be a life-threatening situation and the emotional issues become secondary to the medical emergency.

Several common issues arise in each of these circumstances. The woman will inevitably be admitted to the labor and delivery area and afterward to the postpartum unit. Privacy from normally laboring and delivering women is paramount. If the baby is known to be dead, delivery by the least hazardous means to the woman and attendance of the husband or another person to comfort her is important. To resolve the grieving process, the couple should be allowed to view and handle the body of the baby. This option should be offered if requested and sensitively suggested if not requested. Since an autopsy is often done in these circumstances, it is best for the couple to view the body before it is sent to pathology. The woman who has had a stillbirth is in a postpartum state of recovery, as well as a state of grieving. She will have all the needs of the usual postpartum patient in addition to her emotional needs. Sensitive caretending and nurturing from hospital staff plus unlimited access to her husband will facilitate recovery.

After enduring a miscarriage or stillbirth, the couple still needs to know why. They may fantasize that they did something wrong, which resulted in this event. Anything of medical value that can be learned from the autopsy, especially if it may affect plans for future pregnancies, should be shared with the couple.

THE "NORMAL INFERTILE" COUPLE. For approximately 10% of infertile couples, no cause is ever found to explain why conception has not occurred. The term "normal infertile" has been applied to this group, though the so-called "normal infertile" couple obviously is not normal or they would not have an infertility problem.

Because there is no apparent cause, despite second, third, or more expert opinions, the couple often falls prey to suggestions that the problem may be "all in your heads." The visible signs of anxiety, depression, and frustration may be mistaken for the *cause* instead of the *effect* of the problem. Family and friends encourage the couple to "relax!" The woman is advised to quit her job (if she is working) or to seek employment (if she is sitting at home in despair). These gratuitous psychiatric offerings can be excused from lay persons, but not from physicians and other professionals, who should understand that such comments are of no value and may provoke more anxiety and frustration. It is often presumed that if a couple has no physical pathology to account for infertility, then some mental pathology must be responsible.

One of the most compelling issues for the normal infertile couple is that they never quite give up hope of a pregnancy, though they may make attempts to put infertility out of their minds and go on to adopt their family. Each cycle could be the one; each menstruation proves that it wasn't. Since there is no definitive answer, the couple with this problem has no clear object to grieve. Protracted depressive states may occur in such women and men. The ability to enter into griefwork requires acknowledging a loss, and there is no loss. Such couples may not stop hoping until the menopause heralds the end of the woman's fertile years. For this reason, menopause may be more difficult and laden with meaning for such couples.

Some couples cannot face a life of endless cycles of hope and despair and choose instead to take active control over their situation by practicing contraception or being sterilized. Either of these actions allows the couple to designate an end to hoping, experience their loss, and move on to an alternative.

The normal infertile couple has exaggerated emotional needs caused by these cycles of hope and despair. They are particularly vulnerable to exploitation by fads, quackery, and expensive claims for cure. Couples have resorted to megavitamins, acupuncture, herbal remedies, hypnosis, astrology, faith healers, macrobiotic diets, and other means in the hope of a "cure." The spontaneous conception rate of these couples is about 5%, which probably accounts for the occasional pregnancy that occurs after such measures have been tried.

DONOR INSEMINATION. When infertility rests solely with the male partner, artificial insemination by donor is one possible solution. Donor insemination has become enormously popular and available in the last decade. While statistics are difficult to verify, it is estimated that at least 20,000 babies are conceived by this technique annually in America. The increasing popularity may be caused, in part, by the decreasing supply of healthy young adoptable infants, and also by the increasing acceptability of donor insemination as a medical service. One clinic in the Boston area currently has a 2-year waiting list of people waiting to enter its donor insemination program. This trend is reflected around the country.

Because of the increasing demand for donor insemination, there are a growing number of couples in both counseling and support groups who wish to work through the issues surrounding donor insemination. This alternative offers an excellent solution for appropriate couples since it provides both the longed-for child and the pregnancy experience. Unfortunately, donor insemination is often suggested in a casual manner without proper screening and counseling. Donor insemination should be considered as an alternative to infertility, not as a treatment. The grief and other feelings of both partners need to be dealt with before they are ready to take this step.

Couples considering donor insemination need to work through several important issues. One of the first is their moral, ethical, and philosophic acceptance of the procedure. The Roman Catholic church still views donor insemination as adultery and a child so conceived as illegitimate. Before accepting this means of having children, couples of all religious persuasions need to resolve the potential conflict between their desire for children and their ethical and theologic beliefs. While a counselor cannot offer an opinion about acceptability for a given couple, he or she can often play the role of an objective and nonjudgmental referee as the couple debates their decision. Ultimately, the couple must come to their own unanimous decision, as it is they who must live with the consequences.

Many women feel that it is "selfish" to achieve a pregnancy without the genetic contribution of the husband. This loss of genetic continuity is an important factor for the husband to discuss and to accept. No matter how well the donor is matched to the husband, this loss is real and needs to be grieved over. Some doctors, uncomfortable with donor insemination, play into pretending by mixing donor and husband semen, or by suggesting that the couple have sexual relations immediately after each insemination. I feel this is very unhealthy and should be avoided. However, many husbands participate in the insemination process in other ways. They may be physically present during the procedure, and participate fully in the prenatal period, attending childbirth classes and facilitating labor and delivery, just as any other husband would. Full participation of this kind is healthy and should be encouraged. For couples who have resolved their grief over the loss of genetic continuity, nothing else need be sacrificed in the donor insemination experience.

Both husband and wife may have exaggerated fears as the time of delivery approaches. One fear frequently verbalized is that somehow a mistake in selection of donor may have been made and the resulting baby will have a totally incongruous racial or physical appearance. This fear is the subject of dreams, fantasies, and general anxiety. There may also be more subtle fears regarding the baby's health, intelligence, and attractiveness. To preserve anonymity, very little information is shared about the donor. A great deal of faith must be placed in the hands of the doctor or clinic doing the screening and selecting of donors. This is a sacred trust that no facility offering donor insemination should take lightly. Couples who return for a second or third pregnancy by donor insemination are much more relaxed and unconcerned about the quality of selection and less fearful of mistakes. Many couples are so delighted with the outcome of the first pregnancy that they request the same donor again, if it is possible.

One of the most difficult issues surrounding donor insemination is the issue of confidentiality. Most doctors recommend that the couple keep the procedure secret between them, since in all but a few states, there is no legal definition of the rights of the child born of donor insemination (see Chapter 22). Secrecy also protects the couple from the remarks and reactions of society and friends, and from the possibility that the child might discover his or her origin in a less than desirable way. Every couple I have counseled has struggled to decide whether or not to tell the child about the manner of conception. In making this decision, they also consider whether they wish to share knowledge of the insemination with close friends and family. Confidentiality has always been hotly debated among participants in support groups. There seems to be no right or wrong decision, just a course that each couple can follow comfortably. "You can always decide to tell, but you cannot un-tell" is a frequent remark. This leads most couples to be very discreet in the beginning. One obvious trade-off in choosing secrecy is that the couple is cut off from sources of support. If so, the confidentiality of a support group or counselor may benefit them. Even those couples who are very candid and certain that they want their child or children to know about origins cannot agree on the right age to share this information or the way to impart the information. Donor insemination is clearly different from adoption. The subject is too sophisticated to share with a child when he or she first inquires about where babies come from.

SECONDARY INFERTILITY. Secondary infertility is defined as the inability to achieve a pregnancy after one or more successful pregnancies. Therefore, it can occur after any number of children have already been born. It is always a distressing situation when a couple feels unable to complete their desired family. The most distraught couples are often those who have one child and are unable to conceive a second.

Society has certain expectations of the married adult couple. They are expected to bear children and a single child may not be enough to satisfy societal expectations. The term "only child" and the stereotypes and myths attendant upon it are judgmental at best, punitive at worst. Perhaps the bias against the single child has its roots in the days when families had to be very large to ensure that enough children would survive long enough to have their own children and carry on the family (see Table 1–4). In some developing nations the infant mortality rate still approaches 50% and having only one child creates a great risk to the loss of family continuity.

Couples who have conceived once with relative ease are justifiably baffled when the same good fortune does not hold true the next time. Because they previously controlled their reproductive efforts but now find that fertility eludes them, frustration becomes another common emotion experienced by these couples. They may also feel guilty, especially if contraception had been practiced or a pregnancy terminated since the birth of their child. The rate of cure of secondary infertility is the same as that of primary infertility—approximately 50%. Therefore, the couple should receive the best possible medical investigation. However, there will be those for whom no diagnosis or cure can be found. These couples face the prospect of raising a single child or exploring other options, such as adoption.

One of the most difficult psychosocial pressures in the single child family comes from the child itself. From the time he or she realizes that other friends have brothers and sisters and other mothers have pregnancies, the child may beg, plead, or bargain for a brother or sister. Often the child is too young to grasp the nature of reproduction or understand that a mother and father *cannot* have another baby. Children are more likely to believe that their mothers and fathers *will not* have another baby, because they have behaved so badly that the parents cannot face the prospect of another child.

The parents of a single child often express great fear that something may happen to the one child they have. Overprotection may result and have a negative impact on both child and parents. They may also push their child to be a high achiever, since all their hopes and parental pride rest on the accomplishments of that one child. Each illness, accident, or threat will trigger protective feelings. Each new milestone will be met by a combination of pride, fear, and nostalgia. The first day of school, the first date, driving a car, leaving home—all are moments parents may anticipate but also dread.

The couple who chooses to enlarge their family through adoption or donor insemination faces special concerns. With adoption, parents most often question whether they "will treat an adopted child as second best." This concern is of paramount importance to the counselors of the adoption agency as well. An honest discussion of the difference between birth and adoption should be part of the adoption process. The couple considering donor insemination most often worries that the child so conceived will not resemble them or the sibling and will "stick out like a sore thumb." Any parent of more than one child knows that each child is different. Even among biologic siblings, amazing ranges of physical attributes and other abilities occur. Each child is unique and special. This holds true no matter what the circumstances of its birth and arrival into a family.

HYSTERECTOMY AND PREMATURE OVARIAN FAILURE. Hysterectomy has a profound physical and emotional impact for the woman who has not been able to bear children or who has not completed her desired family. Almost without exception, doctors will strive to preserve both the uterus and ovarian function of a woman still in her childbearing years. Occasionally, a condition so compromises the patient and her health that conservative management is impossible. Among these conditions are severe endometriosis with intractable pain and presumed loss of fertility, cervical or uterine cancer, and recurrent myoma with anemia, or other complications. Because the reason for hysterectomy in the young woman is usually extreme, the woman may be unable to address herself to the issue of the loss of her uterus and childbearing potential until she has physically recovered from what might have been a dangerous or even life-threatening situation. She may be told by those intending to comfort her that she is lucky to have survived and is well rid of an organ that posed such pain or threat to her well-being. This, of course, negates the very real feelings a woman has over the loss of her childbearing potential and of a body organ.

The uterus, while not necessary to life, is very symbolic. To many women, it represents femininity as well as fertility. Though it is internal and invisible, the uterus is not a silent organ like the liver or the spleen (for which most people feel no emotion). The uterus waxes and wanes in hormonal tides. Once a month it declares its presence with the onset of menstruation. Even though many women feel cramps or discomfort accompanying their menstrual period, the loss of cycles is cited as foremost in the physical and emotional adjustment posthysterectomy. Some women describe orgasm as "waves or spasms in the uterus." Therefore, the loss of the uterus has many meanings to a woman: She will not menstruate, she cannot conceive, she may lose some familiar and pleasurable sensations in both foreplay and sexual orgasm. It is normal to grieve for any and all of these losses.

Many young women think about their hysterectomy for years to come, always asking, Was it necessary? Regardless of the answer, the end result is a *fait accompli*. The counselors at RESOLVE recommend a second opinion before a woman consents to a hysterectomy in nonemergency situations. If the opinions concur, the patient seems to undergo the surgery with more equanimity. If the opinions disagree, the woman may be spared unnecessary surgery but faces the dilemma of deciding whose opinion is right.

Feelings about the loss of the uterus may surface at predictable times—on the anniversary of the event, upon being reminded by friends, on seeing advertisements about menstruation or sanitary products, and even monthly, for a time, when the usual event of menstruation fails to occur. Griefwork must be followed by a reworking of her body image and sexuality. She must incorporate a new, adjusted concept of self. With normal grieving and resolution, the new self-concept can be as whole and healthy as the previous state.

Loss of ovarian function by surgical, medical, or unknown factors before the natural cessation of their function at a mean age of 48 years is, unfortunately, often termed "menopause" by members of the medical profession. In the minds of many, menopause has become synonymous with aging, depression, emotional lability, and other negative images. That these images are not true for the great majority of women in natural menopause has not diminished this stereotype.

Like the uterus, the ovaries are symbolic of femininity and fertility. They are, however, silent and unfelt. The loss of fertility when the ovaries fail may be of less concern to women than the loss of femininity caused by the cessation of estrogen production. Many women are merely handed a prescription for estrogen replacement therapy and told that they will feel exactly as they always have. The sudden loss of ovarian function can lead to some common and uncomfortable symptoms, such as "hot flashes," insomnia, and vaginal dryness and atrophy. Estrogen replacement therapy has its staunch proponents and opponents and the reader should refer to other medical literature for their arguments. I have become a proponent of estrogen replacement for women under 40 (who do not smoke) because of the troublesome symptoms of estrogen deprivation, the changes in her psyche and self-image, and because the young woman without ovarian function is more susceptible to osteoporosis and aging of the cardiovascular system. Since most such women are sexually active and hope to be for many more years, the prevention of vaginal atrophy is another benefit of estrogen replacement therapy.

Whether the woman has lost her uterus, her ovarian function, or both, one of the most significant sources of support and recovery to her body image and sexuality will be her partner. Sensitive counseling of the spouse by the physician about how and when to resume sexual activity and what feelings this may trigger in the woman can be most helpful. It is a lucky couple that is able to negotiate honestly and openly their needs and feelings about sexual activity. We must never presume that such communication occurs, nor that a couple cannot learn to communicate if they have not done so in the past. While childbearing may be lost to the couple, a mutually satisfactory sexual relationship is not, and the physician may be the key to helping the couple overcome their fears and reestablishing such a relationship.

How the Health Professional Can Help the Infertile Couple

Infertile couples understand that physicians do not have the knowledge to diagnose and treat every problem. Infertile couples do complain about exclusion of their partners from office visits and procedures, being "worked on" instead of being "worked with," the inability of physicians or their staff to listen to feelings and offer emotional support, the inaccessability of the physician or a member of the staff to discuss important developments by phone, the unwillingness of some physicians to refer them to someone more expert or admit that he or she can do no more for the patient, and a reluctance to refer to and promote community-based support groups for infertile couples.

TREAT INFERTILITY AS THE COUPLE'S PROBLEM. No matter whose body ultimately has the problem, the other partner has a very strong interest in investigation and treatment. The other partner should be involved in the discussion and planning from the beginning. To be seen as a couple has several distinct advantages. When two people visit a physician, power tends to be equalized. They gain courage and assertiveness from each other's presence and will often negotiate their needs more honestly and quickly. Blame is dispelled—not just one person is involved. Both members of the couple will have twice the ability for hearing at a time when they are anxious, and twice the ability for asking questions and seeking clarification.

DEVELOP THE MANAGEMENT PLAN WITH THE COUPLE. The physician is the only one who will know what tests or treatments are indicated for a given couple, but these can be offered as a recommendation, not a mandate. There is room for negotiation in a number of areas. The *sequence* of tests or treatments can often be flexible if there is no contraindication. The *pace* of testing and treatment can be slowed for those who need more time or accelerated for those who feel pressured by an age deadline or who are very highly motivated. The *price* of tests and treatments should be discussed and considered. Many physicians are totally unaware of the discriminatory coverage of "infertility" by third party payors, although some such services are reimbursed by the federal government for patients qualified for Title X or Medicaid.

OFFER EMOTIONAL SUPPORT AND EDUCATION. These should be a responsibility of the physician and his or her staff. Many physicians now employ the services of a nurse or counselor to inform and educate (e.g., describing the usual tests of an infertility investigation), to assist in offering emotional support, and to help in screening couples before proceeding with procedures such as donor insemination. A well-informed couple is much easier to deal with than a partially educated one. Accurate literature, written in lay terms, should be given to the couple at the outset. Since most physicians have limited time for giving emotional support, the counselor becomes an important and necessary adjunct. However, the physician cannot totally abrogate his or her responsibility to provide emotional support because the physical and emotional aspects of infertility are interwoven. The physician, whether or not by intent, becomes an important and powerful figure to the infertile couple. It is very difficult for the couple with an incurable cause of infertility or a couple who has exhausted the physician's expertise to be sent away because "there is nothing more to be done." Offering such couples a chance to return for one or more counseling sessions to discuss their feelings may be very productive and may offer them a lifeline of support until they find new resources.

BE ACCESSIBLE. It is all too common for the infertile person to encounter a "palace guard" when attempting to speak with the physician. It seems reasonable to expect that a physician should be available for brief telephone queries during the day, or at least respond to the patient at another time. It is a tremendous help to the physician and the couple when a nurse or nurse practitioner, not a secretary, can respond to these calls, as most questions are easily answered by someone with this level of expertise. An attitude of reassurance and caring adds a great deal to his or her sense of coping and control.

RESPECT THE LEVEL OF YOUR EXPERTISE. Physicians still do not agree among themselves about who is qualified to conduct the complete infertility investigation and manage its treatment. Not surprisingly, patients are also confused about who possesses the necessary expertise. Since 1973, when I founded RESOLVE, there has been a definite trend toward referral to obstetricians and gynecologists with additional training in reproductive endocrinology and infertility, and to a skilled urologist for any surgery of the male. Recognition that infertility in the male and female requires additional training on the part of physicians in obstetrics and gynecology, urology, and endocrinology has been an important reason for the increased rate of success in recent years. More couples would benefit if the medical profession could agree upon those conditions that are best managed by someone with additional training and experience.

BE AWARE OF RESOLVE'S SUPPORT SERVICES. All infertility specialists should be aware of RESOLVE and its services. This national, nonprofit organization began in 1973 and offers counseling, referral, and support to infertile couples. A national phone line operated at the national headquarters in Boston offers counseling and referral to specialists and to our chapters in more than 30 states. A current listing of these chapters is printed in each issue of the RESOLVE newsletter (available to members for $20.00 per year) or can be requested by phone. On-site, short-term counseling of a crisis intervention type is offered at the national headquarters and several of the more senior chapters (most of which are still staffed by volunteers). Support groups are offered at all chapter sites and consist of approximately 15 weekly sessions geared to working through feelings about infertility. All counseling and support groups are conducted by trained professionals and are confidential. Referral is made to the best source of medical care available (assessed by results of an annual RESOLVE survey) and to sources of alternative help, such as adoption agencies. The staff of RESOLVE publishes a bimonthly newsletter and a wealth of other helpful literature and resources. Through RESOLVE, infertile couples can find others near them who are in similar circumstances and with whom they can share experiences and feelings.

Conclusion

Infertility is a complex life crisis that currently affects 7 million people in the United States. Although new techniques of diagnosis and treatment offer the promise of pregnancy and live birth to 50% to 60% of these, at least 3 to 4 million women will not bear a child and have no easy alternative for family building. Infertility causes profound emotional stresses upon the individual and the couple, and social stresses with family, friends, and colleagues. Medical management has always been seen as the province of the physician. Of equal concern is the provision of psychosocial support.

The feelings of infertile couples range from shock and denial to anger, isolation, guilt, and, ultimately, grief. The process of working through these feelings to a point of resolution may require the assistance of a professional counselor. The physician is in a key position to understand the emotional reactions the couple is experiencing and to facilitate their resolution. By treating the infertile couple as a unit, by involving them in their plan of care, and by being emotionally supportive as well as accessible, the physician can integrate psychosocial support into the total management of infertility.

More information on RESOLVE may be obtained by writing:

RESOLVE, INC.
P. O. Box 474
Belmont, MA. 02178

BIBLIOGRAPHY

Beck W. When therapy fails: artificial insemination. Contemp Obstet Gynecol 1981;17:113–126.

Friedman R, Gradstein B. Surviving pregnancy loss. Boston: Little, Brown & Co., 1982.

MacNamara J. The adoption advisor. New York: Hawthorne Books, 1975.

Mazor M. The problem of infertility. In: Notman M, Nadelson C, eds. The woman patient, vol. 1, ch. 11. New York: Plenum Press, 1978.

Menning B. Donor insemination: the psychosocial issues. Contemp Obstet Gynecol 1981;18:155–172.

Menning B. Emotional needs of infertile couples. Fertil Steril 1980;34:313–319.

Menning B. Infertility: a guide for the childless couple. Englewood Cliffs, N.J.: Prentice-Hall, 1977.

Schiff I, Ryan K. Benefits of estrogen replacement. Obstet Gynecol Surv 1980;35:400–410.

3
The Hypothalamus: Physiology and Pathophysiology

G. William Bates

The hypothalamus has a close functional and anatomic relationship with the pituitary gland. Efferent flow of peptide hormones from the hypothalamus occurs principally by downward extension of the supraoptic and paraventricular nerve tracts into the posterior pituitary and by the portal plexus of the hypophyseal-pituitary circulation.

In 1948, Harris proposed that endocrine secretions of the anterior pituitary gland were regulated by an integrative mechanism located in the neuronal elements of the ventral hypothalamus (1). Earlier, Scharrer proposed the concept of neurosecretion from morphologic studies of hypothalamic cells in fish (2). Hormonal hypothalamic control of anterior pituitary function was ascertained through experiments that combined tissue cultures of fragments of pituitary gland and ventral hypothalamus (3). Guillemin (4) and Schalley (5) identified and subsequently synthesized hypothalamic hormones and were awarded the Nobel prize for their work in 1977. Knobil observed that pulsatile secretion of hypothalamic gonadotropin-releasing hormone (GnRH) is necessary to stimulate pituitary gonadotropin secretion and to initiate and sustain ovulatory menstrual cycles in primates (6,7). Although the human hypothalamus remains inaccessible for tissue study, studies of the synthesis of hypothalamic-releasing hormones and the effects of these hormones on pituitary function have improved our understanding of hypothalamic function and hypothalamic-pituitary disorders.

The demarcation of the hypothalamus from adjacent areas is indistinct; however, the hypothalamus is readily outlined by several landmarks (Fig. 3-1). It is bounded anteriorly by the optic chiasm, laterally by the sulci formed with the temporal lobes, and posteriorly by the mamillary bodies. The smooth, rounded base is termed the *tuber cinereum* (or infundibulum), and the central region (from which descends the pituitary stalk) is termed the *median eminence* (8). Because of its position between the higher central nervous system (CNS) and the brain stem and pituitary gland, the hypothalamus serves as an integrator of CNS neural and endocrine function. Appetite control, thermoregulation, osmoregulation, secondary sexual development, and reproductive function are regulated, in part, by the hypothalamus. Also, the circadian clock may well have its mainspring here.

Neurons innervating the hypothalamus are present at all levels of the brain stem, but no direct input from the spinal cord has been described. Descending input into the hypothalamus originates from the amygdala, hippocampus, and basal forebrain—structures collectively termed the limbic system (9). A direct projection from the retina to the suprachiasmatic nucleus of the hypothalamus has been demonstrated in monkeys, and a similar projection probably exists in the human for the

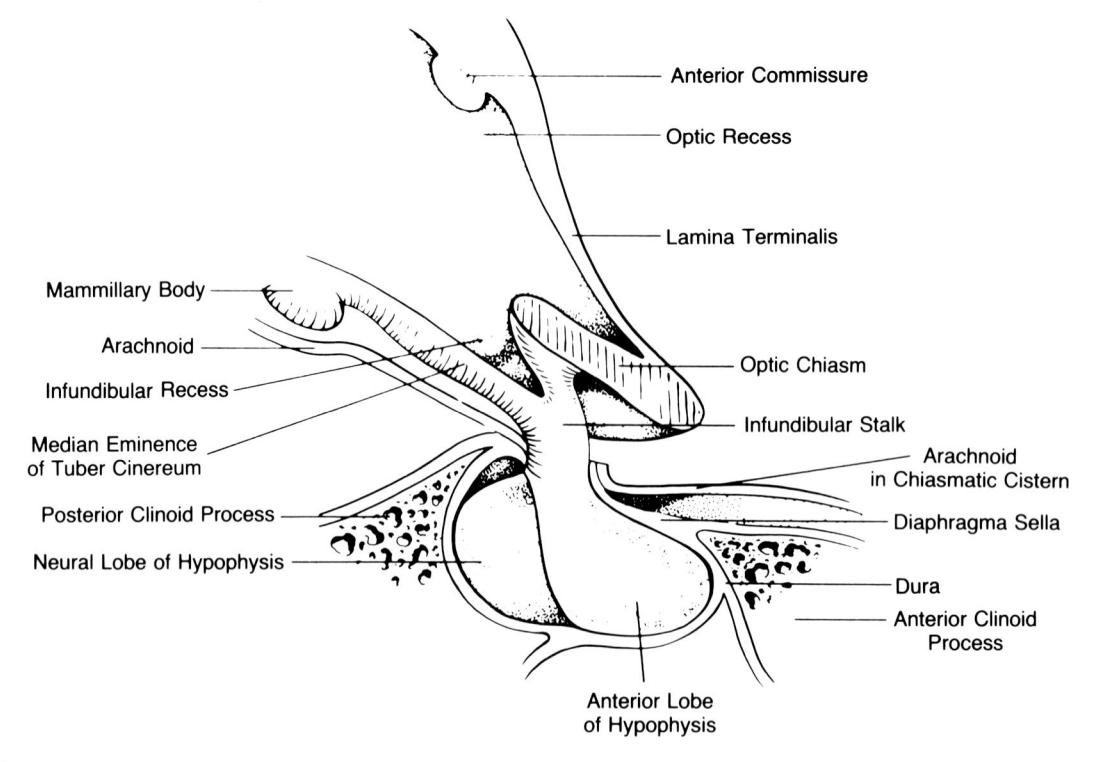

Fig. 3–1. The human hypothalmic-pituitary unit. (Reproduced with permission. Reichlin S. Neuroendocrinology. In: Reichlin S, Williams RH, eds. Textbook of endocrinology, 6th ed. Philadelphia: WB Saunders, 1981:592.)

mediation of visual influences on neuroendocrine function (10).

Hypothalamic Hormones

Hypothalamic hormones can be classified into three categories. First, the posterior pituitary hormones, vasopressin and oxytocin, are synthesized in the cell bodies of the supraoptic and paraventricular nuclei and are bound to neurophysin, a binding protein that transports both hormones. These hormones are carried through the long axons of the pituitary stalk to the neurohypophysis where they are stored for later release. Second, hypothalamic releasing hormones that regulate the release of anterior pituitary hormones are secreted at the median eminence of the hypothalamus and transported through the hypophyseal-pituitary portal circulation into the adenohypophysis where they effect an immediate action. Third, dopamine (a catecholaminergic neurotransmitter) must be considered a hypothalamic hormone because it is secreted in the hypothalamus and acts in the pituitary gland (11).

POSTERIOR PITUITARY HORMONES. Vasopressin secretion is regulated by plasma osmolarity and circulating blood volume. Acute water loading decreases plasma osmolarity and inhibits secretion of vasopressin; this facilitates renal clearance of water. Ingestion or infusion of a hyperosmotic solution stimulates secretion of vasopressin, which causes renal conservation of water.

Vasopressin deficiency gives rise to the clinical syndrome of diabetes insipidus, a condition characterized by the excretion of large volumes of hypotonic urine and ingestion of large volumes of water to prevent dehydration (12). Since diabetes insipidus occurs in 35% of people with hypothalamic disease, it is an important syndrome for the clinician to recognize (13).

Excessive secretion of vasopressin is associated with the syndrome of inappropriate antidiuretic hormone response. This condition is found in association with cerebral trauma, neurosurgical procedures, and a variety of medical conditions that do not directly involve the hypothalamus.

Oxytocin is liberated from the posterior pituitary under the stimulus of suckling and stimulates contraction of the mammary myoepithelial apparatus to cause milk ejection (14). In the latter part of pregnancy, oxytocin stimulates myometrial contraction, but there is no substantial evidence to suggest a physiologic role of oxytocin in the initiation of labor. Oxytocin in pharmacologic doses has antidiuretic properties and may cause water intoxication when large volumes of fluid are administered with it. No clinical disorders have been described resulting from excessive or deficient oxytocin secretion.

HYPOTHALAMIC HORMONES THAT REGULATE ANTERIOR PITUITARY FUNCTION.

Thyrotropin Releasing Hormone (TRH). TRH was the first hormone isolated and structurally identified by Guillemin and Schalley (4,5). TRH is a tripeptide amide that stimulates the release of pituitary thyroid stimulating hormone (TSH). TRH action on pituitary secretion of TSH is modulated by the plasma concentration of thyroxin and the effects of TRH are blocked by prior administration of thyroxin. This suggests that hypothalamic control of pituitary TSH secretion is regulated by the concentration of circulating thyroid hormone (14). TRH also stimulates prolactin release and hyperprolactinemia is often found in men and women with primary hypothyroidism.

Thyroid failure caused by abnormalities of TRH secretion occurs in association with hypothalamic dysfunction (15). When synthetic TRH is given by bolus injection (500 mcg), plasma levels of TSH rise within 3 minutes and reach a peak plasma concentration within 20 minutes. In individuals with suspected hypothalamic hypothyroidism, this test aids in establishing the anatomic site of origin of hypothyroidism.

Gonadotropin Releasing Hormone (GnRH). GnRH is a decapeptide secreted by the arcuate nucleus of the medial basal hypothalamus. The hypothalamus secretes GnRH in rhythmic pulses into the pituitary portal circulation. The hypothalamus must be regulated internally since its isolation from the higher CNS does not interfere with the secretion of GnRH (16,17). Sensory input from other CNS centers, however, modulates the secretion of GnRH in children and adults; blindness, deafness, and anosmia are often associated with precocious or delayed secondary sexual maturation.

The pulsatile release of GnRH is essential to synchronize the pulsatile secretion of pituitary gonadotropins. Knobil observed that continuous infusion of GnRH into female monkeys that had previously undergone ablation of the arcuate nucleus did not reinitiate gonadotropin secretion. When these same monkeys were given GnRH by pulsatile infusion at the rate of one 6 minute pulse/hour, physiologic pulsatile gonadotropin secretion was restored (18). Variation in the concentration of infused GnRH did not influence gonadotropin secretion, but the pulsatile pattern of GnRH seemed to be the critical factor in gonadotropin secretion. Gonadotropin secretion declined when the GnRH pulse frequency was increased to 2, 3, or more per hour (19).

Functional development of the hypothalamus begins with formation of its nuclei by the eighth gestational week (20,21). Biogenic amines have been identified as early as 10 weeks in the human fetus (22), and GnRH is present in fetal blood by 14 weeks (23). Follicle stimulating hormone (FSH) is present in the fetal pituitary by 9 weeks. However, the role of fetal hypothalamic and pituitary hormones in fetal growth, development, and preparation for extrauterine life is not known. Clearly, sex steroid hormones are active in sexual differentiation, but the secretion of sex steroid hormones during the first trimester of pregnancy appears to be under the control of placental tropic hormones rather than fetal pituitary hormones.

Pituitary gonadotropin secretion occurs for several months after birth (24); gonadal secretion of testosterone or estradiol, stimulated by pituitary gonadotoropins, also occurs during the first year of life, then declines to barely detectable concentrations (25). The infusion of GnRH produces a peak response of luteinizing hormone (LH) secretion between 1 and 3 months of age, but the LH response returns to a low prepubertal level between 9 and 12 months of age (26,27). During childhood, there is a diurnal secretion of gonadotropins, a pattern that is peculiar to children (28). At the time of puberty, hypothalamic-pituitary function changes to initiate the gonadotropin secretory pattern necessary to stimulate cyclic gonadal function.

After normal reproductive function has been established, an alteration in the pulsatile secretion of GnRH will cause an abnormality or cessation of reproductive function. Luteal dysfunction, anovulation, galactorrhea, or amenorrhea are each manifestations of changes in GnRH secretion in the female. These alterations occur with anorexia nervosa, simple weight loss and weight control practice, hyperprolactinemia, marijuana use, psychotropic drug use, and idiopathic hypogonadotropic hypogonadism. Although the role of GnRH in these disorders is not clearly established, fragmentary evidence supports the concept that hypothalamic dysfunction is often a principal cause of reproductive failure and other forms of endocrine dysfunction.

Pulsatile gonadotropin secretion is controlled by the feedback action of estradiol (E_2). The preovulatory surge of gonadotropins is the consequence of a positive feedback effect of E_2 on the pituitary. Complete neural disconnection of the hypothalamus from the remainder of the brain does not alter this feedback effect of E_2 (29). Moreover, gonadectomy in the monkey produces a 10-fold increase in plasma LH levels but does not increase portal vein concentrations of GnRH (30). These data suggest that E_2 acts at the pituitary gland rather than at the hypothalamus to modulate gonadotropin surges, while the pulsatile secretion of GnRH serves as the generator for gonadotropin secretion.

Daylight and darkness affect reproductive cycles and may alter the "biologic clock" that produces diurnal variation in the secretion of pituitary and steroid hormones. A direct neural projection from the retina to the suprachiasmatic nucleus of the hypothalamus exists in primates and probably in humans (17). Beyond establishment of circadian cycles, the role of visual input into the hypothalamus remains unknown in humans. Light seems to influence the time of onset of reproductive function—blind girls begin to menstruate at an earlier age than girls with normal sight (31). Light also seems to influence the maintenance of reproductive function. Women of reproductive age who frequently cross several time zones in 1 day (e.g., airline personnel) often experience disruption of cyclic menstruation, whereas those who travel similar distances but cross only 1 time zone retain cyclic menstruation (32). These observations suggest that light influences GnRH secretion.

Neural projections from the olfactory tracts innervate the hypothalamus and modulate, in poorly defined ways, reproductive function. Kallman syndrome is an example of congenital hypothalamic failure associated with an abnormality of olfaction (33,34). In subjects with Kallman syndrome, hypothalamic release of GnRH does not occur. The role of olfaction in the stimulation of GnRH secretion is unknown. The pulsatile administration of GnRH will stimulate pituitary gonadotropin secretion and initate normal reproductive function in affected individuals (35).

Olfaction plays an essential role in the mating behavior of reptiles, insects, lower mammals, and primates. Animals secrete pheromones from specialized secretory glands into the atmosphere or into urine; the pheromones are sensed by a member of the opposite sex of the same species. Induction of mating behavior, nesting behavior, territorial demarcation, and perhaps population control (36,37) are the consequences. Human pheromones have not been identified. However, volatile organic acids have been identified that are unique to the human vagina during the middle of the reproductive cycle (38). If apocrine secretions of the axilla and genitalia play a role in human mating behavior, it is reasonable to expect that the apocrine secretions are mediated through the olfactory-hypothalamic tracts.

Somatostatin and Growth Hormone Releasing Factor. Somatostatin was the third hypothalamic hormone characterized by Guillemin and Schalley (4,5). It is a 14-amino acid peptide that acts in the pituitary gland to suppress growth hormone secretion and acts outside the pituitary to inhibit the secretion of glucagon and insulin by pancreatic alpha and beta cells.

The chemical nature of growth-hormone-releasing factor has not been established. Such a substance must exist because the injection of hypothalamic extracts into the hypophyseal portal plexus stimulates the release of growth hormone.

Dopamine. Dopamine, although classified as a neurotransmitter, must also be considered a hypothalamic hormone. Dopamine is secreted into the portal veins and suppresses prolactin secretion (39). Drugs that block dopamine receptors (e.g., phenothiazines, tricyclic antidepressants, and methyldopa) or deplete catecholamine stores (e.g., reserpine) stimulate prolactin release. Women taking any of these drugs may be anovulatory, oligomenorrheic, or have amenorrhea-galactorrhea (40). Men taking any of these drugs may have loss of libido and decreased frequency of penile erections (41). In both men and women, gonadotropin concentrations are low and the prolactin concentration is high.

Drugs that stimulate dopamine receptors, such as the dopamine agonist bromocriptine, are useful in the management of men and women with reproductive failure brought on by hyperprolactinemia (42). One note of caution must be given. It is not appropriate to treat persons whose reproductive failure is caused by prolactin excess with bromocriptine when the prolactin excess is a result of the use of a dopamine receptor blocking agent (e.g., phenothiazines). The simultaneous use of pharmacologic agents with opposing actions could be hazardous (43).

Hypothalamic Physiology

The hypothalamus is the integrator for a variety of vegetative and endocrine functions. Thermoregulation, satiety, sleep, sexual behavior, and emotional control seem to be modulated in part by the hypothalamus. Puberty is the most dramatic sign of change in hypothalamic function.

INITIATION OF PUBERTY. The hypothalamic-pituitary-gonadal axis matures during fetal life. Soon after birth, the reproductive endocrine system becomes quiescent and remains so until puberty; the mechanism(s) that holds sexual maturation in abeyance until puberty is unknown. However, the hypothalamus, if stimulated, will secrete GnRH during childhood. The pituitary gland, if stimulated by GnRH, will secrete gonadotropins. The gonads, if stimulated by gonadotropins, will secrete sex steroid hormones. The secondary sex target organs (uterus, breasts, vagina, phallus, prostate, etc.), if stimulated by sex steroid hormones, will grow and develop.

The progressive decline in the age of puberty over the past century has been attributed, in part, to improvements in socioeconomic conditions and general health. Recently, body fat has been shown to play a role in the initiation of puberty. Frisch and Revelle postulated that a mean body weight of 86 lbs. is required before breast growth begins and a mean body weight of 106 lbs. is necessary for menstruation to begin (44). The concept that a fixed body weight was the critical event required to initiate a particular phase of pubertal development has been criticized. In clinical practice, however, these weights serve as a useful prognostic guide for evaluating girls with pubertal failure. The prevailing concept of the influence of body weight on puberty and subsequent reproductive function is that a requisite percent of body fat is necessary to initiate and sustain reproductive function. Effects of nutrition and body composition upon the time of onset of puberty are supported by an earlier age of menarche in moderately obese girls (45), by delayed sexual maturation in chronic illness (46), and by the relationship of amenorrhea to such states of diminished body fat as anorexia nervosa (46,47) and voluntary weight loss (48).

The percent of body fat necessary for breast budding, menarche, and maintenance of reproductive function has not been clearly defined. It appears that the body composition in females must be approximately 22% to 24% fat to sustain reproductive function (49). The role of body fat in the initiation of male puberty is not known, but preadolescent males accumulate body fat before testicular function begins and the growth spurt occurs.

How does body fat alter neuroendocrine mechanisms that trigger hypothalamic-pituitary function? There is accumulating evidence that body fat plays both a direct and indirect role in sex-steroid metabolism. Fishman et al. infused radiolabeled estradiol into 3 groups of women (obese women, women of normal body habitus, and women with anorexia nervosa) and found differences in the metabolism of estradiol (50). Obese women excreted estriol as the major estrogen metabolite while women with anorexia nervosa excreted 2-hydroxyestradiol (a catechol estrogen) as the major estrogen metabolite. Catechol estrogens, which compete with catecholamines for metabolism by catechol-o-methyltransferase (51), may inhibit the pulsatile secretion of gonadotropins and may regulate the maturational phase of the LH secretory pattern.

GONADOTROPIN SECRETION DURING PUBERTY. Soon after birth, plasma gonadotropins decrease to low levels and remain so throughout childhood. Plasma concentrations of FSH and LH are low but the concentration of FSH is slightly greater. This results in a ratio of LH:FSH of one or slightly less. Secretory bursts of LH occur during childhood but the amplitude of the secretion is lower than that found in adults (52); the pattern of LH secretion has no relationship to the sleep cycle during childhood.

In the peripubertal period, plasma gonadotropin concentrations rise. In girls, FSH concentrations rise during the early stages of puberty and then plateau; LH levels begin to rise later in puberty and increase sharply at the time of menarche. With the onset of ovulation and the development of predictable reproductive cycles, an adult LH secretory pattern is established. Boyar et al. were the first to note the sleep-associated increase in gonadotropin secretion (both basal levels and secretory pulses) that occurs during early and mid puberty (52). The highest concentration of LH is found during stage IV (anesthetic) sleep. After ovulation is established, prominent LH pulses are noted during the day and the gonadotropin secretory pattern is not entrained to the sleep cycle. A composite diagram of the gonadotropin secretory patterns during the stages of sexual maturation is presented in Fig. 3–2.

Children with idiopathic precocious puberty exhibit the same LH secretory pattern as normal children (52). Children with gonadal dysgenesis have an LH secretory pattern similar to that of normal children at puberty, suggesting that gonadotropin secretion at puberty depends upon hypothalamic function but not gonadal function (53). Sleep-associated LH release appears to correlate with increased sensitivity of pituitary gonadotrophs to the administration of GnRH in the prepubertal period and during puberty (54).

A discussion of the gonadotropin secretory pattern may seem academic for the practicing physician who is treating men and women with reproductive failure. However, an understanding of gonadotropin secretion is essential because gonadotropin secretion reverts to an intrapubertal pattern in a variety of functional hypothalamic disorders, and may even revert to a prepubertal pattern. Recognition of the alterations in LH and FSH secretory patterns and an understanding of the plasma concentrations of these hormones is necessary to diagnose and manage weight-related and drug-induced reproductive failure.

The factors involved in the restraint of the onset of puberty are not well understood. Reiter and Grumbach proposed a dual mechanism to explain the prepubertal restraint (Fig. 3–3) (55). First, there is a sex steroid *dependent* mechanism—a highly sensitive hypothalamic-pituitary-gonadal negative feedback system. Second, there is a sex steroid *independent* mechanism of intrinsic CNS inhibition. Puberty begins when this inhibition is overcome and the arcuate nucleus begins to secrete GnRH (Fig. 3–4).

The prepubertal state is characterized by functional GnRH insufficiency. When Knobil infused prepubertal monkeys with GnRH in a pulsatile manner, he was able to induce cyclic ovulation after an infusion period of 93 to 253 days (7). When the infusion was discontinued, ovulation ceased and the monkeys resumed their prepubertal state. The administration of GnRH to adult humans with hypothalamic failure such as Kallman syndrome (56,57) and anorexia nervosa (58) induces a pubertal-type gonadotropin secretory pattern. These reports enhance our understanding of neuroendocrine physiology, the diagnosis of neuroendocrine disorders, and the treatment of reproductive failure in these individuals.

Marshall and Tanner developed a clinical

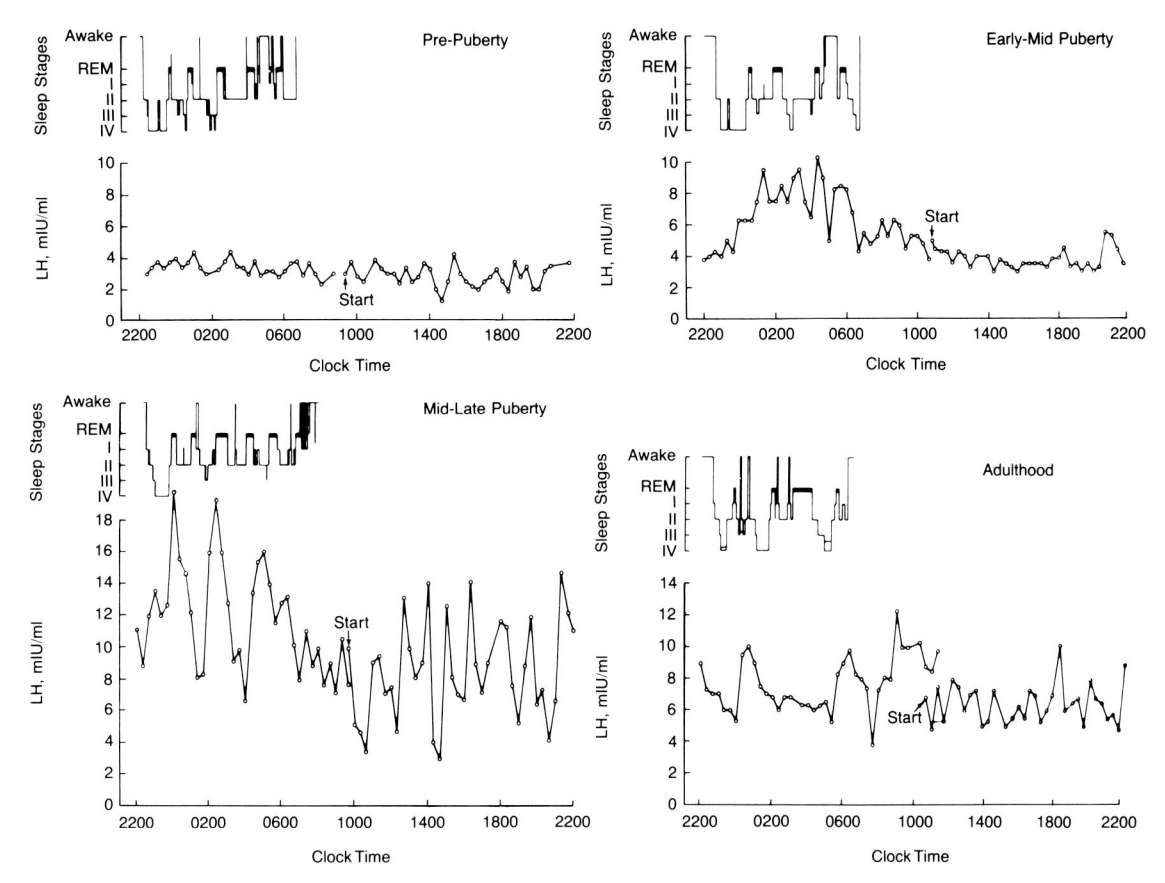

Fig. 3–2. Ontogeny of the human circadian LH secretory pattern from prepuberty, through early and late puberty, into adulthood. (Reproduced with permission. Katz et al. Psychosom Med 1978; 40:555.)

scheme for the progression of secondary sexual development in girls and boys (59). This scheme is useful in evaluating children who present with precocious puberty, incomplete puberty, or sexual infantilism. In girls, the usual progression of sexual maturation is breast budding, sexual hair growth, somatic growth spurt, menarche, and finally development of the adult breast. Deviations from this sequence suggest that an alteration in hypothalamic-pituitary-gonadal function has occurred (60). For example, if a female child presents with pubic hair growth in the absence of breast budding, an extragonadal source of androgens is suggested; or if a female child has breast development in the absence of pubic hair growth, an exogenous source of estrogens or an estrogen-producing ovarian tumor is suggested. When the progression of puberty occurs in the expected sequence, reproductive endocrine function is likely to be normal.

Disorders of Hypothalamic Function

Hypothalamic disease is often associated with disorders of endocrine function, sexual function, and behavior. Bauer found sexual abnormalities (hypogonadism or precocious puberty) in 72% of 60 men and women with autopsy-proven hypothalamic disease (13). Diabetes insipidus and psychic disturbances were present in 35%, obesity or hyperphagia in 33%, and somnolence, anorexia, and alteration in thermoregulation were present in others.

Disorders of sleep, eating, temperature regulation (such as "fever of unknown origin"), sexual behavior, thirst, and recent memory should alert the physician to the possibility of a hypothalamic abnormality. Hypothalamic diseases that alter reproductive function can be classified into one of three major categories: (1) congenital hypothalamic dysfunction such as Kallman syndrome (manifested by anosmia and hypogonadotropic hypogonadism) and Prader-Willi syndrome (manifested by hyperphagia, massive obesity, mental retardation, and hypogonadotropic hypogonadism); (2) functional hypothalamic disorders such as anorexia nervosa, psychogenic amenorrhea, and post-pill amenorrhea; and (3) hypothalamic dysfunction that results from neoplasms or inflammatory lesions that encroach upon or infiltrate the hypothalamus. Functional hypothalamic disorders will be emphasized because they occur most commonly.

CONGENITAL HYPOTHALAMIC DYSFUNCTION. Kallman syndrome (first described in males and referred to as DeMorsier syndrome in females) is characterized by anosmia, varying degrees of hypogonadotropic hypogonadism, color blindness, and eighth nerve deafness. These patients present with sexual infantilism (Fig. 3–5). Males have azoospermia and females have primary amenorrhea. Laboratory evaluation reveals prepubertal levels of FSH, LH, and sex-steroid hormones. Agenesis or dysgenesis of the anterior commissure, the olfactory lobes, the olfactory tracts, and the posterior rhinencephalon causes the anosmia

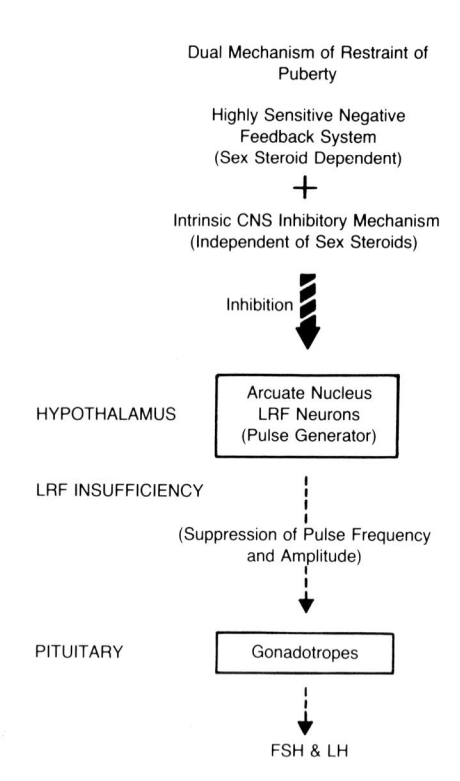

Fig. 3–3. Dual mechanism of restraint of puberty. (Reproduced with permission. Reiter EO, Grumbach MM. Annu Rev Physiol 1982;44:601. Copyright 1982 by Annual Reviews Inc.)

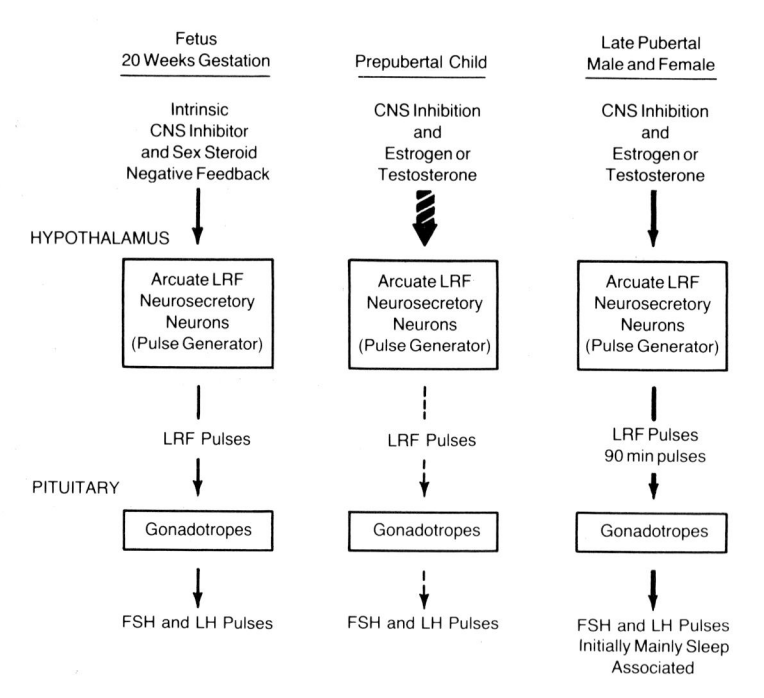

Fig. 3–4. A scheme illustrating the changes in the activity of the arcuate GnRH pulse generator during development. (Reproduced with permission. Reiter EO, Grumbach MM. Annu Rev Physiol 1982;44:603. Copyright 1982 by Annual Reviews Inc.)

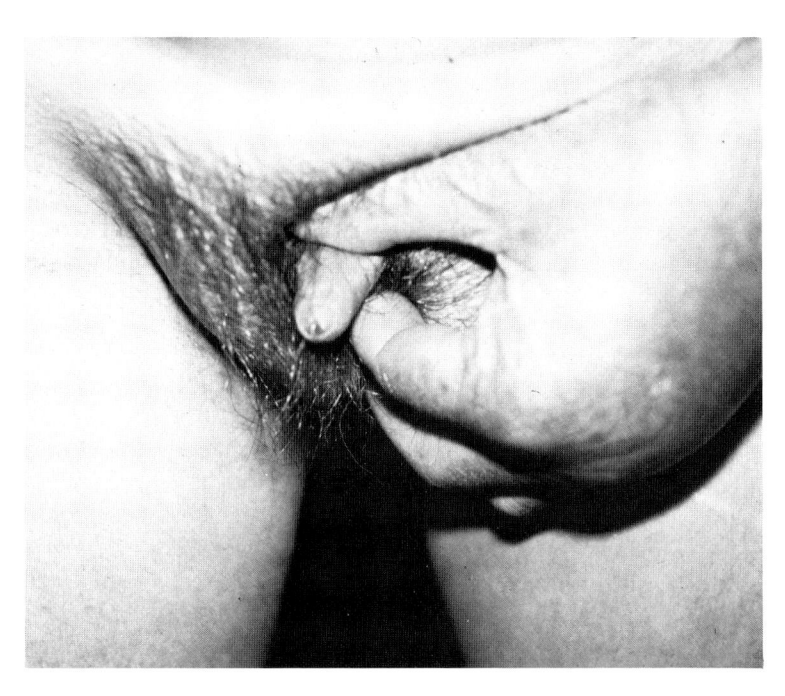

Fig. 3–5. External genitalia of an untreated, middle-aged man with Kallman syndrome. Prepubertal gonads are located in the scrotum. Sexual hair growth was stimulated, presumably, by adrenal androgens.

and failure of hypothalamic secretion of GnRH (34).

The diagnosis of Kallman syndrome should be suspected if a person with pubertal failure is unable to smell an alcohol pledget or freshly brewed coffee. Once anosmia or hyposmia is discovered, the finding of prepubertal plasma concentrations of LH and FSH confirms the diagnosis and an extensive hormonal survey can be avoided.

Persons with this type of pubertal failure have the potential for endogeneous sex steroid secretion and normal reproduction. They should be reassured of this. Puberty can be induced in those with Kallman syndrome by the long-term pulsatile administration of low dose GnRH through a portable infusion pump. Spermatogenesis occurred in 3 of 6 men with hypogonadotropic hypogonadism after 4, 11, and 43 weeks of GnRH therapy (57). Normal menstrual cycles can be induced in women with anosmia who receive GnRH in this manner (61,62). GnRH is available but the cost and route of administration preclude its widespread use at present. The conventional form of management is to induce secondary sexual maturation with sex steroid hormones (63) and then induce spermatogenesis or ovulation with menopausal gonadotropins and human chorionic gonadotropin. This may be replaced by GnRH administration when experience is greater and more convenient routes of administration (e.g., nasal spray) are available.

Hypogonadotropic hypogonadism of hypothalamic origin occurs in disorders associated with massive obesity, mental retardation, and sexual infantilism (Laurence-Moon-Biedl syndrome and Prader-Willi syndrome) (64). Administration of GnRH to pubertal children with this disorder will *not* evoke a normal pubertal response of gonadotropin secretion (65), perhaps because the volume of distribution of GnRH in obese subjects is significantly greater than in normal subjects (66). Weight reduction in massively obese persons has resulted in normal secondary sexual maturation. This suggests that obesity itself may be the cause of hypothalamic-pituitary failure rather than some inherent disorder of hypothalamic function.

A rare cause of hypothalamic failure is a basal encephalocele, which may occur in association with midfacial anomalies including a broad nasal root, hypertelorism, and cleft-lip. In these disorders, the pituitary can herniate through the floor of the sella turcica and secretion of growth hormone, FSH, LH, and prolactin is altered (67).

FUNCTIONAL DISORDERS OF THE HYPOTHALAMUS. Functional disorders of the hypothalamus constitute the most frequently encountered problems of hypothalamic origin in clinical practice and anorexia nervosa is the most extreme example. Other functional disorders are frequently associated with reduced body weight: athletic amenorrhea, infertility secondary to weight control practice, amenorrhea caused by simple weight loss, and post-pill amenorrhea. Precocious puberty is considered in the category of functional hypothalamic disorders because most women with isosexual precocious puberty have no evidence of congenital or anatomic abnormalities. In males with precocious puberty, however, a hypothalamic tumor should be considered first in the differential diagnosis.

Anorexia Nervosa. Anorexia nervosa occurs primarily among adolescent Causcasian females from middle to upper-social-class backgrounds in Western society. The disorder occurs 19 times more frequently in women (68,69) and is rare in males (70). Anorexia nervosa was named by Gull over 100 years ago because of the presence of hyperactivity in emaciated patients whose "want of appetite is due to a morbid mental state" (71). The term, however, is a misnomer as patients with anorexia nervosa are preoccupied with food and have little evidence of loss of appetite.

The anorectic woman is usually the product of older parents, and is an only child or the elder of two daughters in a small, female-dominated family. The family values outward appearance, proper behavior, and outstanding achievement more than mutual understanding, inner contentment, and self-realization. These attitudes make the child eager to please and to achieve perfection. Within this emotional framework, anorectic behavior emerges along with high levels of achievement (68). The development of anorexia nervosa with its attendant sexual infantilism may be a mechanism for avoiding heterosexual relationships and sexual function (72). These and other psychodynamic features must be considered with the neuroendocrine investigation in the evaluation of anorexia nervosa.

The diagnosis of anorexia nervosa is based on (1) unchangeable attitudes toward eating, food, and weight that include denial of illness, apparent enjoyment in losing weight, desire of an extremely thin body image, and (2) profound weight loss (25% or more). The disorder must not be caused by any other known medical or psychiatric disorder (69). The affected woman has a distorted body image; even in her emaciated condition she views herself as having especially large hips and thighs. A useful technique to illustrate this body image distortion is to ask the woman to draw a picture of herself in her present condition and another picture when she has increased her body weight to near ideal proportions (Fig. 3–6). Invariably she will depict herself as obese when she reaches her ideal body weight.

On physical examination the young woman with anorexia nervosa will have a seemingly large face with large eyes that dominate her face (Fig. 3–7). The breasts are atrophic and the external genitalia are withered, like those of an elderly woman. The vagina is atrophic, smooth, and dusky.

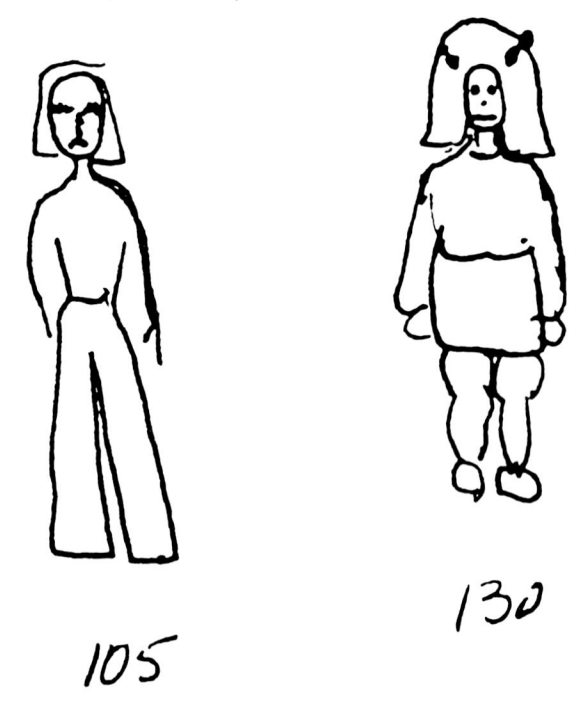

Fig. 3–6. Body proportions as perceived by a young woman who is 68 inches tall and weighs 105 pounds. Note her self-image at ideal body weight (130 pounds).

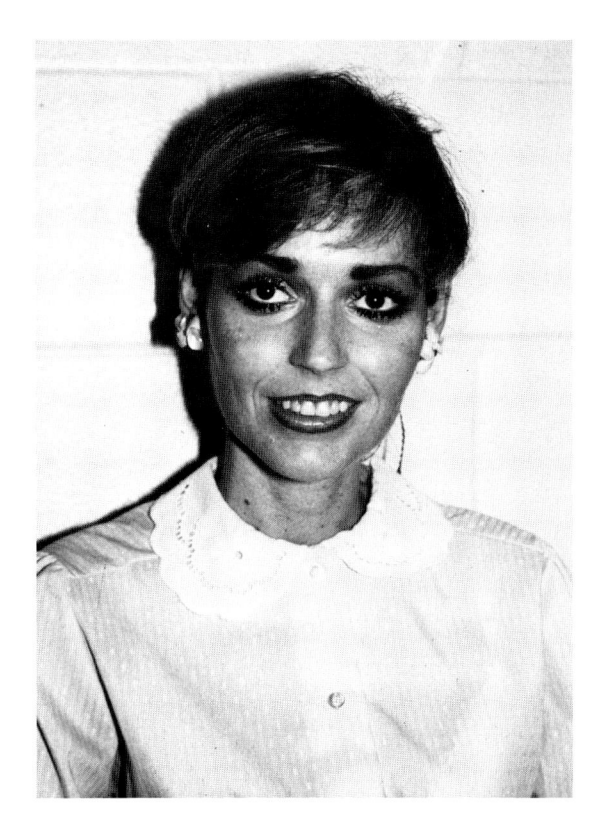

Fig. 3–7. A nineteen year-old woman with anorexia nervosa. Note the dominant eyes.

These women have several clinical features suggestive of hypothalamic and pituitary disease: amenorrhea, functional hypothyroidism, bradycardia, cold intolerance (73), partial diabetes insipidus, and alterations in cortisol metabolism. Amenorrhea is a cardinal feature of anorexia nervosa. Boyar et al. found that the 24-hour secretion of gonadotropins reverts to a prepubertal pattern in women with anorexia nervosa (74) and never returns to an adult pattern, unless the woman restores her body weight and gives up her anorectic behavior (75). Associated with decreased gonadotropin secretion, sex steroid hormone secretion is low.

The LH response to a large single dose of GnRH in women with anorexia nervosa is diminished compared to that observed in normally cycling women in the follicular phase of the menstrual cycle (76). However, pulsatile administration of GnRH over 5 days produces a gonadotropin secretory pattern similar to that found in normal girls at the time of puberty (76). This suggests that the altered reproductive function in women with anorexia nervosa is due to a change in GnRH secretion.

A growing body of evidence indicates that anorexia nervosa is associated with abnormal catecholaminergic activity within the central nervous system (77–79). Animal studies have shown that dopamine and norepinephrine nerve terminals are located near the arcuate nucleus. In humans, LH secretion is inhibited by dopamine, levodopa, and bromocriptine and these observations suggest that dopamine has a direct effect on hypothalamic GnRH release.

Women with anorexia nervosa have functional hypothyroidism. Concentrations of triidothyronine (T_3) are low while thyroxin (T_4) concentrations are normal (79,80). This occurs because of a change in the peripheral deiodination of T_4 to T_3. In extreme weight loss, the inner ring of T_4 is deiodinated to produce reverse T_3—a metabolically inactive form of triidothyronine. Teleologically, this alteration in thyroxin metabolism seems to be protective in that metabolism is slowed and protein utilization is reduced. Although it is tempting to replace T_3 in women with anorexia nervosa because of functional hypothyroidism, such replacement is contraindicated as it will facilitate catabolism. When body weight is restored, there is a transient overproduction of T_3 that results in a temporary state of hyperthyroidism. Thyroxin metabolism returns to normal soon after ideal body weight is achieved (81).

Cortisol metabolism is also altered in anorexia nervosa. The mean plasma cortisol concentration tends to be higher than in normal women but the diurnal variation is normal. The 24-hour cortisol production rate is normal, but the metabolic clearance rate for cortisol is decreased and the plasma half-life is increased (82). ACTH secretion appears to be relatively normal.

The treatment of anorexia nervosa is perplexing because it is difficult to overcome the underlying psychopathology that is so prominent in this disease. Intensive psychotherapy with a goal-oriented weight increase is necessary. Estrogen administration (oral estradiol, 2 mg/day or vaginal estrone, 1.25 mg/day) facilitates weight gain and helps restore secondary sexual characteristics (83,84). This therapy should be continued until body weight approaches 90% of the predicted ideal. Achievement of ideal body weight results in restoration of normal hypothalamic-pituitary-gonadal function. Although the long-term consequences of anorexia nervosa after nutritional rehabilitation has been achieved are unknown, there do not appear to be any lasting sequelae.

Athletic Amenorrhea and Amenorrhea Associated with Simple Weight Loss. Anorexia nervosa is the extreme form of hypothalamic dysfunction and reproductive failure, but simple weight loss, athletic endeavors, and weight control practice are more common causes of amenorrhea and reproductive failure.

Vigersky et al. investigated hypothalamic-pituitary function in 19 women with secondary amenorrhea related to simple weight loss and found alterations in thermoregulation, water metabolism, gonadotropin secretion, and thyrotropin secretion (85). These changes were similar to those found in anorexia nervosa but were less profound. The authors concluded that hypothalamic dysfunction may be caused by weight loss alone. Others have also reported that a loss in body weight of 15% or more is associated with secondary amenorrhea (86,87).

During refeeding of young women with nutritional amenorrhea, plasma LH concentrations increase, menses resume, and ovulation returns (46). When body weight was restored to within 98% of predicted ideal in 29 infertile women who controlled their weight by caloric restriction, 73% conceived spontaneously (88). Knuth et al. advised restoration of weight to normal limits as the primary form of ovulation induction for underweight women (86).

The impact of repeated, prolonged, strenuous exercise on the menstrual cycle of otherwise healthy women is now recognized. Pubertal progression and menarche are delayed in ballet dancers attending professional dancing schools (89–91). When these girls interrupted their training, menses occurred spontaneously. Menstrual dysfunction occurs in distance runners (92). Delayed menarche and amenorrhea are common in college athletes who began training before the onset of puberty (93). The incidence of amenorrhea is less for those who began training after the onset of puberty.

The effects of physical exercise on hypothalamic-pituitary function in males has not been well studied. Morville et al. found decreased concentrations of testicular androgens (testosterone and dihydrotestosterone) and increased adrenal androgens (androstenedione) in highly trained male athletes compared with a control population (94). It is not unreasonable to expect that reproductive dysfunction in male athletes and underweight men will be similar to that found in women, but this has not been established.

The precise endocrine mechanisms underlying the menstrual disturbance in young women athletes are uncertain and the long-term effects of these endocrine abnormalities are unknown. Since these athletes have an altered lean:fat ratio, it is likely that the endocrine dysfunction is similar to that found in anorexia nervosa and other weight-loss disorders. At present, these abnormalities in reproductive function do not seem serious and may be reversed by changes in life style (95).

Marijuana-Induced Amenorrhea. Marijuana (delta-9-tetrahydrocannabinol) decreases the plasma concentration of gonadotropins in males and females of several species (96,97). Men who are heavy users of marijuana have decreased sex hormone secretion and sperm production. Women who are heavy users of marijuana may be anovulatory and amenorrheic. Marijuana blocks reflex ovulation in the rabbit and prevents ovulation in the rhesus monkey (98). When administered to ovariectomized monkeys, marijuana inhibits gonadotropin secretion by 50% to 88%. The mechanism of action of marijuana-induced reproductive failure is unknown, but preliminary studies suggest that this agent blocks the release of GnRH (99).

Delayed puberty, primary amenorrhea, and secondary amenorrhea have been observed in preadolescent, adolescent, and young-adult marijuana users. When the drug is discontinued, menses resume spontaneously within 3 to 6 months (100). Marijuana is widely used in modern Western society; this agent should be considered in evaluating couples with reproductive failure.

Precocious Puberty. The prepubertal child of any age can respond to tropic hormones. Sexual development at puberty progresses in a predictable way in both males and females. Puberty is precocious when any of the pubertal events occurs before the age of 9 years. In evaluating a child with sexual precocity, two questions must be answered: Which hormone(s) is responsible and what is the source of that hormone? Pubic hair growth without breast development in the female or testicular enlargement in the male suggests an extragonadal source of androgens. When there is isosexual precocious puberty (i.e., pubertal development appropriate for the gender) and gametogenesis occurs, a hypothalamic cause should be suspected. Viral encephalitis (Fig. 3–8), craniopharyngiomas, hamartomas, neurofibromatosis, and McCune-Albright syndrome (polyostotic fibrous dysplasia) are the most frequent pathologic causes of precocious puberty of hypothalamic origin.

Children with precocious puberty should have computed axial tomography (CAT scan) of the head to exclude a tumor impinging upon the hypothalamus or pituitary, a skull X-ray to exclude fibrous dysplasia at the base of the skull (McCune-Albright syndrome), a lumbar puncture to exclude viral or bacterial encephalitis, and plasma gonadotropins to evaluate pituitary function. When a neoplasm is encountered it should be managed by radiotherapy or chemotherapy, but when no organic cause for isosexual precocious puberty is found, the disorder is best managed by the administration of a long-acting GnRH agonist. Continuous administration of GnRH or a long-acting analogue of GnRH blocks the release of FSH and LH and arrests further precocious sexual development until the appropriate time for puberty (101,102). This therapy is indicated only in those children with precocious puberty of hypothalamic origin. Chronic administration of a progestin also inhibits gonadotropin secretion and has been the traditional therapy.

An anatomic lesion of the hypothalamus is especially likely when precocious puberty occurs in boys. In Bauer's series of 60 autopsy patients a hypothalamic tumor was the most common finding and 40% had precocious puberty (13).

Post-Pill Amenorrhea. The frequency of post-pill amenorrhea is 0.2% to 3.1% of women stopping oral contraceptives. The variation in the reported frequency is a result of different definitions of the duration of amenorrhea (103). Preexisting menstrual irregularities were present in 37% of women with post-pill amenorrhea studied by Buttram (104). Body weight may be an important factor in the development of post-pill amenorrhea since

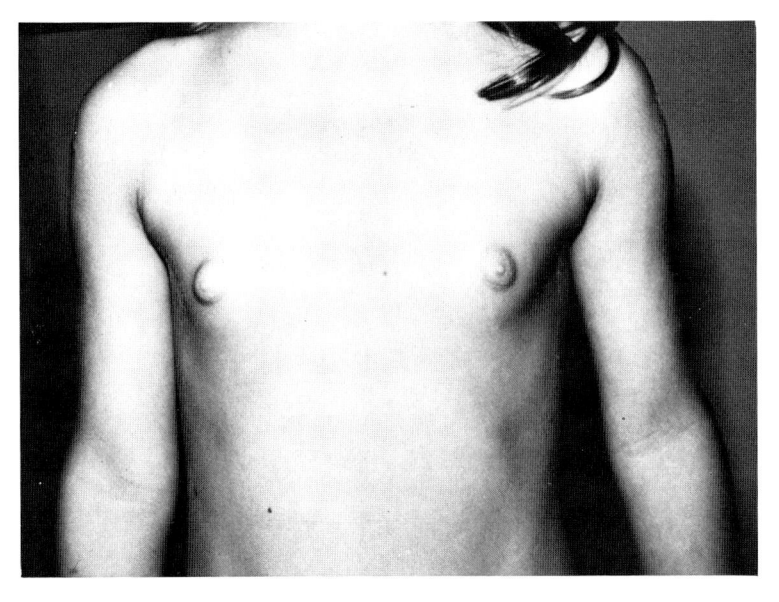

Fig. 3–8. Precocious thelarche in a 5 year-old girl following a short-lived viral encephalitis infection. Plasma gonadotropins were elevated for 2 months after the illness; they returned spontaneously to prepubertal levels.

women who are more than 10% below predicted ideal body weight have an increased incidence of menstrual dysfunction and amenorrhea while taking oral contraceptives (87,105). Moreover, underweight women are more likely than obese women to experience side effects such as headache, nausea, breast discomfort, and fluid retention while on oral contraceptives (106).

Pulsatile patterns of gonadotropin secretion are absent in women with post-pill amenorrhea and the response to GnRH administration is blunted. Approximately 20% of women with this disorder will have hyperprolactinemia with radiologic evidence of a pituitary microadenoma (103). An evaluation of women with post-pill amenorrhea should include a history for possible changes in body weight while taking oral contraceptives, the menstrual history prior to oral contraceptive use, and measurement of gonadotropins and prolactin.

Hypothalamic Dysfunction in Chronic Renal Failure. Gonadal dysfunction in men and menstrual abnormalities in women occur in association with chronic renal failure and uremia. Loss of libido in males and galactorrhea in women are frequent complaints. Pulsatile cyclicity of gonadotropin secretion is lost, the positive feedback response of LH to estradiol administration is lost (107), the pituitary lactotrophs are resistant to dopamine (108), and prolactin is elevated. Hemodialysis will not correct the reproductive endocrinopathy, but bromocriptine administration may improve libidinal desire and restore cyclic menses. Successful renal transplantation, however, will abolish the hypothalamic-pituitary dysfunction (109).

Hypothalamic Dysfunction Resulting from Neoplasms and Inflammatory Infiltrates. Neoplastic tumors and inflammatory infiltrates in, or adjacent to, the hypothalamus may present clinically as an endocrine or neurologic abnormality. The most common neoplasm impinging on the hypothalamus is a craniopharyngioma, which may produce anterior pituitary failure and diabetes insipidus. The tumor usually has its onset before age 15 years. Calcification of the suprasellar region is often noted and enlargement of the sella is common (110).

Inflammatory and granulomatous infiltrates of the hypothalamus produce symptoms of hypothalamic-pituitary failure. The most frequent manifestations of these diseases are reproductive failure (amenorrhea in women, impotence in men) and partial diabetes insipidus. Pituitary function testing may reveal alterations in TSH and growth hormone secretion (see Chapter 4). Hypothalamic endocrinopathies have been reported in sarcoidosis (111,112), Hand-Schuller-Christian disease (113), and infiltrating neoplasms (114). When patients have bizarre symptoms such as fever of unexplained origin (unresponsive to salicylate therapy), bradycardia, somnolence, episodes of uncontrolled laughing or rage, an infiltrating lesion of the hypothalamus should be considered.

Hypothalamic Function Testing

TRH administration is effective in stimulating pituitary TSH release when given intravenously as a bolus or by continuous infusion. It may be given by intramuscular or oral administration as well. A significant increase in TSH is observed within 10 minutes, and a peak level is achieved within 20 to 30 minutes. The response is exaggerated in hypothyroidism and blunted in thyrotoxicosis.

GnRH administration is effective in stimulating gonadotropin release when given intravenously. Doses range from 10 to 25 mcg per test. After a single intravenous injection the peak response occurs 15 to 45 minutes later for LH and 60 to 90 minutes later for FSH (115). The LH response is greater than the FSH response. Plasma estrogen levels modulate the LH response.

Clomiphene citrate acts on the hypothalamus to stimulate FSH release. For clomiphene citrate to be effective, plasma estrogen concentrations must be sufficient to evoke pituitary secretion of gonadotropins. Because the endpoint (ovulation) of clomiphene citrate administration is delayed, it is not an effective test of hypothalamic-pituitary function. Clomiphene is ineffective in hypoestrogenic women.

Computed axial tomography has replaced skull X-rays, arteriograms, and pneumoencephalograms for evaluation of the hypothalamus. Neoplasms invading or impinging upon the hypothalamus or pituitary gland can usually be identified by the procedure. Technique is important to produce optimal results since the volume of the hypothalamic area is small (116).

Summary

The hypothalamus integrates endocrine and vegetative functions through afferent input from neurotransmitters and efferent output by releasing factors and releasing hormones. Satiety, sleep, thermoregulation, water metabolism, growth, adrenal function, thyroid function, reproductive function, and behavior are modulated by the hypothalamus. Therefore, disorders of these body functions suggest a possible hypothalamic origin.

The most frequently encountered disorders of the hypothalamus are functional in origin. In modern Western society, hypothalamic disorders often originate from a particular life style. Marijuana abuse, the projection of a slender body habitus, and avid athletic endeavors may lead to hypothalamic dysfunction. These functional disorders seem to be limited to the continuation of the particular causal life style and they abate rapidly after the life style has been changed.

Tumors and infiltrating lesions of the hypothalamus usually cause insidious changes in hypothalamic function and do not abate with a change in life style. More serious, even life-threatening, symptoms are found in patients with one of these disorders. A disturbance of hypothalamic function may also develop insidiously with many chronic systemic diseases (117).

The key to making a diagnosis of hypothalamic disease is a high index of clinical suspicion. An understanding of hypothalamic-pituitary physiology and hypothalamic-pituitary function testing should lead to the diagnosis of a hypothalamic disorder when one exists.

REFERENCES

1. Harris GW. Neural control of the pituitary gland. Physiol Rev 1948;28:139–179.
2. Scharrer E, Scharrer B. Neuroendocrinology. New York: Columbia University Press, 1973.
3. Guillemin R, Rosenburg B. Hormonal hypothalamic control of anterior pituitary: a study with combined tissue cultures. Endocrinology 1955;57:599–607.
4. Guillemin R. Peptides in the brain: the new endocrinology of the neuron. Science 1978;202:390–402.
5. Schalley AV. Aspects of hypothalamic regulation of the pituitary gland: its implications for the control of the reproductive process. Science 1978;202:18–28.
6. Knobil E, Plant TM, Wildt L, et al. Control of the rhesus monkey menstrual cycle: permissive role of hypothalamic gonadotropin-releasing hormone. Science 1980;207:1371–1373.
7. Wildt L, Marshall G, Knobil E. Experimental induction of puberty in the infantile female rhesus monkey. Science 1980;207:1373–1375.
8. Reichlin S. Neuroendocrinology. In: Williams RH, ed. Textbook of endocrinology. Philadelphia: WB Saunders, 1981:591–594.
9. Moore RY. Neuroendocrine regulation of reproduction. In: Yen SSC, Jaffe, RB, eds. Reproductive endocrinology. Philadelphia: WB Saunders, 1978:3–33.
10. Moore RY. Central neural control of circadian rhythms. In: Martini L, Ganong WF, eds. Frontiers in neuroendocrinology. New York: Raven Press, 1978:185–206.
11. Pohl CR, Knobil E. The role of the central nervous system in the control of ovarian function in higher primates. Annu Rev Physiol 1982;44:583–593.
12. Kleemen CR, Bert T. Neurohypophyseal hormones: vasopressin. In: DeGroot LJ, Cahil GF, Martini L, et al., eds. Endocrinology. New York: Grune & Stratton, 1979:253–275.
13. Bauer HG. Endocrine and other clinical manifestations of hypothalamic disease. A survey of 60 cases with autopsies. J Clin Endocrinol Metab 1954;14:13–31.
14. Reichlin S. Neuroendocrinology. In: Williams RH, ed. Textbook of endocrinology. Philadelphia: WB Saunders, 1981:602.
15. Christy NP, Warren MP. Disease symptoms of the hypothalamus and anterior pituitary. In: DeGroot LJ, Chail GF, Martini L, et al., eds. Endocrinology. New York: Grune & Stratton, 1979:215-252.
16. Krey LC, Butler WR, Knobil E. Surgical disconnection of the medial basal hypothalamus and pituitary function in the rhesus monkey. I. Gonadotropin secretion. Endocrinology 1975;96:1073–1087.
17. Raisman G. Some aspects of the neural connections of the hypothalamus. In: Martini L, Motta M, Frashini F, eds. The hypothalamus. New York: Academic Press, 1970:1–16.
18. Nakai Y, Plant TM, Hess DL, et al. On the

sites of negative and positive feedback action of estradiol in the control of gonadotropin secretion in the rhesus monkey. Endocrinology 1978;102:1008–1014.
19. Wildt L, Hausler A, Marshall G, et al. Frequency and amplitude of gonadotropin-releasing hormone stimulation and gonadotropin secretion in the rhesus monkey. Endocrinology 1981;109:376–385.
20. Fisher DA, Dussault JH, Sack J, Chorpra IJ. Ontogenesis of hypothalamic-pituitary-thyroid function and metabolism in man, sheep, and rat. Recent Prog Horm Res 1977;33:59–116.
21. DeCherney A, Naftolin F. Hypothalamic and pituitary development in the fetus. Clin Obstet Gynecol 1980;23:749-763.
22. Hyyppa M. Hypothalamic monoamines in the human fetus. Neuroendocrinology 1972;9:257–266.
23. Siler-Khodr TM, Morgenstern LL, Greenwood FC. Hormone synthesis and release from human fetal adenohypophyses *in vitro*. J Clin Endocrinol Metab 1974;39:891–905.
24. Penny C, Olambiwonnu NO, Frasier SD. Serum gonadotropin concentrations during the first four years of life. J Clin Endocrinol Metab 1974;38:320–321.
25. Forest MG, Sizenonko PC, Cathiard AM, Bertrand J. Hypophyso-gonadal function in humans during the first year of life. I. Evidence for testicular activity in early infancy. J Clin Invest 1974;53:819–828.
26. Betend B, Claustrat B, Bizillon CA, et al. Etude de la fonction gonadotrope hypophysaire par le test à la LH-RH pendant la première année de la vie. Ann Endocrinol (Paris) 1975;36:325.
27. Tapanaimen J, Koivisto M, Huhtaniemi I, Vihko R. Effect of gonadotropin-releasing hormone on pituitary-gonadal function during the first year of life. J Clin Endocrinol Metab 1982;55:689–692.
28. Beck W, Wutlke W. Diurnal variations of plasma luteinizing hormone, follicle-stimulating hormone, and prolactin in boys and girls from birth to puberty. J Clin Endocrinol Metab 1980;50:635–639.
29. Ferin M, Antunes JL, Zimmerman E, et al. Endocrine function in female rhesus monkeys after hypothalamic disconnection. Endocrinology 1977;101:1611–1620.
30. Neill JD, Patton JM, Dailey RA, et al. Luteinizing hormone-releasing hormone (LH-RH) in pituitary stalk blood of rhesus monkeys: relationship to level of LH release. Endocrinology 1977;101:430–434.

31. Zacharias L, Wurtman RJ. Blindness: its relation to age of menarche. Science 1964;144:1154–1155.
32. Preston FS, Bateman SC, Meichen FW, et al. Effects of time zone changes on performance and physiology on airline personnel. Aviat Space Environ Med 1976;47:763–769.
33. Kallman FJ, Schoenfeld WA, Barrera SE. The genetic aspects of primary eunuchodism. Am J Ment Defic 1944;48:203–236.
34. DeMorsier G. Etudes sur les dysraphies cranio-encéphaliques. Schweiz Arch Neurol Neurochir Psychiatr 1954;74:309–361.
35. Soules MR, Hammond CB. Female Kallman's syndrome: evidence for a hypothalamic luteinizing hormone-releasing hormone deficiency. Fertil Steril 1980;33:82–85.
36. Whitten WK, Champlin AK. The role of olfaction in mammalian reproduction. In: Greep RO, Astwood EB, eds. Handbook of physiology, vol. 2, section 7: endocrinology. Washington, D.C.: American Physiological Society, 1973:109-123.
37. Crews D, Garska WR. The ecological physiology of a garter snake. Sci Am 1982;247:158–168.
38. Huggins GR, Preti G. Volatile constituents of human vaginal secretions. Am J Obstet Gynecol 1976;126:129–136.
39. Kamberi IA, Mical RS, Porter JC. Effect of anterior pituitary perfusion and intraventricular injection of catecholamines on prolactin release. Endocrinology 1971;88:1012–1020.
40. Arze RS, Ramos JM, Rashid HU, Kern DNS. Amenorrhea, galactorrhea, and hyperprolactinemia induced by methyldopa. Br Med J 1981;283:194.
41. Perryman RL, Thorner MD. The effects of hyperprolactinemia on sexual function and reproductive function in men. J Androl 1981;5:233–242.
42. DeBernal M, DeVillamizer M. Restoration of ovarian function by low nocturnal single daily doses of bromocriptine in patients with the galactorrhea-amenorrhea syndrome. Fertil Steril 1982;37:392–396.
43. Yamaji T, Ishibashi M, Kosaka K, et al. Pituitary apoplexy in acromegaly during bromocriptine therapy. Acta Endocrinol (Copenh) 1981;98:171–177.
44. Frisch RE, Revelle R. Height and weight at menarche and a hypothesis of critical body weights and adolescent events. Science 1970;169:397–398.
45. Zacharias L, Wurtman RJ. Age at menarche. N Engl J Med 1969;280:868–875.
46. McArthur JW, O'Loughlin KM, Johnson L, et

al. Endocrine studies during the refeeding of young women with nutritional amenorrhea and infertility. Mayo Clin Proc 1976;51:607–616.
47. Sherman BM, Halmi KA, Zamudio R, et al. LH and FSH response to gonadotropin-releasing hormone in anorexia nervosa: effect of nutritional rehabilitation. J Clin Endocrinol Metab 1975;41:135–142.
48. Graham RL, Grimes DL, Gambrell RD. Amenorrhea secondary to voluntary weight loss. South Med J 1979;72:1259–1261.
49. Frisch RE, McArthur JW. Menstrual cycles: fatness as a determinant of minimum weight for height necessary for their maintenance or onset. Science 1974;185:949–951.
50. Fishman J, Boyar RM, Hellman L. Influence of body weight on estradiol metabolism in young women. J Clin Endocrinol Metab 1975;41:988–991.
51. Bates GW, Edman CD, Porter JC, MacDonald PC. Metabolism of catechol estrogen by human erythrocytes. J Clin Endocrinol Metab 1977;45:1120–1123.
52. Boyar RM, Finkelstein JW, David R, et al. Twenty-four hour patterns of plasma luteinizing hormone and follicle stimulating hormone in sexual precocity. N Engl J Med 1973;289:282–286.
53. Boyar RM, Finkelstein JW, Roffwarg H, et al. Twenty-four hour luteinizing hormone and follicle-stimulating hormone secretory patterns in gonadal dysgenesis. J Clin Endocrinol Metab 1973;37:521–525.
54. Corley KP, Valk TW, Kelch RP, Marshall JC. Estimation of GnRH pulse amplitude during pubertal development. Pediatr Res 1982;15:157–162.
55. Reiter EO, Grumbach MM. Neuroendocrine control mechanisms and the onset of puberty. Annu Rev Physiol 1982;44:595–613.
56. Jacobson RI, Seyler E Jr, Tamborlane WV Jr, et al. Pulsatile subcutaneous nocturnal administration of GnRH by portable infusion pump in hypogonadotropin hypogonadism: initiation of gonadotropic responsiveness. J Clin Endocrinol Metab 1979;49:652–654.
57. Hoffman AR, Crowley WF. Induction of puberty in men by long-term pulsatile administration of low-dose gonadotropin releasing hormone. N Engl J Med 1982;307:1237–1241.
58. Marshall JC, Kelch RP. Low dose pulsatile gonadotropin releasing hormone in anorexia nervosa: a model of human pubertal development. J Clin Endocrinol Metab 1979;49:712–718.
59. Marshall WA, Tanner JM. Variation in pattern of pubertal changes in girls. Arch Dis Child 1979;44:291–303.
60. Bates GW. Precocious puberty. In: Rivlin ME, Morrison JC, Bates GW, eds. Manual of clinical problems in obstetrics and gynecology. Boston: Little, Brown & Co., 1982:358–360.
61. Leyendecker G, Wildt L, Hansmann M. Pregnancies following chronic intermittent (pulsatile) administration of Gn-RH by means of a portable pump ("zyklomat")—a new approach to the treatment of infertility in hypothalamic amenorrhea. J Clin Endocrinol Metab 1980;51:1214–1216.
62. Crowley WF Jr, McArthur JW. Simulation of the normal menstrual cycle in Kallman's syndrome by pulsatile administration of luteinizing hormone-releasing hormone (LHRH). J Clin Endocrinol Metab 1980;51:173–175.
63. Bates GW, Wiser WL. Anosmia and primary amenorrhea in a young woman. J Miss State Med Assoc 1979;20:171–173.
64. Bistrian BR, Blackburn GL, Stanbury JB. Metabolic aspects of a protein-sparing modified diet in the dietary management of Prader-Willi obesity. N Engl J Med 1974;296:774–779.
65. Zarate A, Soria J, Canales ES, Kastin AJ, Schally AV, Toledano RG. Pituitary response to synethetic luteinizing hormone-releasing hormone in Prader-Willi syndrome, prepubertal and pubertal children. Neuroendocrinology 1974;13:321–326.
66. Chikamora K, Suehiro F, Ogawa T, et al. Distribution volume, metabolic clearance and plasma half disappearance time of exogenous luteinizing hormone releasing hormone in normal women and women with obesity and anorexia nervosa. Acta Endocrinol (Copenh) 1981;96:1–6.
67. Ellyin F, Khatir AH, Singh SP. Hypothalamic-pituitary functions in patients with transsphenoidal encephalocele and mid facial anomalies. J Clin Endocrinol Metab 1980;51:854-856.
68. Drossman DA, Ontjes DA, Heizer WD. Anorexia nervosa. Gastroenterology 1979;77:1115–1131.
69. Burks JK, Wetzel RD, Hughes T, et al. Anorexia nervosa. Arch Intern Med 1979;139:352–354.
70. Hay GG, Leonard JC. Anorexia nervosa in males. Lancet 1979;2:574–575.
71. Gull WW. Anorexia nervosa (apepsia, hysterica, anorexia hysterica). Trans Clin Soc Lond 1874;7:22.
72. McAnarney ER, Hoekelman RA. Conflicted

adolescent premarital intercourse: an antecedent of mild anorexia nervosa? Clin Pediatr 1979;18:340–342.
73. Luck P, Wakeling A. Altered thresholds for thermoregulatory sweating and vasodilatation in anorexia nervosa. Br Med J 1980;281:906–908.
74. Boyar RM, Katz J, Finkelstein JW, et al. Anorexia nervosa: immaturity of the 24-hour luteinizing hormone secretory pattern. N Engl J Med 1974;291:861–865.
75. Katz JL, Boyar R, Roffwarg H, et al. Weight and circadian luteinizing hormone secretory pattern in anorexia nervosa. Psychosom Med 1978;40:549–567.
76. Warren MP, Jewelewicz R, Dyrenfurth I, Ans R, Khalaf S, Van de Wiele RL. The significance of weight loss in the evaluation of pituitary response to LH-RH in women with secondary amenorrhea. J Clin Endocrinol Metab 1975;40:601-611.
77. Boyar RM. Endocrine changes in anorexia nervosa. Med Clin North Am 1978;62:297–303.
78. Gross HA, Lake CR, Ebert MH, et al. Catecholamine metabolism in primary anorexia nervosa. J Clin Endocrinol Metab 1979;49:805–809.
79. Jung RT, Shetty PS, James WPT. Nutritional effects on thyroid and catecholamine metabolism. Clin Sci 1980;58:183–191.
80. Moshang T, Parks JS, Baker L, et al. Low serum triiodothyronine in patients with anorexia nervosa. J Clin Endocrinol Metab 1975;40:470–473.
81. Moore R, Mills IH. Serum T_3 and T_4 levels in patients with anorexia nervosa showing transient hyperthyroidism during weight gain. Clin Endocrinol 1979;10:443–449.
82. Boyar RM, Hellman LD, Roffwarg H, et al. Cortisol secretion and metabolism in anorexia nervosa. N Engl J Med 1977;296:190–193.
83. Schwake AD, Lippe BM, Chang J, et al. Anorexia nervosa. Ann Intern Med 1981; 94:371–381.
84. Bates GW. Unpublished data.
85. Vigersky RA, Andersen AE, Thompson RH, Loriaux DL. Hypothalamic dysfunction in secondary amenorrhea associated with simple weight loss. N Engl J Med 1977;297:1141–1145.
86. Knuth WA, Hull MOR, Jacobs HS. Amenorrhea and loss of weight. Br J Obstet Gynaecol 1977;84:801–807.
87. Wentz AC. Body weight and amenorrhea. Obstet Gynecol 1980;56:482–487.
88. Bates GW, Bates SR, Whitworth NS. Reproductive failure in women who practice body weight control. Fertil Steril 1982;37:373–378.
89. Warren MP. The effect of exercise on pubertal progression and reproductive function in girls. J Clin Endocrinol Metab 1980;51:1150–1157.
90. Frisch RE, Wyshak G, Vincent L. Delayed menarche and amenorrhea in ballet dancers. N Engl J Med 1980;303:17–19.
91. Abraham SF, Beumont PJV, Llewellyn-Jones F, Llewellyn-Jones D. Body weight, exercise, and menstrual status among ballet dancers in training. Br J Obstet Gynaecol 1982;89:507–510.
92. Dale E, Gerlach DH, Whilhite AL. Menstrual dysfunction in distance runners. Obstet Gynecol 1979;54:47–53.
93. Frisch RE, Gotz-Welbergen AV, McArthur JW, et al. Delayed menarche and amenorrhea of college athletes in relation to age of onset of training. JAMA 1981;246:1559–1563.
94. Morville R, Pesquies C, Guezennec CY, et al. Plasma variations in testicular and adrenal androgens during prolonged physical exercise in man. Ann Endocrinol (Paris) 1979;40:501–510.
95. Rebar RW, Cumming DC. Reproductive function in women athletes. JAMA 1981;246:1590.
96. Marks BH. Delta-9-tetrahydrocannabinol and luteinizing hormone secretion. Prog Brain Res 1973;39:331–338.
97. Besch NF, Smith CG, Besch PK, Kaufman RH. The effect of marijuana (delta-9-tetrahydrocannabinol) on the secretion of luteinizing hormone on the rhesus monkey. Am J Obstet Gynecol 1977;128:634–642.
98. Asch RH, Smith CG, Siler-Khodr TM, Pauerstein CJ. Effects of delta 9-tetrahydrocannabinol during the follicular phase of the rhesus monkey (macaca mulatta). J Clin Endocrinol Metab 1981;52:50–55.
99. Charavasky I, Sheth PR, Sheth AR, Ghosh JJ. Delta-9-tetrahydro-cannabinol: its effects on hypothalamo-pituitary system in male rats. Arch Androl 1982;8:25–27.
100. Bates GW. Unpublished observations.
101. Crowley WF, Comite F, Vale W, et al. Therapeutic use of desensitization with long-acting LH-RH agonist: a potential new treatment for idiopathic precocious puberty. J Clin Endocrinol Metab 1981;52:370–373.
102. Gonzalez ER. For puberty that comes too soon, new treatment highly effective. JAMA 1982;248:1149–1157.
103. Archer DF, Thomas RL. The fallacy of the post-pill amenorrhea syndrome. Clin Obstet Gynecol 1981;24:943–950.

104. Buttram VC Jr, Vanderheyden JD, Besch PK, Acosta AA. Post "pill" amenorrhea. Int J Fertil 1974;19:37–41.
105. Fries H, Nillius SJ. Dieting, anorexia nervosa, and amenorrhea after contraceptive treatment. Acta Psychiatr Neurol 1973;49:669–679.
106. Talwar PP, Berger GS. The relation of body weight to side effects associated with oral contraceptives. Br Med J 1977;1:1637–1638.
107. Lim VS, Henriquez C, Sievertsen G, Frohman L. Ovarian function in chronic renal failure: evidence suggesting hypothalamic anovulation. Ann Intern Med 1980;93:21–27.
108. Sievertsen GD, Lim VS, Nakawatase C, Frohman LA. Metabolic clearance and secretion rates of human prolactin in normal subjects and in patients with chronic renal failure. J Clin Endocrinol Metab 1980;50:846–852.
109. Cowden EA, Ratcliffe WA, Ratcliffe JG, Kennedy AC. Hypothalamic-pituitary function in uraemia. Acta Endocrinol 1981;98:488–495.
110. Fischer EG, Hedley-White ET. Case records of the Massachusetts General Hospital. N Engl J Med 1982;307:1328-1335.
111. Stuart CA, Neelon FA, Lebovitz HE. Hypothalamic insufficiency: the cause of hypopituitarism in sarcoidosis. Ann Intern Med 1978;88:589–594.
112. Holick MF, Hoffman MA. Case records of the Massachusetts General Hospital. N Engl J Med 1982;307:1257–1264.
113. Rothman JG, Snyder PJ, Utiger RD. Hypothalamic endocrinopathy in Hand-Schuller-Christian disease. Ann Intern Med 1978;88:512–513.
114. Weller RA, Weller EB. Anorexia nervosa in a patient with an infiltrating tumor of the hypothalamus. Am J Psychiatry 1982;139:824–825.
115. Retetoff S, Frank PH, Roubebush C, DeGroot LJ. Evaluation of pituitary function. In: DeGroot LJ, Cahil GF, Martin L, et al., eds. Endocrinology. New York: Grune & Stratton, 1979:175–214.
116. Naidich TP, Pinto RS, Kushner MJ, et al. Evaluation of sellar and parasellar masses by computed tomography. Radiology 1976;120:91–99.
117. Morley JE, Melmed S. Gonadal dysfunction in systemic disorders. Metabolism 1979;28:1051–1073.

The Pituitary: Physiology and Disorders in Infertile Women

Douglas C. Daly and Daniel H. Riddick

The study and understanding of adenohypophyseal (anterior pituitary) function has evolved primarily during the twentieth century. While biblical references indicate that the various authors were aware of some endocrinologic syndromes [("some eunuchs which were so born from their mother's womb," Matthew 19:12) and ("his breasts are full of milk," Job 21:24)] and that they may have been aware of the source of some of the hormones ("He that is wounded in the stones . . . shall not enter into the congregation of the Lord," Deuteronomy 23:1), the early framework for the study of adenohypophysis-peripheral gland relationships did not occur until the nineteenth century. In 1838 Rathke observed that the anterior pituitary arose from an invagination of the roof of the stomodeum and migrated in the early embryologic period to coalesce with the neurohypophysis, which evaginated from the diencephalon. He concluded that the adenohypophysis was not of neural origin (1). By the mid-nineteenth century, it had been demonstrated that the hormonal activity of the testes was not stimulated by its own nerve supply, but rather was maintained by an intact vasculature. However, it was not until the twentieth century that the pituitary-testicular axis was further defined.

Marie was the first to correlate pituitary anatomy and pathophysiology when he described acromegaly in a patient with a pituitary tumor (2). It was not until this century that secretion of a growth-stimulating factor from these tumors was recognized as the cause of acromegaly. Schönenmann, however, deduced the secretory nature of the adenohypophysis in 1892 from the microscopic appearance of pituitary cells (3). Others then observed that the pituitary enlarged after gonadectomy or during pregnancy and that this enlargement was caused by an increase in the number and size of chromophobes, basophils, and eosinophils (4,5). It was then noted that pituitary tumors associated with acromegaly had the same secretory appearance. These discoveries ushered in an era of surgical excision of pituitary adenomas by Harvey, Cushing, and others.

That the pituitary gland was necessary to maintain general health was also recognized in the early years of this century. Growth hormone was isolated in 1921 (6). Over the next 2 decades the relationship between the pituitary and peripheral target glands was studied and then accepted. Left unanswered was the relationship of the adenohypophysis and the central nervous system until a neurovascular connection of the hypothalamus to the pituitary via the portal system was proposed by Green and Harris in the mid 1940s (7). In concert, these observations became the basis for our present concept of hypothalamic-pituitary-peripheral gland function.

In this chapter, we will describe the physiology of the adenohypophysis and the clinical conditions that result when pituitary function is abnormal. The adenohypophysis is an intermediate member in a dynamic relationship between the hypothalamus and peripheral glands. The adenohypophysis modulates the function of the peripheral target glands and the hypothalamus. In turn, the adenohypophysis is affected by humoral signals from the hypothalamus and peripheral target glands. We will define these integrated relationships as a basis for understanding clinical disorders of the anterior pituitary, especially prolactin-secreting pituitary adenomas.

Embryology and Anatomy

During the third week of embryonic development, Rathke's pouch forms as a diverticulum in the primitive oral cavity, the stomodeum, and grows toward the infundibulum of the diencephalon (1). The connection between the oral cavity and Rathke's pouch disappears in the sixth week of embryonic life. Remnants may, however, remain in the oral pharynx. Recent evidence has been presented for another origin of the adenohypophysis—Rathke's pouch may derive from neuroectodermal cells in the caudal region of the ventral neural ridge lying near the stomodeum (8). Both the hypothalamus and adenohypophysis may be of neural origin. The anterior portion of Rathke's pouch proliferates to form the adenohypophysis while the remainder partially surrounds the infundibular stalk to form the pars intermedius. The adenohypophysis secretes its hormones as early as the eighth to twelfth week of gestation (9). The adenohypophyseal portion of the portal system is also developed by this time and its development precedes the secretion of anterior pituitary hormones. By the beginning of the second trimester, functional relationships have been established between the hypothalamus, pituitary, and peripheral target glands, although the portal system is not anatomically mature until 24 weeks (10).

BLOOD SUPPLY. The anterior pituitary derives its blood supply from the superior hypophyseal arteries through the portal veins. Blood flows primarily from the median eminence of the hypothalamus to the adenohypophysis (11), although there may be reverse flow from the pituitary to the hypothalamus through the portal veins. In the body of the adenohypophysis the portal veins disperse to form sinusoidal capillaries that are surrounded by a perisinusoidal space and the parenchymal cells of the pituitary (Fig. 4–1). Releasing factors from the hypothalamus reach the adenohypophysis through the portal veins, diffuse across the perisinusoidal space to the parenchymal cells, and stimulate the target cells to release specific pituitary hormones into the perisinusoidal space. These hormones then diffuse into the sinusoidal capillaries, exit the adenohypophysis via the lateral hypophyseal veins, and enter the systemic circulation. Peripherally produced hormones reach the parenchymal cells via the superior hypophyseal arteries and the long portal vessels. About 15% of the blood supply of the anterior pituitary originates in the short portal vessels from the neurohypophysis. Blood from these vessels, which are branches of the inferior hypophyseal arteries, may contain oxytocin and vasopressin. Whether this blood contains hypothalamic releasing hormones is unclear.

HISTOLOGY. The cells of the anterior pituitary were originally classified as acidophil, basophil, or chromophobe based upon individual histochemical staining characteristics. Presently, the pituitary is understood to be a confederation of 5 cell types producing 6 major hormones and a variety of peptides of undetermined significance. Individual cell types synthesize a single major hormone (12). The gonadotroph cells, which produce luteinizing hormone (LH) and follicle stimulating hormone (FSH), are the exception to this 1 cell/1 hormone rule. Cells producing a given hormone tend to be concentrated in 1 region of the adenohypophysis, although cells for all hormones are present throughout the gland.

MICROANATOMY. The different secretory cells of the adenohypophysis have a common microanatomy specialized for the synthesis and release of proteins (Fig. 4–1). After stimulation, messenger RNA (mRNA) is transcribed from nuclear DNA and binds to ribosomes on the endoplasmic reticulum that are then stimulated to synthesize the amino acid sequences that become the protein hormones of these pituitary cells. The hormone is then transported along the endoplasmic reticulum to the Golgi apparatus where it is condensed and enclosed in a bilaminar lipoprotein membrane to form a secretory granule. Secretory granules bind to the microtubular network that constitutes the

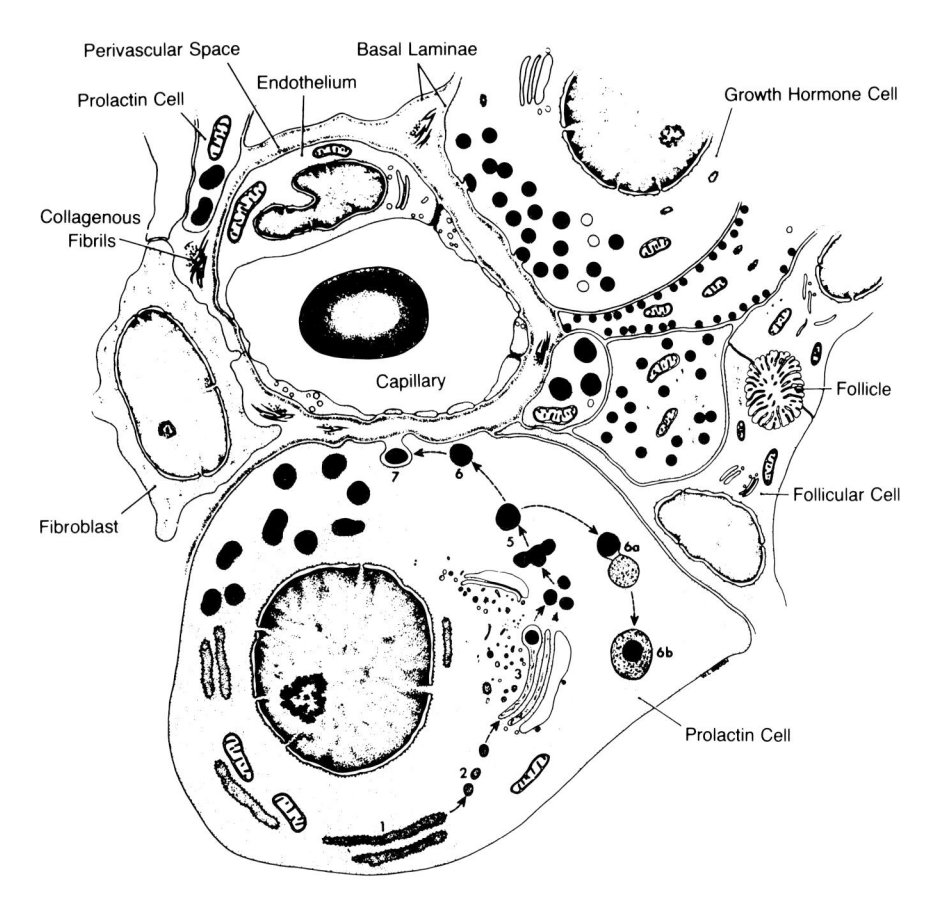

Fig. 4–1. Microanatomy of a portal sinus within the adenohypophysis. Releasing and inhibiting factors diffuse across the capillary membrane and sinusoidal space to affect the appropriate target cells. The microanatomy of the cells reflects their metabolic function. Messenger RNA (mRNA) binds to ribosomes (1) and synthesis of the hormone occurs (e.g., prolactin). The hormone is transported along the endoplasmic reticulum (2) to the Golgi apparatus (3) where it is incorporated into vesicles (4,5). Under appropriate stimulation, the vesicle contents are released into the perisinusoidal space (6,7). If not released, the vesicle undergoes internal degradation by lysosomal digestion (6a,6b). (Reprinted with permission from Baker BL. Functional cytology of the hypophyseal pars distalis and pars intermedia, In: Greep RO, Astwood EB, eds. Endocrinology (section 7, vol. 4). Washington, D.C.: American Physiological Society, 1974:71.)

skeletal framework of the cell, and, under appropriate stimulation, are transported to the cell membrane adjacent to a perisinusoidal space. The contents of the secretory granules are then released by exocytosis, a process by which the granules' bilaminar membrane fuses with that of the cell. Each step in this process can be regulated to control the cellular output of hormone, and each step requires a net energy expenditure by the cell. Granules that are not released undergo internal degradation by membrane fusion with lysosomes and protein digestion.

Receptor Theory

The rate of synthesis and release of adenohypophyseal hormones (like peripheral hormones) is determined by the humoral messages that are received by the cell. The hormones that stimulate or inhibit the adenohypophysis arise primarily from 2 sources: the hypothalamus and the peripheral glands. Three types of hormones modulate pituitary function: peptide-protein hormones, catecholamines, and lipid-soluble steroid and thyroid hormones. The pituitary is also affected by hormones that control overall metabolic functions. Hormones such as insulin, glucagon, intestinal peptides, and others are in this group. The cells of the pituitary recognize these hormones because they possess 1 or both of 2 types of receptors—membrane-associated receptors and cytoplasmic receptors. Each receptor is relatively specific for its respective hormone. Structurally similar hormones may bind to the receptor of another hormone, usually with a lower affinity and less biologic effect. *Agonists* are natural or synthetic analogues that bind to receptors and stimulate hormone synthesis. An *antagonist* binds to a receptor but does not activate it. Therefore, little or no hormone synthesis occurs when a strong antagonist competes with a natural stimulatory hormone for receptor binding sites.

Membrane Receptors

The cell membranes consist of lipid bilayers that join to form a 3-dimensional sheet of phospholipids and cholesterol (Fig. 4–2). Hydrophobic portions of the phospholipids occupy the center of the membrane and the hydrophilic portions occupy the internal and external surfaces. There is little or no molecular binding between phospholipids, and, therefore, lateral movement within each sheet is random and rapid (13). Since the central hydrophobic region repels the surface hydrophilic regions, movement of a phospholipid between the external and internal surfaces is relatively less common. For this reason, the external and internal phospholipid components may not be identical in a particular membrane (14).

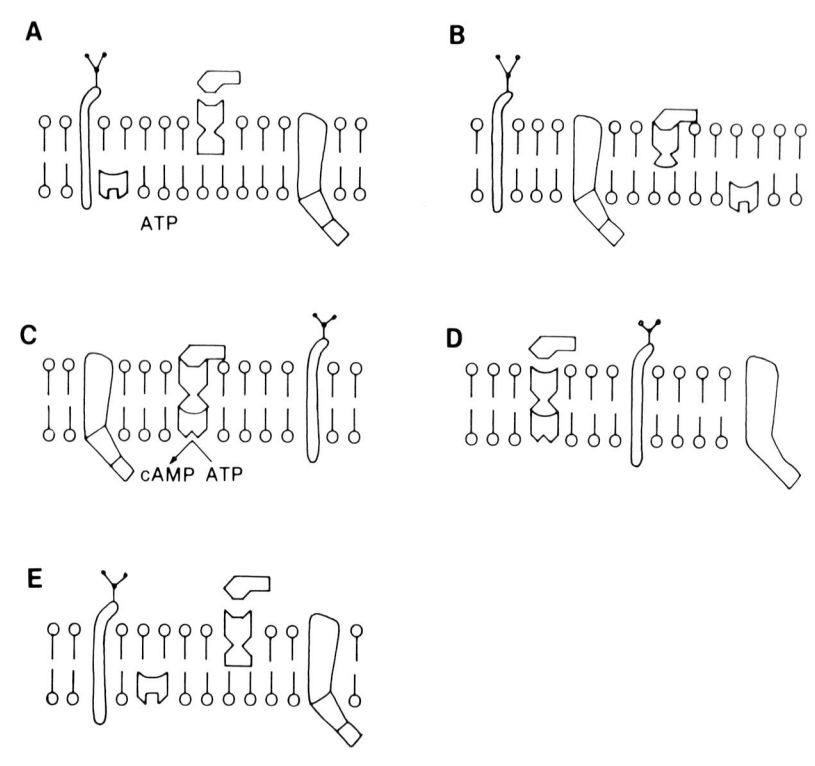

Fig. 4–2. A Bilaminar membrane with a structural protein bound to peripheral proteins on the cytoplasmic surface (structure on the far right), an antigenic protein with carbohydrate moieties (structure on the far left), an enzyme protein on the cytoplasmic surface (structure second from the left), and a receptor protein on the extracellar surface (structure second from the right). All of these proteins move freely throughout the membrane. **B** The hormone, shown above the receptor in **A,** binds to the receptor and causes a conformational change that results in increased affinity for an enzyme protein such as adenyl cyclase. **C** After adenyl cyclase is activated it cleaves a precursor (ATP) to form an active second messenger, cyclic AMP (cAMP). **D** and **E** The hormone-receptor-enzyme complex then dissociates and becomes inactive or is internalized and degraded as illustrated in Fig. 4–5.

Embedded or floating in this lipid bilayer are the integral proteins, which serve at least 4 functions (15):

1. Structural proteins, bound to peripheral proteins on the cytoplasmic side, maintain cell structure.
2. Antigenic proteins containing carbohydrate (i.e., glycoproteins) confer cell-to-cell recognition on the external surface.
3. Receptor proteins bind protein hormones and catecholamines. These are located in the membrane in such a way that they are exposed to the external surface of the cell.
4. Membrane-associated enzymes are positioned so that the active site of the enzyme is exposed predominantly to the cytoplasm (Fig. 4–2A).

Most of these proteins have hydrophobic and hydrophilic regions that maintain their polarity within the membrane. All of these components flow freely in the bilaminar lipid plates and are exposed to one another by random chance. The interaction between any 2 proteins will be a function of the binding affinity between the proteins. For receptor proteins, this binding affinity for other membrane proteins changes when a hormone binds to the receptor. This is 1 mechanism of controlling postreceptor activity.

When a hormone binds to its receptor, conformational changes occur within the receptor that result in increased affinity to a selective population of enzyme proteins within the membrane (Fig. 4–2B). These enzyme proteins temporarily become bound to an activated receptor protein, and a conformational change in the enzyme results in exposure of the active site of the enzyme (Fig. 4–2C). The enzyme proteins are composed of 2 units: a regulator unit that binds to activated receptors and a catalytic unit that determines the activity of the enzyme (16,17). The activity of the regulator unit is GTP (guanosine 5′-triphosphate) dependent and is referred to as the G-protein (18). An example of a membrane hormone is adenyl cyclase. The product of adenyl cyclase activity, cAMP, becomes the internal cytoplasmic messenger (the "second messenger") with cell-specific effects on protein kinase (Figs. 4–3 and 4–4).

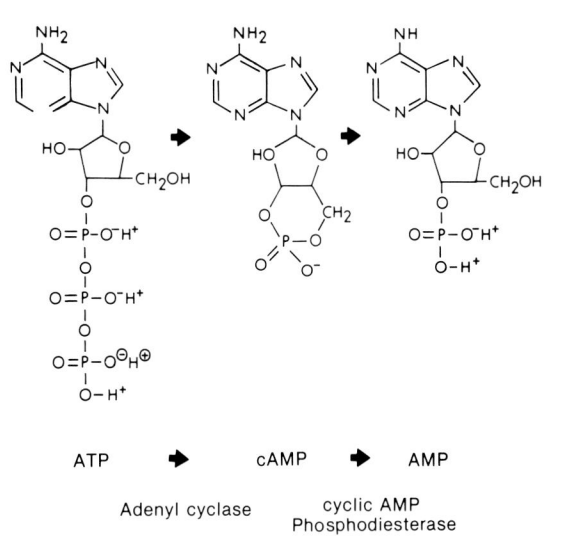

Fig. 4–3. ATP is converted by adenyl cyclase to cyclic AMP (cAMP) by the enzymatic cleavage of 2 phosphate groups. cAMP is subsequently degraded by cAMP phosphodiesterase, which cleaves the phosphate ring and inactivates the second messenger.

The activity of cAMP is calcium and calmodulin dependent. Calmodulin is an intracellular protein that regulates calcium flux and concentration. Prostaglandin effects may be mediated by calmodulin control of free calcium concentrations (19).

The consequence of this second messenger system is the activation (or inactivation) of a large number of cytoplasmic enzymes by a single activated membrane receptor (20). A membrane receptor may also activate (or inhibit) several membrane-associated enzymes, each with its own second messenger and target cytoplasmic proteins. Likewise, a given membrane-associated enzyme protein may be affected by several different activated membrane receptors.

The net activity of an enzyme is the sum of all these inhibitory and stimulatory influences. The hormone-receptor-enzyme complex either dissociates (Figs. 4–2D and E) or is removed from the membrane, internalized, and digested by lysosomal activity (Fig. 4–5). Hormone-receptor activity is limited by either of these mechanisms. Internalization occurs when occupied receptors migrate laterally to regions on the cell membranes called coated pits, which are linked to special proteins called *clathrins*. When the coated pit is occupied by receptor-hormone complexes, the pit invagi-

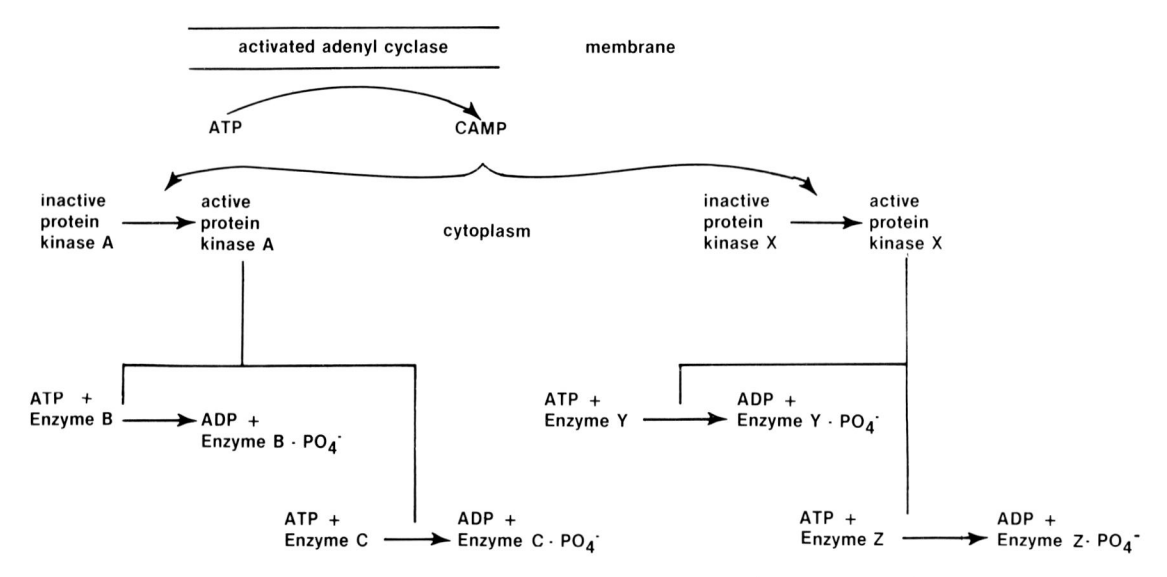

Fig. 4–4. cAMP stimulates 1 or both of the protein kinases within the cytoplasm of the cell. These active protein kinases, in turn, will phosphorylate 1 or more enzymes. These phosphorylated enzymes may be more or less active than the unphosphorylated enzyme. Therefore, a single second messenger, cAMP, effectively stimulates (or inhibits) multiple cytoplasmic enzymes and thereby modifies the cell's metabolic activity.

nates, forms a vesicle within the cytoplasm, and is subsequently digested by lysosomal enzymes (21). For this process to occur the receptors may need to be occupied for several minutes.

Membrane receptors are usually present in excess of the quantity of stimulating hormone and have a relatively constant affinity for that hormone. Therefore, the effect on a responsive cell will be proportional to the hormonal concentration. The number and location of membrane receptors may, however, vary and alter cellular response independent of the circulating hormone concentration. When the number of receptors in a cell or the activity of those receptors is increased, the phenomenon is known as "up-regulation." A decrease in the quantity or activity of a receptor is "down-regulation." Internalization of receptor-hormone complexes and subsequent enzymatic degradation is a major mechanism for down-regulation (22). Exposure to a constant level of a hormone may deplete a cell of its receptors or inactivate postreceptor reactions. Either of these renders the cell less responsive. If the hormone appears at a cell in a pulsate manner, postreceptor activity is maintained, new receptors accumulate between pulses, and sensitivity to the hormone is maintained or enhanced. GnRH receptors in gonadotroph cells are controlled by one or both of these mechanisms. When exposed to pulses of GnRH, GnRH receptor content is maintained or enhanced, possibly because the association time of GnRH with its receptor is short and dissociation occurs before internalization. However, long-acting GnRH agonists, while initially stimulatory, lead to receptor inactivation or depletion and receptor insensitivity to the GnRH agonist. Since these agonists bind more strongly to the receptor and have extended plasma half-lives, the receptors remain occupied and are internalized. This results in depletion of membrane receptors and refractoriness of the cell to GnRH stimulation.

Cytoplasmic Receptors

Receptors for steroid and thyroid hormones are located in the cytoplasm of target cells. Steroids and thyroxine traditionally have been thought to cross the cell membrane by simple diffusion down a concentration gradient. However, specialized regions of steroid binding may exist on the membrane that bind and internalize steroid hormones in a manner similar to coated pits for protein hormone-receptor complexes. The vesicle, once internalized,

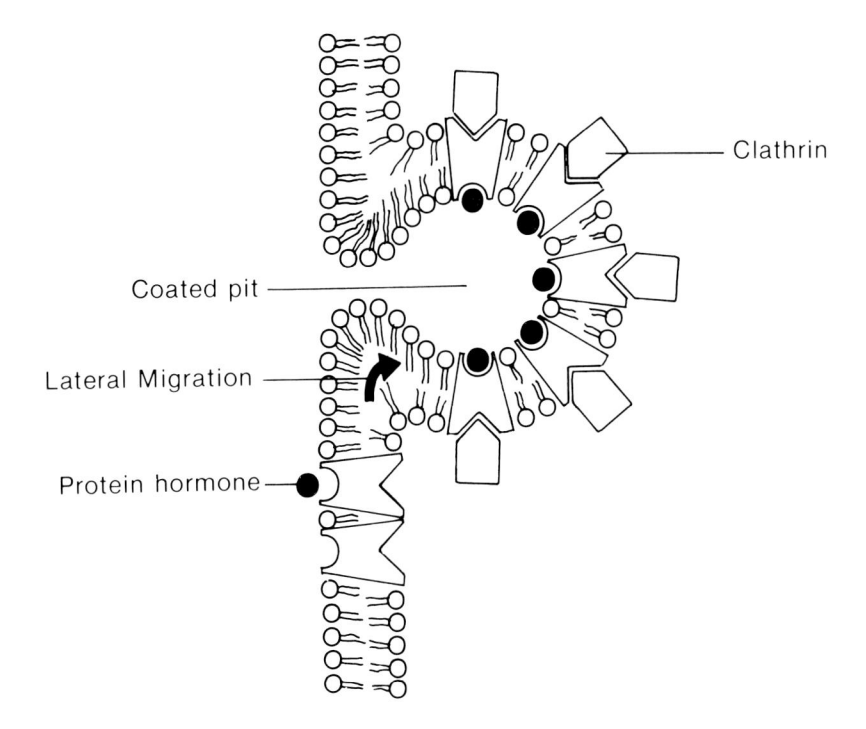

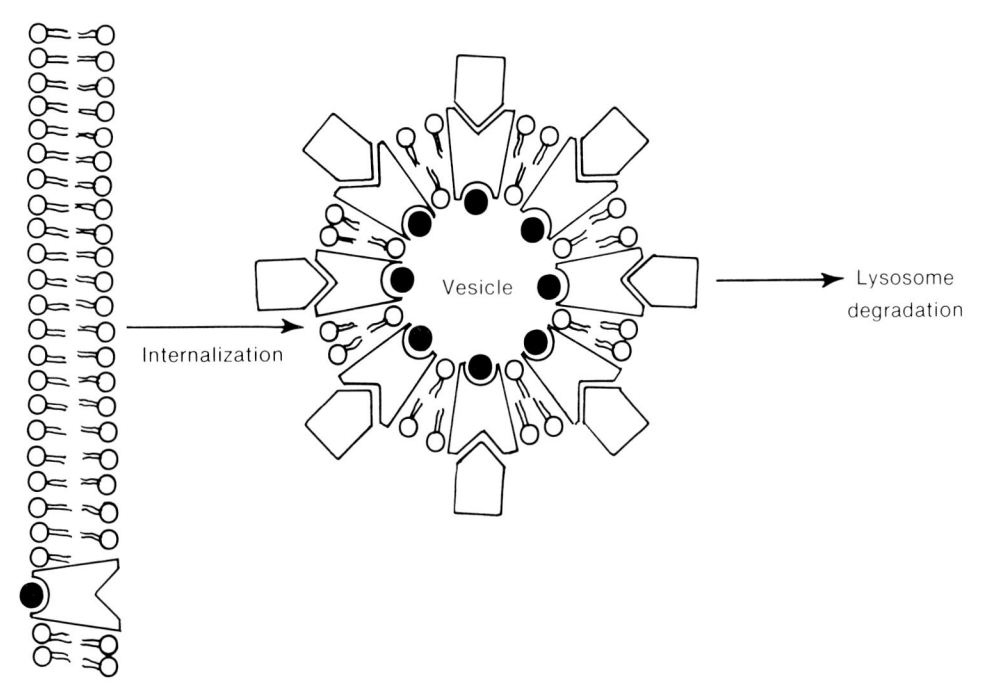

Fig. 4–5. A Membrane receptors, when occupied by a hormone, move by lateral migration along the membrane to coated pits, where cytoplasmic proteins, clathrins, attach. When a coated pit is occupied fully, it is internalized. **B** Internalization of a hormone-receptor-enzyme complex occurs by endocytosis of the coated pit. This terminates the activity of the complex and depletes the membrane of receptors. Temporarily, this depletion may render the cell less responsive to the hormone (down-regulation). Once internalized, the complex is usually degraded by lysosomal enzymes. (Modified and reproduced with permission. Anderson RGW et al. Nature 1977;270:695–699.)

is not digested by lysosomal enzymes, but liberates its steroid hormone into the cytoplasm. Low-density lipoprotein (LDL)-cholesterol complexes enter cells by a similar mechanism (23).

Like membrane receptors, cytoplasmic receptors are relatively specific for individual hormones. Binding of a hormone to its receptor results in a configurational change in the receptor (transformation). Now activated, the hormone-receptor complex crosses the nuclear membrane (translocation), binds to nuclear proteins and DNA, and induces the transcription of mRNA (Fig. 4–6) (22,24). The mRNA produced by transcription of nuclear DNA may code for new gene products and thereby transform a cell (e.g., prolactin synthesis in decidual cells in the endometrium under the stimulation of progesterone) or may stimulate an already expressed gene product (e.g., LH from the gonadotroph under the influence of estradiol).

The hormone-receptor complex may also bind to proteins in the cytoplasm. Such binding changes the activity of these proteins (25).

Steroid receptors are highly regulated within the cytoplasm, usually by inhibition of receptor synthesis by the activated hormone receptor. Estradiol and progesterone receptors are important exceptions to this general rule. Estradiol up-regulates both progesterone and estrogen receptors, while progesterone down-regulates both progesterone and estradiol receptors (26).

Adenohypophyseal Hormones

The hormones produced by the adenohypophysis are all peptides or proteins and are generally divided into 3 groups: corticotropin-related proteins and peptides, glycoprotein hormones, and somatomammotropic hormones. Each group probably evolved from a single ancestral protein since these hormones share certain characteristics.

ACTH. Corticotropin-related proteins are derived from a single prohormone (MW = 31,000) that contains the peptide sequence for

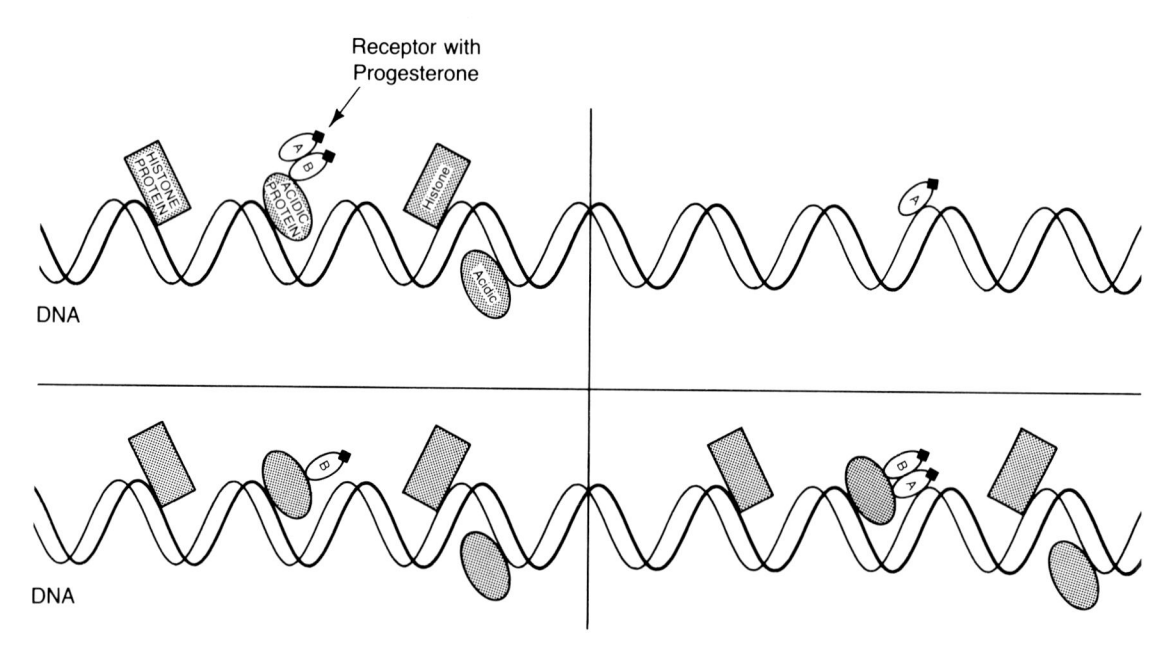

Fig. 4–6. The progesterone receptor consists of paired proteins, each with a binding site for progesterone. The B unit provides specific binding to acidic proteins in the nucleus. The A unit activates mRNA transcription. The A unit alone can activate mRNA transcription when DNA is stripped of acidic proteins and histones; it is inactive when these proteins are present. The B unit alone can bind to acidic proteins but no transcription occurs. Therefore, both units are necessary: the B unit for specificity, the A unit for activity. (Reprinted with permission. Roth J, Grunfeld C. Endocrine systems: mechanisms of disease, target cells, and receptors, In: Williams RH, ed. Textbook of endocrinology, 6th ed. Philadelphia: WB Saunders, 1981:59.)

ACTH and beta-lipotropin (Fig. 4–7). Beta-lipotropin is the precursor for beta-MSH and the endorphin polypeptides. The secretory products of the corticotropin cell are regulated by sequential cleavage from the 31K polypeptide by intracellular enzymes translated from messenger RNA by ribosomes (27). ACTH and beta-lipotropin are the principal secretory products of corticotropin cells. ACTH contains 39 amino acids, although full activity exists in the initial 20 amino acids. This segment binds to and activates ACTH-specific receptors in the cell membranes of the adrenal cortex. As a result, adrenal cortical synthesis of cortisol, dehydroepiandrosterone sulfate, androstenedione, 17-hydroxyprogesterone, and desoxycorticosterone occurs. Aldosterone synthesis is relatively independent of ACTH secretion. The synthesis, storage, and release of ACTH is controlled primarily by hypothalamic corticotropin-releasing hormone (CRF) and the circulating level of cortisol. The diurnal rhythm of ACTH release is regulated by events in the hypothalamus, as is the ACTH-cortisol response to stress and hypoglycemia.

PROLACTIN. Prolactin, growth hormone (GH), and human placental lactogen (HPL) are the somatotropin or growth-stimulating hormones. Each is derived from a distinct cell type, but they all have several common characteristics. They are single chain proteins with many identical amino acid sequences. They contain 191 to 198 amino acids, have similar molecular weights of 21,700 to 23,510, and have intramolecular disulfide bonds at similar locations. The major known function of prolactin in the human is initiation and maintenance of casein synthesis in the breast during the postpartum period. It may have other metabolic functions since many cells possess prolactin receptors (28).

Prolactin is an ancient hormone that regulates electrolyte balance and functions as a growth hormone in a variety of fish and amphibians (29). Prolactin release is not consistently stimulated by any known circulating factor, but its secretion is reduced by a prolactin inhibitory factor (PIF) that is presumed to be dopamine. Sleep, stress, eating, breast stimulation, and hypoglycemia cause an increase in prolactin secretion. A variety of drugs that either decrease dopamine secretion or block dopamine receptors also stimulate prolactin secretion (Table 4–1). Thyrotropin-releasing hormone (TRH) effectively stimulates prolactin release, but is usually present in sufficient concentrations only in subjects with overt hypothyroidism. Prolactin concentrations are increased in both the mother and the fetus during the third trimester of pregnancy, presumably as a result of the increasing estrogen and progesterone secretion from the pla-

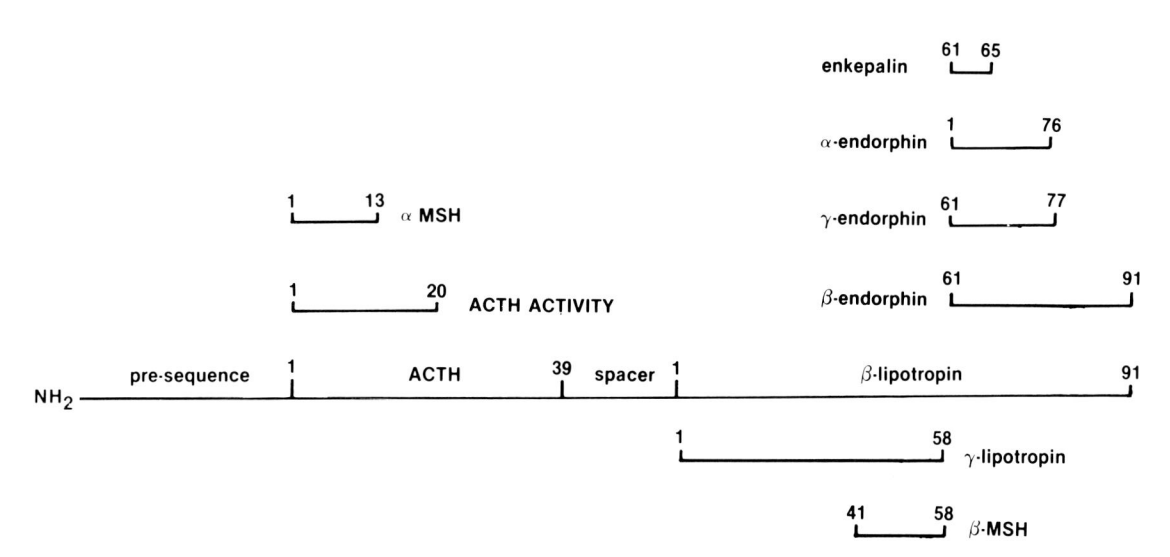

Fig. 4–7. The prohormone for ACTH also contains the sequence for beta-lipotropin. The products of the corticotrophs could be any of the peptide sequences illustrated. However, the protolytic activity of the corticotropin cell results primarily in ACTH and beta-lipotropin release.

TABLE 4–1. Factors Affecting Prolactin Secretion.

	SECRETION INCREASED	SECRETION DECREASED
Hormonal	Estrogens (pregnancy)	Thyroxine Chronic progestin use (?) Glucocorticoids
Neurologic	Stage III & IV sleep Suckling Stress Serotonin (?) TRH	Dopamine Dopamine agonists REM sleep
Metabolic	Exercise Eating Renal failure Hypoglycemia Amino acids	Anorexia nervosa
Medications	Phenothiazines & other tranquilizers Tricyclic antidepressants Methyldopa Reserpine Narcotics	Bromocriptine
Other		Parturition

centa. Prolactin remains elevated in the postpartum period and is important for the initiation of lactation (30).

GROWTH HORMONE (GH). Growth hormone has both direct and indirect effects on body growth and composition (31). The indirect effects are mediated by the somatomedins and insulinlike growth factors that are produced in peripheral tissues, particularly the liver. Many factors influence growth hormone release (Table 4–2). Like prolactin, GH release is markedly affected by hypothalamic catecholamines. In contrast to prolactin, dopamine and norepinephrine probably regulate the release of growth hormone through a releasing

TABLE 4–2. Factors Affecting Growth Hormone Secretion.

	SECRETION INCREASED	SECRETION DECREASED
Hormonal	Estrogen Glucagon Vasopressin	Somatostatin Somatomedin Hypothyroidism Corticosteroids Progestins
Neurologic	Stage III and IV sleep Stress L-Dopa or Dopamine Alpha-adrenergic agonists	REM sleep Emotional deprivation Beta-adrenergic agonists
Metabolic	Hypoglycemia (Insulin tolerance test) Amino acids (Arginine test) Uremia Hepatic failure Acidosis	Hyperglycemia (glucose load) Hyperlipidemia Obesity

factor (GHRF) rather than affect GH secretion directly. Somatomedins function as a circulating factor in the control of growth hormone action (31). Somatostatin, which has been derived from a large number of tissues including the hypothalamus, inhibits GH release.

FSH AND LH. Follicle-stimulating hormone (FSH), luteinizing hormone (LH), thyroid-stimulating hormone (TSH), and placental chorionic gonadotropin (hCG) comprise the glycoprotein hormones. Each of these has an identical alpha subunit, and a beta subunit that is specific for each hormone. These hormones contain 15% to 30% carbohydrate. The carbohydrate composition differs for each hormone and can vary in the same hormone. For example, the carbohydrate content, especially that of sialic acid, is increased in subjects with end-organ failure.

Sialic acid increases the plasma half-life of both FSH and LH (32). The longer half-life of LH and FSH in postmenopausal women is probably the result of an increased sialic acid content. Urinary FSH and LH are less potent than pituitary FSH and LH because of a decreased plasma half-life after injection (as Pergonal® rather than a change in hormone receptor affinity. This appears to be related to a decreased sialic acid content of urinary FSH and LH. Differences in sialic acid content and plasma half-life may account for significant discrepancies in the quantity of FSH and LH measured by bioassay, as compared to that measured by radioimmunoassay. Radioimmunoassays determine the concentration of immunoreactive FSH and LH, whereas bioactivity is a reflection of concentration plus receptor binding, receptor activation, plasma half-life, and the potential action of bioactive metabolic products. Therefore, bioassays and radioimmunoassays are distinctly different measurements of a hormone and may not correlate with each other.

Neither the alpha nor beta subunit is active alone (33). The beta subunit apparently provides cell-specific binding, while the alpha subunit activates adenyl cyclase and the production of the second messenger, cyclic AMP (Fig. 4–8).

FSH and LH are synthesized and secreted within the same cells of the adenohypophysis (34). The primary sites of action of these glyco-

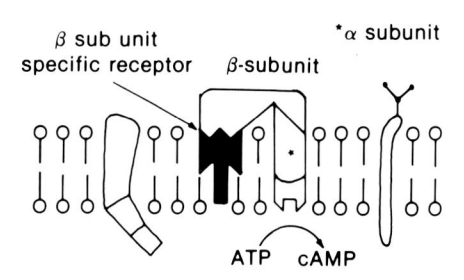

Fig. 4–8. The glycoprotein hormones share a common alpha subunit but have a hormone-specific beta subunit. The beta subunit provides the hormone with cell-specific affinity to hormone receptors while the alpha subunit binds and stimulates adenyl cyclase with resulting cAMP synthesis. Neither subunit is active by itself.

proteins are the ovaries and testes. In the testes, LH stimulates Leydig cells to produce testosterone, while FSH is involved with initiation and maintenance of spermatogenesis by the Sertoli cells (Fig. 4–9) (35). LH stimulates estradiol (E_2), androstenedione, and testosterone (T_1) synthesis in theca and hilar cells of the ovary and progesterone synthesis in granulosa cells after they have acquired or unmasked LH receptors (36).

FSH is the primary stimulant of granulosa cell growth and estrogen synthesis from androgens (Fig. 4–10) (37). FSH synthesis and secre-

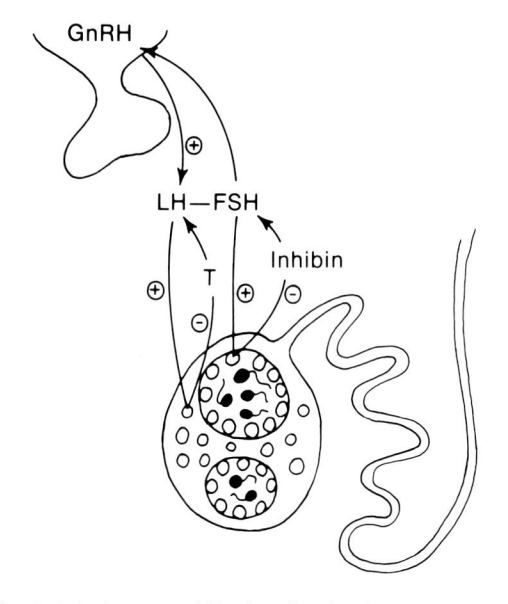

Fig. 4–9. In the testes, LH primarily stimulates testosterone synthesis in Leydig cells. Testosterone, in turn, suppresses LH (negative feedback). FSH stimulates Sertoli cells to initiate processes important for sperm maturation. Inhibin, presumably from the Sertoli cells, suppresses FSH. Without GnRH, both FSH and LH secretion diminish.

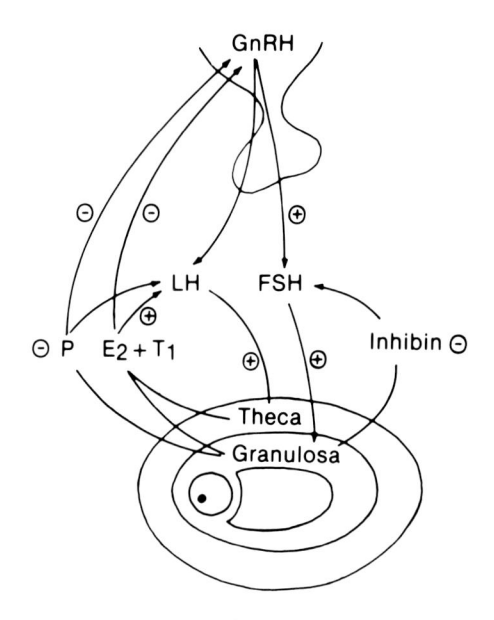

Fig. 4–10. In the ovary, FSH stimulates granulosa cells. Inhibin (presumptively from granulosa cells) has a negative feedback effect on FSH. LH stimulates theca, hilar and, just prior to ovulation, granulosa cells. These cells produce estrogen, androgens, and progesterone, which affect LH synthesis as described in Figs. 4–12 and 4–14. GnRH is required for normal LH and FSH synthesis.

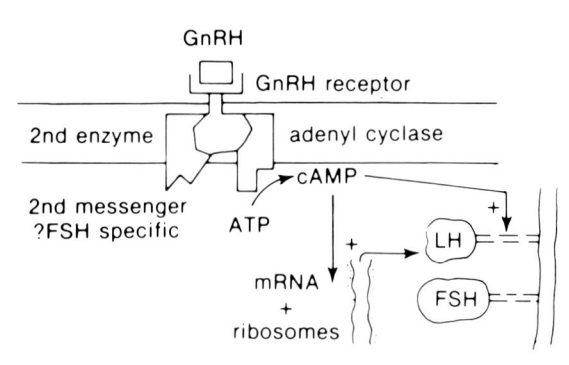

Fig. 4–11. GnRH stimulates the gonadotroph via a membrane receptor and 1 or more membrane-associated enzymes. Adenyl cyclase cleaves ATP to form cAMP, which then stimulates LH and FSH synthesis and release.

tion is suppressed by inhibin, an isolated but unpurified polypeptide produced by both granulosa cells (38) and Sertoli cells (39).

The divergence of FSH and LH secretion from gonadotrophs during the menstrual cycle may be caused by differential stimulation and inhibition by the hormones arising from the FSH and LH target cells. Synthesis and release of FSH and LH are dependent on hypothalamic gonadotropin-releasing hormone (GnRH), but are modulated by the peripheral hormones. The principal hormones affecting LH synthesis and release are GnRH, estradiol, and progesterone. GnRH, inhibin, and progesterone are the hormones that regulate FSH. The interrelationship of these hormones and their receptors is an excellent demonstration of how receptor function integrates a variety of messages and modulates cell function.

GnRH is required for LH and FSH secretion and release (Fig. 4–11). GnRH release is mediated by estradiol and progesterone and by hypothalamic catecholamine secretion from specialized neurons. Released into the portal system in a pulsatile manner, GnRH regulates ovarian function by controlling FSH and LH secretion. Low levels of GnRH (e.g., in prepubertal children) result in low levels of circulating FSH and LH, regardless of the presence or absence of other modulating influences. The high levels of FSH and LH present after the menopause apparently reflect increased GnRH secretion and pituitary stimulation. During the menstrual cycle, however, GnRH may act only in a permissive role and not directly affect the cyclic changes of LH and FSH release. In monkeys and humans, pulsatile injections of a constant dose of GnRH have successfully induced cyclic function in the pituitary-ovarian axis (40,41).

GnRH binds and activates membrane GnRH receptors and the GnRH-receptor complex stimulates adenyl cyclase-mediated cleavage of ATP to form cyclic AMP (see Fig. 4–3). Exposure of the GnRH receptor to long-acting GnRH analogues or to continuous infusion of GnRH results in down-regulation of this response by a process of internalization (Fig. 4–5) (42). Repeated pulsatile exposure to hypothalamic GnRH results in an augmented receptor and cellular response (43,44), which leads to an increased rate of LH and FSH synthesis and release.

Estradiol crosses the lipid bilaminar membrane and binds to cytoplasmic receptors. The bound and activated estradiol-receptor complex then binds to DNA and DNA proteins, and stimulates the synthesis of mRNA. The mRNA then codes for protein products that increase the cell's ability to synthesize and store LH and, probably, FSH (though to a lesser degree) (Fig. 4–12). Estradiol accelerates the pi-

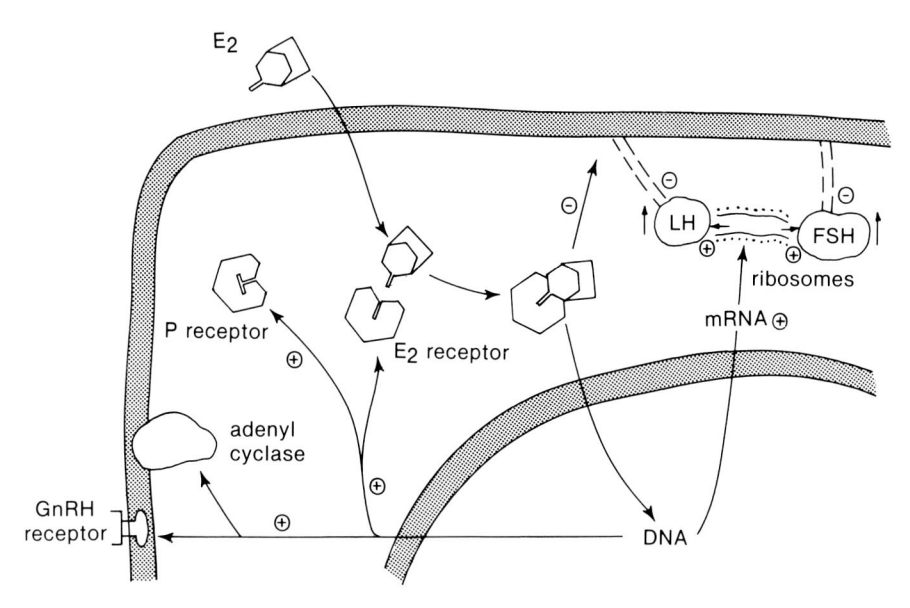

Fig. 4–12. Estradiol (E$_2$) binds to cytoplasmic E$_2$ receptors and is transported to the nucleus of a pituitary gonadotroph. The hormone and receptor complex stimulates the transcription of mRNA and then increased synthesis of LH, FSH, E$_2$ receptors, and progesterone receptors. In addition, GnRH receptor activity is augmented. However, the hormone-receptor complex also decreases the effect of GnRH on LH and FSH release. The net effect is an increase in the amount of LH and FSH stored in gonadotrophs.

tuitary response to GnRH by increasing the number and/or activity of GnRH receptors. Estradiol also partially blocks the effect of GnRH by inhibiting the release of newly synthesized FSH and LH. The net result of these actions is an increase in the intracellular storage of FSH and LH (45). Finally, estradiol also stimulates the synthesis of estradiol and progesterone receptors within the cells of the pituitary. Therefore, the rising level of estradiol in the follicular phase results in an increase in the cell's capacity to synthesize, store, and release FSH and LH in response to a pulse of GnRH. This is an example of the phenomenon of positive feedback.

Inhibin is a peptide hormone produced in granulosa and Sertoli cells. It appears to function by binding to a cellular membrane receptor, which activates a second messenger system to suppress selectively FSH synthesis and release. By inhibiting FSH synthesis, circulating levels of LH and FSH diverge during the follicular phase of the menstrual cycle (Fig. 4–13). Elevated levels of inhibin in the multiple follicles induced by gonadotropin stimulation of ovulation may suppress endogenous secretion of LH and FSH and the midcycle surge of LH (46).

Progesterone affects gonadotrophs by binding to cytoplasmic receptors that were previously induced by estradiol. Progesterone receptor complexes down-regulate estradiol receptor synthesis, decrease LH synthesis, but augment the release of LH and FSH in response to GnRH pulses (47). This facilitates the increase in FSH and LH release from gonadotrophs at the time of the LH surge (Fig. 4–14) (48).

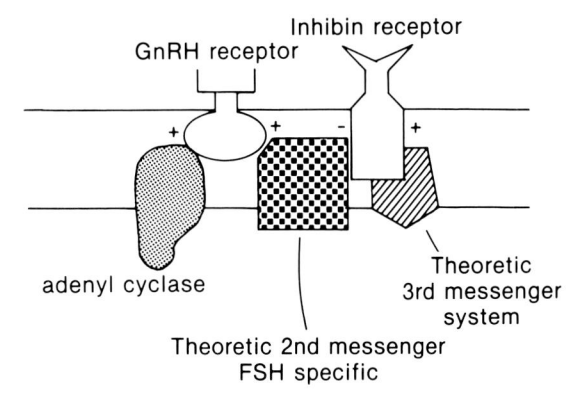

Fig. 4–13. Inhibin is thought to function via a membrane receptor and membrane-associated enzymes. These enzymes may also be affected by the GnRH receptor or may be GnRH receptor independent.

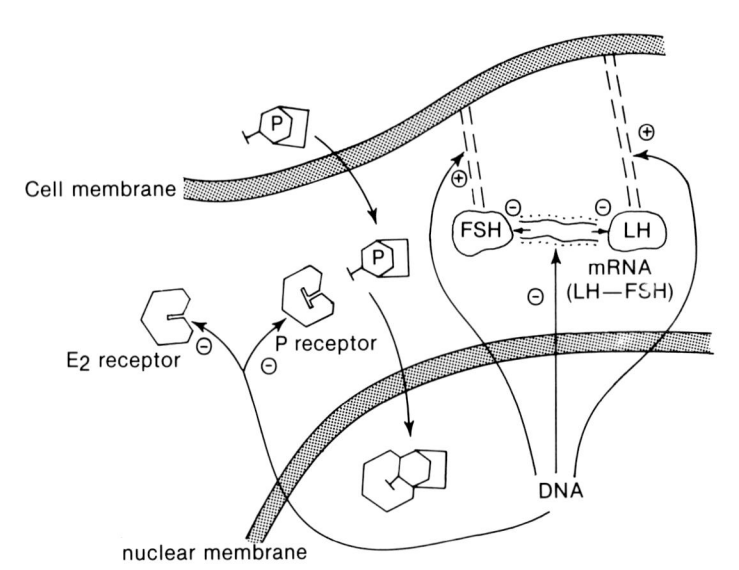

Fig. 4–14. Progesterone (P) binds to a cytoplasmic progesterone receptor that crosses the nuclear membrane and binds to DNA histones in pituitary gonadotrophs. This causes down-regulation in the synthesis of LH and FSH, E_2 receptors, and P receptors. However, the response of FSH and LH to GnRH stimulation is augmented. The net effect is increased secretion of LH and FSH but diminished storage. Continued progesterone action will deplete both synthesis and secretion of LH and FSH and concentrations of these decline.

Together, estradiol and progesterone modulate the effect of GnRH and independently function to control gonadotropin synthesis and secretion. This complex interaction accounts for the positive feedback effect of estradiol during the follicular phase and for the LH surge prior to ovulation. Initiation of 17-hydroxyprogesterone secretion and a decrease in estradiol synthesis by a mature follicle may also signal the gonadotrophs to provide the midcycle LH surge. The LH surge is the result of an increase in both the synthesis and release of LH. In summary, circulating steroid hormone levels affect the ability of gonadotrophs to respond to GnRH. Further, this modulation of gonadotroph function is achieved as much by the regulation of the receptor systems within the gonadotrophs as by the cyclic changes in circulating hormone levels.

THYROID-STIMULATING HORMONE (TSH). TSH stimulates thyroxine (T_4) and triiodothyronine (T_3) synthesis and release from follicular thyroid cells by activation of membrane receptors and the second messenger cAMP (16). These receptors may also be activated by hCG when it is present in high concentrations (e.g., hydatidiform mole). This is an example of a naturally occurring structural analogue of a normal hormone that is capable of inducing a physiologic response, despite low affinity for the receptor, when present in a high concentration. The synthesis and release of TSH is controlled by both thyroid-releasing hormone (TRH) and the circulating concentrations of T_4 and T_3. TSH is elevated in overt primary hypothyroidism. In occult primary hypothyroidism, TSH response to TRH is increased while the response to TRH is blunted in hyperthyroidism. Therefore, TRH infusion tests are capable of diagnosing clinically occult hyper- and hypothyroidism of glandular origin (49).

Pathology and Pathophysiology

The extent to which abnormalities in the hypothalamic-pituitary-peripheral gland axis arise within the anterior pituitary or adenohypophysis has always been and continues to be debated. A small number of women with amenorrhea will have ovarian failure and increased concentrations of FSH and LH. Panhypopituitarism (deficiency of all adenohypophyseal hormones) is rare and usually can be attributed to a specific pituitary or hypothalamic lesion. Women with a pituitary adenoma clearly have a disease process originating in the pituitary.

Until the last decade, however, the origin of an abnormality of menstrual function could not be determined for many women with anovulation and/or amenorrhea. The development of a radioimmunoassay for prolactin led to the recognition that many women are amenorrheic because they have hyperprolactinemia or a pituitary microadenoma. However, the cause of anovulation or amenorrhea is unknown for most women, although a hypothalamic abnormality is likely. Inappropriate androgen or estrogen suppression of hypothalamic function may account for the defect in some of these women (e.g., polycystic ovarian disease).

In this section, the pathophysiology and the clinical management of adenohypophyseal abnormalities will be discussed. Details of the dynamic tests referred to in the text are summarized in an appendix at the end of this chapter.

DEFICIENCY STATES.

Panhypopituitarism. This is a life-threatening condition which usually results from one of two events: Either the gland has been destroyed or communication with the hypothalamus has been lost. All the cells of the adenohypophysis except the lactotrophs are dependent on releasing factors for their function. The result of either of these catastrophic events, therefore, is failure of gonadotroph, thyrotroph, corticotroph, and somatotroph function, and, secondarily, peripheral hormone deficiencies. Since the lactotroph is primarily inhibited rather than stimulated by hypothalamic factors, prolactin is elevated when communication with the hypothalamus is interrupted. When the gland has been destroyed, however, prolactin will be normal or undetectable (Fig. 4–15). The loss of trophic hormones with pituitary failure may occur sequentially. Gonadotropins are frequently the first hormones to be lost and amenorrhea may be the first clinical sign of impending panhypopituitarism.

Women with complete panhypopituitarism also have hypothyroidism or myxedema. They have symptoms of adrenal insufficiency, but may not have significant salt wasting since the renin-aldosterone pathways remain intact. The loss of gonadal steroids results in delayed puberty in adolescents and amenorrhea in adults. Diabetes insipidus may occur if the neurohypophysis (posterior pituitary) is also involved. However, diabetes insipidus is more likely the result of a destructive hypothalamic lesion. Historically, panhypopituitarism was due to tuberculosis, syphilis, or postpartum hemorrhage (Sheehan syndrome [50]), all of which are presently uncommon. In childhood, panhypopituitarism may be the result of Hand-Schuler-Christian disease or other forms of histiocytosis-X. Terminally ill patients, especially those on circulatory or ventilatory support systems, may develop pituitary ischemia that leads to pituitary infarction.

A pituitary adenoma may be a cause of panhypopituitarism. Nonsecreting tumors are rarely detected until symptoms of pituitary deficiency develop. Secretory adenomas usually present with the clinical manifestations of the excessive hormone secretion prior to significant adenohypophyseal destruction. Panhypopituitarism may occur iatrogenically as a result of surgical ablation of a micro- or macroadenoma or as a late consequence of radiation therapy for these disorders.

Hypothalamic panhypopituitarism may be the result of a suprasellar tumor, hydrocephalus, congenital abnormality, meningitis or encephalitis, or traumatic or iatrogenic pituitary stalk section. Patients with head or neck inju-

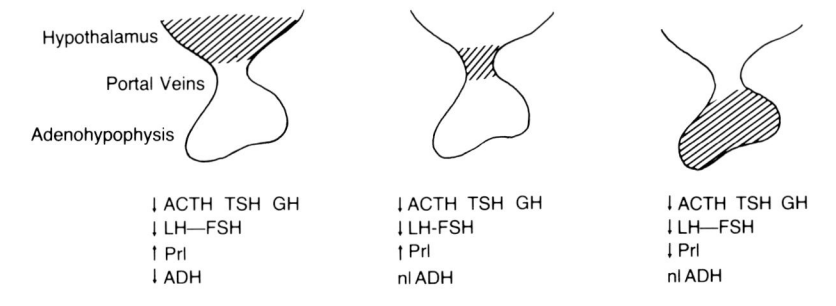

Fig. 4–15. Three potential types of lesions can result in panhypopituitarism. All of these lesions result in loss of LH and FSH, ACTH, TSH, and growth hormone. Loss of hypothalamic control (left) causes prolactin secretion to increase while antidiuretic hormone (ADH) falls. Stalk section (middle) may allow normal ADH activity in the presence of elevated prolactin concentrations. Glandular destruction (right) results in suppressed prolactin secretion, but usually normal ADH secretion.

ries from car accidents are particularly prone to this.

The diagnosis of panhypopituitarism is made by defining secretory abnormalities in each adenohypophyseal-peripheral gland axis. Patients with severe disease present with symptoms of suppressed hypothalamic-pituitary function in the presence of peripheral glandular failure. With a hypothalamic-pituitary abnormality and secondary adrenal failure, ACTH concentrations are low to normal, baseline cortisol concentrations are low, and there is a subnormal rise in plasma cortisol in response to standard doses of ACTH (Cortrosyn stimulation test). In these patients, urinary excretion of free cortisol and 17-hydroxycorticosteroids is also decreased. The diagnostic approach to these patients is summarized in Fig. 4–16. In incipient panhypopituitarism, these tests may be normal and an insulin tolerance test (see Appendix) may be necessary to document suppressed ACTH secretion. Adrenal insufficiency is life threatening, particularly during periods of stress. Therefore, no stress test should be performed when overt adrenal insufficiency exists. These tests should be performed in patients suspected of having latent adrenal insufficiency only if the patients are monitored carefully.

When corticotropin-releasing factor becomes available, direct assessment of corticotroph response and reserve will be possible (51). This will be a welcome replacement for the insulin tolerance test and other stress tests.

Likewise, thyroid or gonadotropin replacement without adrenal replacement is contraindicated in patients with panhypopituitarism. Pituitary hypothyroidism exists when plasma T_4 and T_3 levels are low and the TSH concentration is also low. A TRH infusion test will result in a blunted TSH response when latent pituitary hypothyroidism is present. Patients with well-documented panhypopituitarism should be treated with thyroid, glucocorticoid, estrogen, and progesterone replacement. Ovulation induction with gonadotropins is necessary to restore fertility (see Chapter 6).

Isolated Hormone Deficiencies.

ACTH AND TSH. Isolated deficiency of ACTH (52) or TSH (53) is unusual. The symptoms are those of peripheral gland failure in the presence of low or normal pituitary hormone levels. Function of the hypothalamic-pituitary axis is otherwise normal. The diagnosis of each of these is described in the discussion of panhypopituitarism. When ACTH and

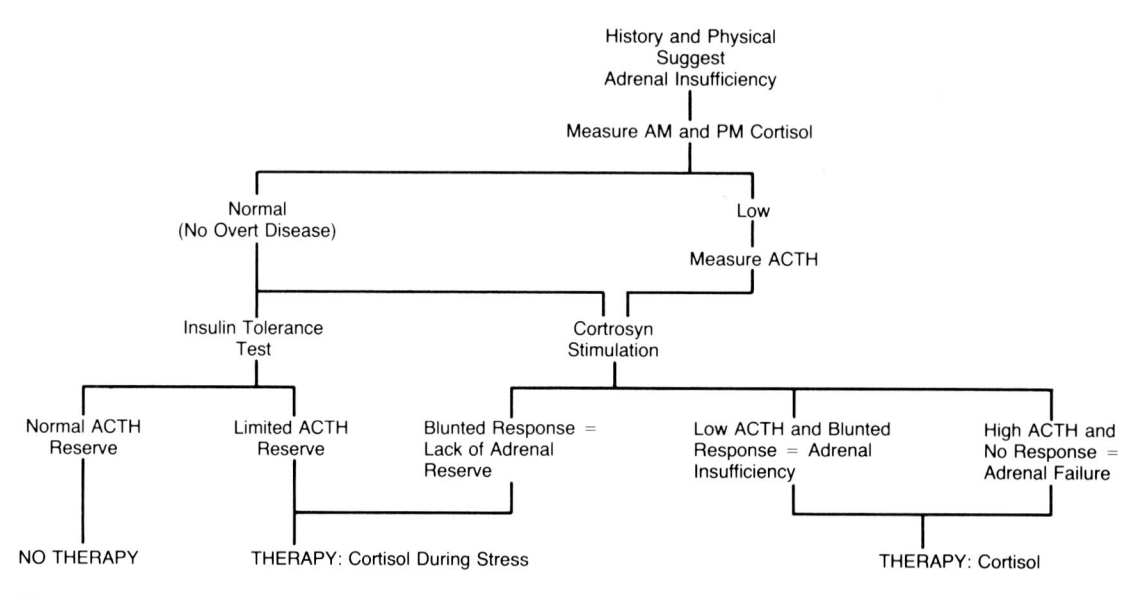

Fig. 4–16. The diagnosis of adrenal and/or ACTH insufficiency must be undertaken with caution. Prior to any stress tests, some evidence of adrenal reserve is necessary. Either normal morning and evening cortisol concentrations or a normal Cortrosyn stimulation test should precede any stress test. Lack of response with the Cortrosyn stimulation test may indicate either adrenal or pituitary insufficiency since the response of the adrenal can become secondarily insufficient when ACTH stimulation has been chronically inadequate. An abnormal insulin tolerance test and a normal Cortrosyn® stimulation test indicates a decreased ACTH reserve.

TSH function is lost, there is usually a primary lesion elsewhere in the hypothalamus or pituitary and deficiency of other pituitary hormones is often present.

GROWTH HORMONE. Growth hormone deficiency may result from a pituitary or hypothalamic disorder. Approximately 10% of subjects have affected family members and are homozygous for this autosomal recessive gene. Thirty percent of patients will have an associated pituitary or suprasellar tumor, and 10% will have an associated midline congenital facial defect. The remaining patients have a pituitary or a combined hypothalamic-pituitary deficiency with no clear etiology. Birth trauma has been suggested as a predisposing cause (54).

Patients with growth hormone deficiency fail to grow, usually from birth, and retain their toddler habitus. However, patients with a pituitary tumor will have a normal growth history until the tumor begins to interfere with growth hormone synthesis or release. Thereafter, there is a sudden deceleration of linear growth. Bone age and puberty will be delayed in all growth hormone deficient children.

Failure of growth hormone function may also occur with a defect in peripheral somatomedin activation that results in low somatomedin C levels (55). Somatomedins are a family of polypeptides that respond to growth hormone and are the immediate cause of growth in responsive tissues. Patients with low levels of somatomedin C have a similar clinical presentation to those with growth hormone deficiency, but will have normal or high circulating growth hormone levels (Fig. 4–17). Some women with isolated growth hormone deficiency will present with primary amenorrhea and/or delayed puberty. Once puberty is complete, gonadotropin secretion will frequently be normal (56).

The diagnosis of growth hormone deficiency often requires the use of provocative tests such as an insulin tolerance test and/or an arginine infusion test to demonstrate a subtle deficiency in growth hormone response (see Appendix). Since an insulin tolerance test also stresses the pituitary-adrenal axis, this must be done with caution. Patients with growth hormone deficiency may also have a deficiency in ACTH secretion and cortisol response. Radiologic studies, particularly computerized tomography (CAT scan), are indicated for patients with growth hormone deficiency to rule out a hypothalamic neoplasm.

Patients with combined hormone deficiencies must receive replacement of all deficient target hormones. Patients with isolated growth hormone deficiency should receive growth hormone only. However, this therapy is inef-

Fig. 4–17. A Normal growth hormone (GH) levels are maintained by the feedback inhibition of somatomedin C, a peripheral effector of GH. Somatomedin C is synthesized primarily in the liver. **B** In GH deficiency, both GH and somatomedin C are low and growth failure occurs. **C** In Laron dwarfism there is a failure in peripheral synthesis of somatomedin C with normal to elevated growth hormone concentrations. These patients are physically identical to those with GH deficiency but will not respond to growth hormone. **D** In gigantism, acromegaly, and puberty, both GH and somatomedin C may be elevated. Provocative tests may be required to distinguish these 3 conditions.

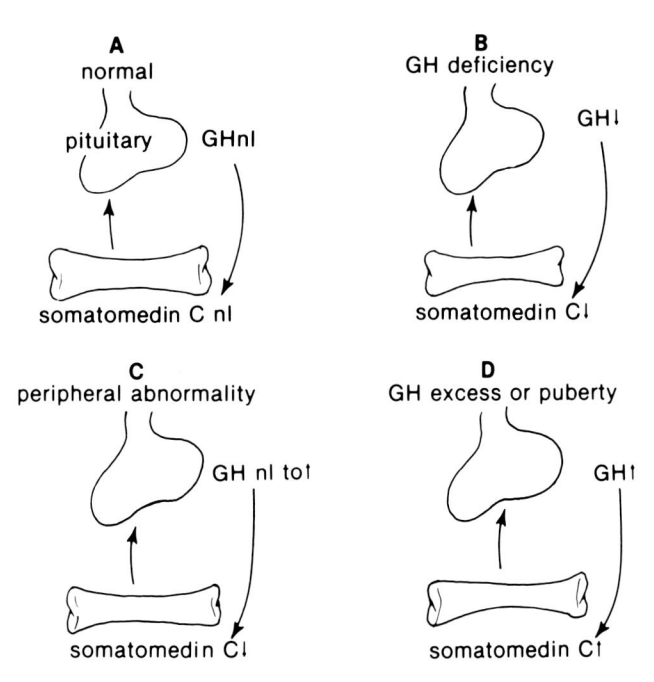

fective for patients with peripheral deficiencies in somatomedin C.

The possibility of Turner's syndrome with a chromosomal variant should be considered in any child whose growth is inadequate. A karyotype is indicated when this is suspected.

FSH AND LH. Hypogonadotrophic eunuchoidism is primarily of hypothalamic origin, although subjects with isolated FSH and/or LH deficiency have been reported (57). When hypothalamic amenorrhea is associated with anosmia, the diagnosis is Kallman's syndrome. These patients will respond to pulsatile GnRH infusions with an increase in both LH and FSH secretion and cyclic ovulatory function returns in the female. Such women can conceive after sexual development has been induced with estrogens and ovulation has been induced with gonadotropins or pulsatile GnRH (see Chapter 6).

Secondary hypothalamic hypogonadotropism may result from sudden weight changes, chronic weight deficiency states (e.g., anorexia nervosa) (58), and from chronic stress in individuals who participate in strenuous physical activities such as distance running, ballet, or gymnastics (59). The mechanisms underlying these secondary hypothalamic states are not completely understood, but have been related to endorphin and/or dopamine function in the hypothalamus. In addition, many women with chronic anovulation may have a mild form of hypothalamic hypogonadism. Secondary hypothalamic hypogonadism is also present in women with increased prolactin secretion. This will be discussed in the next section.

HYPERSECRETION STATES. Hypersecretion of any pituitary trophic hormone can occur. Hypersecretion in the absence of peripheral target gland failure implies the presence of a pituitary adenoma and such tumors have been reported for all of the adenohypophyseal cell types. Functional glycoprotein hormone-secreting tumors are extremely rare and are usually located in the middle of the gland. If the adenoma produces TSH, recurrent goiter and hyperthyroidism will be the primary symptom (60). Usually little or no response to TRF infusions occurs. Since reports of FSH and LH producing adenomas are case studies (61,62), it is impossible to provide general observations and each patient must be approached individually when the possibility of one of these adenomas arises.

ACTH. Adenomas arising from corticotrophin cells are also centrally located and relatively uncommon, but must be considered in any hyperplastic adrenal state. These tumors secrete ACTH and may secrete other corticotrophin-related proteins. Excessive secretion of ACTH causes Cushing's disease. An ACTH-secreting pituitary adenoma should be suspected when clinical Cushingoid features are present (Table 4–3) and the diurnal variation in serum cortisol is lost and/or the morning cortisol concentration is not suppressed below 5 mcg/dl by 1 mg dexamethasone taken at 11:00 P.M. the previous evening (see Appendix). Women whose cortisol concentrations are not suppressed should have additional tests of their pituitary-adrenal axis to distinguish a functional adrenal abnormality from an adrenal tumor or a pituitary adenoma (Fig. 4–18).

A patient whose cortisol concentrations are completely suppressed during a low-dose (0.5 mg 4 times a day) dexamethasone suppression test most likely has a functional adrenal abnormality. Secretion of ACTH from a pituitary

TABLE 4–3. Signs and Symptoms of Cushing's Syndrome or Disease.

AFFECTED AREA	SIGN OR SYMPTOM
Somatic	Obesity (truncal)
	Moon facies (& plethora)
	Weakness & peripheral wasting
	Edema
	"Buffalo hump"
Dermatologic	Striae (purple)
	Bruising
	Poor wound healing
	Pigmentation
	Fungal infections
Systemic	Hypertension
	Renal stones (calcium)
	Polyuria, polydipsia
	Osteoporosis
	Growth failure
Psychiatric	Emotional lability
	Psychosis
	Depression
Endocrine	Glucose intolerance
	Androgen excess (hirsutism, acne)
	Menstrual dysfunction, anovulation

```
                          History and Physical
                          Suggest Cushing's
                              Syndrome
                                 |
                       Measure AM and PM Cortisol;
                       Give 1 mg Dexamethasone @ HS
         ┌───────────────────────┴───────────────────────┐
  Diurnal Cortisol Variation;                    No Diurnal Variation;
  AM Cortisol <5.0 mcg/dl                        AM Cortisol Not
         |                                       Suppressed
   Not Cushing's                                        |
                                            Admit for Workup: 24 hr.
                                            Urine for Creatinine, 17-hydroxy-
                                            steroids, 17-ketosteroids, Free
                                            Cortisol (Days 1 to 3)
                                                       |
                                            0.5 mg Dexamethasone q. 6 hr. X 8.
                                            Repeat Studies on Day 5
         ┌─────────────────────────────────────────────┴──────────┐
  Cortisol Suppressed:                              Cortisol not Suppressed
  17-hydroxysteroids  < 2mg/gm                            |
  Creatinine, Urinary Free                         2 mg Dexamethasone q. 6
  Cortisol < 20 mcg/gm Creatinine                  hr. X 8; Repeat Studies
                                                   on Day 7; Measure ACTH
  ┌──────────────────┬──────────────────────┬──────────────────────┐
 Suppressed ACTH,   Suppressed ACTH,       Unsuppressed ACTH,
 Partially Suppressed Unsuppressed 17-hydroxy- 17-hydroxysteroids, and
 17-hydroxysteroids and steroids and Free Cortisol Free Cortisol
 Free Cortisol
       |                    |                      |
 DIAGNOSIS: Pituitary Adenoma DIAGNOSIS: Adrenal or Ovarian DIAGNOSIS: Ectopic
 (Perform CAT Scan of Sella)  Tumor                          ACTH Secretion
                              (Perform CAT Scan of Abdomen)  (Perform Tumor Workup)
```

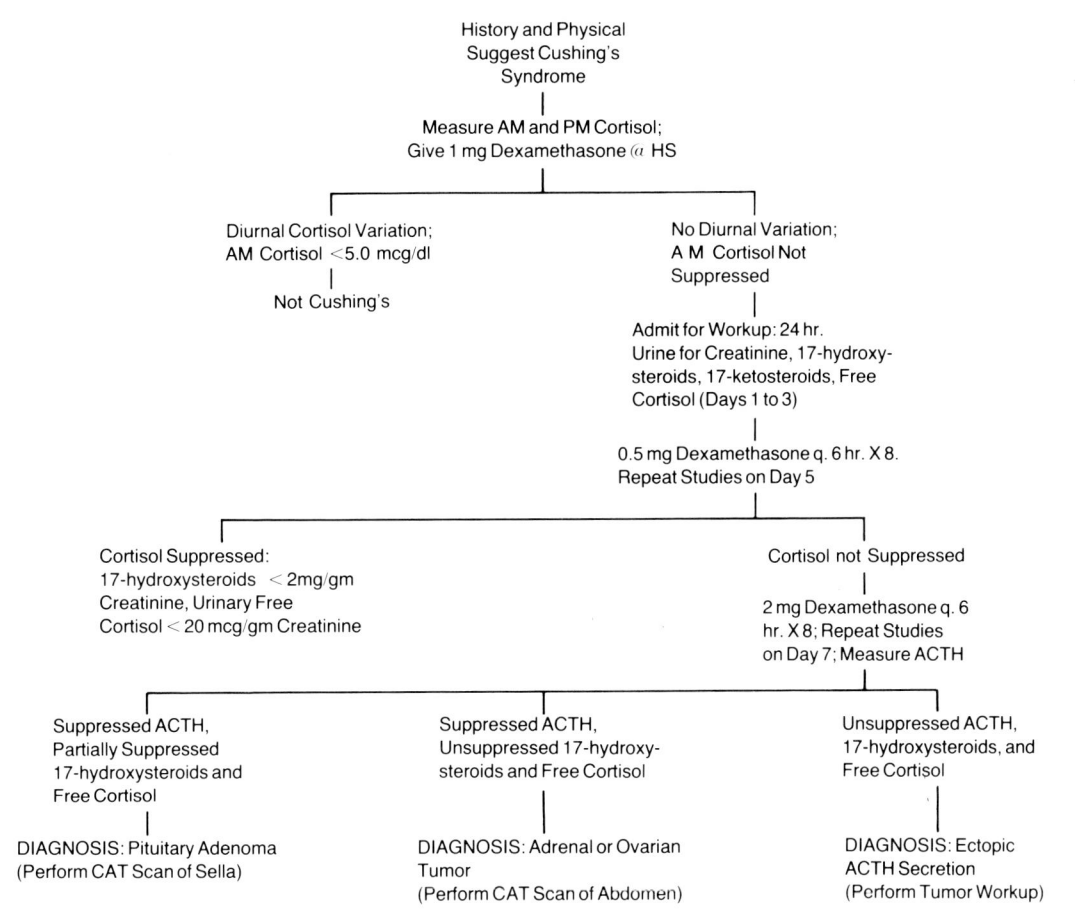

Fig. 4-18. A morning cortisol concentration below 5.0 mcg/dl after an overnight dexamethasone suppression test excludes the diagnosis of Cushing's syndrome. Complete suppression of cortisol synthesis as demonstrated by suppression of urinary 17-hydroxysteroids or free cortisol on a low dose (0.5 mg, 4 times a day) dexamethasone suppression test excludes the possibility of a pituitary adenoma. Failure to suppress after a high dose (2 mg, 4 times a day) dexamethasone suppression test indicates either autonomous adrenal function (implying a tumor) or ectopic ACTH synthesis, which usually occurs in association with a carcinoma. Partial suppression suggests a pituitary adenoma.

adenoma will usually be suppressed partially by high doses (2 mg 4 times a day) of dexamethasone while adrenal tumors will not be suppressed on this dose (63). ACTH levels should also be monitored during these tests, since ectopic sources of ACTH will not be suppressed by either low or high doses of dexamethasone.

High concentrations of ACTH and lack of suppression on high doses of dexamethasone are suggestive of an ectopic source of ACTH. When a pituitary adenoma is suspected, hypocycloidal polytomography or computerized tomography (a CAT scan) should be performed. However, a tumor is found by these procedures in less than 25% of patients with surgically proven adenomas.

In general, the treatment of choice is transphenoidal resection of the adenoma (64). Proton beam radiation (65) or yttrium implantation have also been used (66). Bromocriptine or the serotonin inhibitor, cyproheptadine (Periactin®), may be an effective means of shrinking a tumor (67) and a trial of medical therapy may be indicated prior to surgery.

Growth Hormone. Growth-hormone-producing adenomas result in 2 distinct clinical presentations—gigantism and acromegaly. Growth hormone secretion from an adenoma in a prepubertal child causes gigantism owing to excessive linear growth of the long bones. Development of an adenoma in a postpubertal patient results in continued growth of membranous bones, cartilage, and connective tissue of the skin as well as other changes typical of acromegaly. The adenomas may also secrete significant amounts of prolactin (68). When prolactin hypersecretion occurs, amenorrhea may result. The diagnosis of a growth-hormone-secreting tumor is more likely when concentrations of somatomedin C are elevated (69). This diagnosis is supported by failure of growth hormone concentrations to be suppressed by a glucose infusion and by a lack of response or a paradoxical suppression of growth hormone concentrations during an insulin tolerance test.

During puberty, the concentration of growth hormone may be elevated and somatomedin C concentrations may be high. To distinguish an unusually tall adolescent from one with a growth-hormone-secreting tumor, bone age, pubertal development, parental height, and projected height are important observations. These will be normal for a tall adolescent without a tumor. It may be necessary to monitor patients through puberty to distinguish these possibilities.

If an adenoma is suspected, hypocycloidal polytomography and/or a CAT scan are indicated. Response to bromocriptine has been variable in subjects with a growth-hormone-secreting tumor (70), but more predictable in subjects with an adenoma secreting both prolactin and growth hormone. Radiation has been used with good success, but the risk of panhypopituitarism and optic nerve damage is significant (71). In general, those patients who have failed a medical trial with bromocriptine are best treated with transphenoidal hypophysectomy of the microadenoma.

Prolactin. Prior to 1970, most pituitary adenomas were thought to be nonsecreting. With the isolation, purification, and subsequent development of a radioimmunoassay for prolactin (72), it is now apparent that a majority of these adenomas secrete prolactin (73). The finding of an increased concentration of any of the other adenohypophyseal hormones suggests the presence of a pituitary tumor. This association does not hold for prolactin since hyperprolactinemia does not necessarily indicate the presence of an adenoma.

As previously described, the primary regulator of prolactin secretion is dopamine, which inhibits prolactin secretion. Any hypothalamic abnormality resulting in decreased dopamine release into the portal system will result in hyperprolactinemia. Therefore, any hypothalamic disorder that results in diminished secretion of the other adenohypophyseal hormones will usually cause excessive secretion of prolactin. Moreover, primary hypothyroidism will cause hyperprolactinemia because TRH production by the hypothalamus is excessive. TRH is a potent stimulator of prolactin secretion. In addition, hypothalamic dopamine activity may be suppressed. Correction of the hypothyroidism will cause prolactin secretion to return to normal in most subjects (74).

Vascular abnormalities in the hypothalamus or pituitary may cause hyperprolactinemia. Transection of the pituitary stalk, arteriovenous malformations, and venous thrombosis are examples of such vascular abnormalities. The impact of local venous thrombosis is illustrated in Fig. 4–19. Inhibition of lactotrophs by dopamine and stimulation of the remaining pituitary hormones would be lost. As a conse-

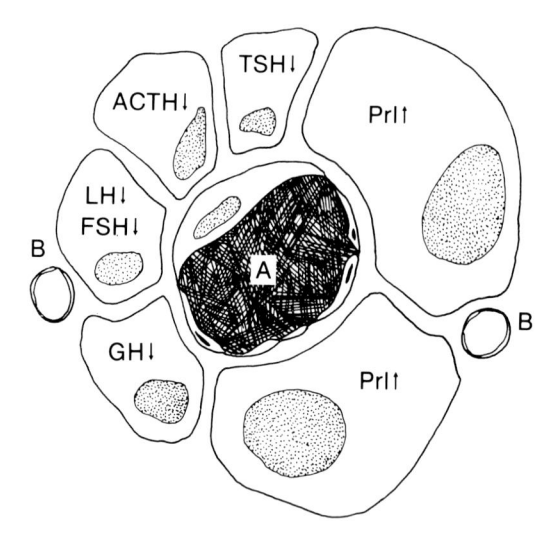

Fig. 4–19. Theoretically, hyperprolactinemia could arise from thrombosis of portal veins or sinusoids. Since the short portal vessels maintain adequate tissue oxygenation, the cells would not undergo infarction. In such a region, the cells synthesizing ACTH, GH, TSH, and LH and FSH would undergo involution from lack of hypothalamic stimulation. Lactotrophs deprived of hypothalamic dopamine would continue to function but in an unsuppressed environment. Such a region eventually may acquire a blood supply from the inferior hypophyseal artery and continue to function independently of hypothalamic control. A = thrombosed sinusoidal capillary, B = patent superior hypophyseal capillaries.

quence, prolactin secretion increases while secretion of the other hormones may decrease. However, secretion of these other trophic hormones would be maintained in viable areas of the pituitary unless necrosis of the pituitary is extensive. Most of the evidence for such an occurrence, however, is circumstantial. The true frequency of vascular abnormalities causing hyperprolactinemia is unknown (75).

Iatrogenic hyperprolactinemia is common. A large number of antihypertensive and psychiatric medications affect either the synthesis or storage of dopamine or block the cell membrane receptor for dopamine (Table 4–1). Phenothiazine derivatives are potent dopamine antagonists as they block dopamine receptors in the central nervous system and pituitary (76).

Women with hyperprolactinemia are frequently anovulatory and amenorrheic because hypothalamic GnRH and, therefore, pituitary FSH and LH secretion are suppressed (77). Hypothalamic inhibition would also account for the decreased growth hormone secretion in women with hyperprolactinemia. The mechanism of this effect appears to be excessive dopaminergic activity within the hypothalamus, which comes about because high prolactin concentrations reach the hypothalamus via retrograde flow through the portal vessels (a "short loop feedback"). High concentrations of prolactin stimulate dopamine secretion in the hypothalamus (a positive feedback). An increased dopamine release would normally inhibit further prolactin synthesis and release (78).

This presumed hypercatecholamine state in the hypothalamus is suggested by results of studies using monoiodotyrosine (MIT) to inhibit dopamine synthesis (Fig. 4–20) (79). LH and growth hormone levels return toward normal but prolactin remains elevated in subjects who receive oral MIT. These findings would further suggest that hyperprolactinemia is not the result of hypothalamic dopaminergic failure, but rather failure of dopamine to reach the lactotroph (vascular theory) or failure of the lactotroph to respond normally to dopamine (theory of decreased receptor activity–cellular autonomy).

Endogenous opioids may also be involved in GnRH supression. They may suppress GnRH secretion directly (80,81); they may also suppress GnRH secretion by altering dopamine metabolism (82).

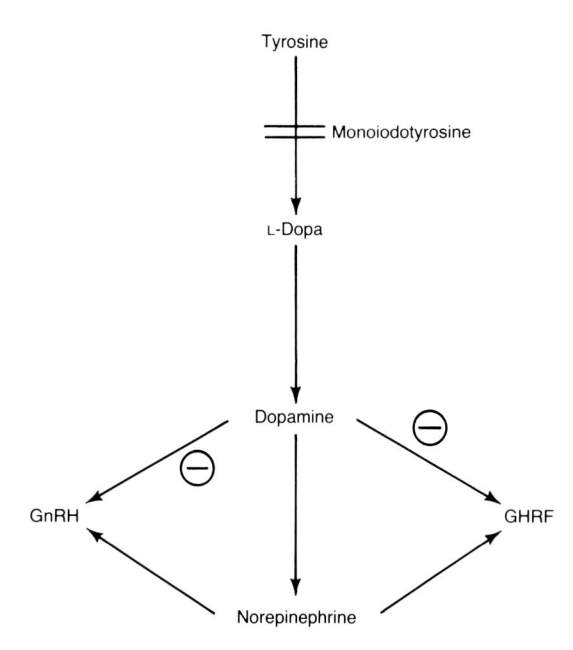

Fig. 4–20. Monoiodotyrosine (MIT) is a competitive inhibitor in the enzymatic conversion of tyrosine to L-Dopa which is the precursor for dopamine. Dopamine suppresses GnRH and growth hormone releasing factor (GHRF). Therefore, decreased dopamine synthesis would result in increased GnRH and GHRF release.

The identification of a hyperprolactinemic woman and the initiation of the workup to diagnose an adenoma depend upon recognizing the woman at risk. A woman with amenorrhea and galactorrhea is most likely to have hyperprolactinemia, which can also be found in women with either amenorrhea or galactorrhea. Women with luteal phase defects may also have hyperprolactinemia (83). Therefore, any woman with an ovulatory defect and/or galactorrhea should have a serum prolactin level measured before treatment is begun (see Chapter 6). In amenorrheic women, measurement of LH and FSH may be necessary to exclude ovarian failure. Other causes of hyperprolactinemia should be sought (e.g., medication, thyroid dysfunction). If a drug history is uninformative and thyroid function is normal, visual field examination and radiologic studies of the pituitary should be performed. Measurement of growth hormone should be considered to eliminate the possibility of a mixed growth hormone-prolactin secreting adenoma (84).

The empty sella syndrome may cause hyperprolactinemia. This abnormality results from invagination of the third ventricle through the diaphragm of the sella turcica. Computerized tomography will usually differentiate this abnormality from a prolactin-secreting pituitary adenoma. The empty sella syndrome is a benign condition that may affect FSH and LH secretion but does not otherwise cause pituitary failure. Treatment of women with the empty sella syndrome and hyperprolactinemia is medical. No therapy is required for affected women who have normal prolactin concentrations and no disturbance of the menstrual cycle (In these women, the empty sella syndrome is often an incidental finding on a skull X-ray done for trauma or headaches.)

Diagnosis of a Prolactinoma. The diagnosis of a prolactinoma is made by demonstrating hyperprolactinemia in a woman with a space-occupying pituitary lesion. Adenomas larger than 10 mm can be demonstrated by any of the radiologic procedures discussed below. However, microadenomas (tumors less than 10 mm) are less easily diagnosed and require sensitive radiologic studies that still may be inconclusive. The presence of amenorrhea and hyperprolactinemia is not diagnostic of an adenoma. Further, since none of the provocative tests of pituitary function have proven to be diagnostic of an adenoma, the distinction between a hypersecretory state and excessive secretion caused by a small microadenoma is not always certain.

RADIOLOGIC STUDIES. Cone-down sella turcica X-rays are capable of demonstrating tumors larger than 10 mm (85). Diagnostic findings include a double sellar floor or upward displacement of the clinoid processes (which indicates suprasellar extension) (Fig. 4–21). It is also useful to identify women with a craniopharyngioma since intra- or suprasellar calcification will be seen. Radiation exposure is less than 0.5 rads. The procedure, however, is inadequate for detecting most microadenomas, although it may be useful to the radiologist as a "scout film" preceding hypocycloidal polytomography and to the clinician as a baseline for future follow-up (86).

Hypocycloidal polytomography shifts the plane of focus 1 mm to 2 mm for each exposure. The result is analogous to depth of field in photography where only a narrow plane is

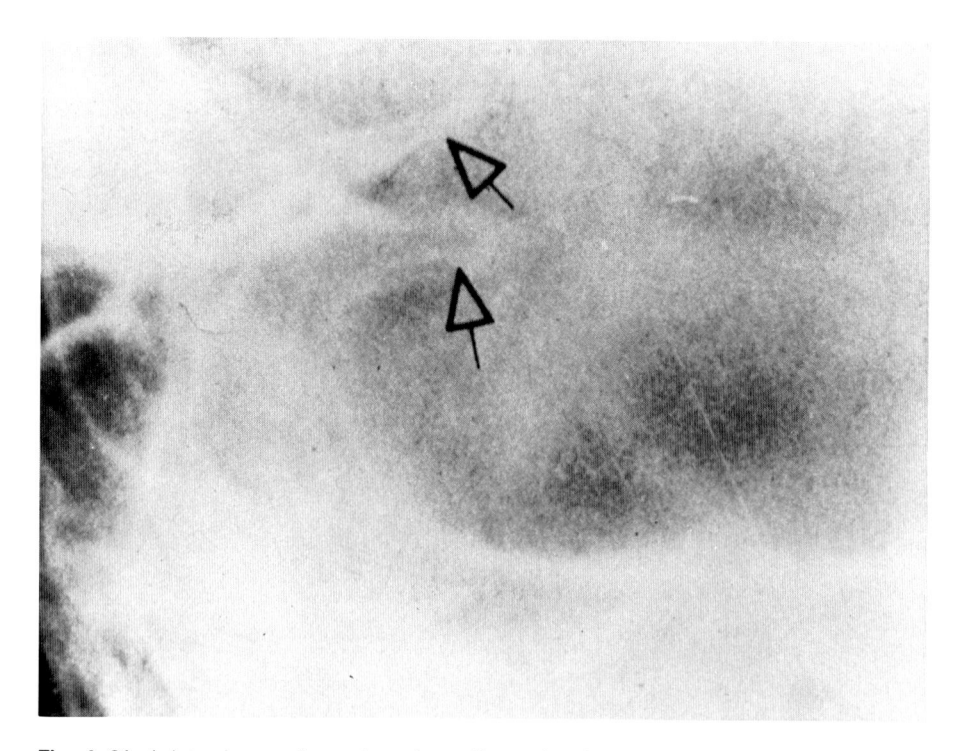

Fig. 4–21. A lateral cone-down view of a sella turcica that reveals elevation of the clinoid processes (arrows) in a patient with a macroadenoma and suprasellar extension of the tumor.

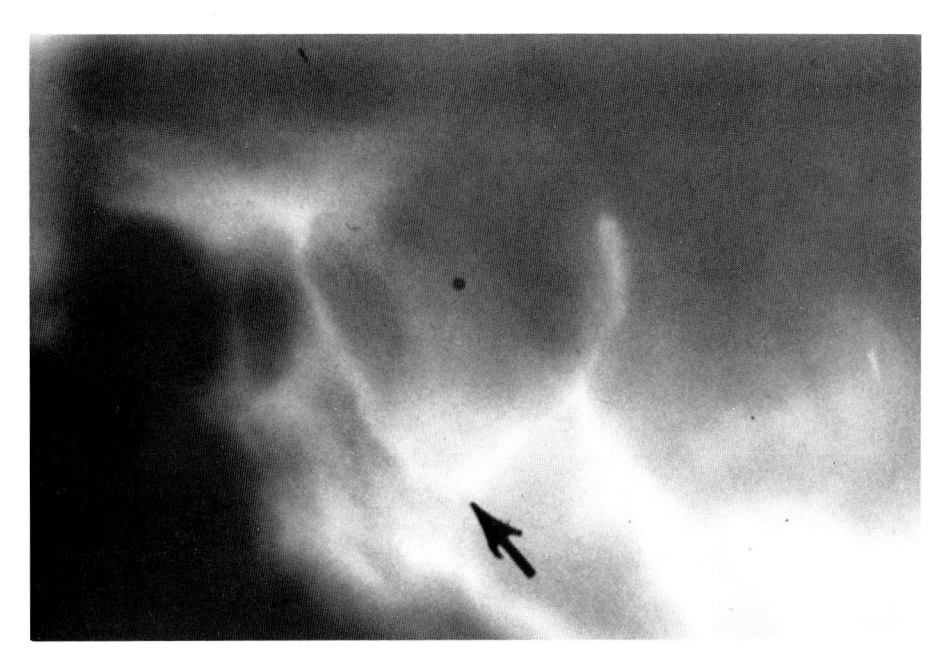

Fig. 4–22. Hypocycloidal polytomography reveals localized "blistering" (arrow) in the floor of the sella turcica. This is consistent with the presence of a microadenoma in a woman with amenorrhea, galactorrhea, and a prolactin concentration of 134 ng/m‹6l.

in focus and any object in front or behind that plane is out of focus. Imaging can be done in the sagittal or coronal planes; the sagittal views usually give better resolution. The technique will show most tumors larger than 4 mm since asymmetry and/or erosion of the floor of the sella will be present (Fig. 4–22). However, identification of smaller adenomas may be confused by the presence of minor anatomic variations in the sella that are observed in approximately 25% of normal women (87,88). Interpretation becomes a difficult problem if polytomography is performed in women with few or no signs of a tumor (e.g., galactorrhea without hyperprolactinemia). Therefore, interpretation of the X-rays must be correlated with the degree of hyperprolactinemia and other clinical features of the woman.

The radiation exposure is relatively high (15 to 25 rads) and repetitive hypocycloidal polytomography has been associated with cataract formation, especially when the eyes have not been shielded. The procedure should not be used for routine follow-up of women with known or suspected microadenomas.

Computerized axial tomography (CAT scan) has become increasingly useful in evaluating the possibility of a tumor in a woman with hyperprolactinemia (89,90). The original scanners were useful only in defining suprasellar extension or the empty sella syndrome. They were a welcome replacement for the painful and hazardous pneumoencephalogram and arteriogram. Newer models achieve a resolution as good or better than hypocycloidal polytomography with a similar radiation exposure. Resolution with the newest models is so great that a CAT scan is probably the procedure of choice to assess the pituitary gland when a tumor is suspected clinically. The scan will reveal both intra- and suprasellar masses (Fig. 4–23).

DYNAMIC PITUITARY TESTING. No dynamic test of pituitary function is consistently useful in differentiating an adenoma from a hypersecretory state. The two most useful tests are an insulin tolerance test and TRH infusion (see Appendix). Some have found that the response of prolactin to TRH infusion has correlated well with the presence of an adenoma (91,92), although others have found no such correlation (93,94).

A scheme to evaluate a woman who may have hyperprolactinemia is illustrated in Fig. 4–24. In general, any woman with a prolactin

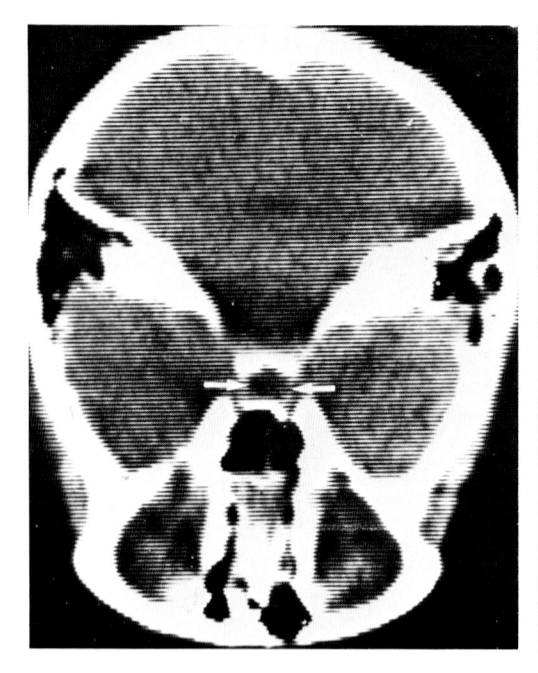

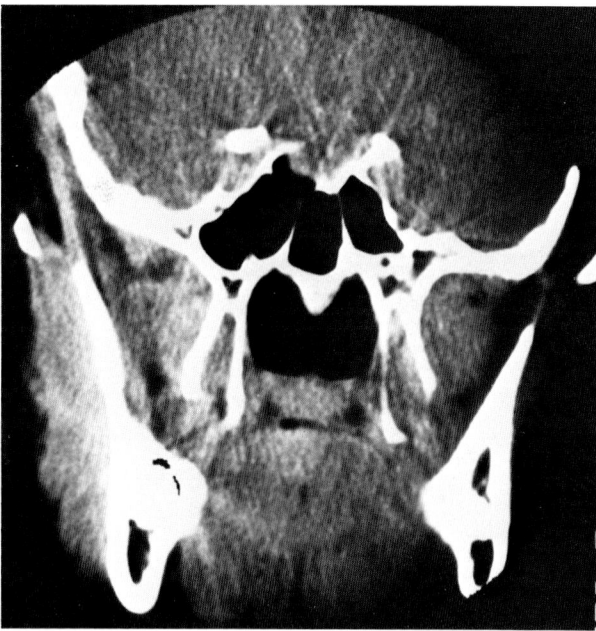

Fig. 4–23. A Unenhanced CAT scan (with a scanner available about 1978) reveals suprasellar extension (arrows) of a microadenoma. **B** With the improved imaging of a current scanner (1982) perforation of the sellar floor by an 8 mm intrasellar adenoma is clearly seen.

concentration over 40 ng/ml that is unchanged after stopping medication (Table 4–1) or becoming euthyroid requires hypocycloidal polytomography or, better, a high-resolution CAT scan and a visual field examination. If polytomography reveals a tumor, a CAT scan is necessary to exclude suprasellar extension of the tumor. In women with a tumor, an insulin tolerance test and TRH infusion are useful to assure normal ACTH and TSH reserve. If hypocycloidal polytomography and/or the CAT scan are negative, then dynamic testing is usually not indicated. In women with a prolactin concentration of less than 100 ng/ml who will accept medical therapy, a single, cone-down view of the sella turcica is adequate to exclude a macroadenoma.

Treatment of a Prolactinoma. Treatment of a prolactin-secreting adenoma depends upon the size of the tumor, the desires of the woman, and, frequently, the past experience of the physician. Four options are available: (1) no treatment, (2) surgical ablation, (3) radiation therapy, and (4) medical suppression.

There is no change in tumor size or severity of symptoms in most untreated subjects (95). Withholding therapy is appropriate only for women with tumors less than 4 mm. Prolactin concentrations should be measured at 6-month intervals. Lateral cone-down X-rays of the sella turcica and visual field examinations should be performed yearly. Microadenomas larger than 4 mm and macroadenomas are usually treated more aggressively. Demonstration of an increasing prolactin concentration, abnormalities of the visual field examination, or progressive radiologic changes are also indications for therapy in a woman previously followed without treatment.

Amenorrheic women with hyperprolactinemia may produce little or no estrogen and be at risk for the development of osteoporosis. Since estrogens may stimulate pituitary lactotrophs, bromocriptine may be the preferred treatment; estrogen-progestin therapy is a reasonable alternative provided serum prolactin concentrations are measured at least every 6 months. Steroid replacement therapy should be stopped if the prolactin concentrations rise. Cyclic progestin therapy is sufficient for hyperprolactinemic women with evidence of es-

Fig. 4–24. In evaluating a patient with a history and physical examination that suggests hyperprolactinemia, the initial step is to document an elevation in prolactin and then eliminate either iatrogenic causes (medications) or other endocrinopathies (e.g., hypothyroidism) as a cause. Once pathologic hyperprolactinemia is established as a diagnosis, visual fields and polytomography, or CAT scan are indicated. If either polytomography or visual fields are abnormal, a CAT scan is necessary. ITT = insulin tolerance test; TRH = stimulation with TSH-releasing hormone.

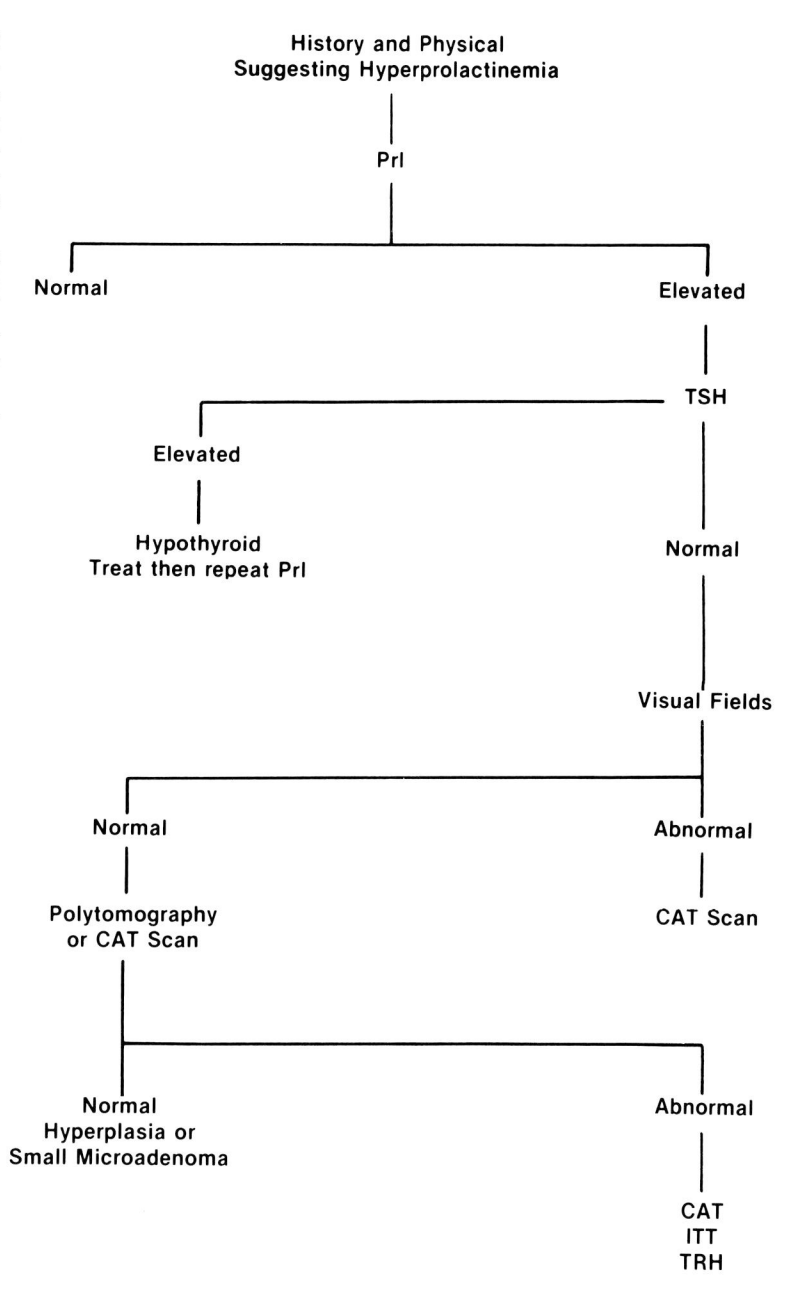

```
          History and Physical
      Suggesting Hyperprolactinemia
                    |
                   Prl
                  /    \
             Normal    Elevated
                          |
                         TSH
                        /    \
                  Elevated   Normal
                     |          |
                Hypothyroid     |
            Treat then repeat Prl
                                |
                          Visual Fields
                           /         \
                       Normal       Abnormal
                         |             |
                   Polytomography   CAT Scan
                    or CAT Scan
                       /      \
                  Normal      Abnormal
              Hyperplasia or     |
              Small Microadenoma CAT
                                 ITT
                                 TRH
```

trogen production (e.g., the presence of cervical mucus or withdrawal bleeding after a progestin).

When performed by a skilled neurosurgeon, transphenoidal resection of a microadenoma is initially successful for many patients (96). LH and FSH secretion and ovulatory menses usually return within 6 to 10 weeks. Macroadenomas are less easily resected by the transsphenoidal route and a frontal craniotomy may be necessary. Adenohypophyseal function is not always maintained in these women, who may develop panhypopituitarism. Hemiparesis and death are also risks, although fortunately these are rare. Recurrence or persistence of a tumor in women with a macroadenoma is frequent, and many eventually require medical or radiation therapy (97,98).

There is a significant recurrence rate after transsphenoidal surgery for a microadenoma

(99,100). Since follow-up of untreated women now indicates that most will have no enlargement of their tumor, transphenoidal hypophysectomy should be reserved for those who demonstrate progressive enlargement and/or have failed medical therapy.

Radiation therapy has been used as an adjunct to pituitary surgery in women who have had either incomplete resections or clinical recurrence. Proton beam therapy is occasionally used as the primary treatment modality and is successful in decreasing the size or eliminating the adenoma in approximately 50% of women. Since adenomas are slow growing and relatively radioresistant, large doses of radiation may be necessary (101,102). Panhypopituitarism is a serious complication of radiation therapy that may not develop for many years. While panhypopituitarism may not be as common as once thought (103,104), radiation should not be the primary mode of therapy because of this complication.

Medical therapy is successful only if the adenoma contains dopamine receptors. Cultured adenoma cells contain receptors that bind dopamine with a normal to slightly diminished affinity (105,106). This is an important observation because ergot alkaloids suppress the growth of adenomas and inhibit prolactin secretion by binding to dopamine receptors (105). Bromocriptine and pergolide are ergot derivatives that function as long-acting dopamine agonists, suppress prolactin secretion from both normal and adenoma cells (107,108), and reduce the size of many tumors (109,110). LH, FSH and growth hormone return to normal during therapy and most women have a return of cyclic pituitary-ovarian function.

Whether therapy for a long period will cure the woman is unknown. It is our experience and that of others (111) that symptoms recur when medication is discontinued, even after 5 years of therapy. Also, the medication is approved for treatment of hyperprolactinemia but not for adenomas. Until adequate clinical trials have been performed to assure women that these drugs are safe and effective for radiologically demonstrated adenomas, they should be informed of the experimental nature of the medication and, ideally, be referred to a research center for treatment and follow-up. Women taking bromocriptine who do not wish to conceive should receive appropriate contraception.

Regardless of the therapy chosen, women with abnormal pituitary-ovarian function should have a prolactin level measured every 6 months and visual field examinations and cone-down views of the sella turcica annually. If cyclic pituitary-ovarian function and ovulation return, a prolactin level measured yearly is adequate. Women treated with extensive surgery or radiation should be monitored annually for the development of panhypopituitarism. The recurrence of amenorrhea and/or a falling prolactin level may be the first sign of impending pituitary failure.

A significant percentage of women with hyperprolactinemia wish to conceive. Bromocriptine is quite successful in inducing ovulation. The subsequent course of pregnancy is rarely complicated by the tumor and both maternal and fetal outcomes are good (112–117). The use of bromocriptine for ovulation induction is discussed in Chapter 6.

For most women with a microadenoma, it is not necessary to restart bromocriptine immediately following delivery. Most newly delivered mothers should be allowed to breast feed unless symptoms of an expanding tumor appear, visual fields constrict, or prolactin concentrations increase significantly. Our experience at the University of Connecticut is that most women do not develop symptoms and prolactin concentrations return to within 150% of the pretreatment, prepregnancy level. We recommend that these women discontinue breast feeding by 4 to 6 months and restart therapy. However, if a woman understands the risks and wishes to continue breast feeding, we delay therapy, provided her postpartum evaluation, including prolactin concentration, is similar to what it was before she began therapy.

Summary

The adenohypophysis is a confederation of trophic cells that include gonadotrophs and lactotrophs. The gonadotrophs, secreting LH and FSH, function as an amplifier of hypothalamic GnRH. This amplification is modulated by estradiol and progesterone and is a major reason for the positive feedback phenomenon and the resulting LH and FSH surge in the preovulatory period. The lactotrophs, negatively inhibited by dopamine, are the major source of pituitary pathology. Prolactin-producing adenomas result in hypothalamic suppression of GnRH and subsequent anovulation and amenorrhea. Bromocriptine suppresses prolactin secretion and permits GnRH function to return to normal. Women with a microadenoma can be followed safely in pregnancy without medication and be allowed to breast feed if they are carefully monitored for evidence of tumor enlargement.

Appendix

INSULIN TOLERANCE TEST (I.T.T.) The woman should fast overnight, be at bed rest, and not smoke prior to or during the test. A 50% solution of glucose should be at the bedside and the woman should be attended throughout the test. Vital signs are recorded every 15 minutes. Regular insulin (0.1 unit/kg of body weight) is injected intravenously at time zero. Venous blood is sampled at −15, 0, 20, 30, 45, 60, and 90 minutes and the concentrations of growth hormone, cortisol, and glucose are measured. At least a 50% fall in serum glucose to less than 40 mg/100 ml is required for a valid test. The test is contraindicated in patients known to have adrenal insufficiency or panhypopituitarism. If there is a suspicion of either, a Cortrosyn stimulation test should be done first and normal results observed.

Normal response to an insulin tolerance test is a rise in the serum cortisol concentration of at least 7 mcg/dl or to a level greater than 20 mcg/dl. Growth hormone concentrations should increase by 5 ng/ml or to a level above 10 ng/ml.

CORTROSYN® STIMULATION TEST.

1. Initial venous blood sample for serum cortisol.
2. 25 USP units of ACTH or 250 mcg of alpha 1-24 corticotropin is given intravenously.
3. Blood for serum cortisol concentrations is obtained at 60, 90, and 120 minutes.

Cortisol concentrations normally should increase by 7 mcg/dl or to a level above 20 mcg/dl. Lack of stimulation suggests adrenal insufficiency.

TRH INFUSION. The patient fasts overnight, stays at bedrest, and may not smoke prior to or during the test infusion. Five hundred mcg of TRH is given intravenously over 30 seconds. Venous blood samples are taken at −30, −15, 0, +5, +30, +45, +60, +120, and +180 minutes in relation to the TRH injection. These samples are assayed for TSH and prolactin. Normal response is a prompt increase in the concentration of both hormones within 30 to 45 minutes of the injection.

An exaggerated TSH response occurs with hypothyroidism while a blunted response indicates hyperthyroidism or inadequate pituitary TSH reserve. Results, therefore, must be interpreted with reference to thyroid function. A lack of a prolactin response is suggestive but not diagnostic of an adenoma.

RAPID SCREENING DEXAMETHASONE SUPPRESSION TEST.

1. Morning and late evening cortisol concentrations are obtained.
2. 1 mg dexamethasone is given orally at bedtime.
3. A cortisol concentration is obtained at 8:00 A.M. the morning after dexamethasone.

Normal response is a morning cortisol concentration less than 5 mcg/dl after dexamethasone. Lack of suppression may be caused by the presence of illnesses other than pituitary or adrenal dysfunction, especially endogenous depression.

DEXAMETHASONE SUPPRESSION TEST. This is indicated only if serum cortisol and dehydroepiandrosterone sulfate concentrations or the 24-hour urinary excretion of 17-ketosteroids, 17-hydroxysteroids, or free cortisol are increased. With low dose suppression, the woman receives 0.5 mg of dexamethasone every 6 hours for 48 hours. The dose is increased to 2 mg every 6 hours for 48 hours for a high dose suppression test. These should usually be done with the patient in the hospital so that sample collections are complete and medications are taken on time.

Normal suppression with a low dose of dexamethasone indicates a functional adrenal disorder. Incomplete suppression on either low or high dose indicates the possibility of a pituitary ACTH-secreting adenoma. Lack of suppression with high dose dexamethasone indicates the presence of an adrenal tumor or an ectopic source of ACTH, such as carcinoma of the lung. A normal response is defined as a decrease in 17-hydroxysteroid excretion to less than 2 mg/gm of creatinine or a decrease in urinary free cortisol excretion to less than 20 mcg/gm of creatinine. Serum cortisol concentrations should drop to less than 5.0 mcg/dl.

REFERENCES

1. Moore KL. The pituitary gland (hypophysis cerebri). In: The developing human: clinically oriented embryology, 5th ed. Philadelphia: WB Saunders, 1982:396–398.
2. Marie P. Sur deux las d'acromégalie. Hypertrophie singulière non congénitale des extrémités supérieures, inférieures et cephaloque. Rev Med (Paris) 1886;6:297–333.
3. Schönenmann A. Hypophysis and thyreoidea. Arch Pathol Anat Physiol Klin Med 1892;129:310–336.
4. Tandler J, Grosz S. Über den einfluss der kastration auf den organismus. Wien Klin Wochschr 1907;20:1596–1597.
5. Erdheim J, Strumme E. Uber die schwangerschaftsveranderung der hypophyse. Beitr Pathol Anat Allgem Pathol 1909;46:1–132.
6. Evans HM, Lang JA. The effect of the anterior lobe of the hypophysis administered intraperitoneally upon growth and maturity and oestrous cycles of the rat. Anat Rec 1921;21:62–63.
7. Green JD, Harris GW. The neurovascular link between the neurohypophysis and adenohypophysis. J Endocrinol 1947;5:136–146.
8. Takor-Takor T, Pearse AGE. Neuroectodermal origin of avian hypothalamohypophyseal complex: the role of the ventral neutral ridge. J Embryol Exp Morphol 1975;34:311–325.
9. Siler-Khodr TM, Morgenstern LL, Greenwood FC. Hormone synthesis and release from human fetal adenohypophyses in vitro. J Clin Endocrinol Metab 1975;39:891–905.
10. Falin LI. The development of human hypophysis and differentiation of cells of its anterior lobe during embryonic life. Acta Anat (Basel) 1961;44:188–205.
11. Stanfield JP. The blood supply of the human pituitary gland. J Anat 1960;94:257–273.
12. Pelletier G, Robert F, Hardy J. Identification of human anterior pituitary cells by immunoelectron microscopy. J Clin Endocrinol Metab 1978;46:534–542.
13. Singer SJ, Nicholson GL. The fluid mosiac model of the structure of all membranes. Science 1972;175:720–731.
14. Rothman JE, Lenard J. Membrane asymmetry. Science 1977;195:743–753.
15. Lodish HF, Rothman JE. The assembly of cell membranes. Sci Am 1979;240:48–63.
16. Catt KJ, Harwood JP, Aquilera G, Dufau ML. Hormonal regulation and peptide receptors and target cell responses. Nature 1979;208:109–116.
17. Baxter JD, Funder W. Hormone receptors. N Engl J Med 1979;301:1149–1161.
18. Rodbell M. The role of hormone receptors and GTP-regulatory proteins in membrane transduction. Nature 1980;284:17–22.
19. Wang JH, Wassman DM. Calmodulin and its role in the second messenger system. Curr Top Cell Regul 1979;15:47–108.
20. Roth J, Lesniak MA, Bar RS, et al. An introduction to receptors and receptor disorders. Proc Soc Exp Biol Med 1979;161:3–12.
21. King AD, Cautrecasas P. Peptide hormone-induced receptor mobility, aggregation, and internalization. N Engl J Med 1981;305:77–82.
22. Lefkaurtz RJ, Wessels MR, Stadd JM. Hormones, receptors and cyclic AMP: their role in target cell refractoriness. Curr Top Cell Regul 1980;17:205–230.
23. Kaplan J. Polypeptide-binding membrane receptors: analysis and classification. Science 1981;212:14.
24. Katzenellenbogen BS. Dynamics of steroid hormone action. Annu Rev Physiol 1980;42:17–35.
25. Rosen JM, Matusik RJ, Richards DA, Gupta P, Rodgers JR. Multihormonal regulation of casein gene expression at the transcriptional and posttranscriptional levels in the mammary gland. Recent Prog Horm Res 1980;36:157–193.
26. Bayand F, Damilano S, Robel P, Baulieu E. Cytoplasmic and nuclear estradiol and progesterone receptors in human endometrium. J Clin Endocrinol Metab 1978;46:635–648.
27. Roberts JL, Herbert E. Characterization of a common precursor to corticotropin and beta-

lipotropin: identification of beta-lipotropin proteins and their arrangement relative to corticotropin in the precursor synthesized in a cell free system. Proc Natl Acad Sci (USA) 1977;74:5300–5304.
28. Frantz AG. Prolactin. N Engl J Med 1978;298:201–207.
29. Bern HA, Nicoll CS. The comparative endocrinology of prolactin. Recent Prog Horm Res 1968;24:681–720.
30. Tyson JE, Hwang P. Studies of prolactin secretion in human pregnancy. Am J Obstet Gynecol 1972;113:14–19.
31. Van Wyk JJ, Underwood LE. The somatomedins and their actions. Biochem Actions Horm 1978;5:101–148.
32. Van Hall EV, Vaitukaitis JL, Ross GT, Hickman JW, Ashwell G. Effects of progressive desialylation on the rate of disappearance of immunoreactive hCG from plasma in rats. Endocrinology 1971;89:11–15.
33. Catt KJ, Dufau ML, Tsuruhara T. Absence of intrinsic biological activity in LH and HCG subunits. J Clin Endocrinol Metab 1973; 36:73–80.
34. Phifer RF, Midgley AR, Spicer SS. Immunohistologic and histologic evidence that follicular stimulating hormone and luteinizing hormone are present in the same cell type in the human pars distalis. J Clin Endocrinol Metab 1973;36:124–141.
35. Dufau ML, Catt KJ. Gonadotropin receptors and regulation of steroidogenesis in the testis and ovary. Vitam Horm 1978;36:461–592.
36. Goodman LA, Nixon WE, Johnson DK, Hodgen GD. Regulation of follicular genesis in cycling rhesus monkey: selection of the dominant follicle. Endocrinology 1977; 100:155–161.
37. Richards JS, Ireland JJ, Rao MC, Bernath GA, Midgley AR Jr, Reichert LE. Ovarian follicular development in the rat: hormone receptor repopulation by estradiol, follicular stimulating hormone and luteinizing hormone. Endocrinology 1976;99:1562–1570.
38. DeJong FH, Sharpe RM. Evidence of inhibin-like activity in bovine follicular fluid. Nature 1976;263:71–72.
39. Franchimont P. Chari S, Demoulin A. Hypothalamus-pituitary-testis interaction. J Reprod Fertil 1975;44:335–350.
40. Knobil E, Plant TM, Wildt L, Belchetz PE, Marshall G. Control of the rhesus monkey menstrual cycle: permissive role of hypothalamic gonadotropin releasing hormone (GnRH). Science 1980;207:1371–1373.
41. Leyendecker G, Wildt L, Hansmann M. Pregnancies following chronic intermittent (pulsatile) administration of GnRH by means of a portable pump ("Zyklomat"). A new approach to the treatment of infertility in hypothalamic amenorrhea. J Clin Endocrinol Metab 1980;51:1214–1216.
42. Heber D, Swerdloff RS. Down regulation of pituitary gonadotropin secretion in postmenopausal females by continuous gonadotropin-releasing hormone administration. J Clin Endocrinol Metab 1981;52:171–172.
43. Crowley WF, Comite F, Vale W, Rivier J, Loraux DL, Cutler GB. Therapeutic use of pituitary desensitization with a long acting LHRH agonist: a potential treatment for idiopathic precocious puberty. J Clin Endocrinol Metab 1981;52:370–372.
44. Smith MA, Vale WW. Desensitization to gonadotropin releasing hormone observed in superfused pituitary cells on cytodex beads. Endocrinology 1981;108:752–759.
45. Hoff JD, Lasley DL, Wang CF, Yen SSC. The two pools of pituitary gonadotropin. Regulation during the menstrual cycle. J Clin Endocrinol Metab 1977;44:302–312.
46. Tanabe K, Channing CP. Observation of a greater concentration of inhibin activity in follicular fluid of preovulatory follicles of human menopausal gonadotropin-hCG treated women compared to untreated women. Endocrine Society 1983;(Abs. 849):293.
47. Leyendecker G, Wildt L, Gips H, Nocke W, Plotz EJ. Experimental studies on the positive feedback effect of progesterone, hydroxyprogesterone, and 20-alpha dihydroprogesterone on the pituitary realse of LH and FSH in the human female. Arch Gynecol 1976;221:29–45.
48. Lasley BL, Wang CF, Yen SSC. The effects of estrogen and progesterone on the functional capacity of the gonadotrophs. J Clin Endocrinol Metab 1975;41:820–826.
49. Hall R, Ormston BJ, Besser GM, Cryer RJ, KcKendrick M. The thyrotophin-releasing hormone test in diseases of the pituitary and hypothalamus. Lancet 1972;1:759–762.
50. Sheehan HL. Post partum necrosis of anterior pituitary. J Pathol Bacteriol 1937;45:189–214. (Reprinted in Am J Obstet Gynecol 1971;111:851–854.)
51. Schulte HM, Booth JD, Oldfield EH. Corticotropin releasing factor (CRF) stimulation test in man: pituitary responses and pharmacokinetics. Endocrine Society 1983;(Abs. 5):82.
52. Cleveland WW, Green IC, Migeon CJ. A case of proven adrenocorticotropin deficiency. J Pediatr 1960;57:376–381.

53. Miyai DM, Azukizaga M, Kumshara Y. Familial isolated thyrotropin deficiency with cretinism. N Engl J Med 1971;285:1043–1048.
54. Goodman HG, Grumbach MM, Kaplan SL. Growth and growth hormone: II. Comparison of isolated growth-hormone deficiency and multiple pituitary hormone deficiencies in 35 patients with idiopathic hypopituitary dwarfism. N Engl J Med 1968;278:57–68.
55. Laron Z. Syndrome of familial dwarfism and high plasma immunoreactive growth hormone. Isr J Med Sci 1974;10:1247–1253.
56. Tanner JM, Whitehouse RH. A note on the bone age at which patients with true isolated growth hormone deficiency enter puberty. J Clin Endocrinol Metab 1975;41:788–790.
57. Bell J, Benvenite R, Spitz I, Rabinowitz D. Isolated deficiency of follicle stimulating hormone: further studies. J Clin Endocrinol Metab 1975;40:790–794.
58. Frankel RJ, Jenkins JS. Hypothalamic-pituitary function in anorexia nervosa. Acta Endocrinol 1975;78:209–221.
59. Frisch RE, Gotz-Welbergen AV, McArthur JW, et al. Delayed menarche and amenorrhea of college athletes in relation to age of onset of training. JAMA 1981;246:159–163.
60. Baylis PH. Case of hyperthyroidism due to a chromophobe adenoma. Clin Endocrinol (Oxf) 1976;5:145–150.
61. Demura R, Kubo O, Demura H, Shizume K. FSH and LH secreting pituitary adenoma. J Clin Endocrinol Metab 1977;45:653–657.
62. Friend JN, Judge OM, Sherman BM, Santen RJ. FSH secreting pituitary adenomas: stimulation and suppression studies in 2 patients. J Clin Endocrinol Metab 1976;43:650–657.
63. Liddle GW. Tests of pituitary-adrenal suppressibility in the diagnosis of Cushing's syndrome. J Clin Endocrinol Metab 1970;20:1539–1560.
64. Tyrrell JA, Brooks RM, Fitzgerald PA, Cofoid PB, Forsham PH, Wilson CB. Cushing's disease, selective transphenoidal resection of pituitary microadenomas. N Engl J Med 1978;298:753–758.
65. Gold EM. The Cushing syndromes: changing views of diagnosis and treatment. Ann Intern Med 1979;90:829–844.
66. Cassar J, Doyle FH, Mashiter K, Joplin GF. Treatment of Cushing's disease in juveniles with interstitial pituitary irradiation. Clin Endocrinol (Oxf) 1979;11:313–321.
67. Kreiger DT, Amorosa L, Linick F. Cyproheptadine-induced remission of Cushing's disease. N Engl J Med 1975;293:893–896.
68. Frank S, Jacobs HS, Nabarro JDN. Prolactin concentrations in patients with acromegaly, clinical significance and response to surgery. Clin Endocrinol (Oxf) 1976;5:63–69.
69. Clemmons DR, VanWyck JJ, Ridgeway EC, Kluman B, Kjellberg RN, Underwood LE. Evaluation of acromegaly by radioimmunoassay of somatomedin-C. N Engl J Med 1979;301:1138–1142.
70. Besser GM, Wass JA. Acromegaly: results of long-term treatment with bromocriptine. Acta Endocrinol (Suppl 216) 1978;88:187–198.
71. Lamberg BA, Kivikangas V, Vartiainen J, Raitta C, Palkonen R. Conventional pituitary irradiation in acromegaly. Effect on growth hormone and TSH secretion. Acta Endocrinol 1976;82:267–281.
72. Huang P, Guyda H, Friesen H. A radioimmunoassay for human prolactin. Proc Natl Acad Sci (USA) 1971;68:1902–1906.
73. Child DF, Naden S, Mashiter K, Jeld MK, Banks L, Fraser TR. Prolactin studies in "functionless" pituitary tumors. Brit Med J 1975;1:604–606.
74. Keye WR, Yuen BH, Knopj RF, Jaffe RB. Amenorrhea, hyperprolactinemia and pituitary enlargement secondary to primary hypothyroidism. Obstet Gynecol 1976;6:697–702.
75. Sherman BM, Harris CE, Schlechte J, et al. Pathogenesis of prolactin-secreting pituitary adenomas. Lancet 1978;2:1019–1021.
76. Kuew-Hsiung L, Amenomori Y, Chen CL, Meites J. Effects of central acting drugs on serum and pituitary prolactin levels in rats. Endocrinology 1970;87:667–672.
77. Hokfelt T, Fuxe K. Effects of prolactin and ergot alkaloids on the tubero-infundibular dopamine (DA) neurons. Neuroendocrinology 1972;9:100–122.
78. Ahren K, Fuxe K. Hamberger L, Hokfelt T. Turnover changes in the tubero-infundibular dopamine neurons during the ovarian cycle of the rat. Endocrinology 1971;88:1415–1424.
79. Ho K, Lazarus L, Smythe GA. Functional disturbance in the regulation of pituitary hormone release in patients with pathologic hyperprolactinemia. Endocrine Society 1982;(Abs. 871):297.
80. Simpkins JW, Taylor ST, Gabriel SM, Katovich MJ. Evidence that chronic hyperprolactinemia produced dependence on endogenously released opioids. Endocrine Society 1983;(Abs. 349):168.
81. Cetel NS, Quigley ME, Yen SSC. The control of prolactin (PRL) secretion by endogenous opioids in man: steroid dependent paradoxical response to naloxone. Endocrine Society 1983;(Abs. 964):321.

82. Farah JM Jr., Sapun-Malcolm D, Touzeau PL, Mueller GP. Regulation of pituitary beta-endorphin secretion by dopamine receptor subtypes. Endocrine Society 1983;(Abs. 956):319.
83. Daly DC, Walters CA, Soto-Albors C, Riddick DH. Multiple therapeutic modalities improve pregnancy rates in luteal phase defects. Fertil Steril 1983;39:393.
84. Cocenblum T, Sirek AMT, Horwath E, Kovacs K, Ezrin C. Human mixed somatotrophic and lactotrophic pituitary adenomas. J Clin Endocrinol Metab 1976;42:857–863.
85. Teasdale E, MacPherson P, Teasdale G. The reliability of radiology in detecting prolactin secreting pituitary microadenomas. Br J Radiol 1981;54:566–571.
86. Marro RP, Kletzky OA, Teul J, Davajan V, Marsh C, Mishell DR. Comparison of serum prolactin, plain radiography and hypocycloidal tomography of the sella turcica in patients with galactorrhea. Am J Obstet Gynecol 1979;135:467–469.
87. Swanson HA, DuBoulany G. Borderline variants of the normal pituitary fossa. Br J Radiol 1975;48:366–369.
88. Burrow GN, Wortzma G, Rewcastle NB, Holgate RC, Kovacs K. Microadenomas of the pituitary and abnormal sellar tomograms in an unselected autopsy series. N Engl J Med 1981;304:156–158.
89. Syvertsen A, Haughton VM, Williams AL, Cusick JF. The computed tomographic appearance of the normal pituitary gland and pituitary microadenomas. Radiology 1979; 133:385–391.
90. Post MJD, David JN, Glaser JS, Safran A. Pituitary apoplexy: diagnosis by computed tomography. Radiology 1980;134:665–670.
91. Marrs RP, Bertolli SJ, Kletzky OA. The use of thyrotropin releasing hormone in distinguishing prolacting-secreting pituitary adenomas. Am J Obstet Gynecol 1980;138:620–625.
92. Assie J, Schellenkens APM, Touber JL. The value of an intravenous TRH test for the diagnosis of tumoral prolactinemia. Acta Endocrinol 1980;94;439–449.
93. Klijn JG, Lamberts SWJ, DeJong FH, Birkenhager JC. The value of the thyrotropin-releasing hormone test in patients with prolactin secreting pituitary tumors and suprasellar non-pituitary tumors. Fertil Steril 1981; 35:155–161.
94. Chang RJ, Keye WR, Monroe SE, Jaffe RB. Prolactin secreting pituitary adenomas in women. IV. Pituitary function in amenorrhea associated with normal or abnormal serum prolactin and sellar polytomography. J Clin Endocrinol Metab 1980;51:830–835.
95. March CM, Kletzky OA, Davajan V, et al. Longitudinal evaluation of patients with untreated prolactin-secreting pituitary adenomas. Am J Obstet Gynecol 1981;139:835–844.
96. Hardy J, Velzina JL. Transphenoidal neurosurgery of intracranial neoplasm. In: Thomson RA, Green JR, eds. Advances in neurology. New York: Raven Press, 1975:261–274.
97. Landolt AM. Surgical treatment of pituitary prolactinomas: postoperative prolactin and fertility in seventy patients. Fertil Steril 1981;35:620–625.
98. Rowe SE, Williams HO, Levine JH, Phamsey SA, Hungerford D, Adkins WY. Prolactinomas: surgical therapy, indications and results. Surg Neurol 1980;14:161–167.
99. Auboury PR, Deroma J, Pullon F, et al. Endocrine outcome after transphenoidal adenomectomy for prolactinoma: prolactin levels and tumor size as predicting factors. Surg Neurol 1980;14:141–143.
100. St. George-Tucker H, Grubb SR, Wigand JP, et al. Galactorrhea-amenorrhea syndrome follow-up of forty-five patients after pituitary tumor removal. Ann Intern Med 1981;94;302–307.
101. Kleinberg DL, Noel GH, Frantz AG. Galactorrhea, a study of 235 cases including 48 with pituitary tumors. N Engl J Med 1977; 296:589–600.
102. DeSchuywer A, Vandekuckhave D, Debuyne G. Prolactin secreting pituitary adenomas, observations in irradiation patients. Acta Radiol Oncol Radiat Phys Biol. 1980;19:169–175.
103. Grossman A, Cohen BL, Plowman N, et al. Long term effects of radiotherapy in patients with prolactin-secreting pituitary adenomas. Endocrine Society 1983;(Abs. 436):189.
104. Mehta AE, Reyes FI, Faiman C. Primary radiotherapy of prolactinoma. Endocrine Society 1983;(Abs. 6):82.
105. Ramsdell JS, Bethea CL, Wilson CB, Jaffe RB, Weiner RI. Dihydroergocryptine binding in human prolactin secreting adenomas. Endocrine Society 1981;(Abs. 600):232.
106. Martin M, Roizen M, Monroe S, Weiner R, Jaffe RB. In vivo potency of dopamine (DA) to suppress prolactin in eu- and hyperprolactinemic subjects. Soc Gynecol Invest 1982; (Abs. 12):8.
107. Thorner MO, McNeilly AS, Hagan C, Besser GM. Long-term treatment of galactorrhea and hypogonadism with bromocriptine. Br Med J 1974;2:419–422.
108. Kinch RA. The use of bromocriptine in obstet-

rics and gynecology. Fertil Steril 1980; 33;463–470.
109. Thorner MO, Martin WH, Rogal AD, et al. Rapid regression of pituitary prolactinomas during bromocriptine treatment. J Clin Endocrinol Metab 1980;51:438–445.
110. Valentzas C, Carras D, Vassilouthis J. Regression of pituitary prolactinoma with bromocriptine administration. JAMA 1981;245:1149–1150.
111. Leiter LA, Burrow GN. Five year follow up of bromocriptine-treated prolactinomas. Endocrine Society 1983;(Abs. 435):189.
112. Turkalj I, Braun P, Krupp P. Surveillance of bromocriptine in pregnancy. JAMA 1982;247:1589–1591.
113. Griffith RW, Turkalj I. Braun P. Outcome of pregnancy in mothers given bromocryptine. Br J Clin Pharmacol 1978;5:227–231.
114. Yuen BH. Bromocryptine, pituitary tumours and pregnancy. Lancet 1978;2:1314.
115. Marshall JR. Pregnancy in patients with prolactin producing tumors. Clin Obstet Gyncol 1980;23:453–463.
116. Magyar DM, Marshall JR. Pituitary tumors and pregnancy. Am J Obstet Gynecol 1978;132:739–751.
117. van Roon E, Vander Vijver JCM, Gerretsen G, Hekster REM, Waltendorff RA. Rapid regression of a suprasellar extending prolactinoma after bromocriptine treatment during pregnancy. Fertil Steril 1981;36:173–177.

The Normal Menstrual Cycle

G. Rodney Meeks

Why do women menstruate? It is my purpose to answer this question and, at the same time, to integrate the physiology of the hypothalamus, pituitary, and ovary discussed in other chapters. By describing the menstrual cycle as a biologic unit, the impact of an abnormality in one part of the reproductive system on the others becomes more apparent. It should also become apparent that the endometrium is a complex, biologically active tissue as well as a tissue that responds to trophic stimuli from the ovaries.

This chapter is divided into 6 major topics. After an introduction, a description of the anatomy and blood supply of the uterus, and the clinical characteristics of the normal menstrual cycle, each phase of the menstrual cycle is discussed. The discussion of each phase is further divided into a description of endometrial, ovarian, and hypothalamic-pituitary events.

Anatomy and Blood Supply of the Uterus

While the epithelium of the vagina, cervix, and fallopian tubes responds to ovarian sex steroid hormones, the response of the endometrium is more dramatic. The endometrium is divided into a basal layer and a functional layer. The basal layer is relatively unresponsive to hormonal stimuli and remains intact following menstruation. Most of the functional layer, which can be subdivided into compacta and spongiosa, is lost during menstruation. The functional layer is very responsive to hormonal stimuli from the ovary.

The uterus receives the major portion of its blood supply from 2 uterine arteries, which are branches of the hypogastric arteries. Each uterine artery divides into an ascending and descending branch at the isthmus of the uterus. The ovarian arteries form an arcade through the mesosalpinx and anastomose with the ascending branches of the uterine arteries in the region of the cornua. Six to 10 arcuate arteries form from the ascending branch of the uterine artery in each uterine quadrant (1). They course parallel to the lumen and form a collateral vascular network with the arcuate arteries from the opposite side of the uterus. Radial arteries branch from the arcuate arteries and supply the myometrium. Small-caliber straight arteries branch from the radial arteries after crossing the myoepithelial junction to supply the basal layer of the endometrium. Radial arteries, unresponsive to hormonal changes, continue as the spiral arteries. These have a corkscrew appearance, supply the functional layer, and are very sensitive to the changing hormonal milieu of the menstrual cycle (2).

Clinical Characteristics of the Menstrual Cycle

Menarche occurs at an average age of 12.7 years, although a range of 9 to 16 years is considered normal (3). Frisch has shown that a critical weight, based on a woman's height, must be achieved before menarche occurs (4).

The age of menarche has been decreasing steadily in the past 80 years, possibly as a result of better nutrition, which allows a woman to achieve the critical weight at a younger age.

Menses following ovulation is the consequence of an orderly withdrawal of estrogen and progesterone, and represents the sloughing of the functional layer of secretory endometrium (5). The average duration of menses is 5.2 days, but may normally last 3 to 8 days (6). Midcycle lower-quadrant pain, premenstrual symptoms, and menstrual discomfort are recurrent symptoms of ovulatory cycles, and should be considered normal (7). Blood loss during menses averages 35 ml to 43 ml, but a loss of 30 ml to 180 ml is normal. Younger women tend to lose lesser amounts while older women lose more (8). Approximately 75% of the blood loss occurs in the first 2 days, and over 90% is lost by the third day (9). The hemoglobin concentration is remarkably stable until menstrual blood loss exceeds 80 ml per day. Daily iron loss is 0.4 mg to 1.0 mg, and anemia may result from normal menstruation if iron loss is not compensated for (10). Menstrual blood loss may be estimated from the number of menstrual pads used and by pre- and postmenstrual hemoglobin determinations (11). Rarely does a woman need more than 4 pads for the heaviest day of flow (12). Endometrial bleeding can also be provoked by withdrawal of estrogens, progesterone, and even androgens (13). Even at steady hormone levels, "breakthrough bleeding" may occur (14). However, such bleeding (associated with anovulation) is usually acyclic and unpredictable.

The length of the menstrual cycle is calculated from the day of onset of 1 menses to the day of onset of the next menses. Only one sixth of ovulatory cycles are 28 days and a cycle length between 25 and 35 days is normal (15). Cycle length may be considerably longer during adolescence and the climacteric than during the reproductive years and is most likely the result of anovulation (16,17). During adolescence and the climacteric, the prevalence rates of anovulation are 6.6% and 34%, respectively, while anovulation comprises only 1.2% of cycles during the reproductive years (12).

Ovulation is followed by a 0.3°C to 0.5°C rise in basal temperature. The rise in basal temperature is useful to define the length of the follicular and luteal phases of the menstrual cycle and the approximate time of ovulation (18). The ascending temperature inflection occurs over a 1- to 3-day period and is preceded by a temperature nadir in approximately one third of ovulatory cycles. The proliferative phase begins on the last day of menses and ends the day before the basal temperature increases above the mean basal body temperature. Variation in cycle length occurs and 92% of cycles are between 21 and 36 days. The secretory phase is remarkably consistent at 14 ± 2 days. Thus, abnormal cycle lengths are the result of differences in the length of the follicular phase, or are caused by anovulation.

The Menstrual Phase

The amount of endometrium lost during menstruation is uncertain. Using a vital dye-staining technique, Flowers and Welborn have shown that regression of metabolic function seems to be the hallmark of menses. They have characterized menstruation as a vigorous attempt by the endometrium to survive with very little loss of tissue (19). Ferenczy, however, has found that most of the functional zone is lost while the basal zone remains intact (5). Repair and regeneration of the endometrial surface may be the result of metaplasia of stromal cells into glandular epithelium (20). Flowers and Welborn, however, believe that the remaining secretory spongiosa is converted to proliferative endometrium (19). Ferenczy has presented evidence that neither of these mechanisms is correct and that the remaining endometrial glands provide replacement epithelium (21).

The menstrual effluvium contains more than blood. Columnar and stromal cells, macrophages, histiocytes, and mast cells of endometrial origin are also present. In addition, menses contains short fusiform cells, stratified squamous epithelium, cornified and noncornified navicular cells, parabasal cells, and metaplastic squamous cells that are not of endometrial origin. Bacteria mixed with polymorphonuclear leukocytes are often seen. Autolyzed tissue, proteolytic enzymes, cervical mucus, vaginal secretions, and vulvar sebaceous secretions add to the menstrual fluid. The menstrual discharge also contains prostaglandins, potent smooth muscle stimulants (12).

Prostaglandins (PG) are synthesized from arachidonic acid in the endometrium (22). Endometrial prostaglandin concentrations are low during the proliferative phase of the menstrual cycle but increase steadily under the influence of estrogen (23,24). There is a linear relationship between the $PGF_{2\alpha}$ content in the endometrium and the log-concentration of estradiol in uterine venous blood (25). Physiologic concentrations of progesterone facilitate prostaglandin synthesis, possibly by release of arachidonic acid (26). Prostaglandin synthesis is increased after ovulation and is maximal just before menstruation. Although $PGF_{2\alpha}$ and PGE_2 are both present, more $PGF_{2\alpha}$ is synthesized (27). Menstrual fluid contains 10 times more $PGF_{2\alpha}$ than the endometrium and release of prostaglandin is maximal during menses (28). The high levels of $PGF_{2\alpha}$ may stimulate the onset of menstrual bleeding by causing constriction of the spiral arterioles and expulsion of degenerated endometrium with myometrial contractions (29).

Spiral arteries are found only in menstruating primates and they appear to play a central role in the process of menstruation (30). Each spiral artery supplies 4 to 9 mm^2 of endometrium. Since no collateral vessels are present, the endometrium is very vulnerable to vascular changes (31). At the endometrial surface the spiral arteries form vascular arcades and subepithelial capillary plexuses. Blood in these vessels drains into venous channels that course parallel to the endometrial glands. Sinusoidal dilatations or venous lakes are found where the veins join with the capillaries and, during menstruation, numerous thrombi are present. Venous blood enters arcuate veins and then empties into the uterine veins.

Fifty percent of the functional zone of endometrium is lost as a result of ischemia and cell regression. Progesterone withdrawal beginning late in the luteal phase initiates tonic contractions and spasmodic constriction of the spiral arterioles; this causes cyclic blanching, decreased endometrial blood flow, stagnation of blood, and tissue hypoxia (32). Uterine contractions in the menstrual phase further diminish blood flow in the straight arteries of the basal endometrium and increase tissue hypoxia (33). Endometrial regression intensifies coiling and compression of spiral arteries, and tissue hypoxia is also intensified.

Menstrual endometrium is further characterized by shrinkage of the stroma and collapse of the exhausted secretory glands (19). The lysosomal membranes of endometrial cells, which had been stabilized by progesterone, become fragile; potent and destructive hydrolytic enzymes leak into the cells and additional cell damage is produced (34). Acid phosphatase, the principal lysosomal enzyme, is intensely active during menses, especially in the functional zone. Acid phosphatase is involved in phagocytosis of the cells' own contents (autophagocytosis), and heterophagocytosis as macrophages migrate through the glandular epithelium (35). Indeed, the earliest evidence of menses is the presence, in the cytoplasm of epithelial cells, of phagocytized basophilic nuclear fragments from stromal cells. Intracellular vesicles, cell membranes, basement membranes, and supporting reticular fibers are also digested by lysosomal enzymes from fragmented cells and leukocytes (34). As a consequence of all these events, hemorrhage, cell fragmentation, neutrophilic infiltration, and areas of tissue necrosis are seen (Fig. 5–1). Nuclear pyknosis, karyorrhexis, and loss of cellular detail are the manifestations of cellular necrosis.

Endothelial hypertrophy of endometrial vessels also occurs in response to hydrolytic enzymes and relaxin (36). Capillary permeability increases, vessels rupture, and erythrocytes escape into the endometrium. Coalescence of blood lakes leads to devitalization and shedding of the compact and spongy layers.

Rapid activation of the fibrinolytic system occurs during menses and clotting factors II, VII, and X are consumed (37). This explains the lack of clot formation in the uterus. By the second day of menstruation, the endometrial surface is rough and hemorrhagic, the functional zone is disorganized, and predecidual cells are admixed with glandular cells; both cell types (glandular and stromal) show marked degrees of degeneration. As on the first day of menses, DNA synthesis in the functional zone is essentially nonexistent. These findings are consistent with ultrastructural observations in-

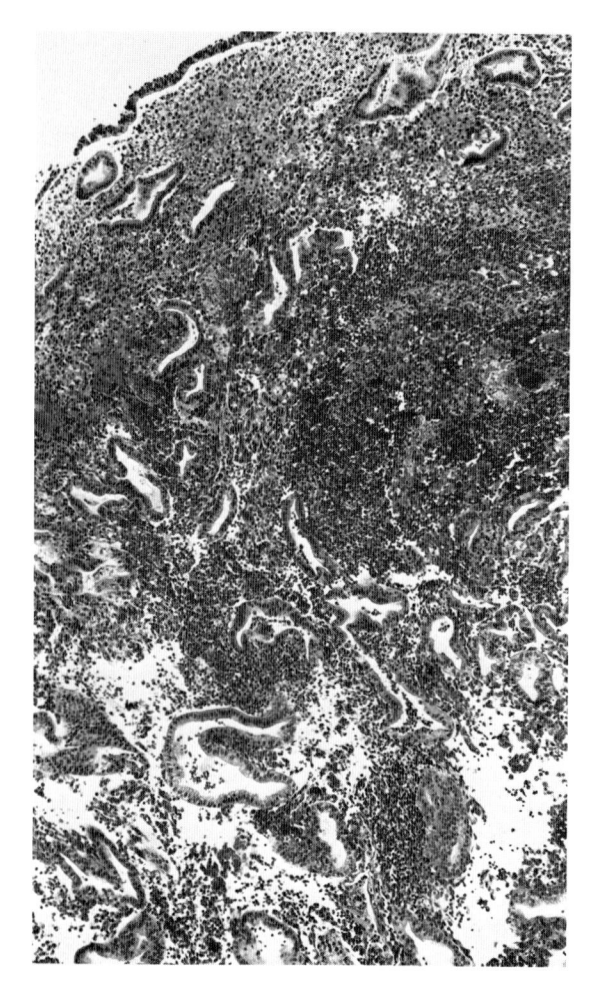

Fig. 5–1. Menstrual endometrium. Collapse of exhausted secretory glands and dissolution of stroma is evident. Hemorrhage produces a shearing effect and fragmentation in the functionalis. Leukocytes and endometrial granulocytes are prominent. The basalis is preserved.

dicating that these cells undergo irreversible injury before being expelled (38). Menstruation is limited by vasospasm and aggregation of platelets at sites of vessel damage (39).

Desquamation is nearly complete by 60 hours when regeneration starts. Repair does not begin until denudation is complete and seems to start only where the basalis is completely denuded of secretory endometrium (21). Loss of surface tissue provides the stimulus for repair and may result in the loss of growth inhibitors such as tissue-specific, species-nonspecific inhibitors of mitosis—the chalones (40). Intact basal glands contain sufficient intracellular organelles and DNA to account for endometrial regeneration from these cells (38).

Endometrial repair begins on the third to fourth day and lasts approximately 48 hours. Reepithelialization may, however, begin as early as 36 hours (41). Thymidine uptake and DNA synthesis is maximal in basal epithelium under denuded areas (38). Basal gland stumps and intact surface endometrium lining denuded areas in the cornual and isthmic regions are the site of repair (Fig. 5–2). First-generation resurfacing cells are spindle shaped, lack mitoses, and expand by ameboid movement. These cells have large flat cytoplasmic surfaces, well-developed microvillous processes, pseudopodal projections, and microfilaments and microtubules, structures necessary for occupying and expanding over large areas faster than cells undergoing maturational replication (42). The lack of mitotic activity may reflect nuclear diploidization (generation of multiples of diploid quantities of DNA), failure of cytokinetics following mitotic division (endomitosis), or fusion of interphase nucei during mitosis, all of which are characteristic of highly active cells. Active DNA and RNA synthesis is demonstrated by nuclear enlargement, a euchromatic nuclear pattern, accumulation of perinuclear chromatin, and abundant cytoplasmic organelles (28).

Despite the increased DNA activity at this time, plasma estrogen and progesterone concentrations are not significantly increased from premenstrual values. Cellular mitoses and ciliogenesis, which are features of estrogen stimulation, are absent (21), implying that endometrial repair is independent of ovarian hormone stimulation. Endometrial regeneration appears to depend solely on tissue repair mechanisms (28).

The stromal cells remain inactive during regeneration of the surface epithelium, resemble immature fibroblasts, and are devoid of mitoses and fibrinogenic activity. Once the surface is restored, the stromal cells mature and demonstrate mitoses and extracellular collagen production (21).

DNA synthesis and cell migration continue simultaneously until a confluent surface is reconstructed, usually by day 5. Cessation of menstrual bleeding coincides with complete reepithelialization (43). Maturation of the flat-

Fig. 5-2. Menstrual endometrium. The functionalis has been lost. Flattened epithelial cells, derived from intact basal gland stumps, recover the denuded surface.

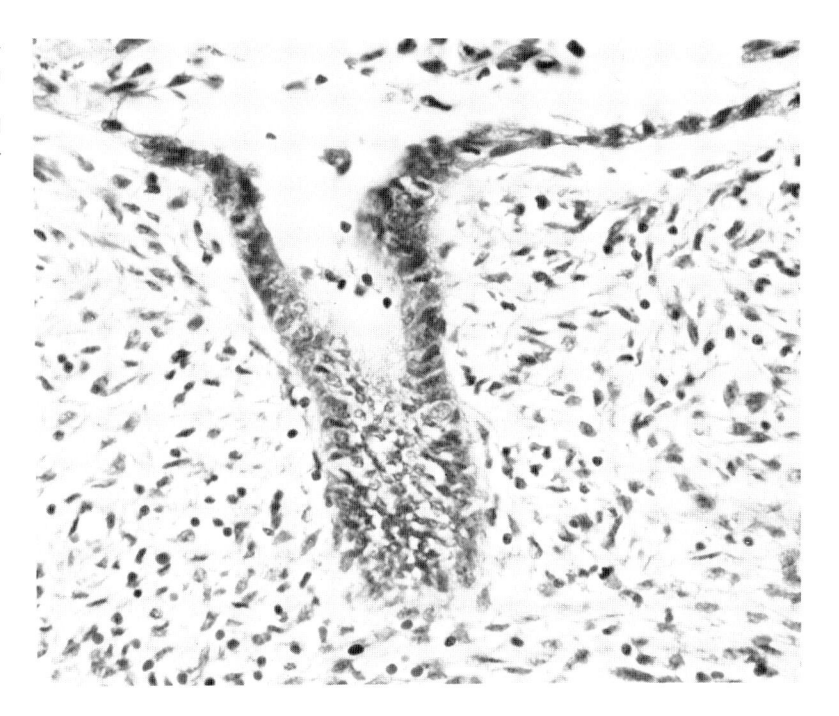

tened, spindle-shaped endometrial surface cells is associated with increased DNA synthesis, mitotic activity, and a change to a cuboidal shape (42). Further growth of endometrium, tissue remodeling, and synthesis of metabolic enzymes are now influenced by estradiol and progesterone (28).

By the fifth day of the menstrual cycle, the Golgi complexes, mitochondria, and free ribosomes undergo hypertrophy and hyperplasia. Alkaline phosphatase concentrates on microvillous surfaces, and acid phosphatase is present in well-developed Golgi complexes, and later in lysosomes (42). Mitoses and cilia are present. Hydrolytic enzymes collect in stromal fibroblasts and fibrillogenesis begins. DNA synthesis and mitoses are present in the vascular stroma, and hydrolytic enzymes appear in the endothelial cells of the vessels (5). These changes continue in the proliferative phase under the influence of increasing estradiol concentrations (38).

Women with hematologic disorders may experience menstrual dysfunction. Disturbances in clot formation cause minimal problems with menstruation, repair, and regeneration. Thus, women who are anticoagulated with coumadin or heparin and those with congenital afibrinoginemia (Factor I), hypoprothrombinemia (Factor II), or deficiencies of Factors III, IV, VI, IX, and XII will have menstrual abnormalities infrequently. Hemostasis is abnormal in women with deficiencies of Factors V, VII, and X, with increased vessel fragility, and with platelet deficiency or dysfunction associated with acute leukemia, systemic lupus erythematosis, or idiopathic thrombocytopenic purpura. These women often have excessive menstrual flow. Women with von Willebrand's disease may have severe menorrhagia (44).

The Proliferative Phase

The proliferative (postmenstrual) phase of the cycle follows the cessation of menses and continues until ovulation. Variation in the length of the menstrual cycle is almost always caused by variation in the length of the proliferative phase, except when pregnancy occurs. This phase can be divided into early, mid, and late on the basis of histologic differences, although the division may not be important. Estrogen stimulates growth of the endometrium; proliferation of the endometrium thus reflects the follicular phase of the ovary.

Early in the proliferative phase (the 2 to 3 days following cessation of menstrual flow), the endometrium is only 1 mm to 2 mm thick. The glands are narrow and straight, contain low columnar or cuboidal epithelial cells, and are widely spaced. The cells have small, oval nuclei but no nucleoli. The nuclei are not stratified and mitotic figures are infrequent. The stroma is dense and compact and is comprised of stellate or spindle-shaped cells with prominent, dark-staining nuclei. The superficial stroma, destined to become the compacta, stains lighter (Fig. 5-3) (45). Blood vessels are inconspicuous, and endometrial granulocytes are present (46). Metabolic activity is minimal.

During the midproliferative phase (days 8 to 10 of the cycle), DNA synthesis is rapid and corresponds to the maximal mitotic activity, a peak in plasma estrogen concentrations, and the greatest number of cytoplasmic and nuclear estrogen receptors (47). Both estrogen and progesterone receptor number increase with increasing estradiol concentrations (48). A 2- to 3-fold increase in DNA content occurs as a result of increasing estradiol concentrations (25). A sudden increase in the incorporation of thymidine into DNA heralds the onset of protein synthesis as well as a rapid increase in cell size, glycogen content, phospholipid metabolism, and synthesis of acid and alkaline phosphatases (5). Free and bound ribosomes, Golgi complexes, primary lysosomes, glandular endoplasmic reticulum, and mitochondria are also stimulated by estradiol (49,50). These organelles provide a protein matrix, energy, and synthesis of enzymes, all of which are important in cell growth. Increased metabolic activity is reflected by an increase in the enzymes that are involved in carbohydrate metabolism (51).

DNA synthesis is maximal in the fundus and body of the uterus and is less in the isthmus and cornual regions. This difference results from a higher concentration of unbound estrogen receptor in the cytosol of the fundus and body than exists in the isthmus (52). Also, DNA synthesis is greater in the functional zone than in the basal zone, a reflection of differences in estrogen receptor content (5). The variation in response of endometrial tissue to hormonal stimulation may be related to differences in blood supply, receptor content, or to different physiologic functions. The upper functional zone facilitates implantation of the blastocyst while the lower functional zone is

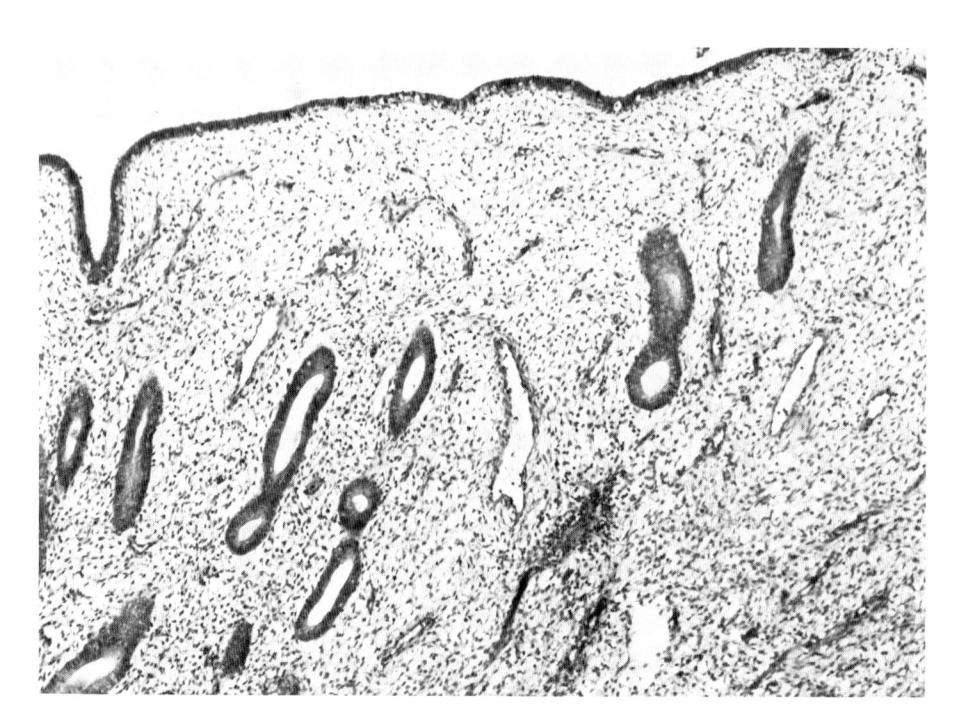

Fig. 5-3. Early proliferative endometrium. The glands are straight and narrow, the stroma is dense, and blood vessels are inconspicuous. Mitotic figures are rare. The thickness of the entire endometrium is 1 mm to 2 mm.

involved in secretory activity. The highest rates of proliferation are seen on days 8 to 10 and in the upper functional zone (5).

The endometrial mucosa becomes considerably thickened as estrogen-stimulated cell growth and proliferation continue. The surface and glandular epithelium becomes columnar, the nuclei become pseudostratified, and nucleoli appear. The glands lengthen, dilate, and become gently curved. More cells are present in the stroma, but the amount of cytoplasm remains scant. The nuclei are prominent and mitoses can be seen. Stromal edema may be present, but to a lesser extent than is found during the midsecretory phase. The dark-staining nuclei, scanty pale-staining cytoplasm, and intracellular edema combine to produce very prominent nuclei (45). Blood vessels, virtually invisible in the early proliferative phase, can now be seen again (53). The midproliferative endometrium has numerous mitoses in glandular, stromal, and vascular components (Figs. 5–4 and 5–5). Cilia can be seen and are especially prominent on the surface epithelium surrounding gland openings. Proliferation of microvilli, synthesis of hydrolytic enzymes and collagen, and vascular growth are maximal at this time (5).

The late proliferative phase, approximately days 11 to 14 of the cycle, is the consequence of stimulation by maximal concentrations of estradiol. DNA activity, however, decreases during this phase, possibly as a result of a growth-inhibiting effect of long-term estrogen stimulation. The decreased DNA synthesis appears to be related to the accumulation of chalone-like inhibitors of DNA synthesis rather than to decreased cytoplasmic estrogen receptors or nuclear translocation of estrogen receptors (40).

The endometrium is now 6 mm to 7 mm thick and develops an undulating surface as a result of rapid growth. The glandular epithelium is comprised of tall columnar cells, and the nuclei remain prominent, although the nuclear chromatin appears less dense. Pseudostratification of the nuclei occurs and nucleoli are prominent. A few subnuclear vacuoles may be present. The glands are dilated and tortuous. The stroma becomes more dense as the edema seen in the midproliferative phase is reabsorbed. The stromal nuclei are less dense but remain prominent. Mitotic figures are easily identified in both glands and stroma. Blood vessels are conspicuous (45) (Fig. 5–6). Just before or at the time of ovulation, hyperemia of

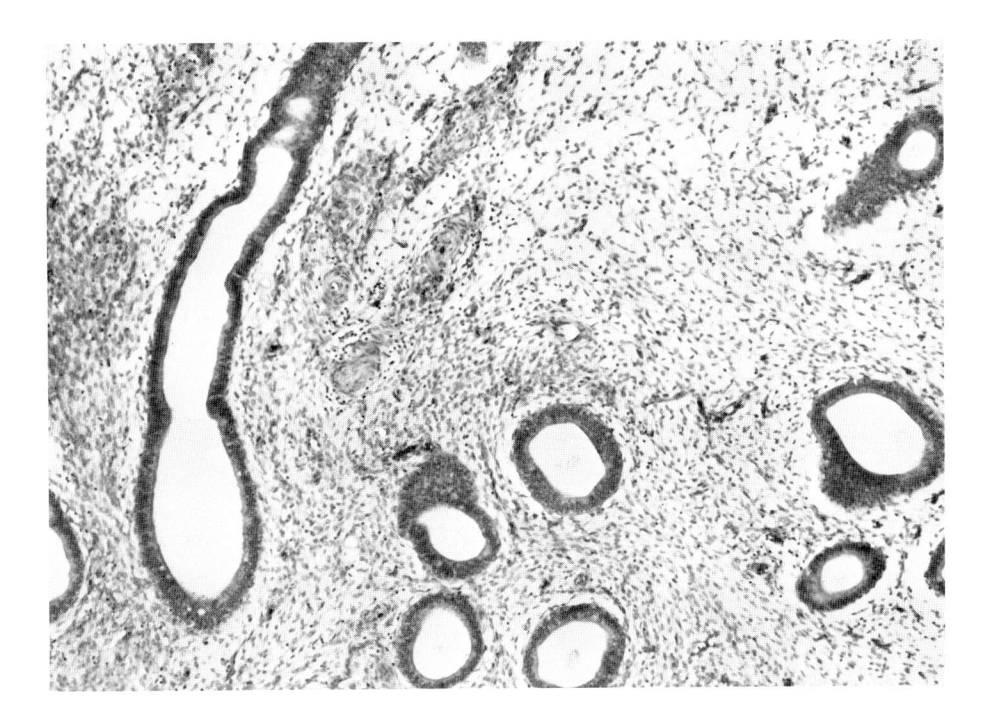

Fig. 5–4. Midproliferative endometrium. The glands enlarge and become gently curved and stromal edema is prominent. Blood vessels can again be seen.

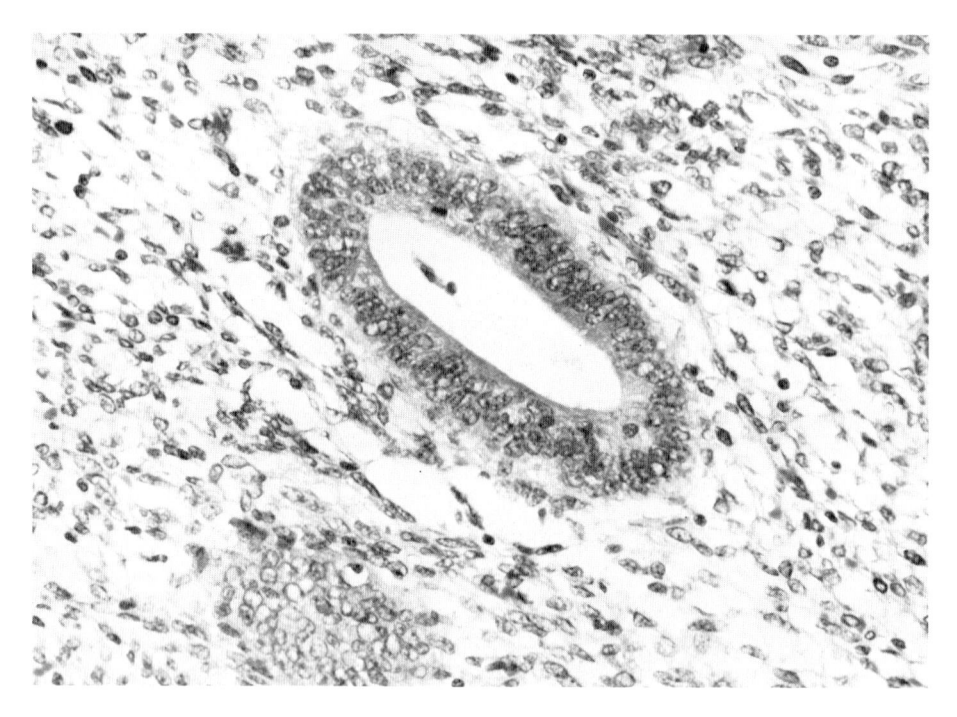

Fig. 5–5. Midproliferative endometrium. Numerous mitoses can be identified within the glands, stroma, and blood vessels.

the stroma can be seen and may result in a few focal areas of hemorrhage, which may produce vaginal spotting for 1 to 2 days at midcycle (33).

Proliferation of the endometrium occurs in response to secretion of estrogen from the ovaries in their follicular phase. The early follicular phase of the ovary actually begins before the onset of menses when FSH concentrations begin to increase in response to decreasing secretion of estrogen from the regressing corpus luteum. As a result, a new cohort of follicles is recruited for the next cycle (54). LH concentrations also increase 1 to 2 days after FSH. Early in the follicular phase, ovarian secretion of estrogen, androgen, and progesterone is relatively low and constant. This suggests that the events of menstruation and the early proliferative phase rely on a minimal concentration of ovarian hormones.

The late follicular phase, beginning approximately on the seventh to eighth day of the menstrual cycle, is characterized by increases in estrogen production and serum concentration. As estrogen secretion increases, FSH concentrations decline. Estrogen concentrations are maximal at the approximate time of the LH surge (55). This preovulatory divergence of FSH and LH concentrations occurs because estradiol may preferentially inhibit FSH release and because production of inhibin by the maturing follicle selectively inhibits FSH (56). Rapid growth of the dominant follicle continues despite declining FSH concentrations. This suggests that follicles are more sensitive to FSH as they mature; however, they still require small amounts of FSH to function normally. The follicle destined to ovulate appears to protect itself from atresia by its own estrogen production, which is much greater than that of less mature follicles. When the intrafollicular estrogen concentration exceeds 1 ng/ml, FSH binding is promoted (57). In smaller, less developed follicles that have a lower intrafollicular estrogen concentration, a decrease in FSH concentrations normally results in loss of growth stimulation. Paradoxically, a wave of atresia parallels the rise in serum estrogen concentration and is the result of a reduction in the number of receptors for estradiol, FSH, and LH. Intraovarian production of androgens may also cause follicular atresia. Atresia insures that the proper number of follicles reach maturity (58).

Theca cells, specialized ovarian stromal cells, are under the influence of LH and are the principal source of estradiol until ovulation (54). LH receptors on the theca cells are in-

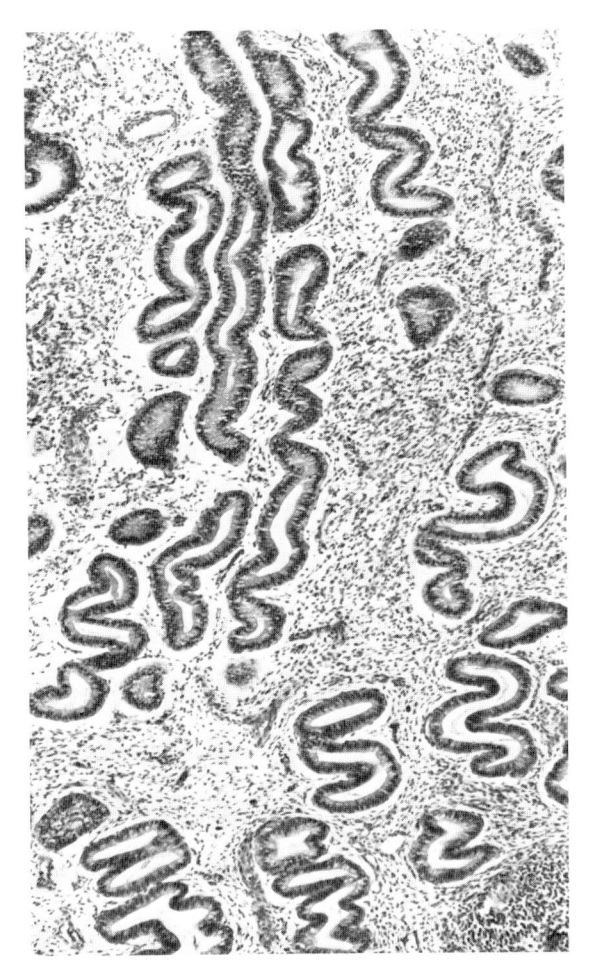

Fig. 5-6. Late proliferative endometrium. The glands are tightly coiled and multiple sections of each gland are seen. The cells are columnar and the nuclei are pseudostratified. The stroma is dense and may resemble predecidual cells.

duced by FSH and enhanced by estradiol. As the concentration of LH and the number of LH receptors increase, luteinization of the granulosa cells begins (24 to 36 hours before the LH surge) and the level of progesterone in the follicle destined to ovulate increases (55). These events within the ovary culminate in ovulation while causing proliferative changes in the endometrium.

Ovulation

Ovulation is the centerpiece of reproduction in all species. In women, it marks the end of the proliferative phase and beginning of the secretory phase of the menstrual cycle. Since no significant changes occur in the endometrium at the moment of ovulation, the endometrium cannot be used to predict the time of ovulation. However, significant changes in ovarian, pituitary, and hypothalamic function do occur. Plasma androgen and 17-hydroxyprogesterone concentrations peak. Progesterone concentrations increase slightly to reflect the increased functional acitvity of the theca and granulosa cells of the ovulating follicle (59). Intraovarian androgens accelerate granulosa cell death and follicular atresia in nonovulatory follicles. Excessive androgen production may cause menstrual cycles to be irregular because of a direct action on the follicles (60). In addition, the midcycle surge of androgens is probably responsible for the increased libido at the time of ovulation. As follicular development progresses, estradiol concentrations increase and trigger a gonadotropin surge. The slight increase in progesterone secretion found at midcycle may enhance this surge (61). Gonadotropin release and ovarian maturity are simultaneous effects of ovarian estradiol production.

A full and proper gonadotropin surge requires an adequate release of gonadotropin-releasing hormone (GnRH) from the hypothalamus and LH from the pituitary. Both are modulated by gonadal steroids. The hypothalamus releases GnRH episodically and causes a pulsatile release of pituitary gonadotropins (62). At midcycle, pituitary response to GnRH is maximal; the surges in FSH and LH are the consequence. Pituitary function is modulated by estradiol, which promotes an enhanced LH response (63). Indeed, the LH surge is the result of a positive feedback stimulus that requires a peripheral estradiol concentration of at least 200 pg/ml and an exposure to this level for at least 50 hours (59). Within hours of the rise in LH, there is a precipitous fall in plasma estrogen concentrations. The subsequent drop in LH concentration may be the result of the loss of estrogen stimulation (64). LH may also regulate its own secretion by inhibiting hypothalamic secretion of GnRH. LH concentrations may also decline because pituitary stores of LH are depleted. The high gonadotropin values persist for approximately 24 hours and then decrease during the luteal phase (65).

The LH surge causes complete maturation of the Graafian follicle and rupture 28 to 32 hours later (64). LH-stimulated increases in follicular blood flow result in increased concentrations of blood constitutents in the antrum. Although antral fluid volume increases, ovulation does not occur because of increased hydrostatic pressure. Rather, degenerative changes in follicular-wall collagen, possibly associated with a sudden increase in prostaglandin, allows for passive expansion and ultimate rupture of the follicle (66). The single ovulating follicle may produce a substance to inhibit growth and maturation of other follicles (67).

Following ovulation, luteinization of the granulosa cells occurs and the follicle changes from a structure that produces predominantly estrogen to one that produces progesterone. This change from follicle to corpus luteum is under the influence of LH. Since LH receptors are under the influence of FSH, the FSH surge may also be necessary for ovulation and the formation of a normal corpus luteum. Although estrogen secretion declines, ovarian stromal cells continue to produce androstenedione and testosterone (64).

Secretory Phase

Accumulation of glycogen, mucopolysaccharides, lipids, and hydrolytic enzymes in endometrial glands and later secretion into the glandular lumen characterizes the secretory phase. Progesterone converts an estrogen-dominated endometrium characterized by a compact stroma and a relatively undeveloped vasculature into the lush, edematous, and biochemically enriched secretory endometrium. In addition, rhythmic uterine contractions are inhibited. Light microscopic changes in the endometrium begin 24 to 48 hours after ovulation. The changes are so uniform and consistent that each of the 14 remaining days of the menstrual cycle can be identified (45).

Ultrastructural changes reflecting increased secretory activity begin with the appearance of glycogen (68) and numerous small secretory vesicles containing acid mucopolysaccharides that originate in the prominent Golgi complex (69). Giant mitochondria, which are involved in steroid metabolism, are now prominent (70). At the time of ovulation, nucleolar channel systems appear that are unique to women, occur only in the postovulatory phase, and are most prominent on day 19 (71). The endoplasmic reticulum is most prominent on day 16 but regresses as a consequence of decreased growth and reduced RNA from the nucleus (72).

The appearance of secretory vacuoles on day 17 to 18 of the cycle is the first light microscopic indication of ovulation. The vacuoles are subnuclear and displace the nuclei toward the glandular lumen. Pseudostratification of nuclei is lost and the nuclei and vacuoles are aligned in 2 orderly rows. These changes are prominent and strikingly uniform in all glands. Similar changes can, at times, be seen with chronic unopposed estrogen stimulation of the endometrium. On day 19, the vacuoles begin to push past the nuclei and, beginning on day 20, they are extruded into the glandular lumina. The luminal surface now becomes very ragged because of detachment of the apical portions of the cells (i.e., apocrine secretion) (Fig. 5–7) (45). Transudation of blood plasma also contributes to the uterine secretory fluids.

The endometrial events of the early luteal phase are associated with an increase in the size of the granulosa cells and penetration of capillaries into the granulosa cell mass. Ultimately, the capillaries reach the central cavity of the corpus luteum and fill it with blood. These events are associated with increasing concentrations of progesterone and estradiol, presumably because blood flow and steroid secretion from the corpus luteum are increased.

The endometrium from day 20 to day 24 is soft, velvety, edematous and 7 mm to 8 mm thick. Glycogen granules are present in the glandular lumina, and the epithelium is a low columnar or cuboidal type. The nuclei have receded to the basal area, and the glandular cell has extruded itself into the lumen. The cytoplasm has a very frayed luminal edge and becomes more eosinophilic. Luminal secretions are abundant and also eosinophilic. The glands are widened and assume a corkscrew pattern. Convolution of the glands is maximal—causing a tuftlike appearance. The glands remain straight and narrow in the compact zone and do not become tortuous until they reach the spongiosa (Fig. 5–8) (45). The surface epithelium remains tall and appears to have less secretory activity than glandular epithelium.

Peak intracellular apocrine secretory activity coincides with the most likely day of implantation, usually day 22 or day 23. The high levels

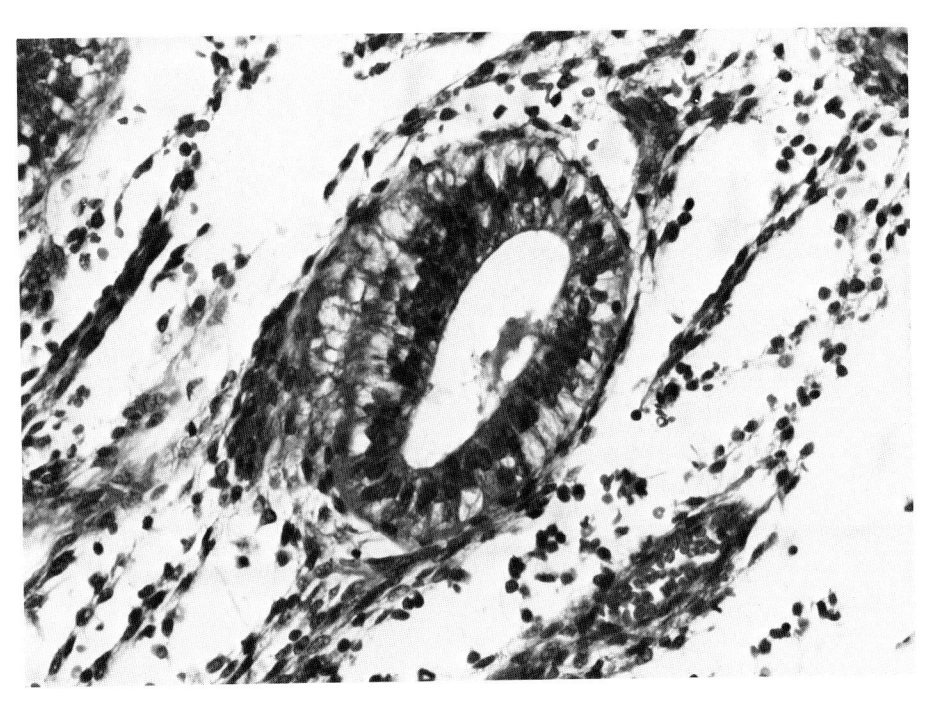

Fig. 5–7. Early secretory endometrium. The glands are comprised of tall columnar cells and vacuoles are prominent. The luminal surfaces of the glands become very ragged and apocrine secretion is evident.

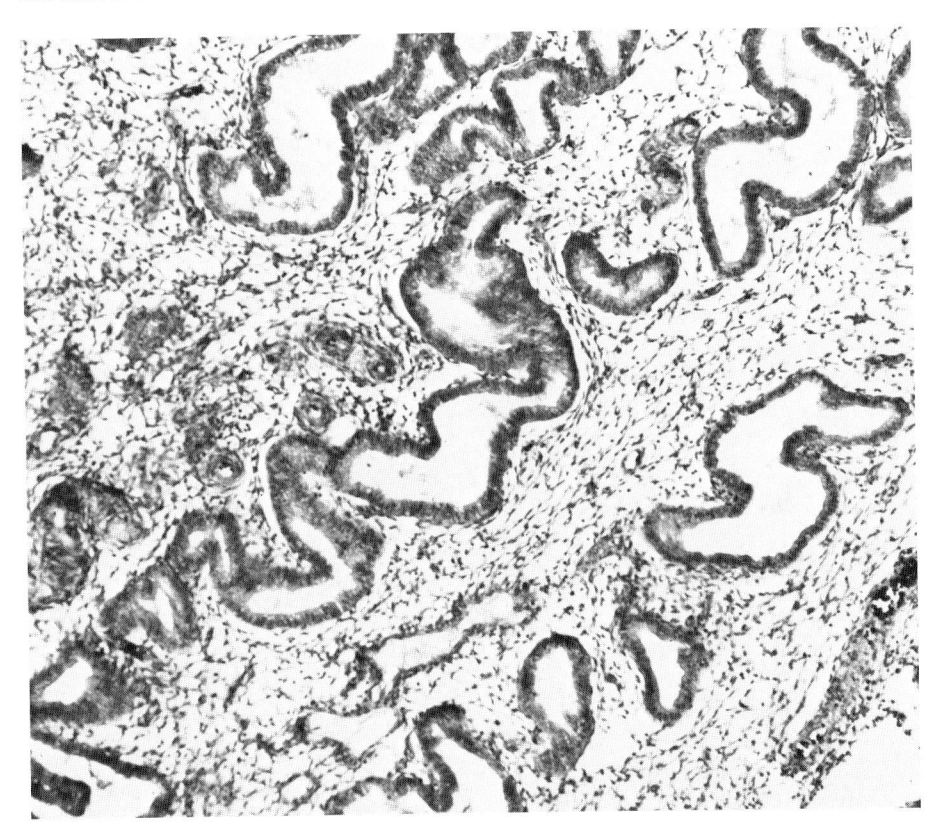

Fig. 5–8. Midsecretory endometrium. The glands are tortuous and dilated, producing a tuftlike appearance. The cells are cuboidal and secretion is present in the glandular lumina. Stromal edema is maximal now and blood vessels are conspicuous.

of progesterone antagonize estradiol effects by reducing the quantity of cytoplasmic and nuclear estradiol receptors and thereby inhibiting mitosis and nucleic acid synthesis (47). Furthermore, progesterone stimulates the synthesis of estradiol-17 beta-dehydrogenase (estradiol dehydrogenase), and conversion of estradiol to estrone is favored. Compared to estradiol, little estrone is translocated to the nucleus and estrogen effects in the luteal phase are further blunted (73).

A prominent increase in stromal fluid is a hallmark of the midsecretory phase and the texture of the stroma is very loose. The edema actually coalesces into lakes that separate individual stromal cells. The scanty cytoplasm and the edema give the cells the appearance of "naked nuclei."

The spiral arteries become more prominent and tightly coiled as they expand into the zona compacta. Their walls are thickened. Occasional mitotic figures are seen in the arterial wall and the endothelium is swollen.

There is an increase in DNA synthesis and mitotic activity in the midsecretory phase of the cycle. This results in an increased number of stromal cells that are, presumably, the result of the midsecretory increase in estradiol concentrations. Growth of stromal cells is independent of the inhibitory effect of estradiol dehydrogenase because this progesterone-dependent enzyme appears to be present only in glandular cells. Progesterone and estrogen are required to transform spindle-shaped stromal cells to predecidual cells. The transformation begins around the spiral arterioles on day 23 and is thought to be mediated by prostaglandins (PG) (45).

PGE_2 promotes capillary permeability and vascular endothelial mitotic activity, which results in stromal edema and coiling of the arterioles, respectively (74). $PGF_{2\alpha}$ is responsible for the predecidual transformation of spindle-shaped stromal fibroblasts (75). Inhibitors of prostaglandin synthesis may, therefore, interfere with the predecidualization process.

The most important ovarian event of the luteal phase is progesterone secretion by the corpus luteum. Progesterone secretion is maximal about 8 days after the LH surge. A parallel but smaller increase in 17 alpha-hydroxyprogesterone, estradiol, and estrone concentrations also occurs as LH and FSH concentrations decline (65).

Beginning on approximately day 24 to day 25 of the cycle, capillary blood flow to the corpus luteum decreases, as does production of estrogen and progesterone. The corpus luteum functions for only 8 days before it begins to regress and the limited life span of the corpus luteum provides the necessary "relaxation oscillation" by which the reproductive system cycles (76). Plasma progesterone concentrations decline from a maximum of 16 ng/ml during the midluteal phase to 0.97 ng/ml on the first day of the next cycle (77). Estradiol concentrations decline to less than 100 pg/ml at the time of menstruation (78). The fixed life span of the corpus luteum is thought to be independent of gonadotropin secretion, although small amounts of LH are required for normal steroidogenesis (79) by the corpus luteum. Pregnancy prolongs the survival of the corpus luteum; placental production of human chorionic gonadotropin (hCG) "rescues" the corpus luteum from luteolysis until the ninth or tenth week of gestation (80).

The glands of the late luteal phase are dilated, markedly convoluted, and lined by a frayed, saw-toothed cuboidal epithelium that indicates secretory exhaustion. In the stroma, edema is reabsorbed and periglandular pseudodecidualization is present. As progesterone secretion declines, glandular secretion stops and the luminal coagulum of secretory products becomes retracted, inspissated, and more intensely stained. The spiral arteries are conspicuous, especially in the spongiosa. Their walls are thick and they extend almost to the surface. The stromal cells undergo hypertrophy, becoming plump with large amounts of pale-staining cytoplasm. These changes are, initially, confined to areas around the spiral arterioles. By day 26, they become widespread and ultimately replace most of the compacta (Fig. 5–9) (45). The exact function of the predecidual cells is unknown. They do, however, contribute to menstrual breakdown by phagocytosis and digestion of extracellular collagen matrix. Following nidation, the predecidual cells seem to prevent too deep an invasion by trophoblastic cells; lack of adequate decidualization may result in myometrial implantation, i.e., placenta accreta.

The spongiosa or middle zone is a lacy labyrinth of dilated and tortuous glands with few stromal cells and little predecidual change. The basalis is in contact with the muscularis

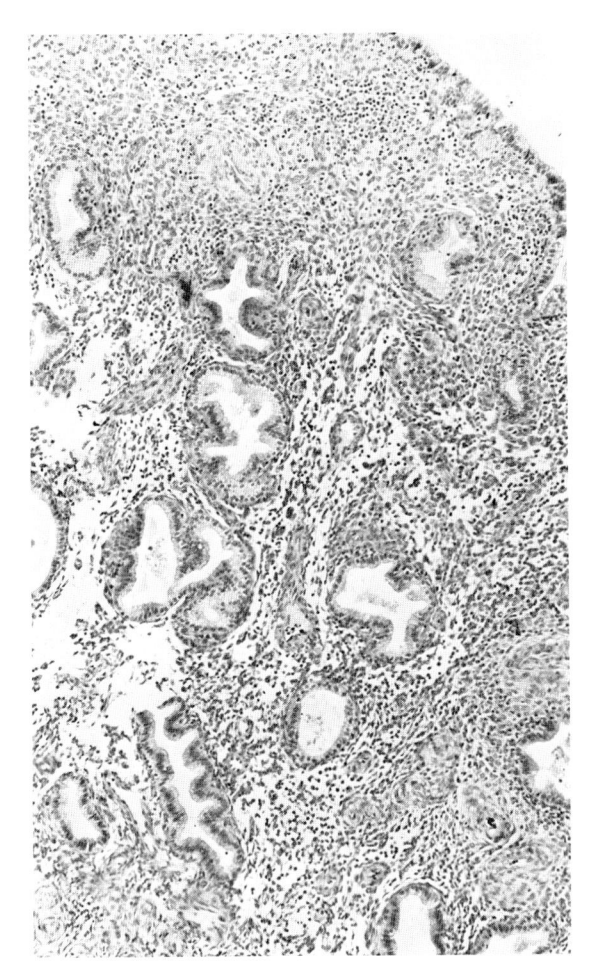

Fig. 5-9. Late secretory endometrium. Exhausted secretory glands are prominent and the luminal secretions are inspissated. Predecidual cells coalesce to form sheets in the compacta. Large numbers of inflammatory cells are present.

and often penetrates it for short distances. Even during intense progesterone stimulation and menstruation, only a proliferative pattern is seen in the compact zone.

On days 26 and 27 of the cycle, small mononuclear cells, lymphocytes, and granulocytes gather in the stroma and produce a pseudoinflammatory response. There is an increased number of extravasated polymorphonuclear leukocytes, so-called metrial cells or menstrual granulocytes. The metrial cells resemble eosinophils except for the presence of a single round nucleus (8). Metrial cells are rich in relaxin, which is believed to play a role in the destruction of the reticulum network of premenstrual and menstrual endometrium. Invariably, the pseudoinflammatory appearance precedes menses by 2 days (81).

The endometrium shrinks by day 28, possibly because of spiral arterial contraction and constriction. Fissures appear in the compact layer that contain edema fluid, red cells, and an acute inflammatory exudate. The staining reaction of the upper layer becomes impaired, suggesting impending dissolution. Areas of degeneration and necrosis appear and are followed by vascular dilatation, focal hemorrhage, and, finally, fragmentation of the endometrium as it is cast off during menstruation (45).

Unless pregnancy occurs, the endometrium gradually involutes, degenerates, and undergoes ischemic necrosis during the last 5 days of the cycle. Golgi-derived primary lysosomes, appearing in the proliferative phase as a result of estrogen stimulation, contain the potent lytic enzyme, acid phosphatase (34). Primary lysosomes are present in the cells of the glands and stroma and in vessel endothelial cells in the functional layer. Because progesterone has a membrane-stabilizing effect, the lytic enzymes are confined within lysosomes during the first half of the luteal phase. With the fall of estrogen and progesterone concentrations in the late secretory phase, lysosomal membranes dissipate and their enzymes are released into the cytoplasm (34). This leads to the digestion of the intracellular elements contained in the autophagic bodies and results in empty vacuoles. A gradual increase in lysosomal permeability may also occur and cause intracellular and extracellular diffusion of the lytic enzymes with a resultant destruction of the glandular epithelium, stromal cells, and vascular endothelium. Endothelial injury promotes platelet deposition, release of prostaglandin, vascular thrombosis, and eventual ischemic tissue necrosis. Many of these events can explain the premenstrual and menstrual cramps common in ovulating women. All of these events cause menstruation.

Summary

Menstruation is a mark of reproductive maturity in women. During the reproductive years, the monthly vaginal discharge of degenerated endometrium occurs at regular intervals with minimal variation. Regular menses document a normal female sex chromatin pattern, a mature hypothalamic-pituitary-ovarian axis, and a responsive end organ with a patent outflow tract. The menstrual cycle is ordinarily judged by its periodicity, duration of flow, and amount of flow. Although the monthly discharge may seem simple, the events portending normal menses are extremely complicated. Normal menstruation requires a highly refined degree of regulation and the intimate interaction of many organ systems.

Stated differently, normal ovulatory menstrual cycles can only occur in women with an intact and normally functioning reproductive system. Any disturbance in the orchestrated and harmonious sequence of hypothalamic, pituitary, and ovarian events may result in anovulation and abnormal menstruation. Beyond serving as an indicator of functional integrity of these glands, the endometrium itself is a complex tissue that can become disrupted despite an otherwise normal reproductive system.

Acknowledgements

I gratefully acknowledge the guidance of G. William Bates in the preparation of this chapter. In addition, Donna Welch and Margaret Taylor prepared the manuscript, and William de Veer provided technical assistance with preparation of photomicrographs. The Department of Pathology allowed the use of tissue slides.

REFERENCES

1. Lundgren N. Studies on the vasculature of the corpus of the human uterus. Acta Obstet Gynecol Scand (Suppl 4) 1957;36:5–115.
2. Bartelmez GW. The form and function of the uterine blood vessels in the rhesus monkey. Contrib Embryol 1957;249:153–181.
3. Stone SC. Physiology of puberty. In: Sciarra JJ, ed. Gynecology and obstetrics, Vol. 5. Philadelphia: Harper & Row, 1983:1–7.
4. Frisch RE, Revelle R. Height and weight at menarche and a hypothesis of critical body weights and adolescent events. Science 1970;169:397–399.
5. Ferenczy A, Bertrand G, Gelfund MM. Proliferation kinetics of human endometrium during the normal menstrual cycle. Am J Obstet Gynecol 1979;133:859–867.
6. Guilleband J, Bonnar J. Longer though lighter menstrual and intermenstrual bleeding with copper as compared to inert intrauterine devices. Br J Obstet Gynaecol 1978;85:707–712.
7. Lahmeyer HW, Miller M, Deleon-Jones F. Anxiety and mood fluctuation during the normal menstrual cycle. Psychosom Med 1982;44:183–194.
8. Rybo G. Menstrual blood loss in relation to parity and menstrual pattern. Acta Obstet Gynecol Scand (Suppl 7) 1966;45:25–41.
9. Hallberg L, Hogelahl A, Nilsson L, Rybo G. Menstrual blood loss—a population study. Acta Obstet Gynecol Scand 1966;45:320–351.
10. Scott DE, Pritchard JA. Iron deficiency in healthy young college women. JAMA 1967;199:897–900.
11. Kempers RD. Menstruation. In: Sciarra JJ, ed. Gynecology and obstetrics, Vol. 1. Philadelphia: Harper & Row, 1983:1–7.
12. Scommegna A, Vorys N, Givens JR. Menstrual dysfunction. In: Gold JJ, Josimovich JB, eds. Gynecologic endocrinology. Hagerstown, Md.: Harper & Row, 1980:290–326.
13. Zuckerman S. The hormonal balance of uterine bleeding. Acta Endocrinol (Copenh) 1957;7:378–388.
14. Zondek B. On the mechanism of uterine bleeding. Am J Obstet Gynecol 1954;68:310–314.
15. Treloar AE, Boynton RE, Benn BG. Variation of human menstrual cycle through reproductive life. Int J Fertil 1970;12:77–126.
16. Fraser IS, Michie EA, Wide L, Baird DT. Pituitary gonadotropins and ovarian function in adolescent dysfunctional uterine bleeding. J Clin Endocrinol Metab 1973;37:407–414.
17. Sherman BM, West JH, Korenman GS. The menopause transition: analysis of LH, FSH, estradiol and progesterone concentration during menstrual cycles of older women. J Clin Endocrinol Metab 1976;42:629–636.
18. Garcia JF, Jones GS, Wright GL, Prediction of the time of ovulation. Fertil Steril 1981;36:308–315.
19. Flowers CE, Welborn WH. New observations on the physiology of menstruation. Obstet Gynecol 1978;51:16–24.
20. Baggish MS, Pauerstein CH, Woodruff JD. Role of stroma in regeneration of endometrial epithelium. Am J Obstet Gynecol 1967;99:459–465.
21. Ferenczy A. Studies on cytodynamics of human endometrial regeneration. I. Scanning electron microscopy. Am J Obstet Gynecol 1976;124:64–74.
22. Moncada S, Vane JR. Arachidonic acid metabolites and the interactions between platelets and

blood vessel walls. N Engl J Med 1979; 300:1142–1147.
23. Jordan VC, Pokoly TB. Steroid and prostaglandin relations during the menstrual cycle. Obstet Gynecol 1977;49:449–453.
24. Abel MH. Production of prostaglandins by the human uterus: are they involved in menstruation? Res Clin Forum 1979;1:33–51.
25. Downie J, Poyser NL, Wunderlich M. Levels of prostaglandins in human endometrium during normal menstrual cycle. J Physiol 1974;236:465–472.
26. Smith SK, Abel MH, Kelley RW. The synthesis of prostaglandin from persistent proliferative endometrium. J Clin Endocrinol Metab 1982;55:284–289.
27. Ferenczy A. Studies on the cytodynamics of human endometrial regeneration. II. Transmission electron microscopy. Am J Obstet Gynecol 1976;124:582–595.
28. Maathuis JB, Kelley RW. Concentration of prostaglandins $F_{2\alpha}$ and E_2 in the endometrium throughout the human menstrual cycle after the administration of clomiphene or an oestrogen-progesterone pill and in early pregnancy. J Endocrinol 1978;77:361–371.
29. Markee JE. Menstruation in intraocular endometrial transplants in the rhesus monkey. Contrib Embryol 1940;177;221–256.
30. Reynolds SRM. The physiologic basis of menstruation: a summary of current concepts. JAMA 1947;135:552-557.
31. Bartelmez GW. Histologic studies on the menstruating mucous membrane of the human uterus. Contrib Embryol 1933;142:142–188.
32. Abell MR. Endometrium. In: Gold JJ, Josimovich JB, eds. Gynecologic endocrinology. Hagerstown, Md.: Harper & Row, 1980:232–270.
33. Okerlund M, Bengtsson L, Ulmsten N. Recording of myometrial activity in the activity in the non-pregnant human uterus by a microtransducer catheter. Acta Obstet Gynecol Scand 1978;57:429–433.
34. Henzl MR, Smith RE, Boost G, Tyler ET. Lysosomal concept of menstrual bleeding in humans. J Clin Endocrinol Metab 1972;34:860–875.
35. Schwabe C, McDonald JK. Relaxin: a disulfide homolog of insulin. Science 1977;197:914–915.
36. Hisaw FL, Hisaw FL Jr, Dawson AB. Effects of relaxin on the endothelium of endometrial blood vessels in monkeys (*Macaca mulatta*). Endocrinology 1967;81:375–385.
37. Hahn L. On fibrinolysis and coagulation during parturition and menstruation. Acta Obstet Gynecol Scand (Suppl) 1974;28:1–25.
38. Ferenczy A, Bertrand G, Gelfand MM. Studies on the cytodynamics of human endometrial regeneration. III. In vitro short term incubation historadioautography. Am J Obstet Gynecol 1979;134:297–304.
39. Sixma JJ, Wester J. The hemostatic plug. Semin Hematol 1977;14:265–299.
40. Gorski J, Stormshak F, Harris J, Wertz N. Hormone regulation of growth: stimulatory and inhibitory influences of estrogens on DNA synthesis. J Toxicol Environ Health 1977;3:371–379.
41. Sturgis SH, Meigs JV. Endometrial cycle and mechanism of normal menstruation. Am J Surg 1936;33:369–384.
42. Ferenczy A. Studies on the cytodynamics of experimental endometrial regeneration in the rabbit. Historadioautography and ultrastructure. Am J Obstet Gynecol 1977;128:536–545.
43. Nogales-Ortiz F, Puerta J, Nogales FF. The normal menstrual cycle. Chronology and mechanism of endometrial desquamation. Obstet Gynecol 1978;51:259–264.
44. Quick AJ. Menstruation in hereditary bleeding disorders. Obstet Gynecol 1966;28:37–48.
45. Noyes RW, Hertig AT, Rock J. Dating the endometrial biopsy. Fertil Steril 1950;1:3–25.
46. van Bogaret LJ. Endometrial granulocytes in proliferative endometrium. Br J Obstet Gynaecol 1975;82:995–998.
47. Natrajan PK, Muldoon TG, Greenblatt RB, Mahesh VB. Estradiol and progesterone receptors in estrogen-primed endometrium. Am J Obstet Gynecol 1982;140:387–392.
48. O'Malley BW, Means AR. Female steroid hormones and target cell nuclei. Science 1974;183:610–620.
49. McLennan CE, Rydell AH. Extent of endometrial shedding during normal menstruation. Obstet Gynecol 1965;26:605–621.
50. MacLennan AH, Harris JA, Wynn RM. Menstrual cycle of the baboon. II. Endometrial ultrastructure. Obstet Gynecol 1971;38:359–374.
51. Sawaragi I, Wynn RM. Ultrastructure localization of metabolic enzymes during the human endometrial cycle. Obstet Gynecol 1969;34:50–61.
52. Tsibris JC, Cazenare CR, Cantor BR, Notelovitz M, Kalra PS, Spellacy WN. Distribution of cytoplasmic estrogen and progesterone receptors in human endometrium. Am J Obstet Gynecol 1978;132:449–454.
53. Friederich ER, Meyer JS. Estrogen-progestin pharmacodynamics of the post-menopausal endometrium studied by thymidine labeling. Am J Obstet Gynecol 1982;143:352–359.
54. di Zerega GS, Nixon WE, Hodgen GD. Intercy-

cle serum follicle-stimulating hormone elevations: significance in recruitment and selection of the dominant follicle and assessment of corpus luteum normalcy. J Clin Endocrinol Metab 1980;50:1046–1048.
55. March CM, Goebelsmann U, Nakamura RM, Mishell DR. Roles of estradiol and progesterone in eliciting the mid-cycle luteinizing hormone and follicle-stimulating hormone surges. J Clin Endocrinol Metab 1979;49:507–513.
56. Channing CP, Schaerf FW, Anderson LD, et al. Ovarian follicular and luteal physiology, Vol. 22. In: Greep RO, ed. Reproductive physiology. III. International review of physiology. Baltimore: University Park Press, 1980:117–135.
57. di Zerega GS, Turner CK, Stouffer RL, Anderson LD, Channing CP, Hodgen GD. Suppression of follicle-stimulating hormone-dependent folliculogenesis during the primate ovarian cycle. J Clin Endocrinol Metab 1981;52:451–456.
58. Readhead C, Lobo RA, Kletzky OA. The activity of 3 beta-hydroxysteroid dehydrogenase and delta 5-isomerase in human follicular tissue. Am J Obstet Gynecol 1983;145:491–495.
59. Young JR, Jaffe RB. Strength-duration characteristics of estrogen effects on gonadotropin response to gonadotropin-releasing hormone in women. II. Effects of varying concentrations of estradiol. J Clin Endocrinol Metab 1976;42:432–442.
60. Yuen BH, Mincey EK. Role of androgens in menstrual disorders of non-hirsute and hirsute women and the effect of glucocorticoid therapy on androgen levels in hirsute and hyperandrogenic women. Am J Obstet Gynecol 1983; 145:152–157.
61. March CM, Marrs RP, Goebelsmann U, Mishell DR. Feedback effects of estradiol and progesterone upon gonadotropin and prolactin release. Obstet Gynecol 1981;58:10–16.
62. Carmel PW, Araki S, Ferin M. Pituitary stalk portal blood collection in rhesus monkeys: evidence of pulsatile release of gonadotropin-releasing hormone (GnRH). Endocrinology 1976;99:243–248.
63. Kao LWL, Gunsalus GL, Williams GH, Weisz J. Response of the perfused anterior pituitaries of rats to synthetic gonadotropin releasing hormone: a comparison with hypothalamic extract and demonstration of a role for potassium in the release of luteinizing hormone and follicle-stimulating hormone. Endocrinology 1977; 101:1444–1454.
64. McNatty KP, Makris A, Osathanondh R, Ryan KJ. Effects of luteinizing hormone on steroidogenesis by theca cells from human ovarian follicles in vitro. Steroids 1980;36:53–63.
65. World Health Organization Task Force Investigators. Temporal relationships between ovulation and defined changes in the concentration of plasma estradiol-17 beta, luteinizing hormone, follicle-stimulating hormone and progesterone. Am J Obstet Gynecol 1980;138:383–390.
66. Weiss TJ, Seamark RF, McIntosh JEA, Moor RM. Cyclic AMP in sheep ovarian follicles: site of production and response to gonadotropins. J Reprod Fertil 1976;46:347–353.
67. di Zerega GS, Marrs RP, Campeau JD, Kling RO. Human granulosa cell secretion of protein(s) which suppress follicular response to gonadotropin. J Clin Endocrinol Metab 1983;56:147–155.
68. Gordon M. Cyclic changes in the fine structure of the epithelial cells of human endometrium. Int Rev Cytol 1975;42:127–172.
69. Coaker T, Downie T, More IAR. Complex giant mitochondria in the human endometrial glandular cell: serial sectioning, high voltage electron microscopic and three-dimensional reconstruction studies. J Ultrastruc Res 1982;78:283–291.
70. Armstrong EM, More IAR, McSeveney D, Carty M. The giant mitochondrion-endoplasmic reticulum unit of the human endometrial glandular cell. J Anat 1973;116:375–383.
71. More IAR, McSeveney D. The three-dimensional structure of the nucleolar channel system in the endometrial glandular cell: serial sectioning and high voltage electron microscopy studies. J Anat 1980;130:673–682.
72. More IAR, Armstrong EM, Carty M, McSeveney D. Cyclic changes in the ultrastructure of normal endometrial stromal cell. J Obstet Gynaecol Brit Comm 1974;81:337–347.
73. King RJB, Townsend PT, Whitehead MI. The role of estradiol dehydrogenase in mediating progestin effects on endometrium from postmenopausal women receiving estrogens and progestins. J Steroid Biochem 1981;14:235–238.
74. Kennedy TG. Prostaglandins and increased endometrial vascular permeability resulting from the application of an artificial stimulus to the uterus of the rat sensitized for the decidual cell reaction. Biol Reprod 1979;20:560–566.
75. Kennedy TG. Estrogen and uterine sensitization for the decidual cell reaction: role of prostaglandins. Biol Reprod 1980;23:955–962.
76. Van de Wiele RL, Bogumil J, Dyrenfurth I, et al. Mechanisms regulating the menstrual cycle in women. Recent Prog Horm Res 1970;26:63–103.
77. Guerro R, Aso T, Brenner PR, et al. Studies on the patterns of circulating steroids in normal

menstrual cycle. I. Simultaneous assays of progesterone, pregnenolone, dehydroepiandrosterone, testosterone, dihydrotestosterone, androstenedione, oestradiol and oestrone. Acta Endocrinol (Copenh) 1976;81:133–149.
78. Landgren BM, Campo S, Cekan SZ, Diczfalusy E. Studies on the patterns of circulating steroid in the normal menstrual cycle. 5. Changes around the onset of menstruation. Acta Endocrinol (Copenh) 1977;86:608–620.
79. Cameron JL, Stouffer RL. Gonadotropin receptors of the primate corpus luteum. II. Changes in available luteinizing hormone and chorionic gonadotropin binding sites in macaque luteal membranes during the non-fertile menstrual cycle. Endocrinology 1982; 110:2068–2073.
80. Laufer N, Navot D, Schenker JG. The pattern of luteal phase plasma progesterone and estradiol in fertile cycles. Am J Obstet Gynecol 1982;143:808–813.
81. Daly DC, Tohan N, Doney TJ, Maslar IA, Riddick DH. The significance of lymphocytic leukocytic infiltrates in interpreting late luteal phase endometrial biopsies. Fertil Steril 1982;37:786–791.

Anovulation and Ovulation Induction

6

Mary G. Hammond

The treatment of anovulation and other forms of ovulatory dysfunction is one of the most successful and rewarding areas of management of the infertile couple. Since the report of conceptions following ovulation induction with human gonadotropin therapy by Gemzell et al. (1) in 1958 and clomiphene citrate (Clomid®) in 1961 by Greenblatt (2), ovulation and pregnancy rates exceeding 80% and 35%, respectively, have been the norm. The increased availability of hormone radioimmunoassay and pelvic ultrasound have increased our understanding of the treatment cycle and improved patient management.

Prior to the introduction of these methods, only 3 treatment regimes were available in the management of the anovulatory woman: rebound ovulation after progestin or estrogen-progestin therapy, ovarian wedge resection for polycystic ovarian disease, and glucocorticoid suppression for adrenal hyperandrogenism.

Women with severe hypothalamic dysfunction or elevated prolactin levels present special problems in ovulation induction. Recent development of suitable infusion systems for gonadotropin-releasing hormone (GnRH) and the availability of bromocriptine (Parlode®) have provided more specific therapy for these problems. The utilization of pure FSH and bromocriptine may improve results in women with polycystic ovarian disease who do not conceive with clomiphene.

In this chapter I will address the pretreatment evaluation of the anovulatory woman, the selection of the appropriate therapy, methods for monitoring ovulation, and the results of specific treatment plans.

Pretreatment Assessment of the Anovulatory Woman

Suitable candidates for ovulation induction include amenorrheic and oligomenorrheic women attempting conception as well as oligoovulatory women (cycles more than 35 days) who have failed to conceive in 1 year. Because of the association of ovulatory dysfunction with systemic disease and the improved pregnancy rates after specific therapy, the etiology of anovulation should be determined prior to initiation of therapy. This evaluation should consist of endocrine assessment as well as identification of other potential subfertility factors in the couple.

ENDOCRINE EVALUATION. Anovulation may result from abnormalities of the hypothalamic-pituitary axis or ovarian dysfunction (Table 6–1). The evaluation of the infertile amenorrheic woman should be as thorough as for the woman presenting with the primary complaint of amenorrhea. History and physical examination should emphasize neurologic symptoms and signs, metabolic disturbances, signs of hyperandrogenism and galactorrhea. Recent changes in weight, activity, or body contour are significant. The possibility of pregnancy should always be considered. Laboratory studies including FSH and prolactin are essential. Thyroid studies and assessment of adrenal and ovarian androgen secretion (dehydroepiandrosterone sulfate, testosterone) should be done if symptoms or signs of thyroid disease or hyperandrogenism are present.

Women with oligomenorrhea should be

TABLE 6-1. Causes of Anovulation

I. Central
  A. Central
    1. Hypothalamic
    2. Abnormalities of feedback
      a. Stress
      b. Weight loss
      c. Cushing's syndrome
      d. Congenital adrenal hyperplasia
      e. Tumors
        i. Ovarian
        ii. Adrenal
  B. Pituitary
    1. Tumors
    2. Abnormalities of feedback
      a. Polycystic ovarian disease
      b. Weight loss
      c. Tumors
        i. Ovarian
        ii. Adrenal
    3. Trauma
    4. Infection
    5. Granulomas (e.g., sarcoidosis)
II. Ovary
  A. Failure
    1. Genetic
    2. Infectious
    3. Surgical
    4. Immunologic
  B. Polycystic ovarian disease
  C. Tumors

evaluated by measurement of FSH, LH, prolactin, and testosterone levels. These studies may aid in selection of the appropriate treatment and exclude women with impending ovarian failure. Demonstration of anovulation by extensive basal body temperature (BBT) charting or endometrial biopsy is not essential in the oligomenorrheic woman, but may reveal anovulation in the eumenorrheic woman.

OTHER FERTILITY FACTORS. The possibility of additional fertility factors should be investigated. A semen analysis and documentation of tubal patency (hysterosalpingography [HSG] and laparoscopy) are advised prior to ovulation induction. Some centers defer an HSG until 3 ovulatory cycles have been completed without conception. Minimal prerequisites for ovulation induction include a motile sperm count greater than 10 million per ejaculate and at least 1 patent tube. Cervical mucus may be difficult to assess in anovulatory women and can be deferred until ovulatory cycles have been established.

SELECTION OF THE APPROPRIATE THERAPY. Women with FSH concentrations greater than 40 mIU/ml are, with few exceptions, resistant to therapy because of absent or resistant ovarian follicles and should not receive ovulation-inducing drugs.

Oligomenorrheic women with normal endocrine results respond well to clomiphene, which is the initial drug of choice.

Women with a demonstrable endocrine abnormality, such as hypothyroidism or one of the various forms of congenital adrenal hyperplasia, should receive specific replacement therapy. Women with hyperprolactinemia who have been judged appropriate for ovulation induction will respond most effectively to bromocriptine. Women who remain anovulatory despite specific hormonal replacement (e.g., thyroid) should be treated with clomiphene.

The mainstay of therapy of the woman with polycystic ovary disease has been clomiphene. Adjuvants to therapy such as prednisone have also been utilized. Women who fail to ovulate with clomiphene present special management problems because of unusual sensitivity to gonadotropins.

The selection of initial therapy for the amenorrheic woman, many of whom fail to respond to clomiphene, has been a source of controversy. Several investigators have recommended a series of simple or more sophisticated tests to guide therapy. These have included withdrawal uterine bleeding after parenteral progestin, gonadotropin-releasing hormone (GnRH) tests, and assessment of positive feedback by administering estradiol (3,4). Many clinicians, including myself, prefer a trial of clomiphene to assess the response of the hypothalamic-pituitary axis before starting other drugs such as GnRH or gonadotropins. Obviously, women with panhypopituitarism, Kallman's syndrome, or specific gonadotropin deficiency (see Chapter 4) will require gonadotropins for ovulation induction.

Drugs in Ovulation Induction

CLOMIPHENE CITRATE.

Indications. Clomiphene is the drug of choice for ovulation induction in anovulatory patients with intact pituitary function. It is marketed as Clomid® and Serophene®).

Pharmacology. Clomiphene is a triphenylethylene compound [2-[p-(chloro-1,2-diphenylvinyl) phenoxyl] triethylamine dihydrogen citrate]. It is a nonsteroidal estrogen with chemical similarity to chlorotrianisene (Tace®, tamoxifen, and diethylstilbestrol (Fig. 6–1).

Clomiphene is water soluble, readily absorbed orally, and is cleared by the liver and excreted in feces. An enterohepatic circulation exists and residual clomiphene is concentrated in liver, gall bladder, and bile. The body half-life of Clomid has been reported as 24 hours after intraperitoneal injection in rats and 48 hours after intravenous injection in monkeys. Eighty-three percent to 90% of clomiphene is excreted in 6.3 days in the monkey (5).

Mode of Action. Uptake studies with radiolabeled clomiphene reveal specific uptake by guinea pig hypothalamus, pituitary, uterus, ovary, adrenal, and liver (6). In estradiol-deficient animals this leads to estrogenic effects such as increased uterine weight. In addition, competition with estradiol for binding to high-affinity estrogen receptors has been demonstrated in human uterine and breast cancer tissue (7), rat uterus, brain and pituitary (8), and chick oviduct (9) with a K_D of $10^{-8}M$ as opposed to a K_D of $10^{-10}M$ for estradiol and $10^{-11}M$ for diethylstilbestrol (8). This competition contributes to the drug's antiestrogenic effects (10). The mode of action of Clomid remains speculative, but increasing evidence supports the original proposal that effects on hypothalamic or pituitary cytosol estrogen receptor binding (11) or replenishment (10) may lead to a decreased negative feedback effect of estradiol (12) that causes increased levels of serum gonadotropins (13,14). An additional estrogenic effect of clomiphene, the sensitization of pituitary cells *in vitro* to GnRH, may amplify gonadotropin release (15).

An alternative hypothesis is that clomiphene affects ovarian steroidogenesis directly by reducing steroid levels and leading to increasing gonadotropin levels (16). This effect on folliculogenesis has recently been confirmed in monkeys. Very high doses of clomiphene administered in the follicular phase to spontaneously ovulating monkeys produced a marked decline in estradiol production (17). In contrast, stimulation of gonadotropin-dependent estradiol production *in vitro* in response to clomiphene therapy has been reported by Zhuang et al. (18), suggesting that clomiphene may increase both sensitivity to FSH and aromatase activity.

Method of Administration.

INDIVIDUALIZED, STEPWISE INCREASES. Clomiphene is administered orally beginning on the third to the fifth day following the onset of a spontaneous menses or progestin-induced withdrawal bleeding. Therapy is started with 50 mg daily for 5 days and the ovulatory response is assessed by basal body temperature and a serum progesterone concentration or endometrial biopsy during the luteal phase. If

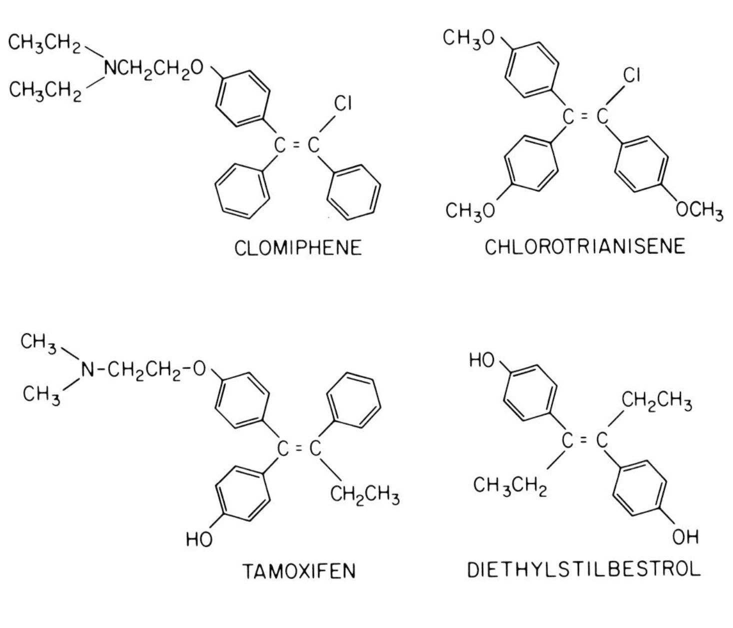

Fig. 6–1. Chemical structures of clomiphene and related drugs.

ovulation does not occur, the dosage is increased to 2 tablets (100 mg) daily for 5 days in the subsequent cycle. Dosage may be increased in this fashion up to a total of 200 mg to 250 mg/day (19).

The addition of 10,000 IU of chorionic gonadotropin (hCG) given intramuscularly 8 to 10 days after a 5-day course of clomiphene improves ovulation rates (20). This drug is useful in women with adequate folliculogenesis (as documented by late follicular phase serum estradiol concentrations greater than 300 pg/ml), but who mount no endogenous midcycle LH peak. The lack of a midcycle LH peak may be caused by failure of positive feedback (3). Repeat injection (5,000 IU) of hCG 1 week later may stimulate the corpus luteum and sustain the luteal phase (21).

A practical approach to the administration of clomiphene is given in Fig. 6–2 (22). This method permits the efficient selection of the suitable ovulatory dose without repetition of doses inadequate to stimulate ovulation or selection of excessive doses.

ALTERNATE ADMINISTRATION PLANS. Approximately 10% to 20% of women treated with the maximal conventional dose of clomiphene, 250 mg/day for 5 days, will not ovulate. Several alterations in the treatment plan have been described. Lobo et al. (23) used 250 mg/day for 8 days. Eight of 13 women ovulated and 3 conceived. Increasing the dosage of clomiphene above 150 mg to 200 mg/day, except in obese subjects (24), may cause significant antiestrogenic effects and abnormal folliculogenesis (17).

Results of Therapy. Ovulation and conception rates in clomiphene-treated women are depicted in Table 6–2. The method of administration and criteria to establish ovulation vary from one series to another; the extent of pretreatment evaluation of other fertility factors also varies. Ovulation rates of 57% to 91% and conception rates of 25% to 49% have been reported (19,21,22,25–29).

A discrepancy between ovulation rates and pregnancy rates is frequently cited, but evaluation of pregnancy rates by the life table method, which corrects for women who discontinue therapy or conceive, reveals that monthly pregnancy rates in ovulating women are comparable to those undergoing artificial insemination by donor (AID) or discontinuing contraception (Fig. 6–3) (22,28,30). In our series, women ovulating on clomiphene have a monthly fecundability rate of 15.7% compared to 24.7% for women terminating diaphragm contraception. In women with no other infertility factors, the fecundability rate is 22% (18).

Metabolic Effects.

ESTROGENIC CHANGES. Clomiphene citrate, 50 mg to 100 mg/day for 14 days, leads to a significant increase in the concentration of thyroxin (T_4), plasminogen (31), cortisol-binding globulin (CBG), and testosterone-estrogen binding globulin (32). The elevation in CBG has been demonstrated in women receiving standard ovulatory doses (33) whose serum cortisol levels were normal. Interpretation of thyroid function tests may be affected (32).

ANTIESTROGENIC EFFECTS. There is considerable debate about the effect of clomiphene on the quality of cervical mucus. Van Campenhout et al. have reported that 25 mg or 50 mg of clomiphene taken daily partially blocked or eliminated the increase in spinnbarkeit of cervical mucus induced in

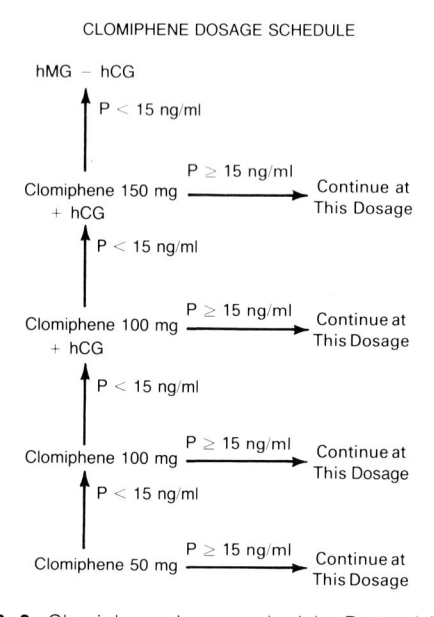

Fig. 6–2. Clomiphene dosage schedule. Protocol for induction of ovulation and criteria for adequate ovulation. P = serum progesterone concentration; hMG = human menopausal gonadotropin; hCG = human chorionic gonadotropin. (Reprinted with permission. Hammond MG, et al. Obstet Gynecol 1983;62:196.)

TABLE 6–2. Clomiphene Citrate: Ovulation and Uncorrected Pregnancy Rates in Women Treated for Anovulation

AUTHOR	NO.	OVULATION (%)	PREGNANCY (%)
Kase et al., 1967 (25)	81	60	25
Karow and Payne, 1968 (26)	410	—	39
MacGregor et al., 1968 (27)	4,098	70	34
Rust et al., 1974 (19)	105	91	38
Garcia et al., 1977 (21)	159	82	40
Gorlitsky et al., 1978 (28)	122	57	37
Gysler et al., 1982 (29)	428	85	43
Hammond et al., 1982 (22)	159	86	49

postmenopausal women by 50 mcg ethinyl estradiol (34).

These findings have also been observed in anovulatory women (22,35,36). In our series of clomiphene-treated women, the cervical mucus of 68 ovulatory women was evaluated by a numerical cervical mucus score based on amount, spinnbarkeit, ferning, cellularity, and viscosity. Thirty-four women (50%) had poor cervical mucous. Gysler et al. found that 15% of 227 cervical mucus samples were abnormal (29). When abnormal mucus is found, Premarin® 0.625 to 2.5 mg/day (22,37,38), Estrace® 75 mcg to 150 mcg/day (39), or diethylstilbestrol (DES) 0.1 mg/day from day 8 to day 15 of the cycle may overcome this effect. Premarin 7.5 mcg daily or Estrace 150 mcg daily has no effect on ovulation in cycles induced with 100 mg clomiphene (37).

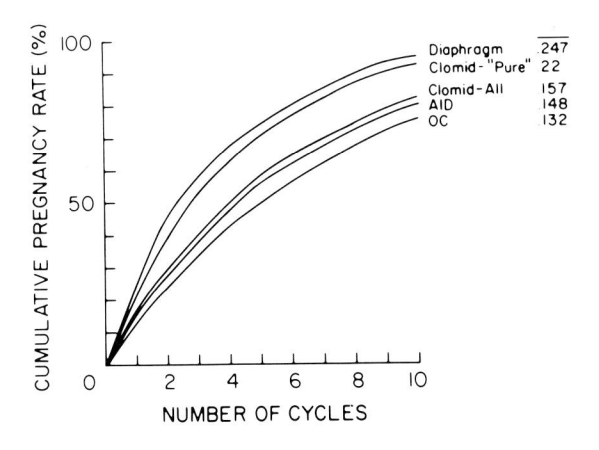

Fig. 6–3. Cumulative pregnancy rates in women undergoing ovulation induction as compared with women discontinuing the use of a diaphragm or oral contraceptives (OC) or undergoing donor insemination (AID). Monthly fecundability rates (f) are shown at the top of each curve. (Reprinted with permission. Hammond MG, et al. Obstet Gynecol 1983;62:196.)

Complications.

1. Ovarian hyperstimulation. Ovarian hyperstimulation occurs infrequently with clomiphene therapy as described and it usually occurs in women with polycystic ovarian disease. Women should be examined before starting clomiphene and monthly until ovulation occurs. If no cysts are noted, no additional exams are necessary unless pain occurs.

2. Multiple gestations. Twins occur in 6.9% of pregnancies, triplets in 0.5%, quadruplets in 0.3%, and quintuplets in 0.13% (5).

3. Birth defects. Offspring of animals that were given large doses of clomiphene during gestation have a dose-dependent increase in the frequency of congenital anomalies (5). In particular, adenosis of the vagina, similar to DES changes, has been noted (40,41).

   One hundred and fifty-eight mothers have been reported who received clomiphene in the first 6 weeks after conception. Eight had unspecified birth defects for a rate of 50/1,000 compared to 23/1,000 in pregnancies in which clomiphene was given only prior to conception. Anomalies reported when clomiphene was administered prior to ovulation are tabulated in Table 6–3. From these data, there appears to be no significant increase in any specific anomaly. A summary of reported malformation rates is given in Table 6–4. Although an increase in the frequency of Down's syndrome (46) and neural tube defects has been reported (47,48), epidemiologic studies offer little support for such a specific effect.

4. Abortion rate. An increased spontaneous abortion rate has been reported for

TABLE 6–3. Clomiphene: Congenital Anomalies in 2,211 Pregnancies

DEFECT	NUMBER
Heart defects	8
Down's syndrome	5
Club foot	4
Gastrointestinal	4
Hemangioma	2
Polydactyly	2
Multiple anomalies	7
Hypospadias	3
Microcephaly	2
Cleft lip and palate	2
Congenital hip dislocation	2
Conjoined twins	2
Spina bifida	1
Other	14

clomiphene-induced pregnancies (49). If so, this may be the result of a specific abnormality of the embryo [an increased incidence of chromosomal anomalies occurs in abortuses from induced cycles—83% vs. 60% from spontaneous cycles (50)] or of endocrine abnormalities of the clomiphene treatment cycle (21). The increased abortion rate does not appear to be an inherent defect in the infertile couple as abortion rates following donor insemination, bromocriptine, or therapy for endometriosis are between 9.3% and 11.8% (49). Reported abortion rates following clomiphene therapy are listed in Table 6–5. The improved results from recent reports are suggestive that the abortion rate may have been overestimated in early studies or that improved methods of therapy may have decreased the rate. In most recent studies, pregnancy losses approach those of normal women.

5. Adverse effects. Significant adverse symptoms reported by 8,029 anovulatory patients are listed in Table 6–6 (5).

HUMAN GONADOTROPINS.

Indications. Gonadotropins are indicated for ovulation induction in women with abnormalities of pituitary function leading to hypogonadotropism such as panhypopituitarism, previous hypophysectomy, pituitary necrosis, or tumor (see Chapter 4). The woman's general medical condition must also be suitable for pregnancy. These drugs may also be used as the initial drug in women with significant hypothalamic dysfunction. In addition, gonadotropins are appropriate for women who fail to ovulate with clomiphene or who develop resistance to that drug.

Pharmacology. Gonadotropins for ovulation induction have been studied in two forms: FSH and LH of pituitary origin (hPG) (1) and from the urine of postmenopausal women (hMG) (52). These preparations differ in that the urinary gonadotropins are partially degraded metabolic products with a lower molecular weight and potency than the pituitary product (53).

Human pituitary gonadotropin, which is not available commercially in the United States, is prepared from acetone-dried human pituitary powder and is standardized to the international reference preparation for hMG. Various ratios of FSH:LH are found in different preparations. Gemzell utilized a preparation with a ratio of 1:2 (FSH:LH).

Human menopausal gonadotropin is available in the United States as Pergonal®.* It is supplied in lyophilized form and each ampule contains 75 IU FSH and 75 IU LH.

HPG and hMG act by direct stimulation of ovarian follicles. FSH stimulates recruitment and development of primary follicles. LH is required for development of the preovulatory

---

* Serono Laboratories, Braintree, Massachusetts.

TABLE 6–4. Malformation Rates after Clomiphene Therapy

AUTHOR	COUNTRY	NO.	MAJOR	MINOR
Hack and Lunenfeld (42)	Israel	344	14.5/1,000	32/1,000
Gysler et al. (29)	United States	193	10.0/1,000	5/1,000
Correy et al. (43)	Tasmania	156	12.8/1,000	19/1,000
Ahlgren et al. (44)	Sweden	148	54.0/1,000	54/1,000
Adashi et al. (45)	United States	86	23.0/1,000	—

TABLE 6–5. Abortion Rates Following Clomiphene Therapy

AUTHOR	YEAR	PREGNANCIES	SPONTANEOUS ABORTION (%)
MacGregor et al. (27)	1967	1744	20.1
Goldfarb et al. (51)	1968	160	10.8*
Ahlgren et al. (44)	1976	159	10.1
Garcia et al. (21)	1977	68	25.3
Correy et al. (43)	1982	156	10.3
Gysler et al. (29)	1982	193	12.9
Hammond et al. (22)	1982	59	15.0

* Used hormonal supplements from weeks 6 to 22.

follicle and estradiol synthesis (54). Development of multiple follicles is common during hMG therapy (55). Injection of human chorionic gonadotropin (hCG) is required to stimulate ovulation and doses from 3,000 to 10,000 IU have been used. A second dose of 5,000 to 6,000 IU hCG may improve luteal function (56). HCG has a half-life of 23.9 hours (57) and LH or hCG may be required to maintain the corpus luteum.

Method of Administration. A variety of dosage schedules has been utlized. These consist of the following (58):

1. Fixed regimens
   a. Daily administration of a fixed dose of hPG or hMG for 8 to 10 days with administration of hCG during or immediately after hMG (59).
   b. hMG on days 1,4, and 8 followed by hCG on day 11 (60,61).
   c. hMG on days 1, 3, and 5 followed by hCG on day 8 if the estrogen level and clinical signs are appropriate (62,63).
2. Individualized regimen
   a. HMG is administered daily. Dosage is increased by 30% to 50% every 4 to 5 days depending on response. HCG is given after adequate response. Subsequent cycles are begun at the daily dose that led to ovulation.

Monitoring of Treatment Cycle.

1. Objective of monitoring
   a. To determine the dose of hMG and the length of therapy. When an individualized adjusted schedule is used, monitoring is done during the actual course of therapy; when a predetermined or fixed schedule is used, the dose of hMG is adjusted after assessing the response in the previous cycle.
   b. To determine when and whether to administer hCG.
   c. To obtain an adequate ovulatory response and to avoid hyperstimulation.
2. Techniques of monitoring
   a. Clinical. Vaginal cytology, cervical mucous quality, and ovarian size have been used extensively to follow patients undergoing ovulation induction (64,65).
   b. Chemical. Measurement of the urinary excretion or serum concentration of estrogen to assess the progression of follicular maturation is presently the preferred method of monitoring. Therapeutic windows for hCG administration have been reported by several authors (Table 6–7). In their hands, achievement of these levels confirms adequate folliculogenesis and reduces the incidence of hyperstimulation. The period from the last hMG injection to hCG varies from 24 to 72 hours.
   c. Ultrasound. Ultrasonic monitoring of follicular development in spontaneous cycles (72) has permitted a far more ac-

TABLE 6–6. Adverse Effects with Clomiphene

ADVERSE EFFECT	%
Ovarian enlargement	13.6
Vasomotor flushes	10.4
Abdominal-pelvic discomfort	5.5
Nausea	2.2
Breast pain	2.0
Visual symptoms	1.5

TABLE 6–7. Acceptable Estrogen Concentrations for Adequate Follicular Development in hMG Therapy

AUTHOR	URINE (MCG/24 HOURS)	SERUM (PG/ML)
Gemzell (66)	60–80	600–800
Lunenfeld (67)	75–150	—
Schwartz et al. (68)	80–250	500–1,500
Karam et al. (69)	50–90	—
March (70)	—	500–1,500
Radwanska et al. (63)	—	300–1,500
Haning et al. (71)	40–100	1,000–2,000

curate assessment of the follicle than clinical evaluation of ovarian size. Preovulatory follicles from spontaneous cycles vary in size from 14 mm to 28 mm. In women undergoing ovulation induction with hPG, follicular growth is more rapid, but the preovulatory follicular size was similar (17 mm to 25 mm) (73). Ultrasound permits the early detection of hyperstimulation and is the first technique available to predict the number of preovulatory follicles and maximum possible number of ova for fertilization.

Practical Regimens for Gonadotropin Use.

1. Individualized method (74). Women with reduced estrogen concentrations are begun at 2 ampules while those with normal estrogen concentrations are begun at 1 ampule. The dosage is administered daily and cervical mucus and ovarian size are evaluated daily. Estrogen monitoring is begun on the first day of hMG therapy or when cervical mucus begins to show the effect of estrogen stimulation. If no response occurs within 4 to 5 days, the dosage is increased by 1 to 2 ampules. When a response occurs, that dose is continued until the serum or urinary estrogen reaches the desired therapeutic window. Ideally, this should occur between 10 to 15 days. Ten thousand IU of hCG is then given. Subsequent treatment cycles are started at the dose that resulted in ovulation in the previous cycle.
2. Standardized method. HMG therapy is begun 3 to 5 days after the onset of induced vaginal bleeding. Three to 5 ampules are given on treatment days 1, 3, and 5. Serum estrogen concentrations are measured on days 3, 5, and 8. On treatment day 8 estrogen status is assessed. If the serum estradiol concentration is 300 to 1,500 pg/ml, cervical mucus is adequate and the diameter of the ovaries is less than 6 cm, then 10,000 IU of hCG is given intramuscularly. The ovulatory dose is repeated in subsequent cycles if pregnancy does not occur. If the serum estradiol concentration is less than 300 pg/ml, then a new treatment cycle is begun by increasing the dose by 2 ampules. If the estradiol concentration is greater than 2,000 pg/ml, but the ovaries are not enlarged, ultrasound is performed. If 3 or fewer preovulatory follicles are seen, then hCG is administered. If the patient is clearly overstimulated, hCG is withheld. After 1 month, a new cycle is begun with a lower dosage.

Results of Therapy. Since the first pregnancy with gonadotropin therapy was reported in 1958, several authors have reported ovulation rates of 73% to 97%. Pregnancy rates have been somewhat lower, 23% to 82%. Ovulation, pregnancy, multiple gestation rates, and the method of administration are listed in Table 6–8.

Lunenfeld and Eshkol have surveyed the recent literature and reported the results of more than 12,000 treatment cycles (75). The overall pregnancy rate was 42.9%. They included an analysis of a group of 1,002 of their own patients treated for 3,234 cycles. The results, evaluated by life table analysis, more closely approached pregnancy rates reported for normally fertile women. In hypoestrogenic women, the cumulative pregnancy rate was 91.2% after 6 cycles. Healy et al. also achieved a very high cumulative pregnancy rate when they treated women for multiple cycles (76).

TABLE 6–8. Results of Gonadotropin Therapy

TREATMENT TYPE	NO. OF WOMEN	% OVULATING	% CONCEIVING	% MULTIPLE GESTATION	REFERENCE
I*	600	"Almost 100"	50	28	66
I	1,002	—	38	32	75
F† (daily)	1,192	77	22	31	58
F (days 1,4,8)	57	61	21	—	58
I	242	97	21	31	68
F	106	77	53	—	61
F (days 3,5,7)	320	80	51	9	77
F	77	—	56	—	79
F (days 1,3,5)	26	85	38	10	63
I	40	93	75	—	76
I	83	76	58	—	69
I	62	—	35	35	80

* I = individualized treatment regimen.
† F = fixed treatment regimen.

Cumulative pregnancy rates are lower in women with oligomenorrhea or other indications of estrogenic activity. Only 41.6% of women with normal estrogen levels who failed to ovulate on clomiphene conceived after 11 cycles of treatment (76). Results of hMG in women with polycystic ovarian disease who failed to ovulate on clomiphene are commonly unsatisfactory (68,75,77,78). The lower pregnancy rates in women with polycystic ovarian disease may be a result of the effects of hyperandrogenism, a variable response to gonadotropin, or the presence of other endocrine or infertility problems. Ninety percent of women who conceive do so within the first 4 treatment cycles. The mean number of hMG ampules per treatment cycle is 40.2 in hypoestrogenic women, but only 18.2 in women with evidence of estrogenic activity (76).

Reported rates of multiple pregnancy with hMG treatment vary. Although a reduction was achieved with the introduction of estrogen monitoring (75), twin and triplet pregnancies are still a frequent result of therapy. Because of this high rate (Table 6–8), ultrasonography should be performed early in pregnancy (74).

Abortion rates following gonadotropin therapy are clearly higher than those after spontaneous conception. Early pregnancy detection and multiple pregnancy may affect this, but normal rates of abortion are found in closely monitored women who received clomiphene. An abnormality of ovulation or inadequate luteal function has been suggested as possible causes. The observed abortion rates of 25% to 30% appear to be fairly uniform in all studies (68). The rate of major (19/1,000) and minor (25.8/1,000) malformations are comparable to those of spontaneously ovulating women (42).

Complications. The primary complication of gonadotropin therapy, ovarian hyperstimulation, has been reported with both hMG and hPG. It usually occurs only in women who ovulate and conceive after treatment (81). Hyperstimulation has been divided into 3 categories and 6 grades as indicated below (69,82,83):

MILD HYPERSTIMULATION.
Grade 1. Chemical hyperstimulation—urinary estrogen excretion exceeds 150 mcg/24 hours.
Grade 2. Chemical hyperstimulation with ovarian enlargement up to 5 cm × 5 cm.
MODERATE HYPERSTIMULATION.
Grade 3. Mild hyperstimulation plus abdominal distention.
Grade 4. Grade 3 hyperstimulation plus nausea and vomiting.
SEVERE HYPERSTIMULATION.
Grade 5. Large cysts and ascites.
Grade 6. Hemoconcentration with coagulation abnormalities.

The extent of hyperstimulation correlates well with urinary estrogen levels (82) and hCG should be withheld if estrogen levels exceed the established therapeutic window. Ovarian hyperstimulation does not usually occur in the absence of ovulation (68), but we have seen an instance of grade 5 hyperstimulation in a woman with polycystic ovarian disease who had an increased serum concentration of LH and a preovulatory estradiol concentration greater than 5,000 pg/ml. Hyperstimulation occurred despite withholding hCG.

Hyperstimulation usually becomes apparent 3 to 7 days after hCG is administered. Women with grades 1 to 3 can be managed without hospital admission. Intercourse and strenuous activity should be avoided. In the absence of pregnancy, symptoms will resolve after menses; however, if pregnancy occurs, symptoms may persist for 6 to 8 weeks.

In women with more severe forms of hyperstimulation, hospitalization is necessary. Since massive fluid shifts occur, fluid intake, urine output, weight, and abdominal girth should be monitored. The hematocrit, coagulation factors, and electrolyte concentrations should also be monitored. Cautious fluid and electrolyte replacement should be started. The role of plasma expanders, paracentesis, and arterial and venous pressure monitoring is, at present, unsettled.

Symptoms are usually transitory, and surgical exploration is indicated only when there is evidence of intraperitoneal hemorrhage or ovarian torsion.

COMBINED CLOMIPHENE-GONADOTROPIN.

Indications. For women with some endogenous estrogenic activity who respond poorly to clomiphene, the combination of clomiphene and hMG has been utilized. This technique was first reported by Kistner (84) and has been utilized by others. A 50% reduction in the required dosage of hMG has been reported (85).

Pharmacology. The apparent mechanism of action is a clomiphene-induced increase in endogeneous FSH and LH levels that reduces the quantity of hMG required to promote follicular maturation.

Method of Administration. Clomiphene, either 200 mg daily from day 5 to day 9 of the cycle or 100 mg daily from day 5 to day 12, is combined with daily injections of hMG. Estrogen response is monitored. HCG is given 24 to 48 hours after adequate stimulation is obtained.

Results. Jarrell et al. reported an increase in the ovulation rate but no increase in the pregnancy rate (86). HMG requirements were reduced 50% (85).

GONADOTROPIN-RELEASING HORMONE (GnRH). Intermittent GnRH therapy for ovulation induction is indicated primarily for women with amenorrhea and intact pituitary function who fail to respond to clomiphene induction of ovulation. GnRH is more physiologic than hMG in women with hypothalamic failure. It stimulates pituitary release of LH and FSH and subsequent folliculogenesis. Since negative feedback at the pituitary level is normal, the incidence of hyperstimulation should be lower than that with hMG. This method of ovulation induction is used extensively in Europe. There are a number of administration systems available and several pregnancies have been reported. Therapy, however, is cumbersome and prolonged.

Pharmacology. GnRH is available as Factrel® (Gonadorelin® HCl) from Ayerst Laboratories. It is a synthetic decapeptide that is identical to the naturally occurring hypothalamic hormone. It is available in 100-mcg and 500-mcg vials. This preparation has been used extensively to distinguish hypothalamic from pituitary disease. Injection of 25 mcg to 100 mcg of GnRH causes a rapid, dose-dependent increase in serum LH and a smaller increase in FSH concentrations.

The drug is essentially devoid of acute toxicity. No symptoms were recorded when it was administered to mice in dosages of 100 mcg/kg and in rats in dosages up to 150 mcg/kg. After 28 consecutive days of GnRH administration to rats, there were no changes in survival, clinical laboratory analyses, physical examination, or postmortem gross and microscopic findings. Secondary changes in male rats consisted of a decreased seminal vesicular and prostatic weight. In female rats, the body and organ weights were unchanged. No histopathologic changes related to the drug occurred in female monkeys treated on days 8 to 15 of the menstrual cycle. No adverse effects were noted in either the fetus or the mother after administration of GnRH to pregnant mice. Litter size, sex distribution, and fetal length and weight were similar in the treatment and control groups. No congenital anomalies were noted (87).

Method of Administration. Schally reviewed the results of therapy of ovulation induction with GnRH in 1975 (88). Of 80 women treated with continuous GnRH therapy, 26 ovulated (32.5%) and 10 conceived (12.5%). Best results were obtained in women with polycystic ovarian disease or anovulatory cyclic bleeding.

Nillius and Wide successfully induced ovulation in amenorrheic women with anorexia nervosa (89). Each woman self-administered 500 mcg GnRH subcutaneously every 8 hours. Estrogen and progesterone concentrations were measured every other day and daily basal body temperatures were recorded. Although normal 28-day cycles resulted from the injection, serum progesterone concentrations were low in the luteal phase, suggesting luteal phase deficiency. This was corrected in subsequent cycles by the injection of hCG when preovulatory estrogen concentrations were adequate and then 1 week following ovulation. With this treatment, luteal phase progesterone concentrations were normal. During the course of therapy, FSH response decreased as estrogen levels increased. This was felt to be an advantage over hMG as it might prevent the development of multiple follicles and hyperstimulation. Pregnancy occurred in the only woman in this study who was attempting to conceive.

The results of these studies demonstrated that high doses of GnRH were required, that GnRH must be continued beyond ovulation into the luteal phase, and that hCG might be required. GnRH has also been given to 13 women who had failed to ovulate with clomiphene (90). These women received 1 mg GnRH or placebo 2 to 3 times daily for 28 days. Ultimately, 61% of the women ovulated and 38% conceived, but only 15% conceived during actual therapy. These results suggest that GnRH might not prove to be useful for ovulation induction.

Subsequently, Knobil et al. demonstrated the importance of the method of administration (91). Knowing that GnRH secretion normally occurs in a pulsatile fashion, they were able to induce ovulation by giving GnRH in pulses to female Rhesus monkeys made GnRH deficient by radiofrequency lesions in the arcuate nucleus. Leyendecker induced ovulation in 2 women by injecting 10 mcg GnRH intravenously every 90 minutes for 17 days. A rise in FSH and LH was followed by a rise in estradiol, which led to a midcycle LH peak and ovulation (92).

GnRH can now be administered by a portable infusion pump with a pulsatile mechanism. Three models are available: Auto Syringe, Inc.,* models AS-2C and AS-BH; and Ferring GMBH,† model Zyklomat. Zyklomat has been specially designed with a pulse frequency of once every 89 minutes. This pump is worn on a belt around the waist. GnRH can also be injected by the woman under sterile conditions through a heparin lock at 2-hour intervals 9 times a day from 7:00 A.M. until 11:00 P.M. Recently, these methods have been modified with subcutaneous needle placement, which eliminates the problems of intravenous needle maintenance (93).

Dosage schedules from 1 mcg to 20 mcg per pulse at 90- to 120-minute intervals have been described. From these studies, it is apparent that there is a dose-response relationship with the preovulatory estrogen level and the midluteal phase progesterone concentration. It also appears that some individualization of doses is required. Ten to 20 mcg per pulse seems to be adequate for women with secondary amenorrhea. Little has been done to determine the optimal pulse frequency. Intervals of 62 to 120 minutes have been used with good results. In the luteal phase a GnRH pulse occurs approximately every 4 hours, so it is likely that less frequent pulses are sufficient after ovulation (94).

Results of Therapy. Results of therapy with intermittent or pulsatile administration of GnRH are still preliminary. Ovulation and conception have been reported in women with secondary amenorrhea. Fifteen of 16 cycles in 6 women treated by Shoemaker et al. were

---

* Auto Syringe, Londonderry Turnpike, Hooksett, New Hampshire.
† D-2300, Kiel, Postfach 2145, Wittland, Germany.

ovulatory and 5 of the women conceived (94). Conception occurred in the first treatment cycle of 2 women, in the third cycle of 2, and in the fifth cycle of 1. One woman had a missed abortion. Leyendecker induced ovulation in 15 women with primary or secondary hypothalamic amenorrhea and 6 pregnancies occurred (95).

Side Effects and Complications. To date, no serious complications of GnRH therapy have been reported, although Shoemaker et al. refer to an occasional patient with phlebitis, ovarian cysts in 2 patients, and 1 instance of bacteremia, which resolved after removal of a heparin lock (94). The potential for bacteremia appears to be the most significant problem associated with the intravenous administration of GnRH.

BROMOCRIPTINE.

Indications. Syndromes of amenorrhea-galactorrhea had been recognized for many years prior to the development of an assay for prolactin or polytomography and other radiographic methods of diagnosis of pituitary microadenomas. Various ovulation-inducing agents have been used with variable results. Surgical removal of small pituitary adenomas has also been recommended.

Hyperprolactinemia is found in 14% to 20% of women with secondary amenorrhea. In addition, it is occasionally noted in women with primary amenorrhea (see Chapter 19) and eumenorrheic women with luteal phase defects. High prolactin concentrations appear to disrupt the menstrual cycle by interfering with hypothalamic, pituitary, and ovarian function. Women with hyperprolactinemia have low levels of LH and estradiol. Administration of estradiol fails to elicit an FSH and LH peak, suggesting that the positive feedback center is unresponsive (96). Lowering the serum prolactin by surgery, radiation, or drug therapy usually corrects any abnormality of the menstrual cycle. Thus, the simplest approach to induction of ovulation is to lower serum prolactin levels with a dopamine agonist such as bromocriptine.

Selection of Women for Ovulation Induction. A serum prolactin concentration should be obtained from all anovulatory women. Unless the level is significantly elevated (greater than 50 ng/ml), the test should be repeated on more than 2 occasions to confirm that an actual elevation does exist. Drugs that cause hyperprolactinemia should be stopped. Tests of thyroid function should be performed since primary hypothyroidism or central hyperthyroidism can cause hyperprolactinemia. If the TSH (thyroid-stimulating hormone) concentration is elevated, therapy with thyroxine (T_4) or triiodothyronine (T_3) should be instituted until the TSH level returns to normal. If the prolactin concentration is still elevated after 3 months of therapy, bromocriptine should be added.

Radiographic assessment of the sella turcica should be performed and baseline visual fields should be obtained if a pituitary adenoma is identified. Some centers prefer surgical excision of pituitary macroadenomas before inducing ovulation (97).

Pharmacology. Bromocriptine (Parlodel®) is a derivative of an ergot alkaloid and acts as a dopamine agonist. It is rapidly and completely absorbed. Peak plasma levels are achieved in 2 to 3 hours and remain detectable in the serum for up to 24 hours (98). Bromocriptine can interact with dopamine receptors in the central nervous system and the anterior lobe of the pituitary gland. Prolactin secretion is reduced because bromocriptine inhibits the mechanisms of its release (99). Bromocriptine, which is supplied in 2.5-mg tablets, is indicated for the therapy of amenorrhea-galactorrhea to restore normal menstrual cycles, to inhibit lactation, and to induce ovulation in hyperprolactinemic infertile women.

Method of Administration. To minimize the side effects, 2.5 mg is administered daily for 1 week. If tolerated, the dosage is increased to 5 mg daily. Basal body temperature charts are maintained to determine if ovulation has occurred. If follicular activity or menstruation has not occurred in 6 to 8 weeks, the prolactin level should be repeated. The dose of bromocriptine is increased to 7.5 mg if the prolactin level is still high. Ovulation is monitored with basal body temperatures and serum progesterone levels. Bromocriptine should be stopped as soon as pregnancy is confirmed (97).

Bromocriptine has also been given in the follicular phase and stopped as soon as ovulation occurs (100). The initial dose is 2.5 mg/day for 2 weeks, then increased to 5 mg/day if ovulation has not occurred. The drug is stopped only when ovulation is confirmed by a rise in the basal temperature.

Results of Therapy. No large series of women treated with bromocriptine for infertility has been reported in the U.S. literature, although the manufacturer reports that 66% of 492 hyperprolactinemic women conceived while taking the drug. Of 187 women with amenorrhea and galactorrhea who were treated with bromocriptine, 80% resumed menses in an average of 5.7 weeks and 76% had decreased galactorrhea in an average of 6.4 weeks (101). Maximum reduction of prolactin levels occurs within 4 weeks. Women who resume ovulation should have normal rates of conception, provided no other cause of infertility is present.

With intermittent therapy, the first ovulation does not occur for 3 to 4 weeks of therapy and the first treatment cycle may be 6 or more weeks. If menstruation occurs, bromocriptine should be started again. Ovulation occurred in all 20 infertile hyperprolactinemic women treated by Bennink in this manner; 13 of these women conceived (100).

Side Effects. Fourteen percent of 226 women had a reduction in blood pressure, although only 6% had a drop exceeding 20 mm Hg (systolic) and 10 mm Hg (diastolic) (101). The most common side effects are listed in Table 6–9. At least 1 adverse reaction occurred in 68% of women and 6% of them withdrew because of symptoms.

Pregnancy Outcomes. Turkalj reported the outcome of 1,410 pregnancies in women taking bromocriptine (102). Fifty percent of women took the drug less than 4 weeks during pregnancy and 77% discontinued the drug within 6 weeks of conception. The rates of ectopic pregnancy and twin gestation were 0.9% and 1.8%, respectively. Although progesterone concentrations are significantly depressed

TABLE 6–9. Adverse Effects of Bromocriptine

EFFECT	FREQUENCY (%)
Nausea	51
Headache	18
Fatigue	8
Abdominal cramps	7
Lightheadedness	6
Vomiting	5
Nasal congestion	5
Constipation	3
Diarrhea	3

from 9 to 12 weeks of pregnancy in women with hyperprolactinemia, abortion rates (11.1%) are not increased (103).

Rates of major and minor congenital anomalies are 10 and 25 per 1,000 pregnancies, respectively. Twenty-one different anomalies have occurred and a hydrocele (with an incidence of 0.9 to 8.2/1,000) is the only malformation that appears to exceed the frequency in a normal population.

Several studies document the outcome of pregnancies induced in the presence of radiologically demonstrable pituitary tumors (104–106). Eighty-one of Gemzell's patients had an untreated prolactin-secreting tumor less than 10 mm in diameter and 65 were treated with bromocriptine. One woman developed headaches and another diabetes insipidus. Both were managed conservatively and delivered at term (105).

Twenty-one women with a prolactin-secreting macroadenoma reported by Gemzell (105) conceived during bromocriptine therapy. One woman developed headaches and 3 developed headaches and visual defects. The women with headaches and visual defects were treated during pregnancy—one with bromocriptine and 2 with hypophysectomy.

Complications during pregnancy occurred in 3% of women with a microadenoma and 19% with a macroadenoma who were treated with bromocriptine. Tumor expansion has not been reported in pregnant women with hyperprolactinemia but normal radiographic studies prior to pregnancy (97).

Use in Pregnancy. Women with hyperprolactinemia require careful observation during pregnancy (97). Those with evidence of a tumor should have monthly visual field examinations and should be questioned about the presence of headaches. Women with no evidence of tumor prior to pregnancy can be monitored by asking if any symptoms occur.

Pregnant women who develop signs of tumor expansion (i.e., visual field changes or diabetes insipidus) have been treated with bromocriptine with a resultant reduction in tumor size (107).

The concentrations of placental steroid and protein hormones are not affected by bromocriptine, although the pregnancy-induced rise in maternal prolactin concentration does not occur (108). Bromocriptine crosses the placenta and fetal concentrations of prolactin are decreased, although amniotic fluid prolactin concentrations are normal. Fetal development is normal (108).

Prophylactic use of bromocriptine during pregnancy has been advocated for women with a pituitary macroadenoma (109). This recommendation is based on the uncomplicated outcome in 4 women treated throughout pregnancy that had been induced with bromocriptine.

GLUCOCORTICOIDS.

Indications. Prior to the availability of clomiphene, glucocorticoids were used to induce ovulation and results were variable. Indications included both anovulatory women with mildly elevated 24-hour urinary 17-ketosteroid excretion and those with hirsutism or congenital adrenal hyperplasia (110). Others used glucocorticoids for any anovulatory woman (111). Best results are clearly obtained in women with carefully characterized adrenal disorders such as congenital adrenal hyperplasia of neonatal or adult onset, and women with hypoadrenalism. In addition to women with congenital adrenal hyperplasia who have basal elevations in 17-hydroxyprogesterone concentrations, a small group of hirsute women have been identified with an exaggerated response to ACTH stimulation who should be included in this category (112,113). Suppression of serum androgen levels with glucocorticoids during clomiphene therapy of women with polycystic ovarian disease may increase pregnancy rates (114,115).

Pharmacology. Elevated levels of serum androgens suppress gonadotropin secretion by suppressing hypothalamic GnRH secretion. This may occur only after the androgens are converted to estrogens (116,117). In addition, acyclic production of estrone in extraglandular tissues exerts a positive feedback on the pituitary and perpetuates a state of chronic anovulation. In subjects with congenital adrenal hyperplasia (neonatal or adult onset), excess androgen secretion is most commonly the result of 21-hydroxylase or 11-hydroxylase deficiency. Lower secretion rates of cortisol lead to increased ACTH secretion, which stimulates the synthesis and secretion of androgenic intermediates. Glucocorticoids suppress ACTH and subsequent adrenal androgen synthesis.

In women with an increased 17-ketosteroid excretion or dehydroepiandrosterone sulfate (DHEAS) concentration in association with a polycystic ovarylike syndrome, glucocorticoid suppression of adrenal androgen secretion may result in the return of ovulation. As an adjunct to clomiphene therapy, glucocorticoids clearly suppress adrenal production of androstendione and testosterone, with a resultant decrease in the circulating testosterone concentration (114).

Method of Administration. The primary ACTH surge is nocturnal so suppressive doses of glucocorticoids should be administered at bedtime to women with congenital adrenal hyperplasia or polycystic ovaries. If an increased dose is required, it should be given in the morning. Equivalent dosage regimens for glucocorticoid replacement are:

Prednisone—5 mg at night and 2.5 mg in the morning (112)

Cortisone acetate—25 mg three times daily (117)

Dexamethasone—0.25 mg to 0.75 mg twice daily (117)

Therapy must be monitored to ensure adequate adrenal suppression. Richards et al. have suggested that serum concentrations of testosterone are more predictive of normal menstrual function than are pregnanetriol or 17-hydroxyprogesterone concentrations (117). The dose of glucocorticoid is increased until testosterone levels return to normal. If women fail to ovulate after 3 months, clomiphene should be added.

Results of Therapy. Kotz and Hermann have summarized reported pregnancy rates (116). The number of women in these reports was small. Jefferies reported a 67% pregnancy rate with small doses of cortisone (5 mg 3 times a day) (111). Similar rates were achieved regardless of the level of 17-ketosteroid excretion. Klingensmith et al. reported a pregnancy rate of 55% in 18 women with congenital adrenal hyperplasia followed from the ages of 1 to 6 months (118). In another report, 33% of women with partial congenital adrenal hyperplasia conceived; this figure became 91% when corrected for other fertility factors (112). Raj and colleagues reported that 65% of women with polycystic ovaries, type II, resumed ovulation with prednisone alone (113). Of these, 17% conceived.

Complications. Low or replacement doses of glucocorticoids rarely cause clinical Cushingoid changes. Adrenal suppression is transient and doses can be discontinued without tapering. Decreased adrenal reserve has been reported, but this was of no clinical significance. No fetal complications were noted with low-dose glucocorticoid therapy during the first half of pregnancy (119).

ESTROGEN AND ESTROGEN/PROGESTERONE. Prior to the availability of other drugs, estrogen or estrogen plus progesterone were used to induce ovulation. Of 352 oligomenorrheic women treated with a placebo, 142 ovulated (40.3%) and 68 conceived (19.3%) (120). Presumably, these 142 women were oligoovulatory. Of the remaining women (presumably anovulatory), only 18.4% ovulated with estrogen and progestin therapy, whereas 27.5% ovulated with clomiphene (a very low ovulation rate for this drug).

Injection of estradiol benzoate has been demonstrated to induce an LH surge (3,4). In certain women with developing preovulatory follicles, ovulation occasionally occurs. Estrogen may also increase the pituitary response to GnRH in hypoestrogenic women.

The popularity of these medications has declined with the appearance of drugs with more predictable success rates.

Ovarian Wedge Resection

INDICATIONS. Surgical therapy for correction of symptoms of polycystic ovarian disease was advocated by Stein in 1939 (121). Regular menses and fertility frequently resulted. The introduction of clomiphene in 1961 has replaced wedge resection in all such women except those who are resistant to clomiphene and who have an erratic response to gonadotropins.

MECHANISM OF ACTION. At least one third to one half of the ovarian cortex is removed to reduce the ovaries to normal size. Originally, disruption of the thickened capsule was thought to be the mechanism for restoration of ovulation. There is now increasing evidence that hormonal alterations are responsible for the effectiveness of wedge resection (122–125). Serum androstenedione concentrations are decreased immediately postoperatively, but eventually return to preoperative levels. Serum testosterone levels are persistently reduced. The mean concentration of testosterone was 65 ng/dl prior to wedge resection and 45 ng/dl at 6 to 16 months following wedge resection (122). Increased basal LH concentrations and LH response to GnRH return to normal after surgery. The variation in response, however, precludes statistical significance.

RESULTS OF THERAPY. Vejlsted and Albrechtsen reported a return of normal menses in 9% and pregnancy in 25% of women (125). Others have reported ovulatory menses in 72% to 80% and pregnancy in 42% to 63% (126,127).

COMPLICATIONS. The primary reported complications of wedge resection are postoperative adhesions and ovarian failure. All women with persistent infertility after wedge resection evaluated by Toaff had significant peritubal and periovarian adhesions (126). Buttram found significant adhesions in 34% of 150 women with persistent infertility (127).

Surgery is recommended only for women resistant to medical management. If performed, the most meticulous microsurgical technique is required.

Problems in Ovulation Induction

CONFIRMATION OF OVULATION. The ability to confirm ovulation and assess luteal function is of paramount importance to the management of women taking ovulation-inducing drugs.

Methods Based on Serum Progesterone Secretion. Until recently, only methods based on progesterone secretion by the corpus luteum have been available. These confirm luteinization but not ovum release. The 3 primary methods are basal temperature, endometrial biopsy, and measurement of serum progesterone concentrations.

The basal temperature is most useful to pinpoint the approximate time of ovulation and to assess the length of the luteal phase. It does not confirm adequate luteal function. The exact relationship of the temperature nadir and rise to the LH peak and ovum release remains controversial (128).

Endometrial biopsy for confirmation of ovulation has been popular in past years. However, the technique is a painful and expensive means to confirm ovulation, and Jacobson and Marshall noted significantly reduced conception rates in biopsied cycles of hMG/hCG-treated women (129).

The use of luteal phase serum progesterone concentrations to confirm ovulation is becoming increasingly common. Physician visits are not required and numerical results are reproducible in different laboratories. Serum progesterone concentrations greater than 3 ng/ml in the midluteal phase of regularly cycling women were reported by Israel et al. (130). We have reported midluteal serum progesterone concentrations greater than 10 ng/ml in all spontaneous conception cycles (131). This value is similar to those reported by Swyer et al. (20) and Hull and co-workers (132). These authors also confirmed our observation that higher progesterone levels (we use 15 ng/ml) are required in clomiphene- or gonadotropin-induced cycles. We measure progesterone on day 21 of clomiphene cycles or 1 week after injection of hCG in gonadotropin-induced cycles.

An endometrial biopsy performed by a skilled person is still required for a thorough evaluation of the luteal phase if pregnancy does not occur. The biopsy should be taken 2 to 3 days prior to expected menses.

Physical Techniques. Both follicular rupture and luteinization of an unruptured ovarian follicle have been detected by ultrasound (133). At present, pregnancy or visualization of an ovarian stigma at laparoscopy are the only direct proof of ovum release.

MANAGEMENT OF WOMEN WHO OVULATE BUT DO NOT CONCEIVE. From a life table analysis of results with clomiphene and other ovulation-inducing drugs, fecundability rates of 12% to 25% per cycle should occur for women who ovulate. Thus, 35% to 65% of women should conceive within 3 months and 60% to 85% within 6 months (134). Monthly fecundability rates remain constant up to 10 ovulatory cycles. Ovulatory women who do not conceive should be reevaluated at 3-month intervals by repeating a postcoital test and a serum progesterone. If no hysterosalpingogram has been done, it is required now. If these are normal, ovulation induction is continued. A woman with abnormal mucus should receive supplemental estrogen. If the progesterone concentration is low, the Clomid dose should be increased. If the serum testosterone concentration is greater than 90 ng/dl, prednisone 5 mg at bedtime is begun. After 6 months, diagnostic laparoscopy should be performed. If all studies are normal, clomiphene should be stopped after 1 year and hMG after 6 to 8 cycles.

POLYCYSTIC OVARIAN DISEASE. Resistance to clomiphene in women with polycystic ovarian disease is occasionally reduced by ancillary prednisone therapy (111,112). Women who do not ovulate on clomiphene are often very sensitive to hMG therapy and Raj et al. (135) and Kamrava et al. (136) reported improved results with supplemental FSH or FSH plus hCG. Bromocriptine has been reported to suppress LH and induce spontaneous ovulation in women with polycystic ovaries (137).

Other Uses for Ovulation-Inducing Drugs

LUTEAL PHASE DYSFUNCTION. Both clomiphene and hMG have been used to enhance follicular maturation and the subsequent luteal phase (131,138). Bromocriptine has also been used to improve the luteal phase of women with a slight increase in prolactin concentration.

POOR QUALITY CERVICAL MUCUS. Sher has recommended the use of hMG to improve cervical mucus in ovulating women. Preovulatory estrogen concentrations greater than 1000 pg/ml are recommended (139).

IN VITRO FERTILIZATION. Both clomiphene and hMG are now being used regularly to induce the development of multiple preovulatory follicles. This has increased the number of ova available for fertilization and has resulted in significantly increased success rates (140). (See chapter 13.)

REFERENCES

1. Gemzell CS, Diczfalusy E, Tillinger G. Clinical effect of human pituitary follicle-stimulating hormone (FSH). J Clin Endocrinol Metab 1958;18:1333–1348.
2. Greenblatt RB, Barfield WE, Jungck EJ, Ray AW. Induction of ovulation with MRL 141. JAMA 1961;178:101–104.
3. Shaw RW, Butt WR, London DR, Marshall J. The oestrogen provocation test: a method of assessing the hypothalamic pituitary axis in patients with amenorrhea. Clin Endocrinol (Oxf) 1975;4:267–276.
4. Weiss G, Nachtigall LE, Ganguly M. Induction of an LH surge with estradiol benzoate. Obstet Gynecol 1976;47:415–418.
5. Merrill Company product information brochure, 1972.
6. Schulz KD, Holzel F, Bettendorf G. Uptake and distribution of ^{14}C-clomiphene citrate in different organs of newborn female guinea pigs. Acta Endocrinol (Copenh) 1972;68:605–613.
7. Hahnel R, Twaddle E, Ratajezah T. Influence of synthetic anti-estrogens on the binding of tritiated estradiol by cytosols of human uterus and human breast carcinoma. J Steroid Biochem 1973;4:687–695.
8. Ginsburg M, Madusky NJ, Morris ID, Thomas PJ. Specificity of oestrogen receptor in brain, pituitary and uterus. Br J Pharmacol 1977;59:397–402.
9. Sutherland RL. Estrogen antagonists in chick oviduct. Endocrinology 1981;109:2061–2068.
10. Clark JH, Peck EJ, Anderson JN. Oestrogen receptors and antagonism of steroid hormone action. Nature 1974;251:446–448.
11. Notides AC. Binding affinity and specificity of the estrogen receptor of the rat uterus and anterior pituitary. Endocrinology 1970; 87:987–992.
12. Vaitukaitis JL, Bermudez JA, Cargille CM, Lipsett MB, Ross GT. New evidence for an anti-estrogenic action of clomiphene in women. J Clin Endocrinol 1971;32:503–508.
13. Ross GT, Cargille CM, Lipsett MB, et al. Pituitary and gonadal hormones in women during spontaneous and induced ovulatory cycles. Recent Prog Horm Res 1970;26:1–62.
14. Wu CH, Prazak LM. Endocrine basis for ovulation induction. Clin Obstet Gynecol 1974;17:65–78.
15. Hsueh AJW, Erickson GF, Yen SSC. Sensitization of pituitary cells to LHRH by clomiphene citrate in vitro. Nature 1978;273:57–59.
16. Hammerstein J. Mode of action of clomiphene I. Inhibitory effect of clomiphene on the formation of progesterone from acetate-1-^{14}C by human corpus luteum slices *in vitro*. Acta Endocrinol 1969;60:635–644.
17. Marut EL, Hodgen GD. Antiestrogenic action of high dose clomiphene in primates: pituitary augmentation with ovarian attentuation. Fertil Steril 1982;38:100–104.
18. Zhuang LZ, Adashi EY, Hsueh AJW. Direct enhancement of gonadotropin-stimulated ovarian estrogen biosynthesis by estrogen and clomiphene citrate. Endocrinology 1982; 110:2219–2221.
19. Rust LA, Israel R, Mishell DR. An individualized graduated therapeutic regime for clomiphene citrate. Am J Obstet Gynecol 1974;120:785–790.
20. Swyer GIM, Radwanska E, McGarrigle HHG. Plasma estradiol and progesterone estimation for the monitoring of induction of ovulation with clomiphene and chorionic gonadotropin. Br J Obstet Gynecol 1975;82:794–804.
21. Garcia J, Jones GS, Wentz AC. The use of clomiphene citrate. Fertil Steril 1977;28:707–717.
22. Hammond MG, Halme JK, Talbert LM. Factors affecting the pregnancy rate in

clomiphene citrate induction of ovulation. Obstet Gynecol 1983;62:196–202.
23. Lobo RA, Granger LR, Davajan V, Mishell DR. An extended regimen of clomiphene in women unresponsive to standard therapy. Fertil Steril 1982;37:762–766.
24. Shepard MK, Balmaceda JP, Leija CG. Relationship of weight to successful induction of ovulation with clomiphene citrate. Fertil Steril 1979;32:641–645.
25. Kase N, Mroueh A, Olson LE. Clomid therapy for anovulatory infertility. Am J Obstet Gynecol 1967;98:1037–1042.
26. Karow MG, Payne SA. Pregnancy after clomiphene citrate treatment. Fertil Steril 1968;19:351–362.
27. MacGregor AH, Johnson JE, Bunde CA. Further clinical experience with clomiphene citrate. Fertil steril 1968;19:616–622.
28. Gorlitsky GA, Kase NG, Speroff L. Ovulation and pregnancy rates with clomiphene citrate. Obstet Gynecol 1978;51:265–269.
29. Gysler M, March LM, Mishell DR, Bailey EJ. A decade's experience with an individualized clomiphene treatment regime including its effect on the post coital test. Fertil Steril 1982;37:161–167.
30. Lamb EJ, Colliflower WW, Williams JW. Endometrial histology and conception rates after clomiphene. Obstet Gynecol 1972;39:389–396.
31. Barbosa J, Seal US, Doe RP. Antiestrogens and plasma proteins. I. Clomiphene and its isomers. J Clin Endocrinol Metab 1973;36:666–678.
32. Marshall JC, Anderson DC, Burke CW, Garbo-Teles A, Fraser TR. Clomiphene in men: increase in cortisol, LH, testosterone and steroid binding globulins. J Endocrinol 1972;53:261–276.
33. Hammond MG, Radwanska E, Talbert LM. Effect of clomiphene citrate on corticosteroid-binding globulin and serum progesterone levels during ovulation induction. Fertil Steril 1980;33:383–386.
34. Van Campenhout JV, Simard R, Leduc B. Antiestrogenic effect of clomiphene in the human being. Fertil Steril 1968;19:700–706.
35. Graff M. Suppression of cervical mucus during clomiphene therapy. Fertil Steril 1971;22:209–215.
36. Lamb EJ, Guderian AM. Clinical effects of clomiphene in anovulation. Obstet Gynecol 1966;28:505–512.
37. Taubert HD, Dericks-Tan JSE. High dose estrogens do not interfere with the ovulation-inducing effect of clomiphene. Fertil Steril 1976;27:375–382.
38. Poliak A, Smith JJ, Romney SL. Clinical evaluation of clomiphene; clomiphene and hCG; and clomiphene hCG and estrogen in anovulatory cycles. Fertil Steril 1973;24:921–925.
39. Insler V, Zakut H, Serr DM. Cyclic pattern and pregnancy rate following combined clomiphene-estrogen therapy. Obstet Gynecol 1973;41:602–607.
40. Gorwill RH, Steele HD, Sarda IR. Heterotopic columnar epithelium and adenosis in the vagina of the mouse after neonatal treatment with clomiphene. Am J Obstet Gynecol 1982;144:529–532.
41. McCormack S, Clark JH. Clomid administration to rats causes abnormalities of the reproductive tracts in offspring and mothers. Science 1979;204:629–631.
42. Hack M, Lunenfeld B. Influence of hormone induction of ovulation on the fetus and newborn. Pediatr Adolesc Endocrinol 1979;5:191–212.
43. Correy JF, Marsden DE, Schokman FCM. The outcome of pregnancy resulting from clomiphene induced ovulation. Aust NZ J Obstet Gynaecol 1982;22:18–21.
44. Ahlgren M, Kallen B, Rannevik G. Outcome of pregnancy after Clomid therapy. Acta Obstet Gynecol Scand 1976;53:371–375.
45. Adashi E, Rock JA, Sapp KC, Martin EJ, Wentz AC, Jones GS. Gestational outcome of clomiphene related conceptions. Fertil Steril 1979;31:620–626.
46. Oakley GP, Flynt JW. Increased prevalence of Down's syndrome (mongolism) among offspring of women treated with ovulation inducing agents. Teratology 1972;(Abs. 5):264.
47. Dyson JL, Kohler HG. Anencephaly and ovulation stimulation. Lancet 1973;1:1256–1257.
48. Biale Y, Leventhal H, Altaras M, Ben-Aderet N. Anencephaly and clomiphene induced pregnancy. Acta Obstet Gynecol Scand 1978;57:483–484.
49. Jansen RPS. Spontaneous abortion incidence in the treatment of infertility. Am J Obstet Gynecol 1982;143:451–473.
50. Boue JG, Boue A. Increased frequency of chromosomal anomalies in abortions after induced ovulation. Lancet 1973;1:679–680.
51. Goldfarb AF, Morales A, Rakoff AE, Protos P. Critical review of 160 clomiphene-related pregnancies. Obstet Gynecol 1968;31:341–345.
52. Donini P, Puzzuoli D, Montezemiola R. Purification of gonadotropins from human menopausal urine. Acta Endocrinol (Copenh) 1964;45:321–328.
53. Roos P. Human follicle-stimulating hormone. Acta Endocrinol (Copenh) 1968;131:1–93.

54. Erickson GF. Normal ovarian function. Clin Obstet Gynecol 1978;21:31–52.
55. Schenken RS, Hodgen GD. FSH ovarian hyperstimulation in monkeys. Society for Gynecologic Investigation 1982;(Abs. 282):163.
56. Johansson EDB, Gemzell C. The relation between plasma progesterone and total urinary oestrogens following induction of ovulation in women. Acta Endocrinol (Copenh) 1969;62:89–97.
57. Rizkallah T, Gurpide E, Vande Wiele RL. Metabolism of hCG in man. J Clin Endocrinol Metab 1969;29:92–100.
58. Thompson CR, Hansen LM. Pergonal: a summary of clinical experience in the induction of ovulation and pregnancy. Fertil Steril 1970;21:844–853.
59. Gemzell C, Roos P. Pregnancies following treatment with human gonadotropins. Am J Obstet Gynecol 1966;94:490–496.
60. Crooke AC, Butt WR, Palmer RF, Norris R, Edwards RL, Anson CJ. Clinical trial of human gonadotropins. Part I. J Obstet Gynaecol Br Commonw 1963;70:604–635.
61. Crooke AC, Butt WR, Palmer RF, et al. Clinical trials of human gonadotropins. Part II. J Obstet Gynaecol Br Commonw 1964;71:571–583.
62. Butler JK. Time course of urinary estrogen excretion after various schemes of therapy with Pergonal. Proc Roy Soc Med 1969;62:34–37.
63. Radwanska E, Hammond J, Hammond M, Smith P. Current experience with a standardized method of HMG/HCG administration. Fertil Steril 1980;33:510–513.
64. Insler V, Melmed H, Eden E, Ser DM, Lunenfeld B. Comparison of various methods used in the monitoring of gonadotropin therapy. In: Beltendorf G, Insler V, eds. Clinical application of human gonadotropins. Stuttgart: Georg Thieme Verlag, 1970:87–101.
65. Taymor ML, Sturgis SH, Leiberman BL, Goldstein DP. Induction of ovulation with human postmenopausal gonadotropin. Fertil Steril 1966;17:731–735.
66. Gemzell CA. Experience with the induction of ovulation. J Reprod Med 1978;21:205–207.
67. Lunenfeld B. Gonadotropins. In: Greenblatt R, ed. Induction of ovulation. Philadelphia: Lea & Febiger, 1979:9–34.
68. Schwartz M, Jewelewicz R, Dyrenfurth I, Tropper, P, Vande Wiele RL. Use of HMG/HCG for induction of ovulation. Am J Obstet Gynecol 1980;138:801–807.
69. Karam KS, Taymor ML, Berger ML. Estrogen monitoring and the prevention of ovarian overstimulation during gonadotropin therapy. Am J Obstet Gynecol 1973;115:972–977.
70. March CM. Therapeutic regimens and monitoring techniques for human menopausal gonadotropin administration. J Reprod Med 1978;21:198–204.
71. Haning RV, Levin RM, Berhman HR, Kase NG, Speroff L. Plasma estradiol window and urinary estriol glucuronide determinations for monitoring menotropin induction of ovulation. Obstet Gynecol 1979;54:442–447.
72. Queenan JT, O'Brien GD, Bains LM, Simpson J, Collins WP, Campbell S. Ultrasound scanning of ovaries to detect ovulation in women. Fertil Steril 1980;34:99–105.
73. O'Herlihy C, Evans JH, Brown JB, de Crespigny LH, Robinson HP. Use of ultrasound in monitoring ovulation induction with human pituitary gonadotropin. Obstet Gynecol 1982;60:577–582.
74. Schwartz M, Jewelewicz R. Use of gonadotropins for induction of ovulation. Fertil Steril 1981;35:3–12.
75. Lunenfeld B, Eshkol A. Induction of ovulation with gonadotropin. In: Rolland R, van Hall EV, Hillier SG, eds. Follicular maturation and ovulation. Amsterdam: Experta Medica, 1982:361–372.
76. Healy DL, Kovacs GJ, Pepperell RJ, Burger HG. A normal cumulative conception rate after HPG. Fertil Steril 1980;34:341–345.
77. Tsapoulis AD, Zourlas PA, Comninos AC. Observations on 320 infertile patients treated with human gonadotropins. Fertil Steril 1978;29:492–495.
78. Goldfarb AF, Schlaff S, Mansi ML. Life table analysis of pregnancy yield in fixed low dose menotropin therapy for patients in whom clomiphene failed to induce ovulation. Fertil Steril 1982;37:639–644.
79. Ellis JD, Williamson JG. Factors influencing the pregnancy and complication rates with human menopausal gonadotropin therapy. Br J Obstet Gynaecol 1975;82:52–57.
80. Spadoni LR, Cox DW, Smith DC. Use of human menopausal gonadotropin for the induction of ovulation. Am J Obstet Gynecol 1974;120:988–993.
81. Schenken JG, Weinstein D. Ovarian hyperstimulation syndrome: a current survey. Fertil Steril 1978;30:225–268.
82. Taymor ML, Berger MJ, Thompson IE. Induction of ovulation with gonadotropins: prevention of ovarian hyperstimulation. In: International symposium on advances in chemistry, biology, immunology of gonadotropins. New York: Academic Press, 1974:512–521.

83. Rabau E, David A, Serr DM, Mashiach S, Lunenfeld B. HMG for anovulation and sterility. Am J Obstet Gynecol 1967;98:92–98.
84. Kistner RW. Use of clomiphene citrate, human chorionic gonadotropin and human menopausal gonadotropin for induction of ovulation in human female. Fertil Steril 1966;17:569–583.
85. March CM, Tredway DR, Mishell DR. Effect of clomiphene on amount and duration of HMG therapy. Am J Obstet Gynecol 1976;125:699–704.
86. Jarrel J, McInnes R, Crooke R, Arronet G. Observations on the combination of clomiphene citrate-HMG-HCG in the management of anovulation. Fertil Steril 1981;35:634–637.
87. Factrel product profile, Ayerst Laboratories, 1983.
88. Schally AV, Kastin AJ, Arimua A. The hypothalamus and reproduction. Am J Obstet Gynecol 1975;122:847–862.
89. Nillius SJ, Wide L. GnRH treatment for induction of follicular maturation and ovulation in amenorrheic women with anorexia nervosa. Br Med J 1975;3:405–408.
90. Hammond CB, Wiebe RH, Haney AF, Yancy SG. Ovulation induction with LHRH in amenorrheic, infertile women. Am J Obstet Gynecol 1979;135:924–939.
91. Knobil E, Plant TM, Wildt L, Belchetz PF, Marshall G. Control of the rhesus monkey menstrual cycle: permissive role of hypothalamic gonadotropin-releasing hormone. Science 1980;207:1371–1373.
92. Leyendecker G. Pathophysiology of hypothalamic ovarian failure. Eur J Obstet Gynaecol Reprod Biol 1979;9:175–186.
93. Shaw R. Personal communication.
94. Shoemaker J, Simons AHM, Burger CM, Delemarre HA, van Kessel H. Induction of ovulation with LHRH. In: Rolland R, ed. Follicular maturation and ovulation. Amsterdam: Excerpta Medica, 1982:373–388.
95. Leyendecker G, Struve T, Nocke W, Hansmann M, Plotz EJ. Induction of ovulation with chronic intermittent administration of LHRH in women with hypothalamic amenorrhea. Endocrine Society 1980;(Abs. 262):140.
96. Glass MR, Shaw RW, Butt WR, Logan-Edwards R, London DR. An abnormality of estrogen feedback in amenorrhea-galactorrhea. Br Med J 1975;3:274–275.
97. Pepperell RJ. Prolactin and reproduction. Fertil Steril 1981;35:267–274.
98. Mehta AE, Tolis G. Pharmacology of bromocriptine in health and disease. Drugs 1979;17:313–325.
99. Hausler A, Rohr HP, Marbach P, Fluckiger E. Changes in prolactin secretion in lactating rats assessed by correlative morphometric and biochemical methods. J Ultrastruct Res 1978;64:74–84.
100. Bennink HJTC. Intermittent bromocriptine treatment for the induction of ovulation in hyperprolactinemic patients. Fertil Steril 1979;31:267–272.
101. Cuellar FG. Bromocriptine mesylate in the management of amenorrhea/galactorrhea associated with hyperprolactinemia. Obstet Gynecol 1980;55:278–284.
102. Turkalj I, Braun P, Krupp P. Surveillance of bromocriptine in pregnancy. JAMA 1982;247:1589–1591.
103. Thomas CMG, Corbey RS, Rolland R. Assessment of estradiol and progesterone serum levels throughout pregnancy in normal women and in women who conceived after bromocriptine. Acta Endocrinol (Copenh) 1977;86:405–414.
104. Magyar DM, Marshall JR. Pituitary tumors and pregnancy. Am J Obstet Gynecol 1978;132:739–751.
105. Gemzell C, Wang CF. Outcome of pregnancy in women with pituitary adenoma. Fertil Steril 1979;31:363–372.
106. Bergh T, Nillius SH, Wide L. Clinical course and outcome of pregnancies in amenorrheic women with hyperprolactinemia and pituitary tumors. Br Med J 1978;1:875–880.
107. McGregor AM, Scanlon MF, Hall K, Cook DB, Hall R. Reduction in size of a pituitary tumor with bromocriptine therapy. New Engl J Med 1979;300:291–293.
108. Bigazzi M, Ronga R, Lancranjan I. A pregnancy in an acromegalic woman during bromocriptine treatment: effects on growth hormone and prolactin in the maternal, fetal and amnionic compartments. J Clin Endocrinol Metab 1979;48:9–12.
109. Canales ES, Garcia IC, Ruiz JE, Zarate A. Bromocriptine as a prophylactic therapy in prolactinemia during pregnancy. Fertil Steril 1981;36:524–528.
110. Jones GES, Howard JE, Langford H. The use of cortisone in follicular phase disturbances. Fertil Steril 1953;4:49–62.
111. Jefferies W McK. Further experience with small doses of cortisone and related steroids in infertility associated with ovarian dysfunction. Fertil Steril 1960;11:100–108.
112. Birnbaum MD, Rose LI. The partial adrenocortical hydroxylase deficiency syndrome in infertile women. Fertil Steril 1979;32:536–541.
113. Raj SG, Thompson IE, Berger MJ, Taymor

ML. Clinical aspects of the polycystic ovary syndrome. Obstet Gynecol 1977;49:552–556.
114. Radwanska E, Sloan C. Serum testosterone levels in infertile women. Int J Fertil 1979;24:176–181.
115. Lawrence DM, McGarrigle HH, Radwanska E, Swyer GIM. Plasma testosterone and androstenedione levels during monitored induction of ovulation in infertile women with "simple" amenorrhea and with the polycystic ovary syndrome. Clin Endocrinol 1976;5:609–618.
116. Kotz HL, Hermann W. A review of the endocrine induction of human ovulation. IV. Cortisone. Fertil Steril 1961;12:299–308.
117. Richards GE, Grumbach MM, Kaplan SL, Conte FA. The effect of long acting glucocorticoids on menstrual abnormalities in patients with virilizing congenital adrenal hyperplasia. J Clin Endocrinol Metab 1978;47:1208–1215.
118. Klingensmith GJ, Garcia SC, Jones HW, Migeon CJ, Blizzard RM. Glucocorticoid treatment of girls with congenital adrenal hyperplasia: effects on height, sexual maturation and fertility. J Pediatr 1977;90:996–1004.
119. Lee F, Nelson N, Faiman C. Low-dose corticoid treatment for anovulation: effect on fetal weight. Obstet Gynecol 1982;60:314–317.
120. Evans J, Townsend L. The induction of ovulation. Am J Obstet Gynecol 1976;125:321–327.
121. Stein IF, Cohen MR. Surgical treatment of bilateral polycystic ovaries—amenorrhea and sterility. Am J Obstet Gynecol 1939;38:465–480.
122. Valkov IM, Dokumov SI. Effect of ovarian wedge resection for the Stein-Leventhal syndrome on FSH, LH, estradiol and testosterone and on the pituitary response to LHRH. Br J Obstet Gynaecol 1977;84:539–542.
123. Mahesh VB, Toledo SPA, Mattar E. Hormone levels following wedge resection in polycystic ovary syndrome. Obstet Gynecol 1978;51:645–695.
124. Judd HL, Rigg LA, Anderson DC, Yen SSC. Effects of ovarian wedge resection on gonadotropin and steroid levels in polycystic ovary syndrome. J Clin Endocrinol Metab 1976;43:347–355.
125. Vejlsted H, Albrechtsen R. Biochemical and clinical effects of ovarian wedge resection in the polycystic ovary syndrome. Obstet Gynecol 1976;47:575–580.
126. Toaff R, Toaff ME, Peyser MR. Infertility following wedge resection of ovaries. Am J Obstet Gynecol 1976;124:92–96.
127. Buttram VC, Vaquero C. Post ovarian wedge resection adhesive disease. Fertil Steril 1975;26:874–876.
128. Brauman JE. Basal body temperature: unreliable method of ovulation detection. Fertil Steril 1981;36:729–733.
129. Jacobson AJ, Marshall JR. Detrimental effect of endometrial biopsies on pregnancy rate following HMG/HCG induced ovulation. Fertil Steril 1980;33:602–604.
130. Israel R, Mishell DR, Stone SC, Thorneycroft, IH, Moyer DL. Single luteal phase serum progesterone assay as an indication of ovulation. Am J Obstet Gynecol 1972;112:1043–1046.
131. Hammond MG, Talbert LM. Clomiphene citrate therapy of infertile women with low luteal phase progesterone levels. Obstet Gynecol 1982;59:275–279.
132. Hull MGR, Savage PE, Bromham DR, Ismail AAA, Morris AF. Value of a single serum progesterone measurement in the midluteal phase as a criterion of potentially fertile cycle derived from treated and untreated conception cycles. Fertil Steril 1982;37:355–360.
133. Coulam CB, Hill LM, Breckle R. Ultrasonic evidence for luteinization of unruptured preovulatory follicles. Fertil Steril 1982;37:524–529.
134. Cramer DW, Walker AM, Schiff I. Statistical methods in evaluating the outcome of infertility therapy. Fertil Steril 1979;32:80–86.
135. Raj SG, Berger MJ, Grimes EM, Taymor ML. Use of gonadotropins for the induction of ovulation in women with polycystic ovary disease. Fertil Steril 1977;28:1280–1284.
136. Kamrava M, Siebel MM, Berger MJ, Thompson IE, Taymor ML. Reversal of persistent anovulation in polycystic ovarian disease by administration of chronic low dose FSH. Fertil Steril 1982;37:520–523.
137. Siebel MM, Taymor ML. New insights into PCO—therapeutic implications. Trans Am Gynecol Obstet Soc 1982;1:145–154.
138. Quagluarello J, Weiss G. Clomiphene citrate in the management of infertility associated with shortened luteal phase. Fertil Steril 1979;31:373–377.
139. Sher G, Katz M. Inadequate cervical mucus—a cause of "idiopathic" infertility. Fertil Steril 1976;27:886–891.
140. Jones HW, Jones GS, Andrews MC, et al. The program for in vitro fertilization at Norfolk. Fertil Steril 1982;38:14–21.

The Cervix in Reproduction

Gilbert G. Haas, Jr. and Phillip C. Galle

The uterine cervix must perform the dichotomous role of providing a barrier to unwanted microbiologic invasion while permitting periovulatory penetration of sperm. On the one hand, the cervical mucus must provide a biochemical milieu that is conducive to spermatozoal survival while inhibiting the passage of abnormal or senescent sperm. Similarly, the immune response of the cervix must be prompt in the face of infection, but it must be damped when presented with equally foreign spermatozoal antigens. Cervical factor infertility occurs when this delicate functional balance goes awry.

Anatomy and Embryology

The character of the cervical epithelium and the increased proportion of fibrous tissue in the cervical stroma distinguishes the thick-walled cylindrical cervix from the uterine corpus. The endocervix is bounded by the portio vaginalis (or ectocervix) and the internal os. The mucosa of the endocervical canal is arranged in a herringbone pattern of ridges called plicae palmatae or arbor vitae (1). These ridges are composed of villous tongues of ciliated columnar epithelium intermingled with nonciliated secretory cells (2). The cilia beat toward the vagina and propel secreted mucus from the external os (3). Although the endocervical canal was once thought to be lined by glands, it has been demonstrated conclusively that the glandlike structures are actually ductless crypts (4).

In a woman of reproductive age, stratified squamous epithelium can be found on the ectocervix from the vagina to the squamocolumnar junction. Prior to adolescence and puberty, however, the ectocervix is covered with tall columnar epithelium. The combined influences of puberty, pregnancy, and sexual activity convert the columnar epithelium to a metaplastic stratified squamous variety. This probably occurs because each of these conditions is associated with an increase in vaginal acidity (1). The erythematous appearance of the ectocervix covered with columnar epithelium can be attributed to the fact that only a single layer of cells overlies the subepithelial capillaries (1). Columnar epithelium is probably less capable of protecting the cervix from infection, and it is more prone to bleed after mild trauma (either coitally induced or following a Pap smear or postcoital retrieval of mucus). Before colposcopy, chronic cervicitis was thought to be the etiology for any increased redness of the cervix. Since bacteriologic examination of "mucopus" frequently yields a normal flora or a sterile culture (5), the infected appearance of the mucus is probably due to the postovulatory influence of progesterone (1). Moreover, "chronic cervicitis" in most women may simply represent the cervix's response to coitally transmitted antigens (6). Singer and Jordan (1) have suggested that leukocytic infiltration of mucus is not usually the result of infection, but is the mechanism for clearing debris or sperm, or an immune response to seminal antigens. They have also noted that the changes that are usually labeled as cervical erosion are probably a result of squamous metaplasia (the replacement of columnar epithelium by squamous cells) that continuously occurs at the transition zone of the cervix (1).

During the seventh week of gestation the paramesonephric (müllerian) ducts are formed lateral but parallel to the mesonephric ducts. These primordial cells migrate caudally through the mesenchyme beneath the coelomic epithelium and cross the mesonephric duct during the eighth week. By the ninth gestational week the paired ducts have fused in the midline and join the posterior wall of the urogenital sinus to form the müllerian tubercle. The unfused paramesonephric ducts form the fallopian tubes; the fused portion becomes the uterus, cervix, and upper portion of the vagina. It is not known at exactly what level epithelium of endodermal origin (the müllerian ducts) ends and epithelium of mesodermal origin (the urogenital sinus) begins (7,8).

The fetal cervix grows more rapidly than the uterine corpus from the twenty-first gestational week until birth (9). The secretion of mucus begins within the caudal portion of the cervix during the twenty-eighth week of gestation, and by the final month of pregnancy the entire endocervix is functional. During the first 2 weeks of neonatal life, the cervix involutes and mucus production decreases as the influence of maternal estrogens diminishes. The menarche is accompanied by a resurgence in circulating estrogens, which rapidly increases both the size of the cervix and the amount of mucus that is produced (7).

Anatomic Abnormalities

Although there are a number of anomalies of the uterine fundus that have been described (10), they usually have little effect upon cervical function (i.e., cervical mucous production or sperm transport). Unification of the 2 cervices of a didelphic uterus is rarely indicated to treat infertility or habitual abortion in a young woman, but such a procedure (accompanied by a metroplasty) may be indicated in the older woman who has otherwise unexplained infertility. Attempts to correct surgically a congenital absence of the cervix have rarely been successful (11).

A variety of benign changes have been reported in some women exposed antenatally to diethylstilbestrol (DES) or other estrogens (12). These anatomic changes are probably not a frequent cause of defective cervical function since a definite relationship between infertility and previous DES exposure remains elusive. However, a correlation between in utero DES exposure and pregnancy wastage has been found (13). A DES-induced increase in the size of the endocervical transition zone may increase the chance of endocervitis simply because there is more columnar epithelium exposed to the vagina, as there is in any woman with cervical ectropion or eversion.

Cervical conization, cryosurgery, or overzealous biopsies can greatly diminish the number of endocervical cells capable of secreting mucus (14). Normally adequate estrogen levels may not induce sufficient mucous secretion, and sperm penetration may be inhibited. Occasionally, even pharmacologic levels of estrogen cannot restore mucous secretion to normal.

Some women have a decreased caliber of their endocervical canal without having had previous cervical surgery. The extent of this diminution in size can be so great that it is impossible to probe the canal. Nonetheless, menstruation usually occurs normally. Dilation of the cervix cannot increase the number of endocervical cells, but it may allow easier identification of the external os when postcoital tests or insemination are attempted.

The Composition and Structure of Cervical Mucus

Although cervical mucus consists primarily of endocervical epithelial secretions, the oviduct, the ovarian follicle, and peritoneal fluid almost certainly contribute to its composition. More than 90% of the content of cervical mucus is water, with the exact proportion being dependent on the phase of the menstrual cycle. Cervical mucus consists of a mucin glycoprotein composed of long polypeptide chains with oligosaccharide side chains. The side chains crosslink to form multichannelled micelles, the basic structural unit of mucus (15).

The two principal types of mucus have been labeled type E and type G. Type E mucus is characteristic of an estrogenic milieu and type G predominates when progesterone or another progestin is present. Immediately prior to ovulation, 97% of the mucus is type E and 3% is type G. The open channels in type E mucus allow maximal sperm penetration. During the luteal phase, however, 90% of the mucus is type G and only 10% is type E. In type G mucus the micellular spaces are irregular and narrow, and the matrix is crosslinked in a manner that inhibits or prevents sperm penetration (16).

Cyclical Changes in Cervical Mucus During the Menstrual Cycle

During the menstrual cycle there are quantitative and qualitative alterations in the cervical mucus as well as variations in the diameter of the external os (17). As a result of the stimulating influence of estrogen before ovulation, the mucus becomes profuse, thin, clear, and acellular; the external os gapes (18). All of these changes result in a material conducive to sperm penetration.

Wolf et al. (19) have shown that the nondialyzable dry weight of mucus (principally mucin) varies little, although there is a midcycle increase in mucous wet weight. This implies that the observed changes in the concentration of mucous solids may reflect the availability of water rather than alterations in the secretory activity of the endocervical epithelium. An interesting (but unproven) hypothesis that follows from this observation is that the primary action of estrogen on the endocervix is to increase the amount of water in the cervical secretions rather than to affect directly the product of the endocervical glands. Previous investigators have reported increases (18) or decreases (19) in the concentration of mucin as ovulation was approached. However, the difference between changes in concentration and nondialyzable dry weight must be understood. Since the volume of mucus varies widely, concentration changes may not be the result of differences in production rates, but merely a reflection of the extent of dilution.

Changes in one of several constituents have been proposed to explain the variation in the physical characteristics of mucus during the menstrual cycle. These include changes in the sialic acid content and, hence, in the net charge of the mucin side chains (20,21), changes in the structure of the mucin molecule (22–24), increased crosslinking between the glycoprotein threads (25,26), and a change in the amount of water within the endocervical secretions. Unfortunately, it has not been possible to isolate the proposed crosslinking proteins (27). The importance of charge differences in changing the biophysical qualities of mucin has also been challenged because mucus shows little alteration when exposed to buffers of different ionic strength (26). Further, removal of sialic acid from mucin does not always change the viscoelasticity of mucus (28). Those proposing that changes in the mucin structure occur during the menstrual cycle minimize the significance of changes in mucous water content and correctly point out that the addition of saline to thick, progestational mucus does not convert it to the thin, clear mucus that is usually associated with ovulation (24). However, the entire range of the viscoelastic properties of mucus can be duplicated by varying the amount of water added to lyophilized mucin (21).

There is evidence that estrogen influences the endocervix by altering the permeability of the vascular epithelium and thereby increasing the availability of water and other constituents. The concentration of mucin changes in relation to changes in serum estrogen concentrations (21). This could lead to changes in the physical and chemical porperties of mucus. Estrogen-induced changes in vascular permeability also result in changes in the concentration of other mucus macromolecular components (although the total amount remains relatively constant) (19,28). Since there is no change in mucin biosynthesis with the addition of estrogen to cultures of rabbit endocervical cells (29), changes in mucin concentrations must be the result of different rates of degradation or, more likely, fluid transudation into the cervix. Estrogen has been shown to increase the permeability of blood vessels in the uterine fundus and result in an increased rate of transudation of intravascular substances (30). The adjacent endocervix may respond in a similar fashion.

The Function of the Cervix and Its Mucus

The cervix functions as a haven for sperm from the hostile vaginal environment, as a mechanical and immunologic barrier to abnormal sperm, as a reservoir for sperm, as an influence for sperm capacitation, and as a filter that allows sperm penetration while maintaining a barrier against the infiltration of microorganisms into the uterine cavity.

The alkalinity (pH = 8.5) of midcycle cervical mucus is more conducive to sperm survival than the acidic environment of the vagina (pH = 3 to 5) (31). The cervical mucus also contains energy substrates (32), which are necessary for sperm survival since the compact sperm cell does not contain its own energy supply. Although sperm can be found in cervical mucus within a few minutes after ejaculation, sperm penetration into cervical mucus continues for 30 to 60 minutes after intercourse (33). Since the sperm remaining in the vagina after this time are destroyed, longer periods of postcoital "bedrest" are probably unnecessary. Anteversion of the uterus positions the external os in the pool of sperm in the posterior vaginal fornix. However, a retroverted uterus also allows adequate sperm-mucus contact, especially if penile withdrawal occurs soon after ejaculation. Thus, restrictions on the couple's coital positioning can usually be avoided without sacrificing normal sperm-cervical mucus interaction. Similarly, pillows placed beneath the female partner's buttocks during coitus only emphasizes the label of a "barren woman" while probably not achieving the desired increase in fertility.

Cervical mucus may aid in the selection of the most fertile sperm by acting as both a mechanical and an immunologic filter (33–36). Sperm recovered from the rabbit fallopian tubes or uterus are more fertile than freshly ejaculated sperm (37), suggesting that sperm with a decreased potential for fertilization have been removed. Women have a higher percentage of motile sperm at the internal os than at the external os (36), and the morphology of sperm found within cervical secretions is significantly better than in the original semen sample (38). *In vitro* ovum fertilization requires a large number of sperm; this implies that only limited numbers of sperm in an ejaculate may be capable of fertilizing the ovum (39). The cervix may be the anatomic site for this selection process.

The cervix provides a reservoir for sperm so that a constant supply is available to ascend the female reproductive tract and cause fertilization (33,36). The cervical crypts are colonized within 2 hours after insemination, and the number of colonized sperm are constant for at least the next 24 hours (40). The number of sperm that can be collected from the fallopian tubes remains stable for 15 to 45 minutes after insemination. If sperm exit from the fimbriated end of the tube, then there must be a continous supply of sperm from the cervical reservoir (41).

Capacitation is the preparative process that allows sperm to undergo the acrosome reaction, penetrate the zona pellucida, and subsequently fertilize the ovum (42). The exact site of sperm capacitation remains controversial. Spermatozoa that remain in cervical mucus for 1 to 56 hours after donor insemination are capable of penetrating the zona pellucida while sperm that were not brought into contact with mucus are not (43). This suggests that the capacitation process is at least facilitated by contact with the cervical environment.

Cervical mucus acts as a protective barrier to the uterine cavity during much of the menstrual cycle and throughout pregnancy (18,44). At these times, the impenetrability of sperm in the mucus is primarily due to the effect of progesterone. These progestational changes provide an effective barrier not only to sperm, but also to bacteria (31).

Hafez has summarized the steps in sperm transport that begin with ejaculation and culminate in ovum fertilization (Fig. 7–1) (33,42). Initial sperm transport is rapid and a few sperm reach the ampulla of the fallopian tube within 5 to 10 minutes after coitus. A slower (10 to 150 minutes) phase of transport then follows, during which the sperm occupy the cervical crypts. Finally, a slow release or escape of sperm from the crypts occurs during the 48 hours subsequent to intercourse. Although some sperm reach the site of fertilization very rapidly, it is not known whether these are the ones most capable of causing fertilization. The speed of sperm transport within the female reproductive tract implies a facilatory effect of the cervix and uterus. In this regard, rhythmical contractions of the myometrium and fallopian tubes may be important. Following the initial phase of rapid transport, the majority of sperm are found within the cervical crypts. The columns of micelles, terminating in individual cervical crypts, provide a pathway for the sperm that creates a reservoir within the endocervix. After establishment of the sperm reservoir, sperm are gradually released or escape (it is not known which) from the endocervix. This assures the continued availability of

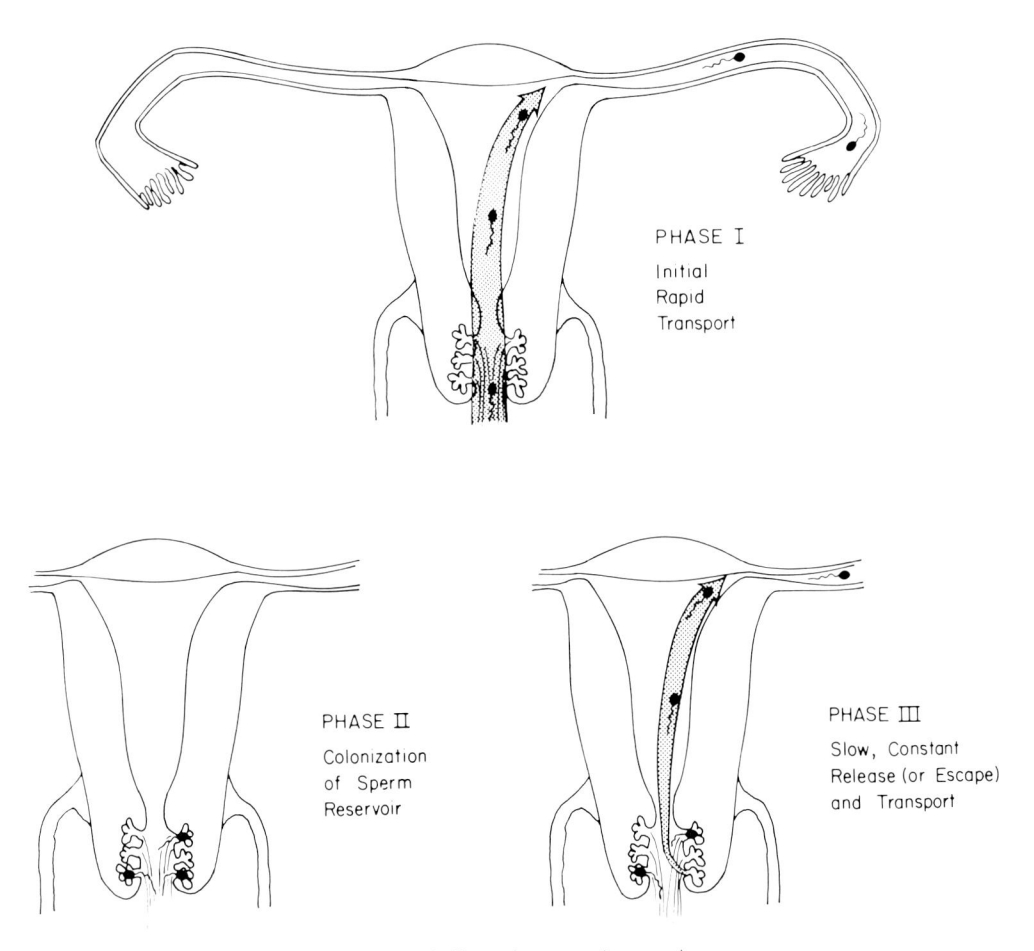

Fig. 7-1. Steps in sperm transport.

sperm for possible fertilization. For this reason, it is not necessary that intercourse be exactly coincident with ovulation.

It is thought that the rhythmic beating of the spermatozoal tail coincides with the oscillation of the micellular network of the mucin molecule (24,36). This permits a minimal expenditure of energy during migration of spermatozoa through the cervical mucus. Inert India ink particles placed in the human cervical canal can be recovered from the oviducts of 30% of women (45). Dead porcine spermatozoa can be transported to the fallopian tube, although to a lesser degree than viable spermatozoa (46). Thus, sperm motility facilitates the progress of sperm into the female genital tract but is not an absolute necessity. It is possible that the departure of sperm from the cervical crypts may be dependent on the release of certain sperm enzymes, which allow the sperm to reach higher levels in the female reproductive tract.

Cervical Infections

Because of its juncture between the upper and lower female genital tract, the cervix is susceptible to infections common to both areas (47). I must reiterate that chronic cervicitis and cervical erosion are excessively diagnosed and are usually not a manifestation of active cervical infection. Gram negative coliform bacteria, anaerobic bacteria, yeast, protozoa (particularly *Trichomonas*), *Gardnerella vaginalis*, *Chlamydia*, and *Mycoplasma* are the more common organisms that infect the cervix. Positive cultures for these organisms do not necessarily indicate that an active infection is present. Their presence may simply be an incidental finding. In most instances, however, it is appropriate to treat an infertile woman whose cervix harbors one of these organisms because the organism may alter the vaginal environment or interfere with fertility in some other manner.

The postmenstrual leukocytic infiltration of cervical mucus slowly diminishes during the proliferative phase amd reaches a nadir at ovulation (18). The number of white blood cells rises sharply in the 2 to 3 days after ovulation and remains high until the onset of menstruation (18). It is unwise to make the diagnosis of endocervicitis unless the leukocytic infiltrate is present in mucus within 2 to 4 days before ovulation (ascertained by basal temperature). In some women, the presence of leukocytes in periovulatory mucus implies that estrogen stimulation or response of the mucus-producing cells to estrogen is inadequate. In these women, small doses of exogenous estrogens or stimulation of endogenous estrogen with gonadotropins may clear the mucus of leukocytes.

The relationship between genital infection with *Mycoplasma* organisms and infertility remains controversial (48). However, a correlation between *Mycoplasma* organisms in the female genital tract and subsequent spontaneous abortion is more certain.

The finding of positive cultures for *Chlamydia trachomatis* in European women with acute salpingitis has led to the assumption that this organism may result in tubal infertility. Inhibition of sperm penetration by chlamydial organisms has not been demonstrated conclusively. Nevertheless, it does appear that chlamydial infections of the lower female genital tract can, if not treated, eventually cause tubal damage (49).

The organisms commonly causing vaginitis (*Candida albicans*, *Trichomonas*, and *Gardnerella vaginalis*) can change the biochemical environment of the vagina (particularly the vaginal pH) (50). However, infected women typically complain of pruritis and discharge early in the acute infection, and are usually treated promptly. The incidence of infertility that is caused by chronic infections with these organisms is unknown. However, 22% of infertile women with presumed endocervicitis subsequently become pregnant after appropriate antibiotic therapy (51). Since senescent sperm are engulfed by macrophages within the endocervix and endometrium (52), anything that increases the number of macrophages (e.g., infection) may increase sperm phagocytosis. Also, enzymes or other substances secreted by white blood cells may decrease mucous penetration by sperm.

Although the most detrimental effect of gonorrhea on fertility is salpingitis, the endocervix is the most common site for the organism (53). Even though the symptoms of vaginal discharge or dysuria may precede acute pelvic pain, three-fourths of women with positive gonnococcal cultures have no symptoms (53). Acute gonorrheal infection of the endocervix probably produces an environment detrimental to sperm survival. However, it is the possibility of salpingitis that necessitates treatment of a woman with a positive culture for gonorrhea, not the effect of the organism on the endocervix. A variety of bacteria, viruses, and protozoa can also inhabit the cervix, but they are infrequently diagnosed and rarely are they the primary cause of infertility.

The Immune Response of the Cervix

The principal role of the immune system is to identify and neutralize foreign antigens that invade the host. Spermatozoa are immunologically foreign to the female and can produce an immune response in some women that is detrimental to their fertility. Studies at the beginning of this century demonstrated that the homologous and heterologous inoculation of sperm could produce a predictable antibody-mediated response in most animals, if the proper adjuvants were employed. In 1922, Meaker reported that the sera from 2 sterile women agglutinated and immobilized their husbands' sperm (54). Franklin and Dukes investigated a group of infertile women whose sera caused a microscopic agglutination of donor sperm and thought that this represented an antibody response to sperm antigens (55). They treated the problem in a novel fashion by prescribing the use of condoms during intercourse in the hope that further antigenic stimulation of the female partner would not occur and that antibody titers would decline. A majority of these women subsequently conceived, and interest in immunologic causes of infertility blossomed.

Nevertheless, the role of antibody-mediated events in infertility remains controversial. In some instances, apparent false negative or false positive results for antisperm antibody activity have been reported, treatment protocols have been implemented without the proper controls, and some assay techniques may not measure immunologically mediated phenomena. There is no experimental evidence that unequivocally proves that a spontaneous antibody response to sperm is a direct cause of infertility. The systemic and local immune response to sperm antigens may be different. Only limited amounts of circulating IgG reach the female reproductive tract (56), and a woman's genital tract (particularly the endocervix) is capable of mounting an isolated local immune response (57). A satisfactory immunoglobulin-specific assay has not been developed that will identify antisperm antibodies in the cervical mucus. It has been difficult to isolate the spermatozoal antigens that are pertinent to antibody-mediated infertility (58). As a result of these problems, it is not possible to state that a positive test for antisperm antibodies can be equated with the presence of an immunoglobulin that actually disturbs fertility. Sperm antigens that elicit a response detrimental to reproduction may eventually be isolated. When this becomes possible, precise radioimmunoassay techniques can be employed to identify antisperm antibodies that truly interfere with reproduction. Finally, the role of the cell-mediated response to sperm antigens remains confusing.

The antithesis to the uncommon problem of antibody-mediated infertility is the ability of sexually active women to inhibit the production of antibodies against sperm. The female reproductive tract is not an immunologically privileged site since vaginally inoculated bacterial toxins (59) and cell wall fragments (60), viral particles (61), and *Candida* organisms (62) will elicit a measurable local and systemic antibody response. Moreover, because multiparous women frequently produce antibodies against their partner's histocompatibility antigens, the afferent limb of a woman's immune response must be damped during pregnancy to prevent a response to the male partner's HLA antigens that interferes with reproduction.

A woman's immune system is not selectively insensitive to spermatozoal antigens since a detectable antibody response accompanied by temporary sterility occurs following parenteral inoculation of human sperm (63). In fact, a U.S. patent was awarded in the 1930s for the injection of semen as a method of contraception (64). Although this study and others in animals provide insight into a female's response to sperm antigens, they are not directly comparable to the spontaneous immune response of infertile men and women with antibody-mediated infertility since adjuvants, repeated inoculations, and large amounts of antigen were usually necessary to obtain a satisfactory immune response.

Some investigators believe that sensitization to sperm is prevented in normally fertile women by the attachment of "natural" antibodies onto sperm that pass through the endocervical canal (65). This may be similar to the protective effect that anti-A or anti-B antibodies have on the Rh-positive fetus born to an Rh-negative mother (66).

Ingerslev (67) has proposed that "naturally occurring" antisperm antibodies are produced because of a nonspecific adjuvant effect of microorganisms on the female reproductive tract. Alternatively, antigens of the infecting organisms could crossreact with those of sperm. An immune response against bacteria, viruses, etc. would also produce immunity against sperm. Indeed, absorption of serum with a variety of bacteria frequently removes naturally occurring antisperm antibodies (65).

It has also been proposed that the cervix protects a distinct subpopulation of sperm while the remaining sperm are coated with antibodies and undergo phagocytosis by endocervical and endometrial macrophages (35). Presumably, this would eliminate the possibility of abnormal sperm fertilizing an ovum. Women with antibody-mediated infertility, however, would also place antibodies on those sperm that had successfully negotiated the cervix. The probability that sperm in the upper levels of the female reproductive tract are a privileged subset is strengthened by the observation that sperm recovered from the mouse and rabbit uterus have immunoglobulins on their surface while those found within the rabbit oviduct do not (37). Because only about 200 of the millions of sperm that are ejaculated eventually reach the site of fertilization in the ampulla of the fallopian tube (42), the inhospitable environment of the uterus may make a large number of sperm necessary for successful reproduction (68). Other investigators (66,69) have argued that sperm are not selected by the cervix, but that the antibody coating of sperm is the result, not the cause, of sperm senescence and death. Thus, the less active sperm that remain (and eventually die) within the endocervix will be coated with antibody and cleared by phagocytes. In this hypothesis, antibodies will attach to sperm that would otherwise have reached the fallopian tube.

Most mucosal surfaces can respond to an antigenic challenge by a localized production of antibodies, particularly secretory IgA (70). In order for local antibody production to occur, plasma cells capable of producing monomeric IgA (the type of IgA usually found in the circulation) must be present beneath the mucosal surface. The IgA molecules, once they are released by the plasma cells, become attached to a small protein called the secretory piece which is found on the adlumenal surface of the mucosal cells. The dimeric (or double) secretory IgA molecule is then transported and secreted into the adjacent lumen. The secretory piece protects the secretory IgA molecule from denaturation by proteolytic enzymes. Although secretory IgA may be found in small amounts throughout the female reproductive tract, the greatest concentration is in the endocervix since the largest number of IgA-producing plasma cells are found there (71). This fact may explain the occasional pregnancy that occurs following intrauterine insemination in antibody-positive women.

The local production of antibodies within the endocervical canal is short lived in comparison to the production of circulating antibodies stimulated by the same antigen (72). For this reason, circulating antisperm antibodies can represent either a concomitant immune response within the genital tract or an antibody response that continues to be measurable within the circulation, but is no longer present locally. These differences may be caused by different classes of antibody response such as IgG systemically (72,73) and secretory IgA locally (Fig. 7–2) (73). Alternately, a systemic response may not occur, and only locally produced antibodies may be identifiable (74,75). IgM is rarely found in the female reproductive tract. It is unable to enter the reproductive secretions because of its large molecular size.

The interaction of complement and antibodies can affect many cell surfaces (76). Complement is a collective term for a series of proteins that are activated in a stepwise manner analogous to the coagulation process. Two molecules of certain classes of cell-associated IgG in close proximity or a single molecule of cell-

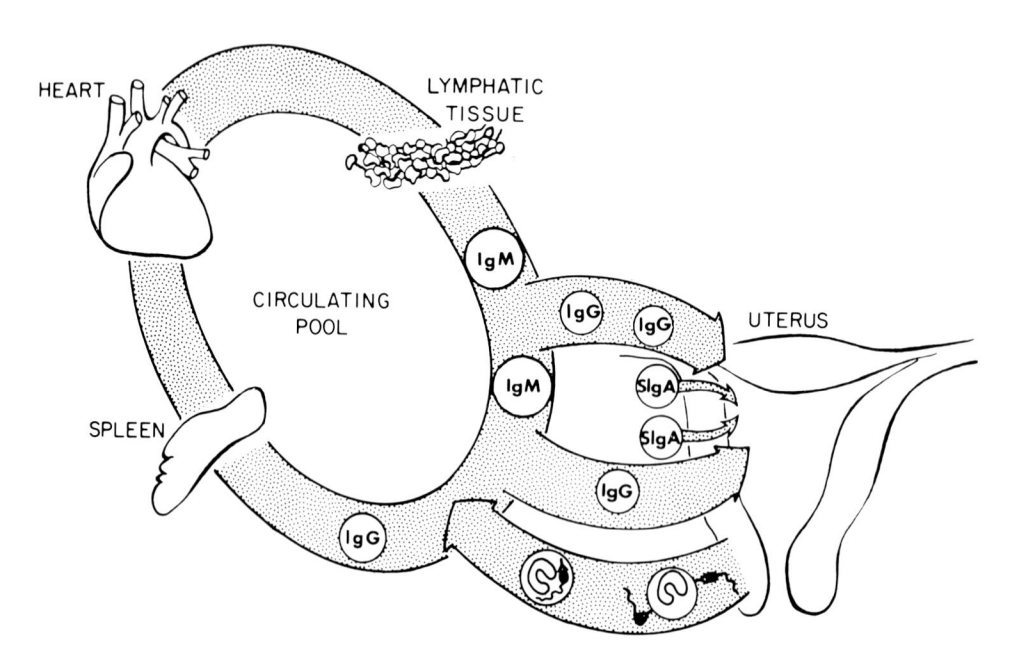

Fig. 7–2. Differences between the systemic and local immune response. Circulating antibodies may persist after local antigenic stimulation and antibody production has ceased.

associated IgM can initiate the complement activation process. Since the female reproductive tract has limited amounts of IgM and only a fraction of the IgG found in the circulation, much of the IgG that is present would have to be directed against sperm surface antigens in order for *in vivo* complement activation to occur. It has been shown *in vitro* that certain sera contain antibodies that, if attached to the sperm surface, can inactivate sperm in the presence of complement (77). Cervical mucous antibodies that can immobilize sperm in the presence of complement are more prevalent than circulating antisperm antibodies (74,78). The effect of these antibodies on sperm *in vivo* is uncertain since cervical mucus contains only about 11.5% of the circulating level of complement (79), an amount insufficient to support complement-dependent red blood cell lysis by antierythrocyte antibodies. This level is not likely to be effective in immobilizing sperm *in vivo* (80). Sudo et al. reported that only a small number of infertile women have agglutinating antisperm antibodies in their cervical mucus (81). It is not clear why there is a greater incidence of immobilizing cervical mucous antibodies than agglutinating antibodies, since it is presumed that fewer immunoglobulin molecules are necessary for agglutination than are necessary to effect immobilization.

There continues to be a number of pitfalls in diagnosing women with antibody-mediated infertility. Agglutination and immobilization assays that measure serum antibodies have been employed without proof that they can detect antibody in mucus. Cervical mucus may not be amenable to some assay techniques because of its increased viscosity, the small volume available for study, the dilute immunoglobulin concentrations, and the possibility that nonspecific immobilizing factors are present. The use of enzymes to liquify mucus may have a detrimental effect on the antigenic structure of the sperm used in the assay; this might also invalidate results. Physical methods of liquification, such as repeated passage of the mucus through a small-bore needle, sonication, or mechanical pulverizing, may be satisfactory alternatives to chemical liquification.

There may be more of a discrepancy between the systemic and local antisperm-antibody response in women (78). Modifications of serum assays for sperm antibodies have been used to show that immobilizing antibodies occur in cervical mucus more frequently than agglutinating or immobilizing antibodies in serum (74,78). Modifications of class-specific assays of immunoglobulin (73) may clarify the antibody-mediated events in female reproduction, particularly the role of locally produced secretory IgA.

Kremer and Jager have observed a shaking phenomenon of sperm when they come in contact with cervical mucus that contains antisperm antibodies (82). The Fc portion of these antibodies (presumably of the IgA class) is thought to attach to the mucin micelles, and inhibit further forward progression of the sperm by producing the shaking motion (82,83). It is difficult to accept this hypothesis completely since some investigators have found that $F(ab)_2$ fragments of antisperm antibodies can also inhibit mucous penetration in spite of the fact that these immunoglobulin fragments lack an Fc piece (84).

The Postcoital Test

Although the postcoital, or Sims-Hühner test is easily performed, it may not reliably assess the cervical factor in infertility (85). If a postcoital test result is obviously acceptable (more than 20 sperm per high power field), then cervical function is probably normal. If the test is obviously poor (absent or only an occasional nonviable sperm), then there is probably an abnormality of sperm-cervical mucus interaction. However, the results of postcoital tests of both fertile and infertile women can fall between these extremes, and corroborative tests must be used to determine if an abnormality of cervical function actually exists.

The lower limit of normal sperm penetration in mucus is between 1 to more than 20 sperm per high power field (86–91). We accept 7 to 10 actively motile sperm with good forward progression per high power field as evidence of adequate mucous penetration. It is essential that couples with an abnormal result have a postcoital test every other day until ovulation is indicated by a rise in the woman's basal temperature. This usually requires only 1 or 2 tests in regularly cycling women, but several return visits may be necessary for an oligoovulatory woman. Regulation of ovulation with clomiphene may be necessary in a few of these women in order to predict ovulation more precisely. Even when clomiphene is used, the periovulatory interval should be monitored with a basal temperature record. Since the time of ovulation may vary (92), judgment and persistence are necessary to ensure that the postcoital test was timed appropriately.

A normal postcoital test may provide good evidence for normal cervical mucus-sperm interaction, but an abnormal test result may be caused by a problem of the semen or mucus. Thus, either spouse or both may require treatment to improve sperm penetration. A semen analysis is probably a logical first step to identify the source of the problem. If the semen analysis is normal, additional studies are necessary. Homologous insemination followed by an evaluation of the adequacy of sperm penetration provides an *in vitro* system to assess sperm-mucus interaction. If the postinsemination examination of the mucus shows an improvement over the postcoital test, homologous insemination may be an appropriate therapy.

The result of a single postcoital test in fertile women does not correlate with the quality of cervical mucus, the number of motile sperm per high power field, the classification of test results, or the occurrence of pregnancy (85). Postcoital tests in 10% of 416 women who became pregnant within 3 months of the test revealed only nonmotile sperm, and in 3% of these women there were no sperm seen (93).

Asch reported that sperm could be recovered from the peritoneal aspirate of 8 of 10 women in whom no sperm were present in the cervical mucus 4 to 8 hours after intercourse (94). Templeton and Mortimer performed laparoscopy and were able to recover sperm from the peritoneal cavity of 4 of 9 women whose postcoital tests showed only nonmotile sperm (95). In women with poor or negative postcoital tests, aspiration of the pouch of Douglas 4 to 7 hours after intercourse may reveal viable sperm (96). These findings are suggestive that the results of postcoital examination of periovulatory cervical mucus may not correlate with the presence of sperm at the site of fertilization—the ampulla of the fallopian tube. Despite these findings, we believe that improvement of an abnormal postcoital test can increase fertility, especially if other aspects of reproductive function are normal.

Women should be scheduled for postcoital testing when the mucous characteristics are thought to be optimal for sperm penetration, usually during the 2 to 3 days prior to ovulation. Since mistiming of the test is the most common cause of an abnormal result, menstrual calendars and adequate basal body temperature charts are mandatory.

The optimal interval from coitus to examination is controversial. Two hours (97), 2.5 hours (98), 8 hours (86–89,99), 10 hours (100), or 24 hours after intercourse (101) have been recommended. Compared with results obtained 2 hours after insemination, there is a significant reduction in the number and motility of sperm after 6 hours (102). Some investigators have recommended that the initial postcoital test should be performed 6 to 8 hours after intercourse, since this interval is usually more convenient for the couple (89). If the results are adequate, no further testing is necessary. However, if the results are abnormal, then a postcoital test should be performed within 2 hours after intercourse since some fertile women have a rapid decline in the number of sperm within the cervical mucus after 2 to 2.5 hours (97). If the results are also abnormal within 2 hours, a cervical cause of infertility should be considered. Postcoital cervical mucus can be collected with a fenestrated forceps, a tuberculin syringe, or a soft catheter. Because there are no standard criteria for a "good" or "poor" postcoital test, multiple aspects of the mucous characteristics and the degree and quality of sperm penetration should be carefully recorded for later reference. The woman's last menstrual period, the number of hours since intercourse, and a brief description of that cycle's basal temperature curve should be noted. The number, percent motility, and grade of motility of the spermatozoa must be described as clearly and accurately as possible. It may be advantageous to divide the sperm into the percentage that are actively motile, that exhibit *in situ* "shaking," and that are immotile. Macroscopic examination of the mucus will provide an estimation of its elasticity, clarity, and spinnbarkeit. Microscopically, the degree of cellularity and ferning will suggest the extent of estrogen stimulation. Although some investigators have advocated the collection of cervical mucous fractions from several levels of the endocervical canal (97,98,103), the data from recent reports are suggestive that this is unnecessary (104).

In Vitro Assessment of Cervical Mucous Function

In vitro studies can be standardized to a greater degree than biologic measurements performed *in vivo*. However, the transfer of a procedure from the body to the laboratory bench introduces a variety of influences that must be considered when interpreting results. *In vitro* cervical mucous penetration assays can help to distinguish whether the male or female partner is the cause of an abnormality of sperm-mucus interaction by substitution of donor mucus for the wife's or donor sperm for the husband's. This is particularly helpful when the male has a normal semen analysis and the gross appearance of the female partner's cervical mucus is satisfactory. Donor mucus from a fertile woman (105), bovine mucus (106), or synthetic mucus (107) can be used to determine whether mucus from an infertile woman is the cause of the impaired sperm penetration.

Kremer described a laboratory technique to measure sperm-cervical mucus interaction (108). Microcapillary tubes filled with the woman's cervical mucus are placed in a reservoir containing the male partner's semen. After a predetermined time interval (usually 30 minutes), the mucous column is inspected for the level of sperm penetration. The mucous column is more easily examined if a flat capillary tube is used (109). Others have mathematically corrected for differences in the concentration and vitality of the husband's sperm in assessing the results of this assay (110). Whether or not such factors should be considered awaits further study.

Other crossed-hostility tests have been devised in which droplets of mucus and sperm are placed in close proximity on a microscope slide (82). A coverslip is placed over the droplets and an interface forms between the 2 reproductive fluids. The mucus is then observed for adequacy of sperm penetration.

Treatment of Cervical Factor Infertility

Therapies that have been used to correct poor sperm penetration and survival in cervical mucus can be divided into those that improve a hostile mucus and those that optimize the penetration of an apparently normal mucus by abnormal sperm (Figs. 7–3 to 7–6).

Estrogen in the absence of progesterone is associated with type E cervical mucus, the type that is the most conducive to sperm penetration (16). Abnormal mucus can be the result of either insufficient estrogen production or a failure of the endocervix to respond to normal estrogen levels (Fig. 7–4). Increases in circulating estrogen can correct this situation in some women. Care must be taken to avoid estrogen dosages that inhibit ovulation. Conjugated estrogens (Premarin®), 0.3 mg, or ethinyl estra-

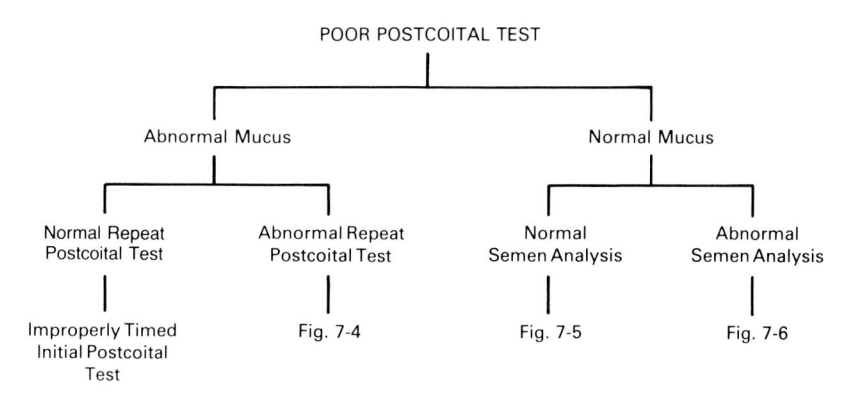

Fig. 7–3. Evaluation of a poor postcoital test. Subsequent assessment depends upon the nature of the initial abnormality and is illustrated in Figs. 7–4 to 7–6.

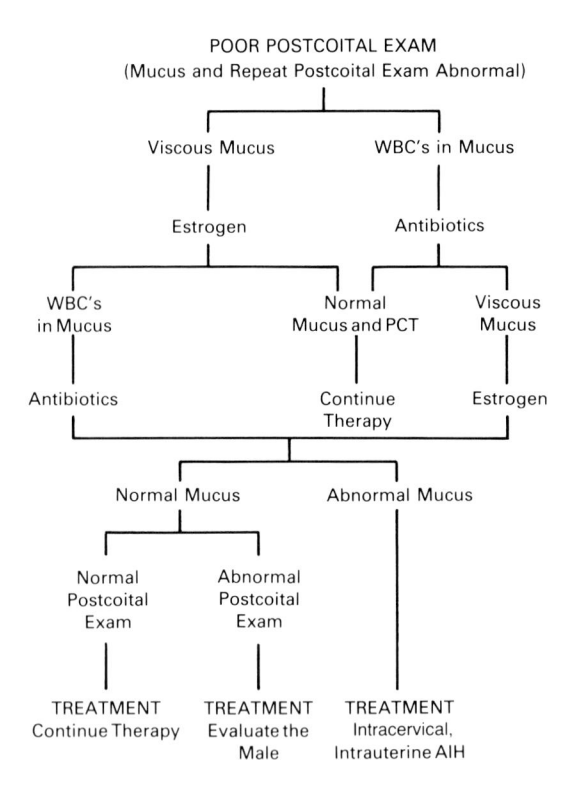

```
POOR POSTCOITAL EXAM
(Mucus and Repeat Postcoital Exam Abnormal)
         |
   ┌─────┴─────┐
Viscous Mucus   WBC's in Mucus
   |              |
Estrogen       Antibiotics
   |              |
┌──┴──────┬───────┴──┐
WBC's    Normal     Viscous
in Mucus Mucus and PCT Mucus
   |       |          |
Antibiotics Continue  Estrogen
           Therapy
              |
        ┌─────┴─────┐
     Normal Mucus  Abnormal Mucus
        |
   ┌────┴────┐
Normal     Abnormal
Postcoital Postcoital
Exam       Exam
   |         |          |
TREATMENT TREATMENT TREATMENT
Continue  Evaluate the Intracervical,
Therapy   Male         Intrauterine AIH
```

Fig. 7–4. Evaluation of a woman with abnormal mucus and persistently abnormal postcoital exams (PCT). AIH = artificial insemination, husband.

diol (Estinyl®), 0.02 mg, daily for the 4 to 5 days prior to ovulation may be effective. Human chorionic gonadotropin (hCG) can be used to stimulate ovulation in women if the estrogen inhibits or delays ovum release. Serial pelvic ultrasounds can monitor follicular development, and the hCG can be given when the diameter of the follicle is greater than 2 cm. If clomiphene is used to stimulate or time ovulation, its antiestrogenic effects may thwart the positive effect of exogenous estrogen therapy.

Human gonadotropins (Pergonal®) can be used to stimulate ovulation when exogenous estrogen therapy inhibits or delays ovulation and clomiphene has exerted an adverse effect on mucous production. Unlike clomiphene, gonadotropins increase mucous production. However, the need to monitor carefully the response to gonadotropin therapy complicates the situation (see Chapter 6).

Antibiotics are useful in treating women with a persistent leukocytic infiltration of their periovulatory cervical mucus (Fig. 7–4). Tetracycline is effective against aerobic and some anaerobic organisms as well as *Chlamydia* and *Mycoplasma* organisms. Doxycycline (Vibramycin®) offers the convenience of a once-a-day dosage regimen while providing a broad spectrum of coverage. Metronidazole (Flagyl®) is highly effective against *Trichomonas* organisms, anaerobic bacteria, and *Gardnerella vaginalis*. When any broad-spectrum antibiotic is used, an opportunistic *Candida* infection can be prevented by the prophylactic use of nystatin (Mycostatin®) vaginal suppositories at one-half the usual daily dosage (1 suppository vaginally each night). This is particularly advantageous for the anxious, infertile woman who fears "wasting" even a single cycle because of the need to treat a secondary yeast infection. The husband should also be treated if *Gardnerella vaginalis* (111), *Mycoplasma* (48), or *Chlamydia* (112) has been diagnosed by microscopic examination, culture, or serologic titer since these organisms frequently infect the male partner. Fourteen days of doxycycline (48,49) (100 mg daily) will effectively treat *Mycoplasma* and *Chlamydia* organisms, while 7 days of metronidazole (1 gm twice a day) is the drug of choice for *G. vaginalis*.

With all therapies for cervical factor infertility, a test-of-cure examination or culture of the cervical mucus must be performed to determine if the abnormality or infecting organism has been eradicated. This sequence of events—diagnosis, therapy, and test-of-cure examination—is the only logical approach to cervical problems. Although tedious both for the physician and the woman, it is necessary to note improvement in sperm-cervical mucous interaction if an empirical therapy is to be continued or adequacy of treatment is to be assured. Many women become frustrated by the length of time necessary to diagnose and treat a cervical problem. Long periods of time are often necessary because the results of a particular therapeutic maneuver can be assessed only in the 2 to 3 days preceding ovulation. If no improvement has occurred, then another month must pass before the results of continued therapy can be reevaluated.

Although a variety of preparations have been heralded as increasing sperm survival in the vagina or mucus, the efficacy of most of these is suspect (17). Guaifenesin® has been reported to improve sperm penetration (113).

7. The Cervix in Reproduction 135

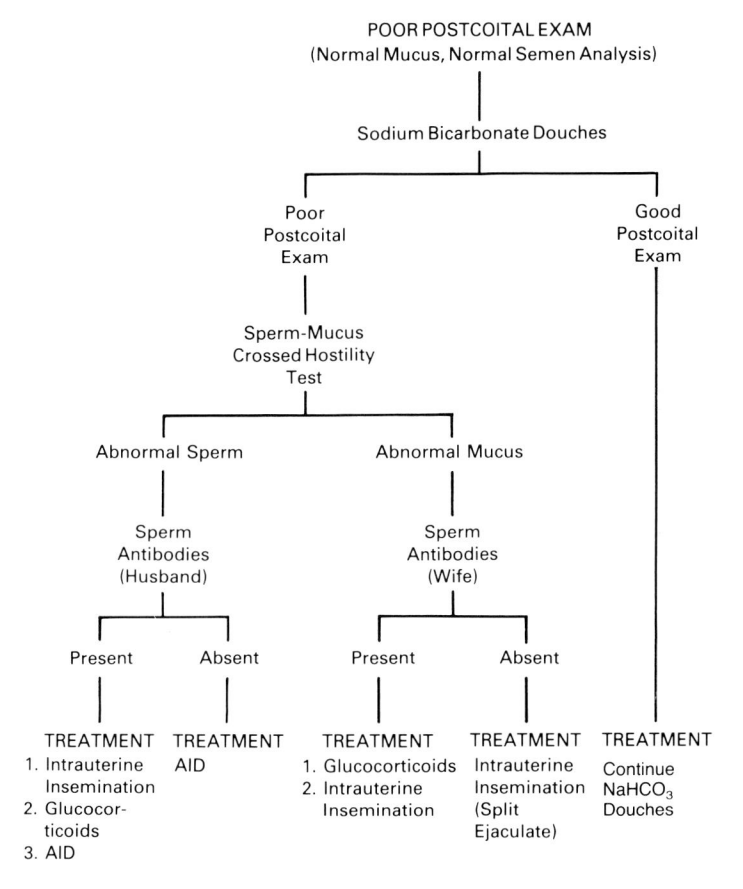

```
                POOR POSTCOITAL EXAM
          (Normal Mucus, Normal Semen Analysis)
                         |
                Sodium Bicarbonate Douches
                         |
              ┌──────────┴──────────┐
            Poor                   Good
         Postcoital             Postcoital
            Exam                   Exam
             |
         Sperm-Mucus
       Crossed Hostility
             Test
             |
    ┌────────┴────────┐
 Abnormal Sperm   Abnormal Mucus
      |                 |
    Sperm             Sperm
  Antibodies        Antibodies
   (Husband)          (Wife)
      |                 |
  ┌───┴───┐         ┌───┴───┐
Present Absent   Present  Absent
```

Present	Absent	Present	Absent	
TREATMENT	TREATMENT	TREATMENT	TREATMENT	TREATMENT
1. Intrauterine Insemination	AID	1. Glucocorticoids	Intrauterine Insemination (Split Ejaculate)	Continue NaHCO₃ Douches
2. Glucocorticoids		2. Intrauterine Insemination		
3. AID				

Fig. 7–5. Evaluation of a woman with normal mucus when the husband's semen analysis is normal. Details of therapy are given in the text. AID = artificial insemination, donor; NaHCO$_3$ = sodium bicarbonate.

```
                  POOR POSTCOITAL TEST
         (Normal Mucus, Abnormal Semen Analysis)
                          |
            ┌─────────────┴─────────────┐
        Abnormal                     Normal
      Urologic Exam              Urologic Exam
                                        |
                              ┌─────────┴─────────┐
                         Normal Sperm        Abnormal Sperm
                        Penetration After    Penetration After
                     Artificial Insemination  Artificial Insemination
```

TREATMENT	TREATMENT	TREATMENT
1. Treat Positive Findings	1. AIH (Split Ejaculate)	1. Intrauterine AIH
2. AID		2. AID

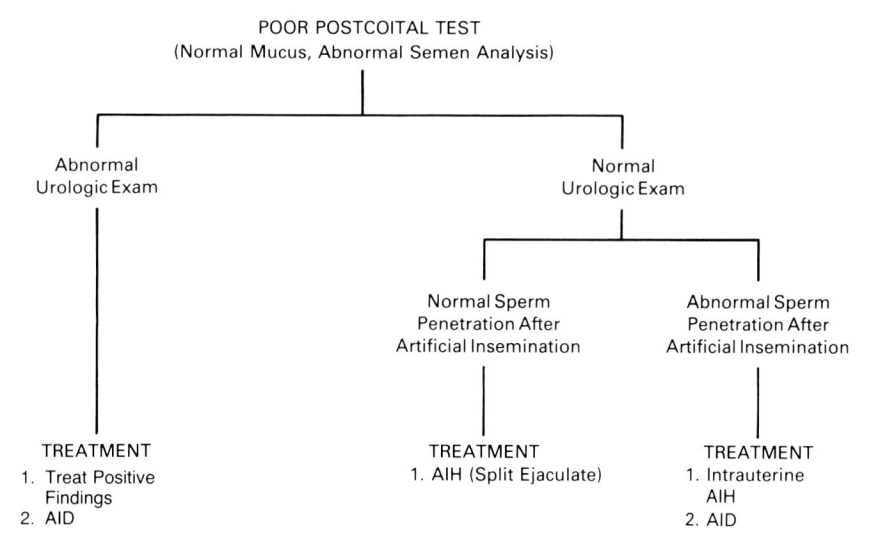

Fig. 7–6. Evaluation of a woman with normal mucus when the husband has an abnormal semen analysis.

However, only a small number of women have been studied. Sodium bicarbonate douches (baking soda, 2 tablespoons per quart of warm H_2O) have been reported to increase the sodium content of cervical mucus and improve sperm penetration (114). It has also been our experience that some women with poor sperm penetration into their mucus, despite normal-appearing mucus and exposure to normal semen, will benefit from precoital $NaHCO_3$ douches. A test-of-cure examination of the postcoital mucus is essential before such an empirical therapy is continued (Fig. 7–5).

We have mentioned that the role of the cervix in the process of capacitation is unclear. Although pregnancies have followed intrauterine or intratubal inseminations, the sperm may still have entered the mucus "through the back door" and come in contact with the mucus at the level of the internal os. Vasovagal reactions and intense uterine contractions can occur after intrauterine instillation of seminal plasma with its high concentration of prostaglandins. Sperm that are washed free of seminal plasma have less chance of producing such a reaction, but such washing can diminish sperm motility. This is particularly important since many men whose wives are candidates for such insemination techniques may have compromised semen parameters.

It is difficult to cannulate the endocervical canal of some women without causing bleeding. Traumatic attempts at endometrial insemination may defeat the purpose of the procedure, since fresh blood may interfere with sperm motility. Some clinicians use the blades of the speculum to close the external os after a cannula is placed high in the endocervix. Attempts are then made to force semen under pressure into the endometrial cavity. The value of this procedure is unproven.

Some investigators believe that the most common cause of cervical factor infertility is the presence of antisperm antibodies within the woman's cervical mucus. This theory is not in accord with our experience, and many women can be treated effectively with antibiotics, estrogen, gonadotropins, or precoital douches. If antisperm antibodies are identified, a variety of therapies have been proposed. These include immunosuppression with corticosteroids (73,115), bypassing abnormal cervical mucus with intrauterine inseminations (116), diluting cervical mucous antibodies by stimulating mucous production with exogenous estrogen (117), and condom therapy to avoid further antigenic stimulation by seminal antigens (55). Freezing of sperm may sufficiently alter the antigenic structure that antisperm antibodies can no longer attach to the sperm surface (118). Some have advocated empirical antibiotic treatment to eliminate a theoretical adjuvant effect of microorganisms within the female genital tract (67).

Some women can experience a true allergic reaction to seminal plasma (not sperm) antigens. The symptoms can range from cardiovascular collapse (119) to postcoital vulvovaginitis (120). Here, condoms are effective, though fertility is obviously reduced if this form of therapy is employed.

We suggest to women with plasma IgG antisperm antibodies (particularly if they have an abnormal postcoital test despite a normal semen analysis) that they receive a short-term course of low-dose corticosteroid therapy. Beginning 3 weeks prior to her expected ovulation, the woman begins methylprednisolone 32 mg 3 times a day for 7 days, followed by 16 mg 3 times a day for another 7 days. The dosage is slowly tapered over the final week of therapy. The level of circulating antisperm IgG and the postcoital test are monitored for improvement. If no improvement occurs, treatment as described is continued for a maximum of 3 cycles. Dyspepsia, symptoms of mild hypoadrenalism upon withdrawal of the drug, transient loss of distant vision, truncal skin rashes, euphoria, depression, unmasking of diabetes mellitus, and muscle and joint pains are some of the side effects of this treatment regimen.

Whether a combination of several therapies (Fig. 7–6) will result in higher pregnancy rates is not known. No study to date has adequately analyzed the value of systemic corticosteroids alone in treating sperm antibodies in cervical mucus. In addition, the dosage and duration of drug therapy remain strictly empirical. There are no controlled studies to define which corticosteroid is best, or whether higher dosages or longer treatment would result in higher pregnancy rates.

As in any disease in which multiple therapies continue to be employed, none has been overwhelmingly successful. Whether types of immunosuppressants other than steroids would be more beneficial is unknown. It is extremely important to monitor the woman's response to therapy, especially when condoms or corticosteroids are used. The decision to continue treatment should be based on both clinical and laboratory data. Levels of antibody in secretions of the reproductive tract may be a more important measure of response to therapy than circulating antibody levels.

The physician and couple attempting to identify and treat cervical factor infertility must be aware of the need for repeated testing that can extend for several months. Apparently effective therapies should be tried for 3 to 4 cycles, but after this time, other causes of the couple's infertility should be sought. If the woman is older or extremely anxious, such investigations should be performed before or during treatment of a cervical factor so that delay is minimal.

REFERENCES

1. Singer A, Jordan JA. The anatomy of the cervix. In: Jordan JA, Singer A, eds. The cervix. Philadelphia: WB Saunders, 1976:13–36.
2. Jordan JA. Scanning electron microscopy of the physiological epithelium. In: Jordan JA, Singer A, eds. The cervix. Philadelphia: WB Saunders, 1976:44–50.
3. Hafez ES, Kanagawa H. Ciliated epithelium in the uterine cervix of the macaque and rabbit. J Reprod Fertil 1972;28:91–94.
4. Fluhmann CF. The nature and development of the so-called glands of the cervix uteri. Am J Obstet Gynecol 1957;74:753–768.
5. Pinkerton JHM, Calman RM, Claireaux AE. The healing of the puerperal cervix: a bacteriological study. Ann NY Acad Sci 1962;97:722–732.
6. Singer A. The uterine cervix from adolescence to the menopause. Br J Obstet Gynaecol 1975;82:81–99.
7. Mossman HW. The embryology of the cervix. In: Blandau RJ, Moghissi K, eds. The biology of the cervix. Chicago: University of Chicago Press, 1973:13–22.
8. Pixley E. Morphology of the fetal and prepubertal cervicovaginal epithelium. In: Jordan JA, Singer A, eds. The cervix. Philadelphia: WB Saunders, 1976:75–87.
9. Hafez ESE. The comparative anatomy of the mammalian cervix. In: Blandau RJ, Moghissi K, eds. The biology of the cervix. Chicago: University of Chicago Press, 1973:23–56.
10. Muckle CW. Developmental abnormalities of the female reproductive organs. In: McElin TW, Droegemueller W, assoc. eds. Sciarra JJ, ed. Gynecology and obstetrics, Vol. 1. Hagerstown, Md.: Harper & Row, 1981:1–22.
11. Niver DH, Barrette G, Jewelewicz R. Congenital atresia of the uterine cervix and vagina: three cases. Fertil Steril 1980;33:25–29.
12. Herbst AL, Ulfelder H, Poskanzer DC. Adenocarcinoma of the vagina. N Engl J Med 1971;284:878–881.
13. Veridiano MP, Delke I, Rogers J, Tancer ML. Reproductive performance of DES-exposed female progeny. Obstet Gynecol 1981;58:58–61.
14. McLaren H. The management of benign cervical abnormalities. In: Jordan JA, Singer A, eds. The cervix. Philadelphia: WB Saunders, 1976:291–305.
15. Elstein M. The biochemistry of cervical mucus. In: Jordan JA, Singer A, eds. The cervix. Philadelphia: WB Saunders, 1976:147–154.
16. Odeblad E. The biophysical aspects of cervical mucus. In: Jordan JA, Singer A, eds. The cervix. Philadelphia: WB Saunders, 1976:155–163.
17. Elstein M. Non-immunological factors in infertility. In: Jordan JA, Singer A, eds. The cervix. Philadelphia: WB Saunders, 1976:175–184.
18. Moghissi KS, Syner FN, Evans TN. A composite picture of the menstrual cycle. Am J Obstet Gynecol 1972;114:405–418.
19. Wolf DP, Blasco L. Khan MA, Litt M. Human cervical mucus. II. Changes in viscoelasticity during the ovulatory menstrual cycle. Fertil Steril 1977;28:47–52.
20. Hatcher VS, Schwarzmann GOH, Jeanloz RW, McArthur JW. Changes in the sialic acid concentration in the major cervical glycoprotein from the bonnet monkey (Macaca radiata) during a hormonally induced cycle. Fertil Steril 1977;28:682–688.
21. Wolf DP, Sokoloski JE, Litt M. Composition and function of human cervical mucus. Biochim Biophys Acta 1980:630:545–548.
22. Schumacher GFB, Strauss EK, Wied GL. Serum proteins in cervical mucus. Am J Obstet Gynecol 1965;91:1035–1049.
23. Elstein M, Pollard AC. Proteins of cervical mucus. Nature 1968;219:612–613.
24. Odeblad E. The functional structure of human cervical mucus. Acta Obstet Gynecol Scand (Suppl 1) 1968;47:57–79.
25. Gibbons RA, Sellwood R. The macromolecular biochemistry of cervical secretions. In: Blandau RJ, Moghissi K, eds. The biology of

26. Gibbons RA. Mucus of the mammalian genital tract. Br Med Bull 1978;34:34–38.
27. Elstein M. The role of cervical mucus in the physiology of sperm transportation and clinical assessment. In: Cohen J, Hendry WF, eds. Spermatozoa, antibodies and infertility. Oxford: Blackwell Scientific Publications, 1978:55–65.
28. Litt M, Khan MA, Shih CK, Wolf DP. The role of sialic acid in determining rheological and transport properties of mucus secretions. Biorheology 1977;14:127–132.
29. Nicosia SV. An in vivo and in vitro structural-function analysis of cervical mucus secretion. Reproduccion 1981;3:261–280.
30. Ham KN, Hurley JV, Lopata A, Ryan GB. A combined isotopic and electron microscopic study of the response of the rat uterus to exogenous oestradiol. J Endocrinol 1970:46:71–81.
31. Moghissi KS. Sperm migration through the human cervix. In: Blandau RJ, Moghissi K, eds. The biology of the cervix. Chicago: University of Chicago Press, 1973;305–327.
32. Mann T. Energy requirements of spermatozoa and the cervical environment. In: Blandau RJ, Moghissi K, eds. The biology of the cervix. Chicago: University of Chicago Press, 1973;329-338.
33. Hafez ESE. Transport of spermatozoa in the female reproductive tract. Am J Obstet Gynecol 1973;115:703–717.
34. Joyce D, Vassilopoulos D. Sperm-mucus interaction and artificial insemination. Clin Obstet Gynaecol 1981;8:587–610.
35. Cohen J, Gregson SH. Antibodies and sperm survival in the female genital tract. In: Cohen J, Hendry WF, eds. Spermatozoa, antibodies and infertility. Oxford: Blackwell Scientific Publications, 1978:11–29.
36. Davajan V, Nakamura M, Kharma K. Spermatozoal transport in cervical mucus. Obstet Gynecol Surv 1970;25:1–43.
37. Cohen J, McNaughton DC. Spermatozoa: the probable selection of a small population by the genital tract of the female rabbit. J Reprod Fertil 1974;39:297–310.
38. Fredricsson B, Bjork G. Morphology of postcoital spermatozoa in the cervical secretion and its clinical significance. Fertil Steril 1977;28:841–845.
39. Wolf DP. The block to sperm penetration in zona-free mouse eggs. Dev Biol 1978;64:1–10.
40. Insler V, Glezerman M, Zeidel L, Bernstein D, Misgav N. Sperm storage in the human cervix: a quantitative study. Fertil Steril 1980;33:288–293.
41. Settlage DSF, Motoshima M, Tredway DR. Sperm transport from the external os to the fallopian tubes in women: a time and quantitation study. Fertil Steril 1973;24:655–661.
42. Hafez ESE. Transport and survival of spermatozoa in the female reproductive tract. In: Hafez ESE, ed. Human semen and fertility regulation in men. St. Louis: CV Mosby, 1976:107–129.
43. Gould JE, Overstreet JW, Hanson FW. Assessment of human sperm function after aging in vivo. Fertil Steril 1981;35:240.
44. Iacobelli S, Garcea N, Angeloni C. Biochemistry of cervical mucus: a comparative analysis of the secretion from preovulatory, postovulatory, and pregnancy periods. Fertil Steril 1971;22:727–734.
45. de Boer CH. Transport of particulate matter through the human female genital tract. J Reprod Fertil 1972;28:295–297.
46. Baker RD, Degen AA. Transport of live and dead boar spermatozoa within the reproductive tract of gilts. J Reprod Fertil 1972;28:369–377.
47. Slavin G. The pathology of cervical inflammatory disease. In: Jordan JA, Singer A, eds. The cervix. Philadelphia: WB Saunders, 1976:251–269.
48. Friberg J. Mycoplasmas and ureaplasmas in infertility and abortion. Fertil Steril 1980;33:351–359.
49. Sweet RL. Chlamydial salpingitis and infertility. Fertil Steril 1982;38:530–533.
50. Novy MJ. Infections as a cause of infertility. In: Simpson JL, asst. ed., Speroff L, assoc. ed., Sciarra JJ, ed. Gynecology and Obstetrics, Vol. 5, Chap. 57. Hagerstown, Md.: Harper & Row, 1982.
51. Hafez ESE. Sperm transport in the human and mammalian cervix. In: Jordan JA, Singer A, eds. The cervix. Philadephia: WB Saunders, 1976:164–175.
52. Howe GR. Leukocytic response to spermatozoa in ligated segments of the rabbit vagina, uterus and oviduct. J Reprod Fertil 1967;13:563–566.
53. Morton RS. The clinical features of venereal disease. In: Jordan JA, Singer A, eds. The cervix. Philadelphia: WB Saunders, 1976:251–269.
54. Meaker SR. Some aspects of the problem of sterility. Boston Med Surg J 1922;187–535-539.
55. Franklin RR, Dukes CD. Antispermatozoal activity and unexplained infertility. Am J Obstet Gynecol 1964;89:6–9.

56. Schumacher GFB. Soluble proteins in cervical mucus. In: Blandau RJ, Moghissi K, eds. The biology of the cervix. Chicago: University of Chicago Press, 1973:201–233.
57. Omran KF, Hulka JF. Infertility associated with induced local antibody secretion against sperm in the bovine uterine cervix. Int J Fertil 1971;16:195–199.
58. Mettler L, Gradl T, Scheidel P. Humoral and cellular response to sperm components. In: Hafez ESE, ed. Human semen and fertility regulation in men. St. Louis: CV Mosby Co., 1976:268–275.
59. Batty I, Warrack GH. Local antibody production in mammary gland, spleen, uterus, vagina, and appendix of rabbit. J Pathol Bact 1955;70:355–363.
60. Yang SL, Schumacher GFB. Immune response after vaginal application of antigens in the rhesus monkey. Fertil Steril 1979;32:588–598.
61. Ogra PL, Ogra SS. Local antibody response to polio vaccine in the human female genital tract. J Immunol 1973;110:1307–1311.
62. Waldman RH, Cruz JM, Rowe DS. Intravaginal immunization of humans with candida albicans. J Immunol 1972;109:662–664.
63. Baskin MJ. Temporary sterilization by injection of human spermatozoa. A preliminary report. Am J Obstet Gynecol 1932;24:892–897.
64. Shulman S. Reproduction and antibody response. Cleveland: CRC Press, 1975:103.
65. Tung KSK, Cooke WD, McCarty TA, Robitaille P. Human sperm antigens and antisperm antibodies. II. Age-related incidence of antisperm antibodies. Clin Exp Immunol 1976;25:73–79.
66. Hancock RJT. Sperm antigens and sperm immunogenicity. In: Cohen J, Hendry WF, eds. Spermatozoa, antibodies and infertility. Oxford: Blackwell Scientific Publications, 1978:1–9.
67. Ingerslev HJ. Antibodies against spermatozoal surface-membrane antigens in female infertility. Acta Obstet Gynecol Scand 1981;100:1–52.
68. Kaye M. Immunological relationship between mother and fetus during pregnancy. In: Hearn JP, ed. Immunological aspects of reproduction and fertility control. Baltimore: University Park Press, 1980:3–31.
69. Symons DBA. Reaction of sperm with uterine and serum globulin determined by immunofluorescence. J Reprod Fertil 1967;14:163–165.
70. Tomasi TB Jr. The secretory immune system. In: Dhindsa DS, Schumacher GFB, eds. Immunological aspects of infertility and fertility regulation. New York: Elsevier/North Holland, 1980:23–31.
71. Tourville DR, Ogra SS, Lippes J, Tomas TB Jr. The female reproductive tract: immunohistological localization of gamma A, gamma G, gamma M, secretory "piece," and lactoferrin. Am J Obstet Gynecol 1970;108:1102–1108.
72. O'Reilly RJ, Lee L, Welch BG. Secondary IgA responses to *Neisseria gonnorrhoeae* in the genital secretions of infected females. J Infect Dis 1976;133:113–125.
73. Haas GG Jr, Cines DB, Schreiber AD. Immunologic infertility: identification of patients with antisperm antibody. N Engl J Med 1980;303:722–727.
74. Moghissi KS, Sacco AG, Borin K. Immunologic infertility. I. Cervical mucus antibodies and postcoital test. Am J Obstet Gynecol 1980;136:941–948.
75. Ingerslev HJ, Moller NPH, Jager S, Kremer J. Immunoglobulin class of sperm antibodies in cervical mucus from infertile women. Am J Reprod Immunol 1982;2:296–300.
76. Lint TF. Complement. In: Dhindsa DS, Schumacher GFB, eds. Immunological aspects of infertility and fertility regulation. New York: Elsevier/North-Holland, 1980:13–21.
77. Isojima S, Tsuchiya K, Koyama K, Tanaka C, Naka O, Haruo A. Further studies on sperm-immobilizing antibody found in sera of unexplained cases of sterility in women. Am J Obstet Gynecol 1972;112:199–207.
78. Menge AC, Medley NE, Mangione CM, Dietrich JW. The incidence and influence of antisperm antibodies in infertile human couples on sperm-cervical mucus interactions and subsequent fertility. Fertil Steril 1982;38:439–446.
79. Price RJ, Boettcher B. The presence of complement in human cervical mucus and its possible relevance to infertility in women with complement-dependent sperm-immobilizing antibodies. Fertil Steril 1979;32:61–66.
80. Schumacher GFB. Humoral immune factors in the female reproductive tract and their changes during the cycle. In: Dhindsa DS, Schumacher GFB, eds. Immunological aspects of infertility and fertility regulation. New York: Elsevier/North-Holland, 1980;93–141.
81. Sudo N, Shulman S, Stone ML. Antibodies to spermatozoa. IX. Sperm-agglutination phenomenon in cervical mucus in vitro: a possible cause of infertility. Am J Obstet Gynecol 1977;129:360–367.
82. Kremer J, Jager S. The sperm cervical mucus

contact test: a preliminary report. Fertil Steril 1976;27:335–340.
83. Jager S, Kremer J, Kuiken J, Mulder I. The significance of the Fc part of antispermatozoal antibodies for the shaking phenomenon in the sperm-cervical mucus contact test. Fertil Steril 1981;36:792–797.
84. Hjort T, Hansen KB, Poulsen F. The reactivity of F(ab)$_2$ fragments of sperm antibodies and their use in the investigation of antigen-antibody systems. In: Cohen J, Hendry WF, eds. Spermatozoa, antibodies and infertility. Oxford: Blackwell Scientific Publications, 1978:101–115.
85. Giner J, Merino G, Luna J, Aznar R. Evaluation of the Sims-Huhner test in fertile couples. Fertil Steril 1974;25:145-148.
86. Moghissi K. The functions of the cervix in fertility. Fertil Steril 1972;23:295–306.
87. Danezis J, Sujan S, Sobrero AF. Evaluation of the postcoital test. Fertil Steril 1962;13:559–574.
88. Harrison RF. The diagnostic and therapeutic potential of the postcoital test. Fertil Steril 1981;36:71–75.
89. Moghissi K. Postcoital test: physiological basis, technique, and interpretation. Fertil Steril 1976;27:117–129.
90. Kovacs GT, Newman GB, Henson GL. The postcoital test: what is normal? Br Med J 1978;1:818.
91. Blasco L. Clinical approach to the evaluation of sperm-cervical mucus interactions. Fertil Steril 1977;28:1133-1145.
92. Newill RGD, Katz M. The basal body temperature chart in artificial insemination by donor pregnancy cycles. Fertil Steril 1982;38:431–438.
93. Grant A. Cervical hostility—incidence, diagnosis, and prognosis. Fertil Steril 1958;9:321–333.
94. Asch RH. Sperm recovery in peritoneal aspirate after negative Sims-Huhner test. Int J Fertil 1978;23:57–60.
95. Templeton AA, Mortimer D. The development of a clinical test of sperm migration to the site of fertilization. Fertil Steril 1982;37:410–415.
96. Hafez ESE, Dellepiane G, Aref I. Functional evaluation of the human oviduct for egg and sperm transport. Fertil Steril 1982;37:293.
97. Davajan V, Kunitake GM. Fractional *in vivo* and *in vitro* examination of postcoital cervical mucus in the human. Fertil Steril 1969;20:197–210.
98. Tredway DR, Settlage DSF, Nakamura RM, Motoshima M, Umezaki CU, Mishell DR. Significance of timing for the postcoital evaluation of cervical mucus. Am J Obstet Gynecol 1975;121:387–415.
99. Jette NT, Glass RH. Prognostic value of the postcoital test. Fertil Steril 1972;23:29–32.
100. Mastroianni LM Jr. Female infertility. In: Conn RB Jr, ed. Current therapy. Philadelphia: WB Saunders, 1966:731–735.
101. Gibor Y, Garcia JC Jr, Cohen MR, Scommegna A. The cyclical changes in the physical properties of the cervical mucus and the results of the postcoital test. Fertil Steril 1970;21:20–27.
102. Galle PC, Beauchamp PC, Blasco L. An evaluation of 115 artificial inseminations with post-insemination testing. unpublished results.
103. Moran J, Davajan V, Nakamura R. Comparison of the fractional post-coital test with the Sims-Huhner post-coital test. Int J Fertil 1974;19:93–96.
104. Versteegh LR, Shade AR. The fractional post-coital test: a reappraisal. Fertil Steril 1979;31:40–44.
105. Check JH, Rakoff AE. Treatment of cervical factor by donor mucus insemination. Fertil Steril 1977;28:113–114.
106. Gaddum-Rosse P, Blandau RJ, Lee WI. Sperm penetration into cervical mucus in vitro. II. Human spermatozoa in bovine mucus. Fertil Steril 1980;33:644–648.
107. Bissett DL. Development of a model of human cervical mucus. Fertil Steril 1980;33:211–212.
108. Kremer J. A simple sperm penetration test. Int J Fertil 1965;10:209–215.
109. Mills RN, Katz DE. A flat capillary tube system for assessment of sperm movement in cervical mucus. Fertil Steril 1978;29:43–47.
110. Katz DF, Overstreet JW, Hanson FW. A new quantitative test for sperm penetration into cervical mucus. Fertil Steril 1980;33:179–186.
111. Gardner HL, Dukes CD. *Haemophilus vaginalis* vaginitis, a newly defined specific infection previously classified "nonspecific" vaginitis. Am J Obstet Gynecol 1955;69:962–976.
112. Jones RB, Ardery BR, Hui SL, Cleary RE. Correlation between serum antichlamydial antibodies and tubal factor as a cause of infertility. Fertil Steril 1982;38:553–558.
113. Check J, Adelson HG, Wu CH. Improvement of cervical factor with guaifenesin. Fertil Steril 1982;37:707–708.
114. Ansari AH, Gould KG, Ansari VM. Sodium bicarbonate douching for improvement of the postcoital test. Fertil Steril 1980;33:608–612.
115. Bassili F, El-Alfi OS. Immunological aspermatogenesis in man. II. Response to corticosteroids in cases of nonobstructive azoosper-

mia with a positive blastoid transformation test. J Reprod Fertil 1970;21:29–35.
116. Kremer J, Jager S, Kierkin J, van Slochteren-Draaisma T. Recent advances in diagnosis and treatment of infertility due to antisperm antibodies and infertility. In: Cohen J, Hendry WF, eds. Spermatozoa, antibodies and infertility. Oxford: Blackwell Scientific Publications, 1978:117–127.
117. Ingerslev HJ. Spermagglutinating antibodies and sperm penetration of cervical mucus from infertile women with spermagglutinating antibodies in serum. Fertil Steril 1980;34:561–568.
118. Alexander NJ, Kay R. Antigenicity of frozen and fresh spermatozoa. Fertil Steril 1977;28:1234–1237.
119. Halpern BN, Ky T, Robert B. Clinical and immunological study of an exceptional case of reaginic type sensitization to human seminal fluid. Immunology 1967;12:247–258.
120. Chang TW. Familial allergic seminal vulvovaginitis. Am J Obstet Gynecol 1976;126:442–444.

8
Uterine Function and Abnormalities Causing Infertility

G. William Bates and Winfred L. Wiser

The uterus fulfills a number of roles in reproduction. At the cervix, the uterus traps seminal fluid in the cervical secretions where spermatozoa are either stored in crypts for later use or immediately swim cephalad into the fallopian tubes. With ejaculation of semen into the posterior fornix of the vagina, the uterus begins a series of rhythmic contractions that aid the transport of spermatozoa to the fallopian tubes. This process is mediated by prostaglandins contained within the seminal fluid (1) and sperm can be found in the human fallopian tubes as early as 5 minutes after insemination (2).

The endometrium is the site of nidation for the blastocyst. The endometrium undergoes a series of exquisite morphologic changes in response to hormonal stimuli during the reproductive cycle (3), and the uterus is the compartment within which the fetus grows to maturity. Prior to pregnancy, uterine blood flow is approximately 1% to 2% of cardiac output, but in the latter months of pregnancy 25% of the cardiac output serves the uterus. During pregnancy the uterus remains quiescent until term and then begins a series of repetitive contractions that culminate in the expulsion of the fetus.

The uterus accomplishes a variety of functions but not autonomously. It requires hormonal signals from the pituitary gland, ovaries, seminal fluid, and placenta. Thus, abnormalities of sperm penetration and transport (see Chapter 7), nidation, pregnancy, and labor may be the result of endocrine dysfunction and not inherent abnormalities of the uterus. Given the number and variety of its functions, it is surprising that intrinsic abnormalities of the uterus are not frequent causes of reproductive failure.

Most uterine causes of reproductive failure result from abnormalities of uterine formation during fetal life, or from neoplastic or inflammatory changes that occur during a woman's reproductive years. In this chapter we will discuss congenital uterine malformations, acquired uterine abnormalities, and inflammatory lesions of the uterus. Endocrine causes of uterine failure such as hostile cervical mucus, luteal phase insufficiency, and premature expulsion of a fetus are discussed elsewhere in this book.

Embryology of the Female Genital Tract

Development of the female genital tract begins in the abdominal cavity and proceeds downward. The mesonephros appears at its subdiaphragmatic location at approximately 4 weeks of gestation. The mesonephric duct, also called the wolffian duct, is the framework for formation of the male internal genitalia (vas deferens, epididymis, and seminal vesicles). The mesonephric duct joins the rete complex of the developing gonad and is later used exclusively to transport sperm from the testes to the exterior if the fetus is genetically destined to be a male (4). In a fetus destined to be a female, the mesonephros regresses but remnants may persist to appear later as hydatids of Morgagni, paraovarian cysts, and Gartner's duct cysts. The mesonephros may, however, be appropriated to form part of the vagina or it may serve as a guide for vaginal development since formation of a vagina cannot occur in its absence (5).

The primordial female reproductive ducts, the paramesonephric or müllerian ducts, arise exclusively for the purpose of forming the female genital tract. Müllerian ducts appear in human embryos 37 days after fertilization as indentations of coelomic mesodermal downgrowths along the wolffian ducts (6). The epithelium in the base of the müllerian ducts proliferates to form a solid, blind cord that grows downward to the pelvis. Later, they become canalized. The upper parts of the müllerian ducts grow lateral to the wolffian ducts to form the fallopian tubes while the lower parts grow ventral and medial to the wolffian ducts. They fuse in the midline to form the uterus. By continued downward growth, the müllerian ducts progress to the posterior wall of the urogenital sinus (Fig. 8–1).

Formation of the internal and external genitalia in males is modulated by hormonal secretions from the fetal gonads during the process of reproductive organogenesis (7). The Sertoli cells of the testis secrete a peptide hormone, müllerian duct inhibiting factor (MIF), which acts locally on the müllerian ducts to cause their involution. Presence of this fetal testicular hormone precludes formation of the female internal genitalia in the male. Soon after the Sertoli cells begin to secrete MIF, the Leydig cells differentiate from mesenchymal cells in the testes and begin to secrete testosterone. Testosterone acts locally on the wolffian ducts to stimulate their differentiation into male internal genital structures (a vas deferens, epididymis, and seminal vesicle on each side) and acts systemically to stimulate growth of the phallus, fusion of the labial-scrotal folds, and infolding of the genital folds to form the penile urethra (8,9). Failure of the testis to secrete MIF results in persistence of the müllerian ducts with resulting formation of female internal genitalia in the male. Failure of the testis to secrete testosterone results in formation of female external genitalia or ambiguous genitalia in an otherwise normal 46,XY male.

The fetal ovary has no defined role in the development of the female reproductive tract. In women with congenital ovarian dysgenesis, the reproductive tract is normal. However, exposure of the fetus to diethylstilbestrol (DES), a synthetic estrogen, during the period of reproductive organogenesis causes morphologic changes in the male and female reproductive tracts (10–12). Males exposed to DES may have epididymal cysts or develop a testicular neoplasm, while exposed females may have structural deformities of the cervix, uterus, and fallopian tubes.

Congenital Anomalies of Müllerian Ducts

Abnormalities of the uterus that lead to reproductive impairment result most often from defects in the downgrowth, fusion, or canalization of the müllerian ducts. At any stage during the course of normal downgrowth or fusion, an impediment may occur. Resultant conditions range from the extreme form of uterine and vaginal agenesis (Rokitansky-Küster-Hauser syndrome) to an inconspicuous notching of the uterine fundus. Moreover, the entire female reproductive tract may be duplicated because of failure of fusion of the müllerian ducts. In this instance a woman would have a double uterus, cervix, and vagina.

MÜLLERIAN AGENESIS. Women with agenesis of the uterus and vagina have no reproductive potential. This condition is the second most common cause of primary amenorrhea and must be managed appropriately if a young woman so afflicted is to make a healthy heterosexual adjustment. Vaginal agenesis occurs once in every 4,000 to 5,000 female births (5,13); approximately 8% of these women will have a functional uterus and cervix that can be salvaged for future reproduction (14,15).

Women with müllerian agenesis have normal ovarian function. Thus, they experience normal secondary sexual maturation at the expected time of puberty and ovulate once the hypothalamic-pituitary-ovarian axis matures. Abnormal findings include absence of the vaginal opening (Fig. 8–2) and absence of the uterus on rectal palpation. Approximately 30% of these women will have a renal anomaly (e.g., unilateral renal agenesis, horseshoe kidney, or a pelvic kidney, and 25% will have an

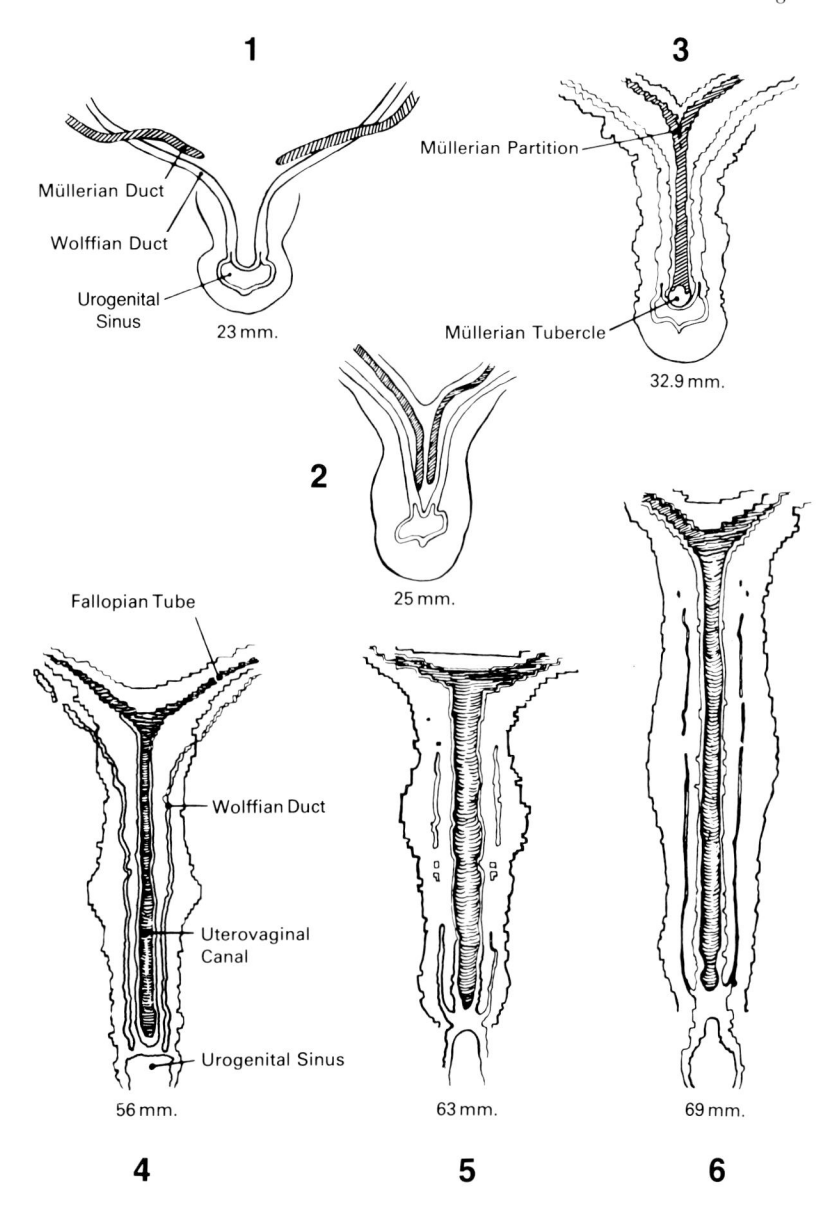

Fig. 8–1. Reconstructions of müllerian and wolffian ducts in female embryos at 8 to 14 weeks of development. (Reproduced with permission. Ramsey EM. Embryology and developmental defects of the female reproductive tract. In: Danforth DN, ed. Obstetrics and gynecology, 4th. ed. Philadelphia: Harper and Row, 1982:119. [Originally published by Didusch JF, Koff AK. Contrib Embryol 1933;24:61.])

occult or overt skeletal anomaly such as spina bifida occulta, scoliosis, or wedge vertebrae.

Young women with complete müllerian agenesis usually present to their physician by the age of 15 to 17 years with a complaint of failure to menstruate. Young women who have vaginal agenesis but a functional uterus present earlier (age 12 to 13 years) and complain of pelvic pain stemming from the hematometra that results from obstruction of the lower genital tract.

The diagnosis of müllerian agenesis should present no problem. Secondary sexual features develop normally and ovulation occurs. The only disorder that could mimic vaginal agenesis is the syndrome of complete androgen insensitivity, which is the most common cause of genital ambiguity in a genetic male. Women with androgen insensitivity also present during their mid teens with primary amenorrhea and full breast development but, because of the lack of receptors for testosterone and dihydro-

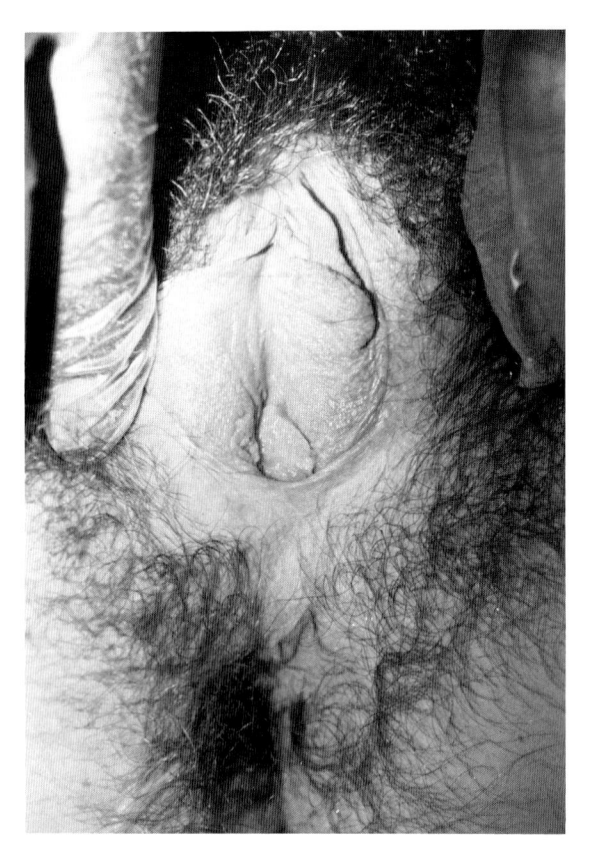

Fig. 8–2. The perineum in a woman with vaginal agenesis. Note that pubic hair growth is normal. This distinguishes women with vaginal agenesis from those with complete androgen insensitivity.

testosterone in androgen target tissues, axillary and pubic hair is absent or sparse. Moreover, evidence of ovulation, such as a biphasic basal temperature graph or luteal phase concentrations of progesterone, is lacking in these male pseudohermaphrodites. Serum testosterone concentrations are normal in women with müllerian agenesis, but are increased to adult male levels in subjects with androgen insensitivity.

Congenital absence of the vagina was first described by Realdus Columbus in 1572. Since the nineteenth century, many different surgical procedures have been devised to create a vagina: the application of pressure to the perineal space (Frank technique) (16), the inlay of a split-thickness skin graft into a surgically created vaginal space (McIndoe technique) (17), the implantation of an isolated segment of bowel into the vaginal space, and creation of an epidermal pouch in the perineum.

We prefer a modification of the McIndoe split-thickness skin graft vaginoplasty for management of vaginal agenesis because the vaginal canal can be dissected to the level of the peritoneal reflection. This allows the creation of a vagina of adequate depth. Further, the neovagina will assume the secretory and contractile functions of the natural vagina. We perform the operation when the woman is 16 to 18 years old—at a time when she is becoming fully aware of her sexual function and her need for heterosexual relationships. If the procedure is performed just prior to marriage, the young woman with vaginal agenesis may never establish a comfortable and lasting heterosexual relationship. These women tend to be emotionally immature and sexually inhibited, but they mature rapidly after the surgery. This transformation is not as striking if the surgery is delayed beyond the teenage years (18).

The modified McIndoe vaginoplasty is performed by obtaining a 4 inch × 8 inch sheet of skin, 0.016 inch thick, from a buttock. After making a semilunar incision in the perineum, a vaginal space is opened between the bladder and rectum by blunt dissection with narrow Deaver retractors. The space is extended to the peritoneal reflection. The perineal muscles and levator ani muscles are not transected but are preserved for later vaginal function. A mold is carved in the operating room from a block of Styrofoam and shaped to conform to the vaginal space in order to maintain depth and cylindrical volume of the neovagina. The split-thickness skin graft is sutured over the condom-covered mold (Fig. 8–3) and inserted into the vaginal space. The external edges of the skin graft are sutured to the perineal margins of the vaginal space with simple stitches using a fine, absorbable material.

One week later, the mold is removed, the vaginal vault is inspected, irrigated, and a balsa-wood (condom-covered) mold is replaced in the vagina. We carve a longitudinal groove in the anterior surface of the mold to relieve pressure on the urethra. Our patients wear the mold continuously for 4 months to maintain vaginal depth and caliber. They remove the mold daily to irrigate the vagina with a mixture of hydrogen peroxide and saline. After 4 months they begin wearing the mold for shorter periods of time until they become sexually active.

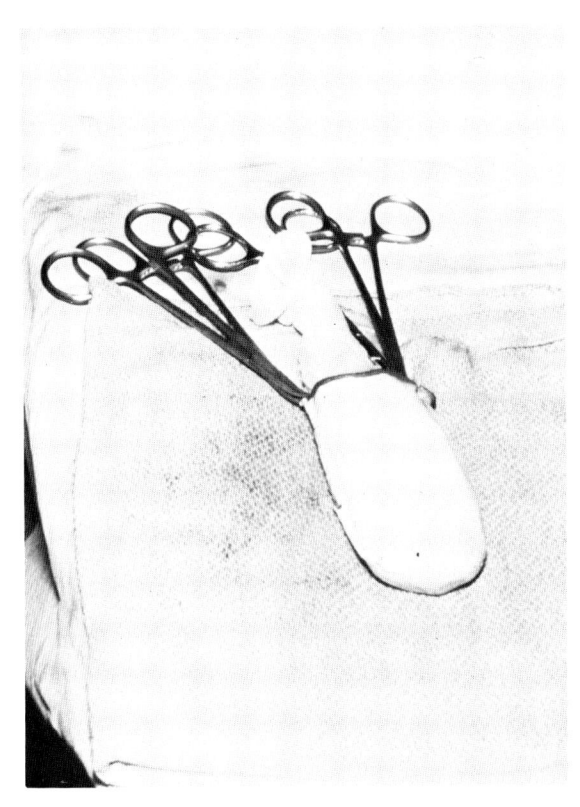

Fig. 8–3. Split-thickness skin graft sutured over a condom-covered mold. The skin graft is ready for insertion into the newly created vaginal space.

The anatomic and functional results are excellent. Only 1 of 92 women developed a vaginal stricture that required reoperation. One woman developed an intraoperative rectal fistula that required repair. Hecker and McGuire point out that the sensitivity of a young woman's family, and the counselling and advice of her physician take precedence over anatomic results in the eventual outcome of this disorder (19).

Recently, Ingram (20) has advocated a modification of the Frank nonoperative technique for creating a vaginal space. He developed a bicycle seat with a perineal dilator mounted to the seat. The patient sits upon the seat and applies pressure to the perineal area daily. As progress is made with dilation, the dilator is gradually lengthened until a vagina of adequate depth and caliber has been obtained.

In those women with vaginal agenesis and a functional uterus (8%), the surgeon should preserve the uterus by performing a vaginoplasty and attaching the neovagina to any remnant of original vagina or cervix (14,15). Pregnancies have occurred in women after this procedure was performed. If, however, the cervix is atretic, a hysterectomy should be performed because of the unacceptable morbidity and risk of death associated with the attempt to preserve the uterus in this unusual condition (21,22).

ANOMALIES OF UTERINE DEVELOPMENT. It has long been recognized that congenital anomalies of the uterus resulting from abnormal fusion of the müllerian ducts or from failure of absorption of the septum have been responsible for some instances of reproductive failure. A variety of abnormalities of the uterus can result from failure of fusion or absorption of the septum; these are depicted in Fig. 8–4. Most of these uterine anomalies are not suspected or discovered until a woman presents with a history of recurrent pregnancy wastage (either habitual abortion or premature labor). An anomaly is occasionally discovered at the time of uterine exploration following the birth of a child with an abnormal presentation, such as a transverse lie or breech presentation. Rarely is a uterine anomaly the cause of primary infertility. If an occult uterine anomaly is discovered in the course of an evaluation of a woman with primary infertility, a search for some other abnormality should be made before a metroplasty (uterine unification) is performed. When the müllerian anomaly results in a rudimentary uterine horn not connected to the cervix or vagina (Fig. 8–5) or an obstructed hemivagina with a double uterus (23), the young woman may present to the physician during her late adolescent years with a complaint of pelvic pain or a recurring vaginal mass. In these instances, surgery to alleviate vaginal obstruction or to remove a blind uterine horn may be necessary to relieve pain and preserve reproductive potential.

Habitual abortion and premature labor associated with a double uterus may be caused by a variety of factors. Moreover, the type of uterine anomaly affects the prognosis for successful reproductive outcome. A didelphic uterus (Fig. 8–6) is rarely associated with early pregnancy wastage, but has a 95% chance of causing premature labor prior to the thirty-eighth gestational week. Women with a unicornuate uterus (Fig. 8–7) have a moderate incidence of

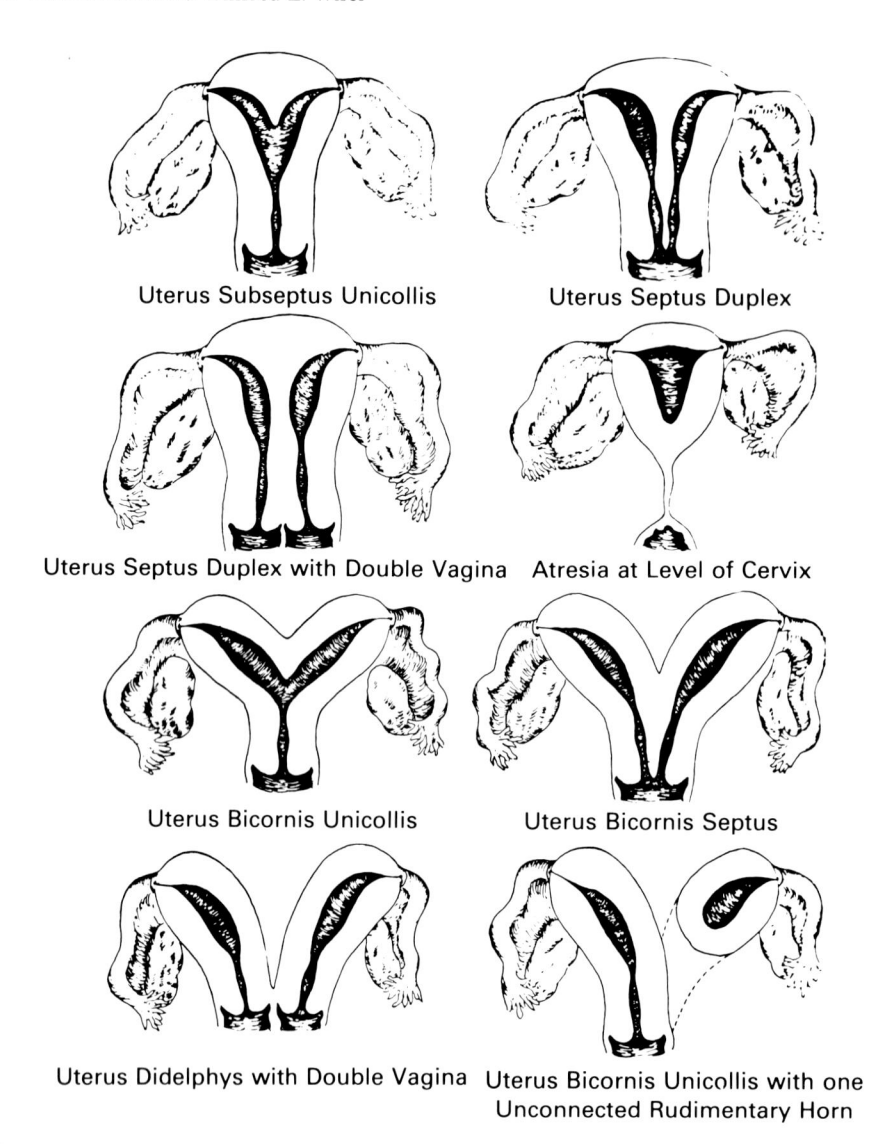

Fig. 8–4. Schematic diagrams of the various types of abnormal uteri. (From Patten BM. Human embryology, 3rd ed. New York: McGraw-Hill, 1968:482. As adapted from Stander HJ: Williams Obstetrics, 7th ed., New York, D. Appleton-Century Company, 1936: 791, 792. Used with permission.)

early pregnancy wastage but have an increased incidence of cesarean section (24).

The risk of reproductive failure is greater in women with a bicornuate uterus (Fig. 8–8) and greatest in those women with a septate uterus. In general, women with a septate or bicornuate uterus have no difficulty becoming pregnant. However, the incidence of early pregnancy loss in women with a septate uterus is 85% to 90% (25–28).

There is no indication for surgical intervention in a woman with a didelphic uterus except for the removal of a vaginal septum if it causes dyspareunia. However, surgical reconstruction of the septate uterus is indicated when it is considered to be the cause of habitual abortion (see Chapter 15). Unification of a septate uterus is also indicated in women who have never conceived if no other cause of infertility can be found or if the infertility is of long duration.

SURGICAL MANAGEMENT OF UTERINE ANOMALIES. Following a uterine unification procedure, 77% to 87% of women will deliver a viable infant (29–32). Not only is pregnancy outcome greatly improved, but the incidence of fetal malpresentation is also reduced. The

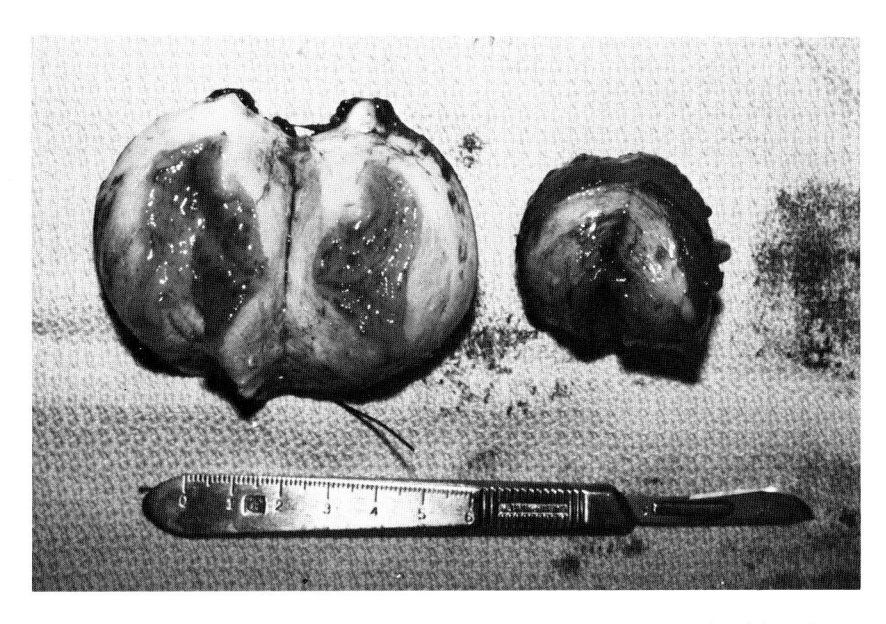

Fig. 8–5. Rudimentary uterine horns. These were removed because of pelvic pain.

latter may be a moot point, however, as most authors recommend a cesarean section following a uterine unification procedure.

Several techniques have been developed for correction of a bicornuate or septate uterus. Strassmann (33) developed the first modern procedure for uterine unification and his technique is still used for correction of a complete bicornuate uterus. Tompkins (34) described a technique for enlarging the septate uterine cavity by opening the uterus vertically, dividing the septum, and reapproximating the septum in an opposite plane. Jones and Jones (35) developed the method of excising a wedge of myometrium that includes the septum and unifying the two halves of the uterus. The surgical principles of these techniques are presented in Fig. 8–9. Criteria to select the opti-

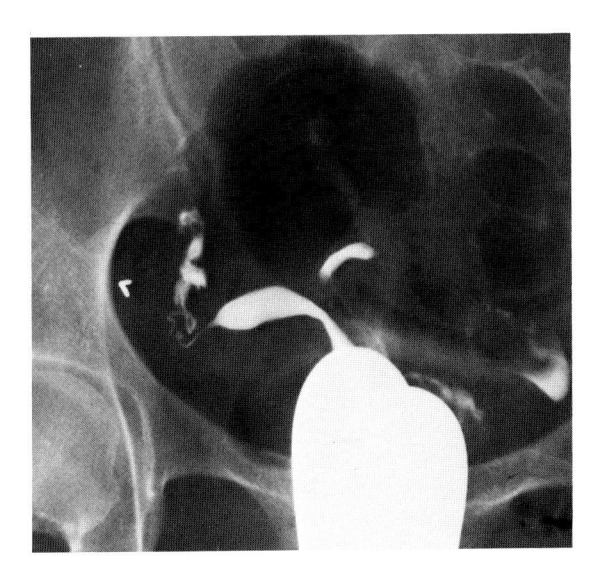

Fig. 8–6. Uterus didelphys with complete reduplication of the vagina. Note the rudimentary right uterine horn. (Courtesy of Dr. Royice Everett.)

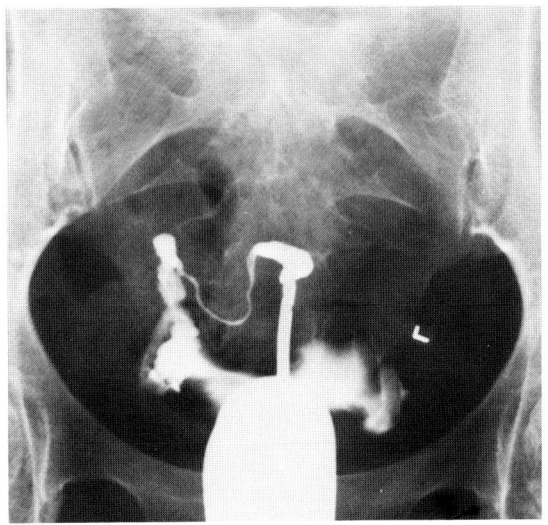

Fig. 8–7. Uterus unicornis in a woman with midtrimester reproductive failure.

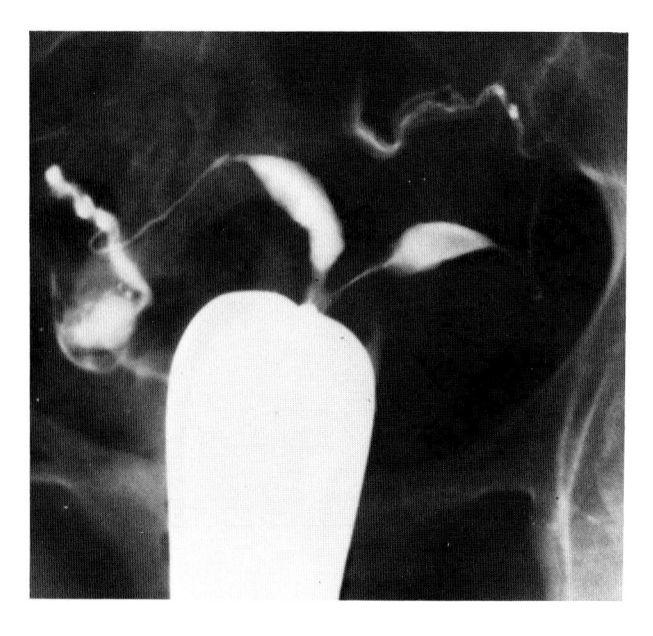

Fig. 8–8. Bicornuate uterus in a woman with early pregnancy wastage.

mal procedure are not well defined (26). Regardless of the technique, properly selected women can anticipate a 70% to 80% chance of conceiving and delivering a living child.

The original Strassman procedure is unsuitable for correcting the septate uterus and should be reserved exclusively for women with a complete bicornuate uterus (36). For correction of a septate uterus, we prefer the Tompkins operation because of the simplicity of the surgery, the minimal amount of bleeding associated with the procedure, and the postoperative configuration of the uterine cavity.

TOMPKINS METROPLASTY. The Tompkins metroplasty is illustrated in Figs. 8–10 and 8–11. The uterus is packed through the cervix with iodoform gauze saturated with methylene blue. A polyglycolic acid suture (#0) is placed on either side of the midline of the uterus for elevation. Care must be taken not to place these retraction sutures into the uterotubal junction. The uterus is bisected in the midline with a scalpel until the uterine cavity (or upper cervical canal) is reached. The uterine septum is opened vertically with a knife or dissecting scissors in a plane 90° to the original incision. This incision is carried to the superior pole of the uterine cavity. The uterine cavity is reapproximated by first suturing the anterior halves of the septum together and then the posterior halves (Fig. 8–12). All sutures are placed before they are tied so access to the uterine cavity is not compromised. After the sutures are tied, the myometrium is closed in 2 layers.

The woman should take oral contraceptives for 3 months after the Tompkins procedure to allow the uterus adequate time to heal. We per-

Fig. 8–9. Surgical methods of uterine unification: **A** Wedge technique of Jones and Jones, **B** Transverse incision of Strassman, **C** Technique of Tompkins. (Reproduced with permission. Rock JA, Jones HW Jr. Fertil Steril 1977;28:804.)

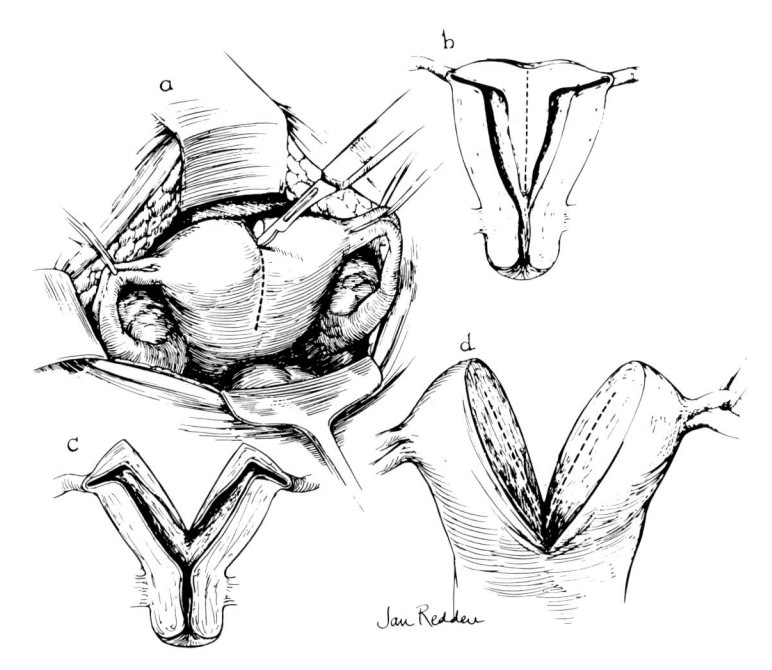

Fig. 8–10. Steps in the surgical correction of the septate uterus according to the method of Tompkins. (From Buttram VC, et al. Fertil Steril 1974;25:374. Figs. 8–9, 8–10, and 8–11 are reproduced with permission of the publisher, The American Fertility Society.)

form a hysterosalpingogram (Fig. 8–13) at the end of 90 days to evaluate the endometrial cavity. In a fertile couple, conception should occur within a few months after oral contraception is discontinued. As these couples have a history of pregnancy wastage, they will require a great deal of personal attention and reassurance during the first half of gestation. The physician can offer a positive, encouraging attitude to women following a metroplasty because the outcome with the procedure is so favorable. We deliver these women by cesarean section.

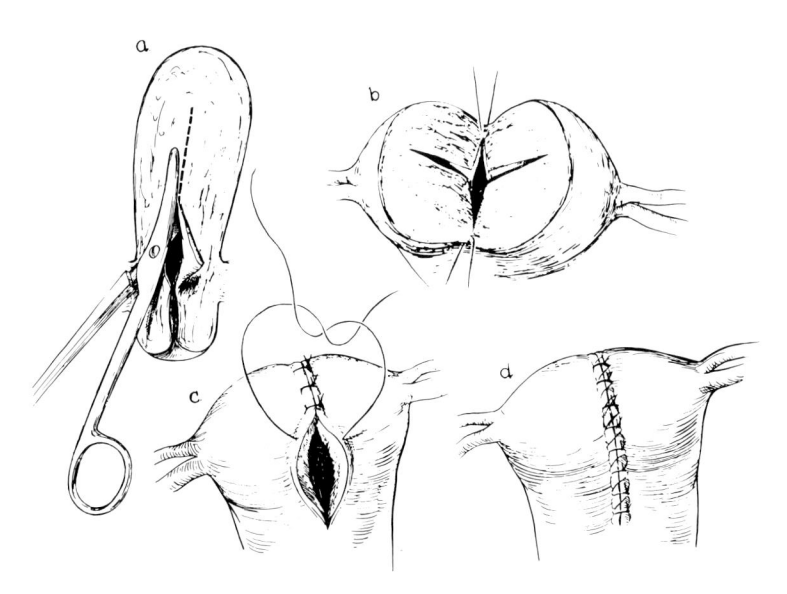

Fig. 8–11. Steps in the completion of a Tompkins metroplasty. (Reproduced with permission. Buttram VC, et al. Fertil Steril 1974;25:375.)

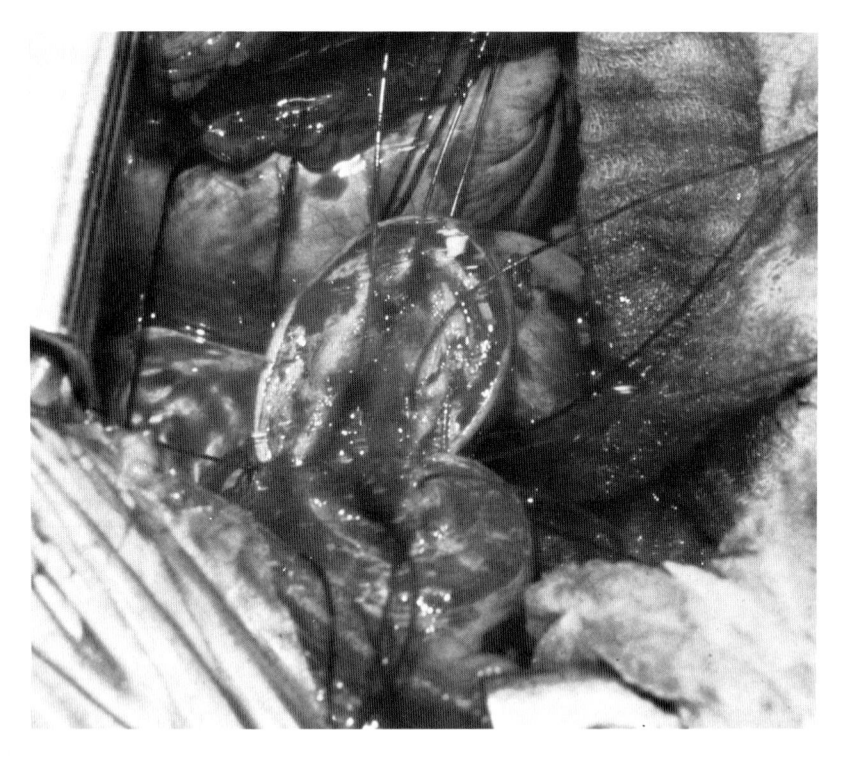

Fig. 8–12. Reunification of the septate uterus.

Acquired Uterine Abnormalities

DIETHYLSTILBESTROL (DES). *In utero* exposure to DES with its consequent effects on the male and female genital tract is a tragedy of modern medicine. The use of DES was advised in 1946 as a therapeutic agent to prevent habitual abortion and complications of pregnancy such as prematurity, intrauterine death, and toxemia (37). In 1953, Dieckmann et al. (38) reported that DES was of no benefit in preventing early or late pregnancy complica-

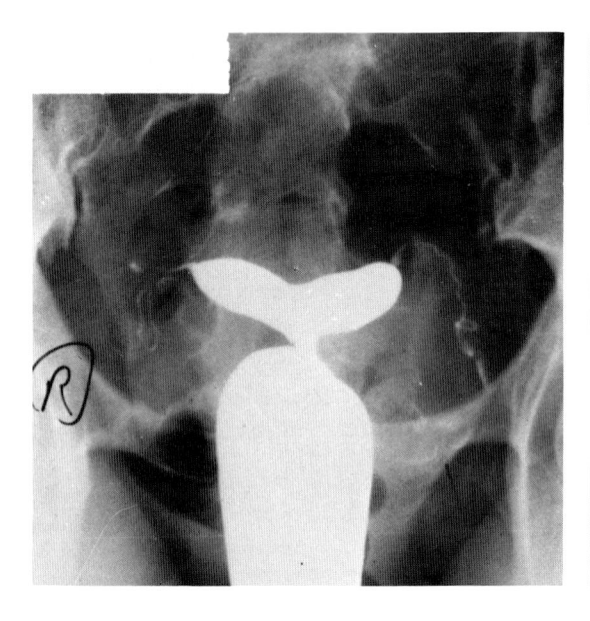

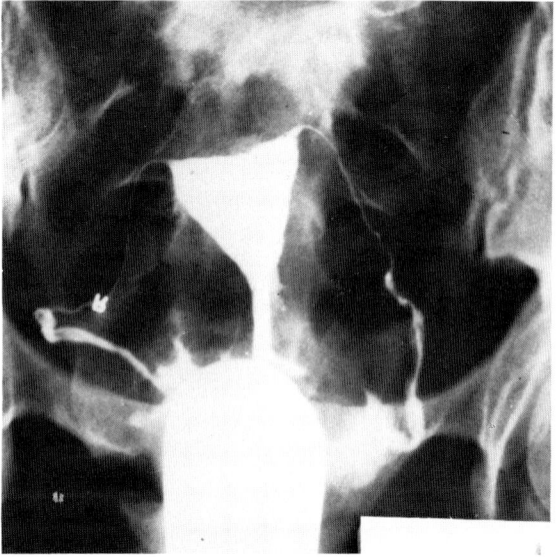

Fig. 8–13. Hysterosalpingogram prior to (left panel) and following (right panel) a Tompkins uterine unification.

tions. However, millions of pregnant women were given DES during the 1950s and 1960s. Despite reports indicating that DES was of no therapeutic value, clinicians continued to prescribe the drug in an effort to "do something" for the pregnant woman with a history of pregnancy loss. The first group to question the effects of DES on the fetus was Herbst et al. (10), who reported that 7 of 8 young women with clear-cell adenocarcinoma of the vagina had been exposed to DES *in utero*. Following this report, a number of reports followed that linked DES exposure to cervical abnormalities such as transverse ridges, a cockscomb deformity of the anterior cervical lip, and cervical ectropion.

An association of upper genital tract anomalies and DES exposure was first made in 1977 when Kaufman et al. described hysterographic changes of the endometrial cavity (12). In a subsequent study, Kaufman et al. (39) found a T-shaped endometrial cavity in 69% of 267 women with known DES exposure. Other uterine deformities such as uterine filling defects, synechiae, diverticulae, constriction rings, myometrial bands, uterine hypoplasia, and abnormalities of müllerian fusion were also noted frequently in DES-exposed women (Fig. 8–14). In an extensive study of the upper genital tract in DES-exposed women, Haney and co-workers found that the intrauterine volume was significantly reduced compared to that of women not exposed to DES and that the abnormalities of the uterus were unique to DES-exposed women (40).

The effect of DES exposure on conception rates and the outcome of pregnancy is an unsettled issue. Initial reports that addressed this question suggested that the prognosis for successful reproduction is sharply compromised. Bibbo et al. found that only 18% of women exposed to DES had ever conceived whereas 33% of the control women had conceived at least once (41). Other authors contradict these findings, but suggest that the risk of early or midtrimester abortion and the risk of prematurity is slightly increased (39,42,43). Goldstein suggested that an incompetent cervix may be the cause of pregnancy wastage in DES-exposed women and recommended that these women have a cervical cerclage (44). However, Noller et al. have recommended that a cerclage be performed only for established obstetric indications (45). From our experience and review of the current literature, DES-exposed women have a reasonable chance of a successful pregnancy without surgery.

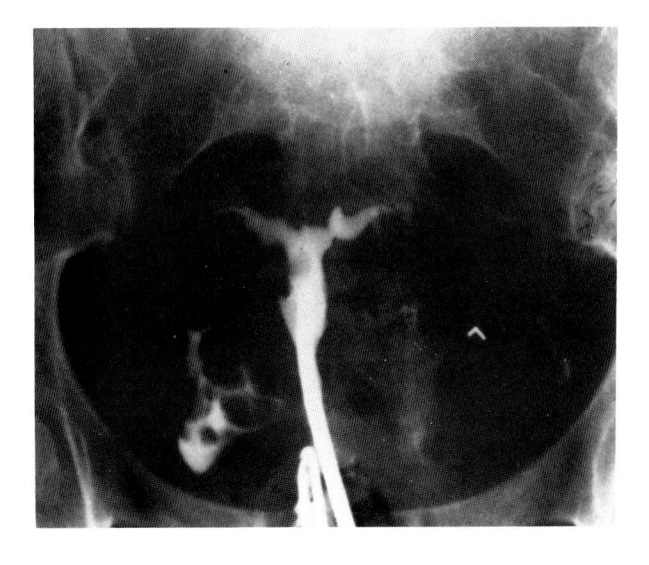

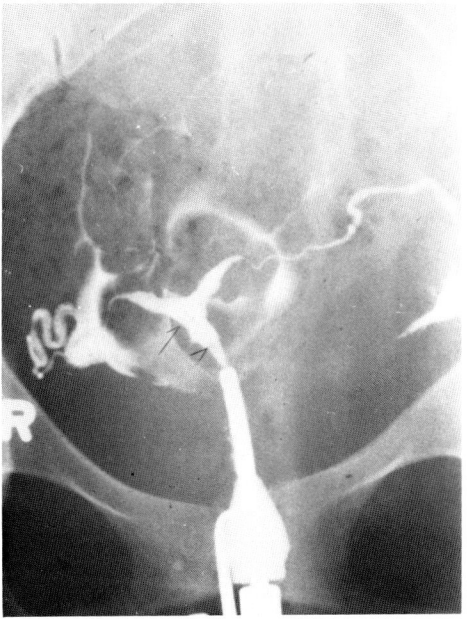

Fig. 8–14. The endometrial cavities of 2 women with *in utero* DES exposure. The left panel demonstrates filling defects, diverticulae, and constriction rings in a woman with habitual abortion. The right panel demonstrates minor uterine deformities in a woman who carried 2 pregnancies to term.

UTERINE LEIOMYOMATA. Uterine leiomyomata develop in 20% of women during their reproductive life (46) but only 5% of women will require a myomectomy for treatment of infertility (47). The mechanism by which a leiomyoma produces infertility is unknown, but the following have been suggested: alterations in blood flow to the endometrium, mechanical compromise of the endometrial cavity, distortion of uterine configuration, occlusion of the uterotubal junction, and prevention of implantation of the blastocyst. Malone and Ingersoll reported a 50% pregnancy rate with a successful outcome in 75 women after myomectomy (48). Buttram and Reiter reviewed 18 studies of 1,193 women in whom myomectomy was performed for infertility (46). They found 480 (40%) pregnancies after surgery. They also found that the spontaneous abortion rate was reduced from 41% to 19% in another 1,941 women after myomectomy.

A complete evaluation for infertility should be performed in a woman with uterine leiomyomata before myomectomy is contemplated. In addition to documentation of ovulation and measurement of sperm density, a hysterosalpingogram is necessary to ascertain the presence of filling defects in the endometrial cavity or obstruction of the uterotubal junction. If the endometrial cavity is normal in size, shape, and configuration, it is unlikely that leiomyomata are the cause of infertility. A history of recurrent early abortion suggests that leiomyomata may be the cause of infertility; infertility resulting from failure of conception is infrequently due to leiomyomata, especially if the endometrial cavity is normal.

The technique of myomectomy is described in detail elsewhere (46,49). We perform this procedure through a vertical abdominal incision and make a vertical incision in the uterine fundus to minimize blood loss. After the uterus is closed, we irrigate the pelvic cavity copiously with 0.9% saline and instill 100 ml of 32% dextran into the pelvis to prevent the formation of adhesions.

The etiology of uterine leiomyomata is unknown but there is compelling teleologic evidence to suggest that estrogen plays a role in the formation and growth of leiomyoma. These benign tumors arise during a woman's reproductive years, enlarge during pregnancy, and regress at menopause. Wilson et al. found a greater concentration of 7S estrogen receptors in leiomyomata than in normal myometrium from the same uterus (50). This finding has not been confirmed by other investigators, but it suggests the possibility that uterine leiomyomata can be managed by the administration of estrogen-receptor binding agents (e.g., tamoxifen).

ABNORMAL UTERINE POSITIONS. Uterine retroversion, of itself, rarely causes infertility (51). Occasionally a cervix that is positioned sharply anterior may be unable to receive the ejaculate. In an earlier era, the finding of a retroflexed uterus was indication (even in young women who had not tested their reproductive potential) for a uterine suspension. In modern infertility practice, this is not warranted.

However, when the uterus is retroflexed and fixed into an immobile position (or displaced and fixed laterally), there may be underlying pelvic adhesions, endometriosis, or an adnexal mass responsible for the uterine displacement. This finding demands further diagnostic investigation by X-ray evaluation and laparoscopy.

Diseases of the Endometrium Causing Infertility

INTRAUTERINE ADHESIONS (ASHERMAN SYNDROME). Intrauterine adhesions were described first by Fritsch in 1894. In 1950, Asherman described the cause, diagnostic clinical features, and therapy (52). Intrauterine adhesions usually result from vigorous curettage of the uterine cavity following obstetric delivery or abortion. The basal layer of the endometrium is especially susceptible to being denuded during pregnancy because the underlying myometrium is soft and the "grating" sensation that is felt when the surgeon scrapes the basal layer of the endometrium is lost. Endometritis further increases the susceptibility for creating intrauterine adhesions. An awareness that vigorous curettage increases the risk for creating intrauterine adhesions should reduce the incidence of this disorder. However, most physicians tend to curette more vigorously when confronted with a woman who has a massive obstetric hemorrhage. Klein has noted the irony of this—pregnancy, when complicated by hemorrhage, can be a contributing cause of infertility (53).

The diagnosis of intrauterine adhesions is usually simple to make. Amenorrhea after a puerperal curettage is the most useful clue, especially if there was a coincident episode of uterine infection. Since women with this disorder have normal ovarian function, they continue to experience cyclic breast changes and premenstrual molimina. This is an important diagnostic point since failure to obtain a history of uterine curettage immediately prior to the onset of amenorrhea may mislead the clinician into pursuing an expensive endocrine investigation that ultimately will be normal. A basal temperature record for 4 to 6 weeks is also useful. Evidence of ovulation excludes an endocrine disorder as the cause of amenorrhea.

When the woman's history suggests intrauterine adhesions as the cause of amenorrhea, a uterine sound should be inserted into the uterine cavity to evaluate its configuration. A hysterosalpingogram should also be obtained. If adhesions extend to the lower uterine segment, it may be impossible to sound the uterine cavity or obtain a hysterosalpingogram without general anesthesia. The hysterosalpingogram reveals filling defects at the sites of uterine adhesions (Fig. 8–15).

Management of the woman with intrauterine adhesions has changed during the past decade. In 1968, Loures et al. recommended endometrial curettage and insertion of 1 or more intrauterine devices (IUD) into the uterine cavity to prevent agglutination of the uterine walls (54). In a group of 60 women, all had resumption of menses, 93% had restoration of a patent endometrial cavity, but only 17% became pregnant. In 1978, March et al. (55) and Sugimoto (56) reported a higher pregnancy rate (70% and 41%, respectively) by performing hysteroscopy and lysis of intrauterine adhesions under direct vision. Both groups placed a pediatric Foley catheter or IUD in the endometrial cavity at surgery to prevent endometrial agglutination. March et al. administered exogenous estrogen for 60 days after lysis of adhesions to stimulate endometrial growth (55).

ENDOMETRIAL INFECTIONS. Endometritis may result from inflammation of the fallopian tubes or cervix, from hematogenous dissemination, or by direct inoculation into the endometrial cavity. Under ordinary circumstances, the endometrium is sterile (57), but may become infected by a virulent organism such as

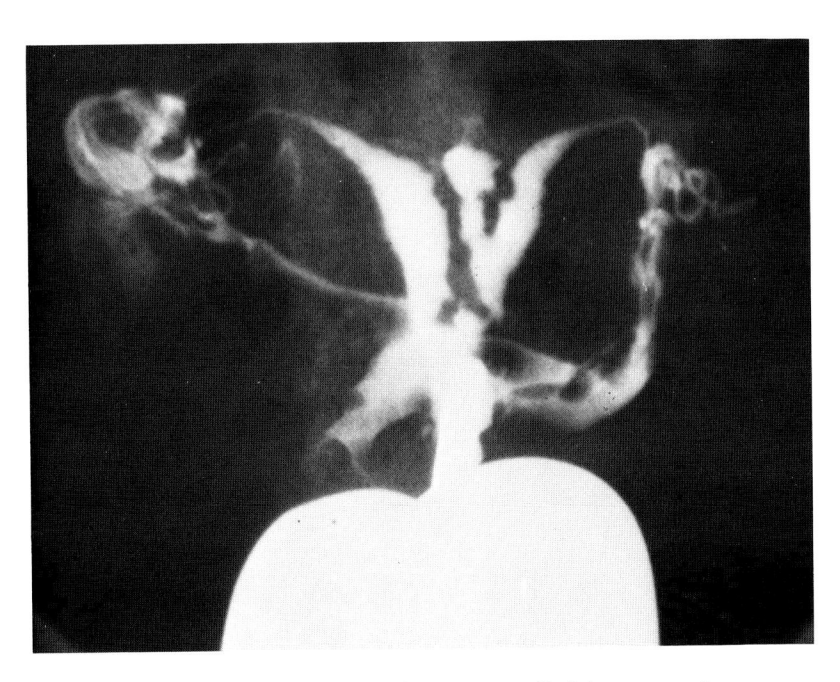

Fig. 8–15. Intrauterine adhesions in a woman with Asherman syndrome.

Neisseria gonorrheae or by an indolent mycotic infection such as *Actinomyces israelii* (58).

Women with acute endometritis have pelvic tenderness, fever, and a purulent vaginal exudate. Fertility is frequently impaired or ablated because these infections cause occlusion of the fallopian tubes or impair tubal motion and contact with the ovary. Acute endometritis may occur in the immediate postpartum period and produce secondary infertility. This may go undiscovered because women often do not remember a postpartum infection. To minimize the risk of infertility, women with acute endometritis should be treated with broad-spectrum antibiotics. For a comprehensive discussion of the management of endometritis the text by Monif is recommended (59).

Chronic endometritis may cause infertility by inhibiting implantation of the blastocyst. As this disorder may be elusive, the clinician should include this in the differential diagnosis of a couple with unexplained infertility. Women with endometritis may be asymptomatic, but some will have unexplained dysfunctional uterine bleeding, pelvic pain, or increased vaginal exudate. Recently, *Chlamydia trachomatis* has been recognized as a cause of endometrial and tubal disease (60).

The treatment of chronic endometritis consists of broad-spectrum antibiotics before, during, and after curettage of the endometrium (51). After curettage, the administration of conjugated estrogens (5.0 mg to 7.5 mg per day, for 60 days) may induce endometrial shedding of necrotic endometrium and rapid regeneration of healthy endometrium (51).

Tuberculous endometritis is rare in the United States, but it accounts for 14.5% of primary infertility in India (61). The menstrual cycle may become irregular and secondary amenorrhea is common. The diagnosis is suggested when Langhans' giant cells are found in the endometrium.

OCCLUSION OF THE UTEROTUBAL JUNCTION. The uterotubal junction is an ill-defined anatomic unit that separates the tubal isthmus from the uterus. It is thought to control sperm transport from the uterus to the fallopian tube and egg transport in the opposite direction (62). Structural abnormalities of the uterotubal junction may cause reproductive failure. Obstruction may result from hypertrophy of the endometrium, endometriosis, endometrial polyps, or salpingitis isthmica nodosa. Like other parts of the female reproductive tract, the uterotubal junction responds to hormonal stimulation. Just prior to menstruation a pressure of 180 to 200 mm Hg is required to force gas into the fallopian tubes whereas the required pressure decreases to 80 to 100 mm Hg just after menstruation (63).

Although abnormalities of the uterotubal junction are rare, apparent occlusion of the uterotubal junction is more commonly seen at hysterosalpingography. If the hysterosalpingogram is performed in the mid- or late luteal phase of the menstrual cycle, the thickened endometrium may obstruct the flow of dye into the tubes or increase the pressure required to pass the dye or carbon dioxide through the tubes. Endometriosis, leiomyomata, or adhesions can obstruct the uterotubal junction.

To distinguish an apparent from an actual cornual obstruction we perform the hysterosalpingogram only during the midfollicular phase of the menstrual cycle. If filling defects, characteristic of endometriosis, are present, we treat the women with danazol, 800 mg/day for 4 months. After the danazol therapy is completed, the hysterosalpingogram is repeated to evaluate the response to therapy.

Diagnostic Methods for Evaluating the Uterus

ENDOMETRIAL BIOPSY. After the dynamic changes of the endometrium were described by Noyes et al. (3), endometrial biopsy became the most frequently used diagnostic test to evaluate the endometrial response to ovarian hormones. Endometrial biopsy is used to date the endometrium, evaluate the endometrial response to endogenous and exogenous hormones, and search for endometrial inflammation. Of the diagnostic tests employed by physicians caring for infertile women, this one is most dreaded by women. Because of the extreme pain, an endometrial biopsy should be performed sparingly and judiciously.

We obtain an endometrial biopsy by inserting a Novak curette into the endometrial cavity and taking a single sample of tissue from the anterior uterine wall. Aspiration with a syringe is not necessary to obtain an adequate tissue

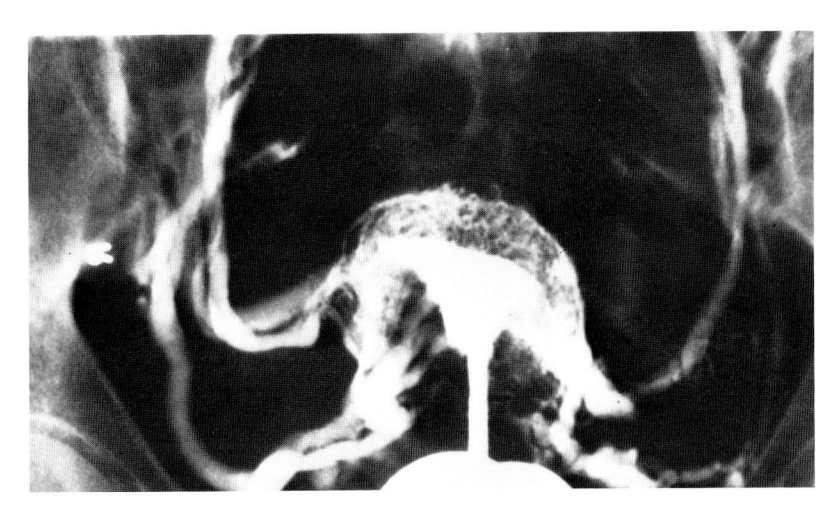

Fig. 8–16. A pelvic venogram that was produced on day 5 of the menstrual cycle.

sample for histologic interpretation. We schedule the endometrial biopsy on day 25 of a 28-day menstrual cycle.

HYSTEROSALPINGOGRAPHY. A hysterosalpingogram done in the midproliferative phase of the menstrual cycle is the primary diagnostic test for evaluating the uterine cavity, and the configuration and patency of the fallopian tubes. If done too early in the cycle, a pelvic venogram may be obtained (Fig. 8–16).

A variety of techniques and instruments have been used in performing a hysterosalpingogram. Instillation of dye through a pediatric Foley catheter has been advocated (65), but we prefer a rigid Cohen cannula attached to a plastic "acorn" tip. This allows manipulation of the uterus to ascertain spatial relationships and visualization of the lower uterine segment. With every technique, the dye should be introduced *slowly* to permit visualization of the contour of the uterine cavity and the architecture of the fallopian tubes. By injecting the dye slowly, uterotubal spasm and pain almost never occur.

The hysterosalpingogram is an essential diagnostic test in an infertility evaluation. It has not been supplanted by diagnostic laparoscopy because the intrinsic configuration of the genital tract cannot be evaluated by endoscopy alone.

HYSTEROSCOPY. Introduction of fiberoptics and development of effective media for uterine distention have made hysteroscopy possible. The contour and configuration of the uterine cavity and the surface texture of the endometrial cavity are assessed (66). Hysteroscopy is performed with a rigid endoscope (modified from the design of a cystoscope) that is introduced into the uterine cavity after the cervical canal has been dilated to accept the sheath of the endoscope. We instill high-molecular-weight dextran* (Hyskon®) through the hysteroscope to distend the uterine cavity and provide an optically clear field. High-mo-

---

* Pharmacia Laboratories Inc., Piscataway, N.J.

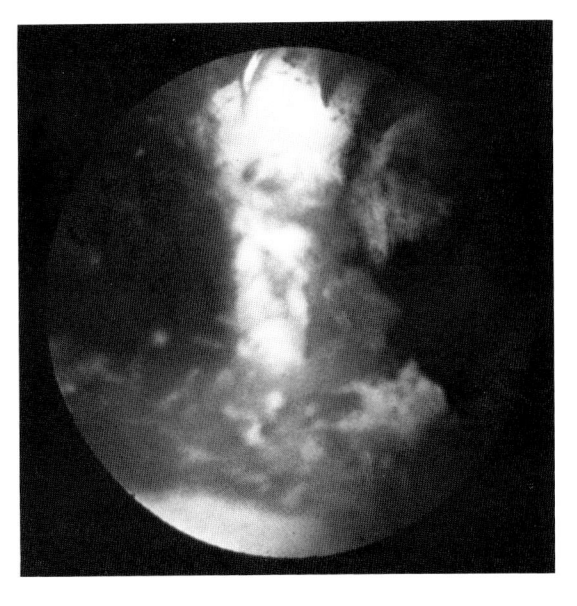

Fig. 8–17. A hysteroscopic photograph of a uterine septum. (Courtesy of Dr. J. A. Daniell.)

lecular-weight dextran is immiscible with blood.

As a technique for evaluating infertile women, hysteroscopy is indicated when structural defects of the endometrial cavity are identified on hysterosalpingogram, to evaluate submucous leiomyomata, to cut intrauterine adhesions, and to resect pedunculated leiomyomata or endometrial polyps. A uterine septum, as seen through the hysteroscope, is shown in Fig. 8–17.

Summary

Although the uterus is essential to successful reproduction, abnormalities of the uterus are infrequent causes of reproductive failure. Structural abnormalities of the uterus are the most common uterine disorders that lead to infertility. Acquired disorders such as leiomyomata, intrauterine adhesions, and inflammation occur less frequently.

The uterus is evaluated best by bimanual pelvic examination and hysterosalpingography. When a uterine abnormality is discovered, it may not be the cause of reproductive failure. Other causes should be sought before a woman is subjected to surgical revision of the uterus. When a uterine abnormality is the cause of reproductive failure, the prognosis for successful pregnancy following surgical revision is excellent.

REFERENCES

1. Coutinho EM, Maia HS. The contractile response of the human uterus, fallopian tubes, and ovary to prostaglandins in vivo. Fertil Steril 1971;22:539–543.
2. Settlage DSF, Motoshima M, Tredway DS. Sperm transport from the external cervical os to the fallopian tubes in women: a time and quantitation study. Fertil Steril 1973;24:655–661.
3. Noyes RW, Hertig AT, Rock J. Dating the endometrial biopsy. Fertil Steril 1950;1:3–25.
4. Ramsey EM. Embryology and developmental defects of the female genital tract. In: Danforth DN, ed. Obstetrics and gynecology. Philadelphia: Harper and Row, 1982:112–126.
5. Griffin JE, Edwards C, Madden JD, Harrod MJ, Wilson JD. Congenital absence of the vagina: the Mayer-Rokitansky-Küster-Hauser syndrome. Ann Intern Med 1976;85:244–236.
6. Evans TN, Poland ML, Boving RL. Vaginal malformations. Am J Obstet Gynecol 1981;141:910–920.
7. Jost A. Problems of fetal endocrinology: the gonadal and hypophyseal hormones. Recent Prog Horm Res 1953;8:379–418.
8. Serra GB, Perez-Palacios G, Jaffe RB. De novo testosterone biosynthesis in human fetal testes. J Clin Endocrinol Metab 1970;30:128–130.
9. Wilson JD. Recent studies on the mechanism of action of testosterone. N Engl J Med 1972;287:1284–1292.
10. Herbst AL, Ulfelder H, Pockanger DC. Adenocarcinoma of the vagina: association of maternal stilbestrol therapy with tumor appearance in young women. N Engl J Med 1971;284:878–881.
11. Gill WB, Schumacher FB, Bibbo M. Structural and functional abnormalities in the sex organs of male offspring of mothers treated with diethylstilbestrol (DES). J Reprod Med 1976;16:147–153.
12. Kaufman RH, Binder GL, Gray PM Jr, Adam E. Upper genital tract changes associated with exposure in utero to diethylstilbestrol. Am J Obstet Gynecol 1977;128:51–59.
13. Bryan AL, Nigro JA, Counseller VS. One hundred cases of congenital absence of the vagina. Surg Gynecol Obstet 1949;88:79–86.
14. Jeffcoate TNA. Advancement of the upper vagina in the treatment of hematocolpos and hematometra caused by vaginal aplasia. Pregnancy following the construction of an artificial vagina. J Obstet Gynaecol Br Commonw 1969;76:961–968.
15. Musset R. Aplasia vaginale avec uterus fonctionnel résultats operatoires et commentaires: à propos de 10 observations. J Gynecol Obstet Biol Reprod (Paris) 1978;7:316–333.
16. Frank RT. The formation of an artificial vagina without operation. Am J Obstet Gynecol 1938;35:1053–1055.
17. McIndoe AH, Banister JB. An operation for the cure of congenital absence of the vagina. J Obstet Gynaecol Br Emp 1938;45:490–494.
18. Wiser WL, Bates GW. Management of vaginal agenesis: a report of 92 cases. Surg Gynecol Obstet (In press, February, 1984).
19. Hecker BR, McGuire LS. Psychosocial function in women treated for vaginal agenesis. Am J Obstet Gynecol 1977;129:543–547.
20. Ingram JM. The bicycle seat stool in the treatment of vaginal agenesis and stenosis: a preliminary report. Am J Obstet Gynecol 1981;140:867–873.
21. Niver DH, Barrett G, Jewelewicz R. Congenital

atresia of the uterine cervix and vagina: three cases. Fertil Steril 1980;33:25–29.
22. Geary WL, Weed JC. Congenital atresia of the uterine cervix. Obstet Gynecol 1973;42:213–217.
23. Rock JA, Jones HW Jr. The double uterus associated with an obstructed hemivagina and ipsilateral renal agenesis. Am J Obstet Gynecol 1980;138:339–342.
24. Green LK, Harris RE. Uterine anomalies. Frequency of diagnosis and associated obstetric complications. Obstet Gynecol 1976;46:427–429.
25. Musich Jr, Behrman SJ. Obstetric outcome before and after metroplasty in women with uterine anomalies. Obstet Gynecol 1978;52:63–66.
26. Rock JA, Jones HW Jr. The clinical management of the double uterus. Fertil Steril 1977;28:798–806.
27. Jones HW Jr. Reproductive impairment and the malformed uterus. Fertil Steril 1981;36:137–148.
28. Craig CJT. Congenital abnormalities of the uterus and foetal wastage. S Afr Med J 1973;47:2000–2005.
29. Strassmann EO. Fertility and unification of the double uterus. Fertil Steril 1966;17:165–176.
30. Capraro KJ, Chuang JT, Randall CL. Improved fetal salvage after metroplasty. Obstet Gynecol 1968;31:97–103.
31. Buttram VC, Zanotti L, Acosta AA, Vanderheyden JS, Besch PK, Franklin RR. Surgical correction of the septate uterus. Fertil Steril 1974;25:373–379.
32. Jones HW Jr, Wheeless CR. Salvage of the reproductive potential of women with anomalous development of the müllerian ducts, 1868-1968-2068. Am J Obstet Gynecol 1969;104:348–364.
33. Strassmann P. Die operative Vereinizing eines doppelten uterus. Zentralbl Gynaekol 1907;43:1322.
34. Tompkins P. Comments on the bicornuate uterus and twinning. Surg Clin North Am 1962;42:1049–1062.
35. Jones HW Jr, Jones GES. Double uterus as an etiological factor of repeated abortion, indication for surgical repair. Am J Obstet Gynecol 1953;65:325–339.
36. Jones HW Jr, Rock JA. Anomalies of the müllerian ducts. In: Reparative and constructive surgery of the female generative tract. Baltimore: Williams & Wilkins, 1982:146–185.
37. Smith OW, Smith GV, Hurwitz D. Increased execretion of pregnanediol in pregnancy from diethylstilbestrol with special reference to late pregnancy accidents. Am J Obstet Gynecol 1946;51:411–415.
38. Dieckmann WJ, Davis ME, Rynkiewicz IM, Pottinger RE. Does the administration of diethylstilbestrol during pregnancy have therapeutic value? Am J Obstet Gynecol 1953:66:1062–1081.
39. Kaufman RH, Adam E, Binder GL, Gerthoffer E. Upper genital tract changes and pregnancy outcome in offspring exposed in utero to diethylstilbestrol. Am J Obstet Gynecol 1980;137:299–308.
40. Haney AF, Hammond CB, Soules MR, Creasman WT. Diethylstilbestrol-induced genital tract abnormalities. Fertil Steril 1979;31:142–146.
41. Bibbo M, Gill WB, Azizi F, et al. Follow-up study of male and female offspring of DES-exposed mothers. Obstet Gynecol 1977;49:1–8.
42. Barnes AB, Colton T, Gundersen J, et al. Fertility and outcome of pregnancy in women exposed in utero to diethylstilbestrol. N Engl J Med 1980;302:609–613.
43. Berger MJ, Goldstein DP. Impaired reproductive performance in DES-exposed women. Obstet Gynecol 1980;55:25–27.
44. Goldstein DP. Incompetent cervix in offspring exposed to diethylstilbestrol in utero. Obstet Gynecol 1978;52:73S-75S.
45. Noller KL, Townsend DE, Kaufman RH. Genital findings, colposcopic evaluation, and current management of the diethylstilbestrol-exposed female. In: Herbert AL, Bern HA, eds. Developmental effects of diethylstilbestrol (DES) in pregnancy. New York: Thieme-Stratton, 1981:81–102.
46. Buttram VC, Reiter RC. Uterine leiomyomata: etiology, symptomatology, and management. Fertil Steril 1981;36:433–445.
47. Ranney B, Frederick I. The occasional need for myomectomy. Obstet Gynecol 1979;53:437–441.
48. Malone LF, Ingersoll FM. Myomectomy in infertility. In: Behrman SJ, Kistner RW, eds. Progress in Infertility. Boston: Little, Brown & Co., 1975:85–90.
49. Jones HW Jr, Rock JA. Surgery of the body of the uterus. In: Reparative and constructive surgery of the female generative tract. Baltimore: Williams & Wilkins, 1983;61–71.
50. Wilson EA, Yang F, Rees ED. Estradiol and progesterone binding in uterine leiomyomata and in normal uterine tissues. Obstet Gynecol 1980;55:20–24.
51. Hunt JE, Wallach EE. Uterine factors in infertility—an overview. Clin Obstet Gynecol 1974;17:44–64.
52. Asherman JG. Traumatic intrauterine adhesions. J Obstet Gynaecol Br Empire 1950;57:892–896.

53. Klein SM. Asherman's syndrome. In: Sciarra JJ, ed. Gynecology and obstetrics, Vol. 5, Chap. 24. Philadelphia: Harper & Row, 1982:1–8.
54. Loures NC, Danezis JM, Potifix G. Use of intrauterine devices in the treatment of intrauterine adhesions. Fertil Steril 1968;19:509–528.
55. March CM, Israel R, March AD. Hysteroscopic management of intrauterine adhesions. Am J Obstet Gynecol 1978;130:653–657.
56. Sugimoto O. Diagnostic and therapeutic hysteroscopy for traumatic intrauterine adhesions. Am J Obstet Gynecol 1978;131:539–547.
57. Mishell DR, Moyer DL. Association of pelvic inflammatory disease with the intrauterine device. Clin Obstet Gynecol 1969;12:179–197.
58. Schiffer MA, Elguezabal A, Sultana M, Allen AC. Actinomycosis infections associated with intrauterine contraceptive devices. Obstet Gynecol 1975;45:67–72.
59. Monif GRG. Infectious diseases in obstetrics and gynecology. Philadelphia: Harper & Row, 1982.
60. Mordh PA, Ripe T, Svensson L, Westrom L. *Chlamydia trachomatis* in patients with acute salpingitis. N Engl J Med 1977;296:1377–1379.
61. Rozin S. Genital tuberculosis. In: Behrman SJ, Kistner RW, eds. Progress in infertility. Boston: Little, Brown & Co., 1975:189–206.
62. Hafez ESE. Anatomy and physiology of the mammalian uterotubal junction. In: Greep RO, Astwood EB, eds. Handbook of physiology, Vol 7. Washington, D.C.: American Physiological Society, 1973:87–95.
63. Lisa JR, Giola JD, Rubin IC. Observations on the interstitial portion of the fallopian tube. Surg Gynecol Obstet 1954;99:159–169.
64. Ayres JWT. Hormonal therapy for tubal occlusion: danazol and tubal endometriosis. Fertil Steril 1982;38:748–750.
65. Ansari AH, Nagamani M. Foley catheter for salpingography, pneumography, tubal insufflation, and hydrotubation. Obstet Gynecol 1977;50:108–112.
66. Valle RF, Sciarra JJ. Current states of hysteroscopy in gynecologic practice. In: Wallach EE, Kempers RD, eds. Modern trends in infertility and conception control. Philadelphia: Harper & Row, 1982:210–223.

The Fallopian Tube: Physiology and Pathology

Carlton A. Eddy

The importance of the fallopian tube in reproduction has been recognized almost from the time this organ was first described as a distinct anatomic entity. Despite early and continuing insight and interest in the function of the fallopian tube and in the consequence of its malfunction, successful clinical management of the "tubal factor" in involuntary female infertility remains an important but all too often elusive goal. Because at present we do not possess the means with which to measure objectively and accurately a single physiologic function of the fallopian tube, treatment of the tubal factor is undertaken in the absence of knowledge regarding its functional status and is aimed primarily, if not exclusively, toward reestablishing patency. That infertility can persist in concert with restored patency underlines the complexity of this organ and the need to restore its function if fertility is to follow.

The systematic investigation of tubal physiology in the laboratory, coupled with the emergence and dramatic success of gynecologic microsurgery in reversing elective tubal sterilization, has generated a resurgence of interest in reconstructive tubal surgery. Each year postgraduate courses in gynecologic microsurgery expose hundreds of gynecologists to this new modality of treating tubal infertility. Operating microscopes, loupes, a wide variety of gynecologic microsurgical instruments, nonreactive inert or absorbable microsutures, tissue adhesives, lasers, microcautery units, antibiotics, antiinflammatory agents and other adjunctive measures have arrived on the gynecologic scene. Tubal surgery has undergone dramatic change and currently embraces techniques of precise hemostasis, atraumatic tissue manipulation, meticulous restoration of anatomy and, most significantly, an appreciation for the need to reestablish physiologic function.

Despite advances in our understanding of tubal physiology and pathophysiology and in the technical armamentarium available to the gynecologist, success in overcoming tubal infertility is significantly higher in women who have previously undergone elective tubal sterilization or who suffer minimal tubal disease. It is almost axiomatic that the success of tubal reconstructive surgery is related to the amount of healthy tube present and in the ability of the diseased tube to heal and resume normal function.

Two groups of women suffering tubal infertility can therefore be described: those who have undergone elective tubal sterilization with minimal tissue destruction in whom the prognosis for success can be quite high, approaching 80% in the hands of the skilled surgeon, and those with congenital or disease-induced tubal malfunction, in whom the prognosis is often far less favorable. In this chapter I will review the physiology and pathology of the fallopian tube and the management of tubal dysfunction in female infertility.

Physiologic Function of the Normal Fallopian Tube

The birth of an individual is the culmination of a temporally well-defined and integrated series of complex physiologic functions, many of which occur within and require the active participation of the fallopian tube. The female reproductive tract constitutes a direct passage from the peritoneal cavity, into which the egg is released, to the outside world, from whence come spermatozoa. It is within the tube that the male and female determinants of each new individual are first brought together and where the embryo undergoes its initial development. When the fallopian tube is incapable of performing any or all of its functions, infertility results.

SPERM TRANSPORT. The oviduct has the task of bringing the ovum and spermatozoa together so that fertilization can occur. Several biologic curiosities are associated with the transport of spermatozoa from the site of insemination to the site of fertilization. First, although the normal ejaculate must contain many millions of spermatozoa to be considered normal, far fewer than 1% reach the site of fertilization, and only a single sperm ultimately participates in fertilization. Second, the tube must be capable of transporting the egg and spermatozoa in opposite directions. Third, the transport of spermatozoa from the site of insemination to the site of fertilization occurs more rapidly than can be accounted for by the intrinsic motility of the sperm.

In current clinical practice, the only assessments of the interaction between spermatozoa and the female genital tract are the Sims-Hühner (postcoital) test, which assesses the ability of sperm to penetrate cervical mucus and presumably to enter the cervical canal, and laparoscopic aspiration of peritoneal fluid following coitus or donor insemination. The recovery of spermatozoa indicates the ability of spermatozoa to traverse the female genital tract (1). Despite the limited assessment possibilities, many important observations concerning sperm transport have been documented and allow a tentative description of the process to be made.

The average normal human ejaculate is deposited at the cervix and may contain more than 100 million spermatozoa, a significant percentage of which are morphologically and, possibly, functionally abnormal. Of this large and heterogeneous population of spermatozoa, most, including may abnormal forms, remain in the vagina or lower reproductive tract to be later expelled or undergo phagocytosis (2). The remaining small percentage undergo a selective filtering process as they sequentially ascend the female reproductive tract in order to ensure that an optimum number of normal, highly fertile spermatozoa reach the ovum.

Two phases of sperm transport appear to occur: an initial short phase in which spermatozoa are rapidly transported to the ampulla and a subsequent sustained phase in which spermatozoa are less rapidly transported to the site of fertilization. The rapid phase of transport, which requires only minutes, is primarily the consequence of the contractile activity of the reproductive tract (3). Experiments with live and dead spermatozoa, radiopaque solutions, and inert particles indicate that sperm motility is not a requisite for this initial rapid phase of transport (4). However, the sustained phase of transport, including entrance of spermatozoa into the cervix, requires or is associated with normal sperm motility. Moreover, detailed evaluation of the morphology of sperm recovered from the various parts of the female tract shows that the selection of sperm is largely achieved by a reduction in the number of abnormal sperm that would be expected to exhibit abnormal motility (5).

Sperm are distributed along the female genital tract in a concentration gradient from the site of insemination to the tubal ampulla. Following colonization of the cervix, sperm continually ascend, enter the fallopian tube, colonize the tubal isthmus and establish an optimum population of sperm in the ampulla consisting of a high proportion of morphologically normal, motile forms (6). Spermatozoa are constantly cleared to the peritoneal cavity and replaced by others from reservoirs below.

The mechanism of sustained transport of spermatozoa following colonization of the isthmus has not been defined, but may include intrinsic motility of the sperm and tubal muscular, ciliary, or secretory activity. The segmental contraction of the oviduct may compartmentalize the lumen and cause a turbulent movement of the tubal fluid. This would tend to cause a reflux of suspended spermatozoa throughout the segment. Successive segmental contractions could result in continuous, random transport of spermatozoa throughout the oviduct.

Sperm transport proceeds opposite to the direction of ciliary beating. If sperm are deposited on the tubal mucosa of a freshly opened oviduct *in vitro*, the strong ciliary currents rapidly transport spermatozoa toward the uterus, completely independent of their own flagellar activity (7). It would therefore appear that spermatozoa would have to be protected from this directionally inappropriate ciliary beating in order to be transported to the site of fertilization. Contraction-induced compartmentalization of the tube may integrate with ciliary activity to create the countercurrent pattern of fluid flow previously described.

SPERM CAPACITATION. Spermatozoa undergo final maturation within the epididymis and are stored in this location until expelled during ejaculation. Freshly ejaculated sperm or those surgically removed from the epididymis are incapable of penetrating the ovum and fertilizing it. Sperm must first undergo a physiologic change, ideally within the female reproductive tract, which is called capacitation. Capacitation renders sperm capable of penetrating the zona pellucida, an acellular mucopolysaccharide layer surrounding the egg. As a result, fertilization can occur (8,9). Capacitation appears to be a general prerequisite for fertilization in all mammals, including the human.

Initially it was believed that capacitation entailed loss of the acrosome, a caplike structure covering the anterior portion of the sperm head. This concept has been abandoned because no morphologic changes in capacitated sperm have been observed. In addition, capacitated sperm recovered from the female tract lose their ability to fertilize the egg when they are returned to seminal plasma. Capacitation therefore involves changes at the molecular level. It would appear that 1 or more substances contained in the seminal plasma inhibits the ability of sperm to fertilize the egg. Since little or no seminal plasma enters the uterus and fallopian tubes, it is appealing to speculate that removal of sperm from the seminal plasma and bathing them within the fluid of the uterus and fallopian tube would dilute the seminal decapacitating factor and expose sperm to a capacitating factor(s) within the female tract.

Sperm recovered from the uterus and tubes appear to be more vigorous than those in the ejaculate or those recovered from the vagina. It is not clear if the endocrine status exerts any effect on the reproductive tract's ability to induce capacitation.

OVUM PICKUP. The transfer of the newly ovulated egg from the surface of the ovary to the interior of the oviduct is crucial to fertility. It is commonly assumed that ovum pickup requires the fimbria to be positioned so that the mucosal surface with its dense complement of cilia beating toward the tubal ostium and uterus can physically contact the cumulus mass and the ovum contained within it. The fimbriae are aided in their function by their attachment to the ovary via an elongated fimbrial fold, the fimbria ovarica, and through their ability to cover a large area of the ovarian surface (10).

As ovulation approaches, the fimbria is brought into contact with the ovary through the contractions of the fimbria ovarica and other folds, and through contractions of the mesovarium, mesosalpinx, oviduct, and the ovary itself to ensure that when the egg is released from the ovary it will enter the tubal lumen.

Ova may be recovered from the oviduct opposite the ovary containing the corpus luteum (11) and pregnancy can result in women with only a single ovary and oviduct located contralateral to each other (12). Under such circumstances, ovum pickup may simply result from the chance encounter of ovum and fimbria, perhaps in the cul-de-sac, or it may reflect the ability of the fimbriae to locate ova successfully within the peritoneal cavity.

FERTILIZATION. Fertilization is the process in which the chromosomes of the male and female gametes unite to form a new and genetically unique individual. Since ovulation occurs spontaneously, regardless of whether coitus has taken place, there must be a mechanism to ensure that normal fertilization can occur despite long intervals of time between ovulation and the occurrence of coitus. During coitus, spermatozoa are deposited in the vagina, an environment relatively hostile to spermatozoa, but soon colonize the cervix and upper female tract, where their survival is prolonged. A relatively constant number of morphologically normal, highly motile spermatozoa are maintained in the ampulla of the tube. This constancy reflects a balance between constant loss of sperm into the peritoneal cavity and replacement from below. Spermatozoa, therefore, await the arrival of the ovum in the oviduct. The fertile life of spermatozoa within the female genital tract is at least 48 hours, but may be as long as 120 hours (13). In contrast, the fertilizable life span of the egg is probably less than 24 hours.

Fertilization occurs in the fallopian tube, most probably in the distal ampulla. When the egg arrives in the tube it is surrounded by the zona pellucida and an aggregation of cumulus cells densely adherent to each other and to the zona pellucida adjacent to the egg. These barriers must be penetrated by the spermatozoa before fertilization can occur. The head of spermatozoa contains enzymes located on the outer and inner acrosomal membranes. Among these enzymes are hyaluronidase, thought to be responsible for cumulus dispersion, and acrosin, necessary for zona penetration. The lytic action of these enzymes creates a tunnel or path for the vigorously motile spermatozoa (14). While both motile and immotile spermatozoa may be transported through the female genital tract, penetration of the egg requires sperm motility.

After penetrating the zona, the fertilizing sperm crosses the perivitelline space and contacts the vitelline membrane with which it fuses. This results in biochemical activation of the egg so that it undergoes final maturation and releases cortical granules from the peripheral cytoplasm into the perivitelline space. The liberated material from the granules alters the physicochemical properties of the zona, rendering it impermeable to further sperm penetration and, thereby, preventing polyspermic fertilization. The sperm head sinks into the egg cytoplasm, undergoes decondensation of its chromatin, and forms the male pronucleus, which then fuses with the egg pronucleus. The result is a genetically complete and new individual (15).

EMBRYRO TRANSPORT. Detailed information on tubal transport of the egg or embryo has been complicated by the difficulty of determining accurately the time of ovulation and of executing appropriate clinical studies. Using serial estrogen and LH determinations to approximate the time of ovulation, eggs have been recovered from the tubes and uteri of women operated upon at various intervals after ovulation and their location within the genital tract has been related to the time interval. The detailed pattern of transport through the fallopian tube is characterized by slow passage through the isthmus so that the egg, and presumably the embryo if fertilization had occurred, enters the endometrial cavity approximately 80 hours after ovulation (16).

Egg transport is thought to be the result of the interaction of tubal contractility, ciliary activity, tubal secretion, and changes in mucosal fold erectile activity (17). The degree to which each of these functional components contributes to or is necessary for successful transport of the developing embryo to the uterus is unknown. Several theories have been offered to explain the process (18,19). Secretory material is made to flow toward the uterus by the persistent, aduterine beat of the cilia. The sphincterlike closure of the circular muscle of the tubal isthmus at midcycle prevents entrance of the luminal contents into the uterus. The production of thick, glycoproteinaceous secretions may contribute to functional occlusion of the isthmus and arrest transport of the embryo in the ampulla or at the ampullary-isthmic junction. This mucus-like material forms a matrix that masks the inappropriately beating cilia, which would otherwise impede sperm movement toward the ampulla, and constitutes a medium comparable to cervical mucus through which sperm easily pass, but not the egg or embryo. This mucus, produced in response to the midcycle peak in estrogen, persists for several days after ovulation. In response to the postovulatory rise in progesterone, tubal secretion of a thick mucuslike fluid stops. Secretory material disappears from the lumen, the cilia once again become free and prominent, and resume their ability to assist in transporting the embryo toward the uterus. The isthmic musculature decreases its sphincterlike activity and increases its segmental contractility in a uterine direction. These, and possibly other mechanisms, ultimately deliver the embryo into the uterus.

EARLY EMBRYO DEVELOPMENT. The fertilized ovum begins to cleave while it is still in the oviduct. Between ovulation and implantation, a period of approximately 1 week, the developing embryo exists in a free-living state suspended in the fluids of the genital tract. It must obtain its metabolic support from these tubal and uterine fluids.

In order to cleave and develop, the fertilized ovum requires both a source of energy and a source of biosynthetic precursors. At ovulation, the ovum contains a wide variety of enzymes capable of catalyzing the necessary metabolic reactions in support of embryonic development. The types, amounts, and activities of these enzymes reflect the progressive changes in metabolic activities of the developing embryo. Early embryos are much more fastidious in their requirements than embryos in later stages of development (20).

Unlike the embryos of lower forms, which rely on stored nutrients in an otherwise hostile environment, the mammalian embryo is dependent on continuing support from the maternal environment. The oviduct, therefore, provides ideal conditions for early embryo development. Although the oviductal lumen does supply such an environment, the necessity of normal tubal epithelial function for embryo development remains to be proved. The human embryo is capable of implanting and developing to advanced stages in the oviduct. Because ectopic implantation often occurs in tubes that have been previously damaged by infection or previous elective sterilization and subsequent surgical repair, it is likely that functional tubal mucosa is not essential for survival of the early human embryo. In contrast, a normal and functional tubal mucosa is almost certainly necessary for proper embryo transport, particularly through the ampulla.

Abnormalities of the Fallopian Tubes

PELVIC SURGERY. Pelvic surgery in women of reproductive age carries with it the possibility of inadvertent but devastating trauma to the ovaries, fallopian tubes, and pelvic peritoneum that may lead to formation of adhesions and loss of fertility through interference with ovulation, ovum pickup, and gamete transport. Pelvic surgery, ideally, should be undertaken only when a clear indication exists. In an era when noninvasive diagnostic procedures and medical management of gynecologic disorders obviate many of the historic indications for "exploratory" or elective pelvic surgery, such indications appear to be on the decline. For example, ovarian cystectomy for functional cysts of unknown origin can often be avoided by monitoring their growth sonographically and allowing spontaneous or progestationally induced resolution to occur. Malignant ovarian tumors are likely to be solid rather than cystic, a distinction that can be made clinically or ultrasonographically (21). Similarly, ovarian wedge resection as treatment of anovulation associated with the polycystic ovary syndrome has largely been replaced with the use of clomiphene or gonadotropins for hormonal induction of ovulation (Chapter 6).

When pelvic surgery is indicated, it should be undertaken as if it were primarily a tuboplastic operation to preserve or restore fertility. Every precaution should be taken to preserve normal function and avoid trauma. All the ancillary techniques that have come to be associated with gynecologic microsurgery should be used, including an appreciation of the ease with which the ovarian and tubal surfaces may be damaged.

The peritoneum should be handled with gloves washed free of starch or talcum. The upper abdomen should be gently packed away with soft, moistened sponges. The uterus should be elevated by packing the posterior vaginal fornix prior to laparotomy or the cul-de-sac after opening the abdomen. The adnexa are placed on a suitable platform, such as one made of a Silastic® sheet. The tubes and ovaries will therefore lie on an elevated, flat plane. All exposed tissues should be kept continually moist with a balanced salt solution such as lactated Ringer's, to which some surgeons add heparin to prevent fibrin formation and avoid the formation of adhesions. The adnexa should not be grasped and clamped with instruments. The historically established use of forceps or Babcock clamps in order to manipulate the adnexa "atraumatically" should be restricted to those tissues scheduled to be resected. The gloved finger or rods made of glass or of Silastic-coated malleable metal are far more appropriate and considerably less traumatic.

Blunt or sharp dissection of adhesions should be avoided. Cutting diathermy delivered with a microneedle electrode, in concert

TABLE 9–1. Restoration of Fertility According to the Site of Surgery

	SITE OF SURGERY					
	Ampullary-Ampullary	Isthmic-Ampullary	Isthmic-Isthmic	Cornual-Ampullary	Cornual-Isthmic	TOTAL
Number of women	30	72	28	39	19	204
Number pregnant	15	40	19	21	14	117
Number ectopic	—	3	—	1	—	5
Pregnancy rate (%)	50	55	68	54	74	57

Data from Rock et al. (23), Silber and Cohen (24), and Winston et al. (25).

with nonconducting glass or Silastic rods used to place adhesions on tension and define planes of dissection, gives far superior results and, together with bipolar coagulation, allows meticulous hemostasis to be achieved. The use of catgut suture should be avoided in the pelvis of the female who wishes to remain fertile. Nonreactive absorbable (Dexon® and Vicryl®) or non-absorbable (Nylon and Prolene®) sutures should instead be used. The risk versus benefit of incidental appendectomy performed by the gynecologist or general practitioner should be weighed carefully, particularly in the woman whose pelvis already may be traumatized and predisposed to postoperative adhesion formation. The recognition and use of sound diagnostic, therapeutic, and technical principles, together with meticulous attention to surgical details and the needs of the woman, will aid greatly in providing quality health care while minimizing the risk and compromise to future fertility.

TUBAL STERILIZATION AND ITS REVERSAL. By far the most frequent iatrogenic tubal trauma is that performed in response to the wishes of the woman who requests a surgical end to her reproductive ability. More than 60 million women worldwide rely on tubal sterilization to control their fertility. In the United States, more than 5 million women have undergone tubal sterilization, and currently as many as 700,000 women are sterilized each year. If this trend continues, over 15% of women in the United States will undergo tubal sterilization before they reach the end of their reproductive life spans (22).

While the majority of women who elect to be sterilized remain pleased with their decision, the demand for reversal is substantial. If only 1% of women annually sterilized request a reversal, this would yield a population of 7,000 candidates each year. Successful reversal of tubal sterilization reflects the complex interaction of numerous factors, many of which remain undefined or incapable of manipulation. Few clinical studies presently exist that objectively document the condition of the oviduct following surgical repair or determine its bearing on subsequent fertility. It is, therefore, difficult to establish a correlation between structure and function or determine with accuracy the feasibility of surgically restoring fertility to a particular woman. It would appear that lesser degrees of tubal damage improve the prognosis for reversibility and that some sterilization techniques are more reversible than others. The intrauterine pregnancy rate following reversal of the major tubal sterilization techniques is not known. However, a growing body of clinical data is making it possible to evaluate the importance or dispensibility of various portions of the fallopian tube (Table 9–1).

Ampullary-Isthmic Junction. Ovum transport, and presumably embryo transport, through the fallopian tube is characterized by a pause at the ampullary-isthmic junction. The functional significance of this pause is unknown, but may be important in synchronizing the endometrial maturation and embryo development that is necessary for successful implantation. The mechanism responsible for the pause remains undefined and may be more functional than anatomic since no sphincterlike arrangement of muscle fibers can be demonstrated.

Clinically, surgical reversal of tubal sterilization in which the ampullary-isthmic junction has been destroyed, necessitating an isthmic-ampullary anastomosis, has resulted in a term

TABLE 9-2. Relationship of Ampullary Length to Pregnancy

	LENGTH OF AMPULLA (cm)				
	0–1	1–2	2–3	3–4	>4
Number of women	2	5	8	5	5
Number of pregnancies	1	2	3	4	5
Pregnancy rate (%)	50	40	36	80	100

From Silber and Cohen (24).

intrauterine pregnancy in up to 55% of women (Table 9–1). It would thus appear that the ampullary-isthmic junction either has little functional significance or that, in performing an isthmic-ampullary anastomosis, a new and functional ampullary-isthmic junction is created.

Uterotubal Junction. The uterotubal junction is the region of transition between the fallopian tube and the uterus. It includes the most proximal portion of the isthmus and the muscular components of the uterus that surround the fallopian tube. Among the various functions ascribed to the uterotubal junction is the control of gamete transport between the uterus and fallopian tube. It has been hypothesized that the uterotubal junction is a hormonally controlled physiologic sphincter that retards passage of eggs into the uterus, thereby preventing premature entry of fertilized eggs into the uterus.

Successful pregnancy in about half of women with bilateral proximal tubal blockage treated with bilateral uterotubal implantation on the posterior aspect of the uterus suggests that the uterotubal junction is not critical to human reproduction (26). Microsurgical tubocornual anastomosis has been associated with a pregnancy rate of 54% to 74% (Table 9–1). Such a technique, unlike uterotubal implantation, maintains the anatomic integrity of the uterus. Women who undergo this type of sterilization reversal need not necessarily have a Cesarean section for delivery since uterine rupture is not likely to occur during normal labor and vaginal delivery.

Tubal Length. The existence of a "shortened tube syndrome" or, specifically, the importance of a minimum length of oviduct necessary for fertility is gaining increasing acceptance. The length of residual (and presumably functional) tube deemed necessary before sterilization reversal is more likely to be successful in ranges from 3 cm to 5 cm for end-to-end anastomosis when the fimbria are normal (27,28) to as much as 8 cm for salpingostomy after sterilization by fimbriectomy (29).

Not only is the length of tube remaining of importance, but also the site of tubal damage. Results of anastomoses performed between isthmus and isthmus or isthmus and uterus gave better results than those that involved the ampulla (Table 9–1). This may indicate that a critical length of ampulla is necessary for normal fertility. There appears to be a positive correlation between the length of ampulla remaining after sterilization reversal and subsequent pregnancy rates (Table 9–2). Since pregnancy is possible when only 1 cm of ampulla remains, the length of the entire tube may be of paramount importance (Table 9–3). Reliance on tubal length as a criterion for patient selection must be tempered by other factors such as associated tubal pathology and the portion of tube remaining.

It would appear from limited data that the following must be present in order for surgical repair of a sterilized fallopian tube to be successful:

1. An ovum pickup mechanism consisting of either an intact fimbria or a mobile neostomy. Either must be in proximity to the

TABLE 9-3. Relationship of Total Tubal Length to Pregnancy

	TUBAL LENGTH (cm)			
	<3	3–4	4–6	>6
Number of women	7	18	26	9
Number of pregnancies	0	7	19	7
Pregnancy rate (%)	0	39	73	78

From Silber and Cohen (24), Wilson (30), and Winston (31).

ovary and possess a normal endosalpinx capable of transferring the ovum into the lumen.
2. A length of tube capable of transporting sperm and ova into proximity with each other. This presupposes some degree of ciliary and myocontractile activity. Such a tube must also possess sufficient secretory activity to provide proper conditions for capacitation, fertilization, and early embryo development.
3. Finally, the reconstructed tube must successfully transport the developing embryo to the uterus. Without this capability, ectopic pregnancy will occur.

It is apparent that no particular segment of the fallopian tube has a unique and indispensable secretory, ciliary, or contractile function. The tube demonstrates a high degree of functional redundancy so that normal pregnancy is possible despite partial resection or damage associated with tubal disease. The gynecologic surgeon exploits this reserve in undertaking tubal repair. Only when tubal anatomy is meticulously restored and sufficient reserve function remains will normal pregnancy occur.

ECTOPIC PREGNANCY. Ectopic pregnancy is a phenomenon essentially unique to the human. By far the most common site of ectopic implantation is the fallopian tube, an organ poorly equipped to support such a pregnancy. The causes of a tubal pregnancy remain obscure but are thought to include (1) mechanical blockage of the tubal lumen brought on by antecedent or coincident salpingitis that allows passage of spermatozoa but not of the fertilized ovum; (2) functional inability of the tube to effect timely pickup of the ovum or embryo transport into the endometrial cavity; and (3) cytogenetic abnormality of the developing embryo that may predispose to tubal implantation.

The incidence of tubal ectopic pregnancy varies and is affected by socioeconomic and geographic factors. Reported figures vary from 0.3% to 3% of all conceptions. If the conservative estimate of 1% of conceptions is used, approximately 30,000 ectopic pregnancies occur in the United States each year. Widespread use of the IUD (32), liberalization of therapeutic abortion (33), and a dramatic increase in sexually transmitted pelvic inflammatory disease with delayed, or inadequate treatment (34) appear to increase the incidence of ectopic pregnancy. Although some tubal ectopic pregnancies resolve spontaneously, tubal abortion or rupture is almost inevitable without intervention. Because of the difficulty in making the diagnosis early, a woman with a tubal ectopic pregnancy most often presents in an acutely ill situation following tubal rupture. The resulting hemorrhage is a life-threatening emergency that accounts for up to 10% of maternal deaths when diagnosis and treatment are delayed.

Traditionally, aggressive surgical management, including ablation of the affected tube and adnexa, has been the treatment of choice. The advent of better diagnostic techniques, including highly sensitive and specific radioimmunoassay of the beta subunit of human chorionic gonadotropin, ultrasonography, and more liberal use of diagnostic laparoscopy, is making early diagnosis of ectopic pregnancy possible. Increasingly, women are seen prior to tubal rupture, in stable condition, with minimal or no demonstrable blood loss. Although surgical intervention is required, a more conservative approach, compatible with the woman's desire to retain her reproductive potential, is being adopted.

In the past, radical and conservative surgery resulted in a low rate of subsequent intrauterine pregnancy and a high rate of repeat ectopic pregnancy (35). Only one third to one half of women who have had an ectopic pregnancy will subsequently give birth to a living infant and 6% to 20% will have another ectopic pregnancy (36,37). However, the evolution of better surgical techniques, such as the use of magnification to visualize the tube and its anatomy, as well as conservative and meticulous handling of the tissues, improves the potential of achieving a subsequent term intrauterine pregnancy.

The goal of conservative surgery is to preserve as much of the affected tube as possible. To acommplish this, it is necessary to understand the histopathology of a tubal gestation. Implantation in the fallopian tube begins intraluminally at the surface of the endosalpinx. The trophoblast, which is highly invasive, quickly penetrates the myosalpinx in a process that may be enhanced by the tube's inability to mount a decidual response to the initial trophoblastic attachment. Following penetration of the endosalpinx, growth of the trophoblast and conceptus is largely extraluminal within the tube. Continued trophoblastic growth involves increasing amounts of the tubal wall adjacent and lateral to the site of implantation (38). Retroperitoneal and intramural hemorrhage result as erosion of tubal arterioles progresses in what normally would be the formation of functional lacunar spaces in the uterus. The resulting stretching of the tubal peritoneum causes the clinical symptoms of pelvic pain and fullness and causes the woman to seek medical consultation. Ideally, the diagnosis is made prior to tubal rupture, loss of the tamponading effect of the surrounding tissue, and massive intraperitoneal hemorrhage. Obviously, the earlier a tubal gestation is diagnosed, the more stable the woman will be, the less damage will have occurred to the tube, and the easier will be its surgical management.

With conservative surgery, only the portion of oviduct containing the ectopic gestation is resected. Alternatively, an incision of the tube over the gestational sac is made and the products of conception are removed. Some surgeons elect to perform an end-to-end anastomosis at the time of segmental resection in order to spare the woman a second major operation (39). Often it is better to defer an anastomosis until the changes of pregnancy have resolved, especially if the tissue is hyperemic, edematous, and fragile. When the tube is incised, subsequent pregnancy rates may be higher if the incision is made in the anterior, not antimesenteric, surface (40). In so doing, entry into the lumen of an uninvolved segment of tube is avoided, as is iatrogenic trauma to the endosalpinx of the lumen. Because of the extensive lateral spread of the trophoblast away from the implantation site and its intimate maternal vascular involvement, great care must be taken to achieve hemostasis. The inability of maternal arterioles invaded by trophoblast to constrict and the ineffectiveness of the myosalpinx to compress them, can lead to intraoperative hemorrhage when the conception is removed, or to delayed bleeding after surgery as residual trophoblast sloughs. Vigorous debridement of the site of implantation should not be attempted because of the difficulty of differentiating between trophoblastic and tubal tissue. Bleeding sites should be carefully identified by liberally irrigating the area and applying pinpoint microelectrocautery. Alternatively, hemostatic sutures may be placed using 6–0 to 9–0 sutures. Repair of the incised tube can be accomplished by first intention, using interrupted or continously placed sutures of 6–0 to 9–0 inert material or may be allowed to occur without primary closure.

When implantation has taken place in the distal ampulla or infundibulum, the pregnancy may be enucleated or "shelled out" without incising the tube. Conversely, when implantation is adjacent to the uterus or within the intramural portion of the tube, simple resection of the involved segment should be performed, if possible, without performing a cornual wedge resection, since this procedure may lead to extensive operative hemorrhage, which, if intractable, may require hysterectomy. Cornual wedge resection also increases the risk of uterine rupture during labor should an intrauterine pregnancy subsequently be achieved.

Because of the disparity between characteristics of women and operative techniques in published studies, it is difficult to assess the impact of conservative management on subsequent fertility. Two recent studies, in which an ectopic pregnancy in women with a single tube was treated conservatively, provide useful insight since the presence of a potentially normal contralateral tube was not a confounding factor in the outcome. In the first study, 15 women underwent tubal incision with removal of the conception and closure by secondary intention. The overall term intrauterine pregnancy rate was 53% and the recurrent ectopic pregnancy rate was 20% (41). In the second study, 13 women underwent a similar procedure. Of the 11 women actively attempting pregnancy, all experienced at least 1 term delivery and none has had a repeat ectopic pregnancy (42).

Clearly, ectopic pregnancy is a manifestation of abnormal reproductive function and, regardless of its etiology and management, women who experience such a gestation remain at risk of experiencing another. Yet its treatment need not automatically entail radical excision that further compromises an already suboptimally fertile woman. While the gynecologic surgeon may consider the 20% risk of recurrent ectopic pregnancy unacceptable, his patient may not. The increasing incidence of ectopic pregnancy within the general population, coupled with its diagnosis prior to tubal abortion or rupture, provides the opportunity to consult with the woman and to provide treatment consistent with sound medical practice and her desire for future fertility.

DIETHYLSTILBESTROL. The widespread use of diethylstilbestrol (DES), a nonsteroidal, orally effective synthetic estrogen, to support a high-risk pregnancy began in the mid 1940s and continued until the 1960s (43,44). A decade ago, epidemiologic studies initially suggested an association of *in utero* exposure to DES and subsequent vaginal and cervical adenocarcinoma (45). Fortunately, the incidence of DES-related malignant neoplastic disease has proved to be considerably less than originally feared. That risk is now estimated to be 1.4 to 14 women through age 24 per 10,000 exposed to DES (46).

Benign abnormalities of the lower genital tract, however, have been described in these women and include vaginal septa, hypoplasia and adenosis of the cervix, and morphologic and cytologic anomalies of the cervix (47). When lower genital tract anomalies are present, a significant number of women will also exhibit upper genital tract anomalies, including those of the fallopian tube. These include the now classic T-shaped uterine endometrial cavity with widening of its lower two thirds and an irregular, "shaggy" contour of the walls (48). Changes in the fallopian tubes include widening and elongation of the intramural portion that extend to the proximal isthmus, with or without bandlike constrictions (48). Shortened, thin-walled, sacculated, convoluted tubes with thinning of the endosalpinx and increased connective tissue, atrophic fimbriae, and marked phimoses or occlusion have also been described (49).

Between 1 and 2 million live female births are estimated to have occurred in the United States following chronic *in utero* exposure to DES (50,51). The incidence of genital anomalies in women exposed to DES is difficult to determine owing to the self- or physician-selected patient population and the uncontrolled, retrospective nature of most studies.

While lower genital tract anomalies are often apparent, the diagnosis of uterine anomalies requires hysterosalpingography. Unfortunately, hysterosalpingography is a crude way of acquiring information about tubal morphology. The tubes may appear patent and normal yet exhibit extensive morphologic abnormality when viewed at laparoscopy (49).

The association between DES exposure and infertility is similarly difficult to define. The generation of women exposed *in utero* to DES is now reaching its peak reproductive years. While it appears that many of these women are free of the genital stigmata of DES exposure and exhibit normal reproductive performance, others manifest varying degrees of anatomic change in müllerian derivatives and suffer a resultant impairment of fertility. The degree of infertility is generally related to the extent and severity of the morphologic abnormality. The cervical and uterine anomalies may increase spontaneous abortion rates to as high as 32% of the number of intrauterine pregnancies (52). Women with documented or suspected DES-induced tubal anomalies may have a rate of tubal gestation at least 5 times that of unexposed women (49,52). Despite these statistics, normal pregnancy and delivery have been achieved in women with severe anomalies, including those of the fallopian tube. Because of the inability to correct DES-induced malformations surgically, particularly those of the tube (49), the management of infertile women who present with classic DES-induced genital anomalies is largely medical and expectant. Because so many DES-exposed women are presently using contraception and because the cause-and-effect relationship between DES exposure and subsequent impairment of fertility has not been fully defined, the full impact of DES on reproduction is yet to be seen.

SALPINGITIS. The number of women who have been electively sterilized and subsequently seek restoration of their fertility is significant and has provided much of the impetus for the current interest in fertility surgery, particularly that undertaken with the operating microscope. To the approximately 7,000 women each year who are potential candidates for surgical reversal of their elective tubal sterilizations must be added a considerably larger number who suffer involuntary infertility. Pathologically induced tubal damage accounts for 30% to 50% of female infertility (53); most of this is due to salpingitis. Although pelvic inflammatory disease (PID) may be the result of postoperative, postabortal, or puerperal infection, the prevalent view considers sexually transmitted microorganisms as the primary causative agents. Salpingitis caused by genital tuberculosis, leprosy, parasites, or fungal infections is uncommon in developed countries.

Gonorrhea. The gonococcus (*Neisseria gonorrhoeae*) has traditionally been considered the causative organism of most cases of acute, nongranulomatous salpingitis. There were more than 1 million reported and 4 million unreported cases of gonorrhea in the United States in 1975 and it is estimated that the incidence of this disease is increasing by 15% each year (54). Gonorrhea predisposes the woman to subsequent episodes of salpingitis, which will be bilateral in 90%. Salpingitis affects more than 500,000 women in the United States each year, half of whom require hospitalization.

Not all pelvic inflammatory disease is gonococcal in origin. The microbiology and clinical course of salpingitis is complex and poorly documented because the tube is inaccessible for bacterial sampling and because it is difficult to culture some of the more fastidious pathogens. Commonly, the etiology of PID is defined by the potential pathogens isolated from the endocervix. The cervix of healthy women normally may contain all of the species of opportunistic pathogenic organisms associated with intraabdominal infections in a nonpathologic host-organism relationship. The recovery of a potential pathogen from the cervix of an infected woman, therefore, is only presumptive evidence that the organism caused the disease in the fallopian tube or that it is the only infectious agent present in the tube. Only an estimated 10% to 17% of women with positive isolates of gonococci from the endocervix develop salpingitis (55), while 10% to 90% of women with acute pelvic inflammatory disease have positive endocervical cultures for *Neisseria* (56,57). Culture of tubal aspirates or peritoneal exudate obtained at laparoscopy, culdoscopy, or laparotomy may give more definitive evidence of the causative agent(s). *Chlamydia trachomatis* is now thought to be an important cause of both acute and chronic salpingitis (58). In some parts of the world it is recovered from inflamed tubes more often than *Neisseria*, which may be recovered only from the cervix of some women with salpingitis. The primary etiologic role of *Neisseria* in salpingitis may be to induce acute disease and cause limited or reversible tubal damage that predisposes the woman to reinfection, or to enhance the virulence of nongonococcal facultative pathogens.

Salpingitis results from the direct ascent of organisms, usually along mucosal surfaces from the cervix, through the endometrium, and into the tubes. This ascent is brought about by altered host-organism relationships and occurs most often during or immediately after menstruation. Lymphatic or hematogenous spread may occur during pregnancy, but is otherwise uncommon (59). Acute gonococcal salpingitis is primarily an endosalpingitis and results in destruction of the mucosa with partial or complete occlusion of the tube and attenuation or obliteration of the fimbria and tubal abdominal ostium. The endosalpinx undergoes an intense inflammatory reaction characterized by tissue infiltration with polymorphonuclear leukocytes, focal necrosis and epithelial deciliation, and filling of the tubal lumen with a purulent exudate composed of pus, desquamated epithelium, and necrotic material. If spontaneous or antibiotic-induced resolution does not occur, inflammatory changes continue and often lead to the accumulation of a purulent exudate, chronic infection, the formation of a pyosalpinx, and tubal obstruction. In chronic infection, with frequent episodes of acute exacerbation, all anatomic layers of the tube become involved in the inflammatory changes; infiltration of the endosalpinx extends to the myosalpinx and serosa. The involvement of the serosa generally produces a perisalpingitis, which may, in time, result in the formation of peritubal adhesions. The tubes become moderately enlarged, primarily as a result of interstitial thickening and edema. They may retain some semblance of their normal shape and position.

Resolution of occlusive, polymicrobial, pyogenic salpingitis with resorption of the purulent exudate and its replacement with a watery or serouslike fluid gives rise to a hydrosalpinx, the size of which may vary from the enormous, retort-shaped entity referred to in Europe as a "sactosalpinx" to a tube only slightly enlarged from normal. Peritubal adhesions are generally present and may greatly distort the relationship of the tube to the other pelvic organs, particularly the ovary. The tubal walls are thin and are often translucent in the grossly distended hydrosalpinx. The hydrosalpinx may have a single lumen, which is a gaping, hollow space into which project a few sparse, atrophic mucosal plicae instead of the normal virtual space of the healthy tube that is filled with a branched and folded mucosa. Alternately, the mucosa may undergo extensive agglutination of adjacent folds, which results in a lumen filled with a complex, multiloculated system of gutterlike compartments, many of which end blindly.

Women with a hydrosalpinx present with a cystic, nontender mass that is asymptomatic or associated with only mild pelvic pressure or pain. It is quite common for women seeking consultation for involuntary infertility to deny a history of pelvic infection and to have bilateral hydrosalpinges as an incidental finding on hysterosalpingography.

Because of its widespread occurrence, frequently nonspecific symptomatology, difficult differential diagnosis, and consequent delayed or absent treatment, salpingitis can have a devastating effect on subsequent fertility. In a study of women who had been treated for pelvic inflammatory disease, about 21% were involuntarily infertile, in contrast to 3% of matched control subjects who had not had PID. Tubal occlusion develops in 12.8% of women following 1 episode of PID, in 35.5% of women following 2 episodes, and in 75% of women following 3 or more episodes (60).

Salpingoplasty

Involuntary infertility caused by tubal pathologic changes following acute or chronic salpingitis remains one of the most prevalent conditions and the least amenable to surgical correction. The natural history of salpingitis and its effect on the fallopian tube may vary dramatically. In many women bilateral distal tubal occlusion occurs and is accompanied by loss of the fimbria, peritubal and ovarian adhesions, and marked alteration in the architecture of the tubal wall. Salpingitis leads to multicentric disease with diffuse loss of function. Unfortunately, the histology and functional impact of these changes have not been separated from that resulting from varying loss of epithelial architecture and deciliation and subjective changes in the thickness of the tubal wall.

The prognosis for fertility following reconstructive surgery of tubes damaged by infection is essentially determined by: (1) the degree of deciliation in the endosalpinx, and (2) the extent of thickening and fibrosis of the tubal wall, which seems to reflect changes in the myosalpinx and its ability to undergo normal functional contractile activity (61). Such anatomic abnormalities are slow to regress following tubal surgery, if, in fact, the endosalpinx and myosalpinx are capable of regenerating at all. In this regard, it is noteworthy that conception following salpingostomy for postinfectious disease often requires 1 to 2 years and conceptions more than 4 years after surgery are not unusual. In contrast, a significant number of women who undergo end-to-end anastomosis for reversal of elective tubal sterilization conceive within a year of surgery—as early as the first cycle following reversal and occasionally in the same cycle in which surgery is performed. These differences reflect the fact that elective tubal sterilization is performed on a normal organ resulting in conservation of functionally normal residual portions of fallopian tube. Such a tube simply lacks continuity between the ovary and uterus. In contrast, disease-induced changes following salpingitis entail loss of structure and function throughout much or all of the fallopian tube.

Representative results of conventional macrosurgical repair of distal occlusion following tubal disease are listed in Table 9–4. Of 653 women who underwent salpingostomy, only 62, or 9.5%, achieved a term pregnancy with the birth of a live infant. The spontaneous abortion and ectopic pregnancy rates were in excess of 3.1% and 4.5%, respectively, for all women who underwent surgery. Approximately 83% of the women never conceived after their surgery.

Table 9–5 lists the results of a similar group of women who underwent salpingostomy with microsurgical techniques, techniques that have been shown to give excellent results for rever-

TABLE 9–4. Macrosurgical Salpingostomy of Postinfectious Tubes

AUTHOR (REF.)	YEAR	NO. OF PATIENTS	TERM PREGNANCY		SPONTANEOUS ABORTION (No.)	ECTOPIC PREGNANCY (No.)
			No.	%		
Mulligan (62)	1966	66	11	17	3	6
Rock et al. (63)	1978	99	16	16	N.S.	6
Clyman (64)	1968	27	5	18	N.S.	N.S
Jessen (65)	1971	25	5	20	5	3
Lamb and Moscovitz (66)	1972	35	2	6	N.S.	3
Ozaras (67)	1968	106	2	2	N.S.	0
Siegler (68)	1969	27	2	7	0	0
Foix (69)	1974	12	1	8	0	1
Young et al. (70)	1970	18	3	17	0	3
Boyd and Holt (71)	1973	77	5	6.5	2	2
Mroueh and Hajj (72)	1968	60	1	2	0	0
Fjallbrant (73)	1975	35	6	17	2	3
Hanton et al. (74)	1964	32	1	3	4	1
Crane and Woodruff (75)	1968	34	2	6	4	2
Total		653	62	9.5	20	30

N.S. = Not stated.
Modified from Winston (76).

sal of elective sterilization. Of 448 women operated on, 94 (21%) achieved a term pregnancy. Although this is double the percentage of women who achieved a term live birth after a macrosurgical procedure, the majority of women remained infertile. Moreover, the spontaneous abortion and ectopic pregnancy rates, 5.8% and 9.4%, respectively, were also double those in the group of women who underwent conventional macrosurgical salpingostomy. The poor results in both groups of women reflect the extent of tubal damage beyond loss of the fimbria and distal occlusion, and the inability of surgery to restore patency and function.

The outcome of salpingostomy in women in whom loss of the tubal fimbria and distal occlusion were not the result of tubal disease but rather of elective sterilization by fimbriectomy is summarized in Table 9–6. Of the 34 women so sterilized, 17 achieved an intrauterine pregnancy following microsurgical reversal. This is a 6-fold improvement over conventional surgery and a 3-fold improvement over microsurgical repair of postinfectious distal tubal occlusion. The spontaneous abortion and ectopic pregnancy rates were at least 5.8% and 2.9%, respectively. These rates are comparable to those following salpingostomy of post-infectious tubes. Although a mechanically induced hydrosalpinx may occur following fimbriectomy sterilization, no disease is present and the tube appears to remain morphologically and, presumably, functionally normal in most women. Because the major portion of the tube is conserved, attempts at reversal may be quite successful. It would, therefore, appear that absence of the fimbria does not mean absolute infertility. The ideal candidate for fimbriectomy reversal has an oviduct of approximately

TABLE 9–5. Microsurgical Salpingostomy of Postinfectious Tubes

AUTHOR (REF.)	YEAR	NO. OF PATIENTS	TERM PREGNANCY		SPONTANEOUS ABORTION		ECTOPIC PREGNANCY	
			No.	%	No.	%	No.	%
Swolin (77)	1975	33	8	24	0	0	8	24
Winston (25)	1980	241	42	17	18	7.5	23	9.5
Frantzen and Schlösser (61)	1982	85	12	14	4	4.7	3	3.5
Gomel (78)	1983	89	28	32	4	4.5	8	9
Total		448	94	21	26	5.8	42	9.4

TABLE 9-6. Salpingostomy for Reversal of Fimbriectomy Sterilization

AUTHOR (REF.)	YEAR	NO. OF PATIENTS	INTRAUTERINE PREGNANCY No.	%	SPONTANEOUS ABORTION (No.)	ECTOPIC PREGNANCY (No.)
Novy (29)	1980	9	4	44	1	0
Betz et al. (79)	1980	7	4	57	N.S.	1
Gomel (80)	1980	14	6	43	1	N.S.
Verhoeven (81)	1983	4	3	75	—*	0
Total		34	17	50	2	1

N.S. = Not stated.
* All 3 patients still pregnant.

normal length, an ampulla at least 1 cm in diameter, rugal patterns discernable on hysterosalpingography, and no or few peritubal adhesions. Most notably, successful reversal appears to be associated with spontaneous eversion of the endosalpinx at the time of surgery, and a tendency to form a neofimbria-like structure that may substitute for the excised normal fimbria (79).

Summary

Intuitively, most physicians (but few infertile couples) understand that the fallopian tubes are much more than passive conduits for the passage of spermatozoa and ova. The tubes are complex structures that actively participate, even regulate, transport of germ cells, fertilization, and embryo migration. Anatomic and functional integrity of the fallopian tubes is impaired easily by injudicious surgical techniques, medication, and infection.

The most effective treatment of tubal disease is prevention—pelvic surgery only for established indications, observation of microsurgical principles such as gentle handling of tissues, stringent hemostasis and copious irrigation, and prompt antibiotic therapy of acute pelvic infections.

When prevention of disease fails, microsurgery of the fallopian tubes has improved term pregnancy rates in women with tubes damaged by infection. Microsurgery restores fertility in more than 50% of women who request reversal of tubal sterilization.

REFERENCES

1. Asch RH. Laparoscopic recovery of sperm from peritoneal fluid in patients with negative or poor Sims-Hühner test. Fertil Steril 1976;27:1111-1114.
2. Moyer DL, Rimdusit S, Mishell DR Jr. Sperm distribution and degradation in the human female reproductive tract. Obstet Gynecol 1970;35:831-840.
3. Settlage DSF, Motoshima M, Tredway DR. Sperm transport from the external cervical os to the fallopian tubes in women: a time and quantitation study. Fertil Steril 1973;24:655-661.
4. DeBoer CH. Transport of particulate matter through the human female genital tract. J Reprod Fertil 1972;28:295-297.
5. Mortimer D, Leslie EE, Kelly RW, et al. Morphological selection of human spermatozoa *in vivo* and *in vitro*. J Reprod Fertil 1982;64:391-399.
6. Ahlgren M, Bostrom K, Malmqvist R. Sperm transport and survival in women with special reference to the fallopian tube. In: Hafez ESE, Thibault CG, eds. Sperm transport, survival and fertilizing ability in vertebrates, Vol. 26. Paris, INSERM, 1974:183-200.
7. Blandau RJ. Gamete transport: comparative aspects. In: Hafez ESE, Blandau RJ, eds. The mammalian oviduct. Chicago: University of Chicago Press, 1969:129-162.
8. Chang MC. Fertilizing capacity of spermatozoa deposited into the fallopian tubes. Nature 1951;168:697.
9. Austin CR. The capacitation of mammalian sperm. Nature 1952;170:326.
10. Okamura H, Morikawa H, Oshima M, et al. A morphological and physiological study of mesotubarium ovarica in humans. Int J Fertil 1972;22:179-183.
11. Doyle LL, Lippes J, Winters HS. Human ova in the fallopian tube. Am J Obstet Gynecol 1966;95:115-117.
12. First A. Transperitoneal migration of ovum or spermatozoon. Obstet Gynecol 1954;4:431-434.
13. Ferin J, Thomas K, Johansson ED. Ovulation detection. In: Hafez ESE, Evans T, eds. Human reproduction: conception and contraception. New York: Harper & Row, 1973:261-283.

14. Allison AC, Hartree EF. Lysosomal enzymes in the acrosome and their possible role in fertilization. J Reprod Fertil 1970;21:501–515.
15. Fawcett DW. The male reproductive system. In: Greep RO, Koblinsky MA, Jaffe FS, eds. Reproduction and human welfare: a challenge to research. Cambridge: MIT Press, 1976:165–277.
16. Croxatto HB, Ortiz ME, Diaz S, et al. Studies on the duration of egg transport by the human oviduct. II. Ovum location at various intervals following luteinizing hormone peak. Am J Obstet Gynecol 1978;132:629–634.
17. Croxatto HB. The duration of egg transport and its regulation in mammals. In: Coutinho EM, Fuchs F, eds. Physiology and genetics of reproduction, part B. New York: Plenum Press, 1974:159–166.
18. Jansen RPS. Fallopian tube isthmic mucus and ovum transport. Science 1978;201:349–351.
19. Jansen RPS. Cyclic changes in the human fallopian tube isthmus and their functional importance. Am J Obstet Gynecol 1980;136:292–308.
20. Whitten WK. Culture of tubal ova. Nature 1957;179:1081.
21. Jansen RPS. Pelvic surgery in young women. Med J Aust 1982;1:525–526.
22. Population Reports. Law and policy: legal trends and issues in voluntary sterilization. Baltimore, Md.: Population Information Program, Series E, 1981, No. 6.
23. Rock JA, Katayama KP, Jones HW Jr. Tubal reanastomosis: a comparison of Hellman's technique without magnification and a microsurgical technique. In: Population Reports. Female sterilization: reversing female sterilization. Baltimore, Md.: Population Information Program, Series C, 1980, No. 8.
24. Silber SJ, Cohen RS. Microsurgical reversal of female sterilization: the role of tubal length. Fertil Steril 1980;33:598–601.
25. Winston RML. Microsurgery of the fallopian tube: from fantasy to reality. Fertil Steril 1980;34:521–530.
26. Peterson EP, Musich JR, Behrman SJ. Uterotubal implantation and obstetric outcome after previous sterilization. Am J Obstet Gynecol 1977;128:662–667.
27. Cantor B, Riggall FC. The choice of sterilizing procedure according to its potential reversibility with microsurgery. Fertil Steril 1979;31:9–12.
28. Diamond E. Microsurgical reconstruction of the uterine tube in sterilized patients. Fertil Steril 1977;28:1203–1210.
29. Novy MJ. Reversal of Kroener fimbriectomy sterilization. Am J Obstet Gynecol 1980;137:198–206.
30. Wilson PCM. Results of Australia sterilization reversal series. In: Population Reports. Female sterilization: reversing female sterilization. Baltimore, Md.: Population Information Program, Series C, 1980, No. 8.
31. Winston RML. Microsurgery in the treatment of female infertility. In: Population Reports. Female sterilization: reversing female sterilization. Baltimore, Md.: Population Information Program, Series C, 1980, No. 8.
32. Seward PH, Israel R, Ballard CA. Ectopic pregnancy and intrauterine contraception. A definite relationship. Obstet Gynecol 1972;40:214–217.
33. Panayotou PP, Kaskarelis DB, Miettinen OS, et al. Induced abortion and ectopic pregnancy. Am J Obstet Gynecol 1972;114:507–510.
34. Persaud V. Etiology of tubal ectopic pregnancy, radiologic and pathologic studies. Obstet Gynecol 1970;36:257–263.
35. Thimonen S, Nieminen U. Tubal pregnancy, choice of operative method of treatment. Acta Obstet Gynecol Scand 1967;46:327–339.
36. Bronson RA. Tubal pregnancy and infertility. Fertil Steril 1977;28:221–228.
37. Kitchen JD, Wein RM, Nunley WC Jr, et al. Ectopic pregnancy: current clinical trends. Am J Obstet Gynecol 1979;134:870–876.
38. Budowick M, Johnson TRB Jr, Genadry R, et al. The histopathology of the developing tubal ectopic pregnancy. Fertil Steril 1980;34:169–171.
39. Stangel JJ, Reyniack V, Stone ML. Conservative surgical management of tubal pregnancy. Obstet Gynecol 1976;48:241–244.
40. Brosens IA, Gordts S, Boeckx W. Tubal pregnancy: salpingostomy versus salpingotomy. Fertil Steril 1983;39:384 (letter).
41. DeCherney AH, Maheaux R, Naftolin F. Salpingostomy for ectopic pregnancy in the sole patent oviduct: reproductive outcome. Fertil Steril 1982;37:619–622.
42. Valle JA, Lifchez AS. Reproductive outcome following conservative surgery for tubal pregnancy in women with a single fallopian tube. Fertil Steril 1983;39:316–320.
43. Smith OW, Smith GV, Hurwitz D. Increased excretion of pregnanediol in pregnancy from diethylstilbestrol with special reference to the problem of late pregnancy accidents. Am J Obstet Gynecol 1946;51:411–415.
44. Smith OW. Diethylstilbestrol in the prevention and treatment of complications of pregnancy. Am J Obstet Gynecol 1948;56:821–834.
45. Herbst AL, Ulfelder H, Poskanzer DC. Adenocarcinoma of the vagina: association of maternal stilbestrol therapy with tumor appearance in young women. N Engl J Med 1971;284:878–881.
46. DES Task Force Summary Report. Washing-

ton, D.C.: United States Department of Health, Education, and Welfare, 1978.
47. Herbst AL, Kurman RJ, Scully RE. Vaginal and cervical abnormalities after exposure to stilbestrol *in utero*. Obstet Gynecol 1972;40:287–298.
48. Kaufman RH, Binder GL, Gray PM, et al. Upper genital tract changes associated with exposure *in utero* to diethylstilbestrol. Am J Obstet Gynecol 1977;128:51–56.
49. DeCherney AH, Cholst I, Naftolin F. Structure and function of the fallopian tubes following exposure to diethylstilbestrol (DES) during gestation. Fertil Steril 1981;36:741–745.
50. Kaufman RH. Structural changes of the genital tract associated with in utero exposure to diethylstilbestrol. In: Wynn RM, ed. Obstet Gynecol Annu. Norwalk, Ct.: Appleton-Century-Crofts, 1982:187–202.
51. Glebatis DM, Janerich DT. A statewide approach to diethylstilbestrol—the New York program. N Engl J Med 1981;304:47–50.
52. Schmidt G, Fowler WC Jr, Talbert LM, et al. Reproductive history of women exposed to diethylstilbestrol *in utero*. Fertil Steril 1980;33:21–24.
53. O'Brien JR, Arromet GH, Eduljee SY. Operative treatment of fallopian tube pathology in human fertility. Am J Obstet Gynecol 1969;103:520–531.
54. Spence MR. The role of gonococcus in salpingitis. J Reprod Med 1977;19:31–35.
55. Sweet RL. Diagnosis and treatment of acute salpingitis. J Reprod Med 1977;19:21–29.
56. Curtis AH. Bacteriology and pathology of fallopian tubes removed at operation. Surg Gynecol Obstet 1921;33:621–631.
57. Rendtorff RC, Curran JW, Chandler RW. Economic consequences of gonorrhea in women: experience from an urban hospital. J Am Vener Dis Assoc 1974;1:40–47.
58. Mardh PA, Ripa T, Svensson L, et al. Chlamydia trachomatis infection in patients with acute salpingitis. N Engl J Med 1977;296:1377–1379.
59. Hedberg E, Spetz SO. Acute salpingitis, views on prognosis and treatment. Acta Obstet Gynecol Scand 1958;37:131–154.
60. Westrom L. Effect of acute pelvic inflammatory disease on fertility. Am J Obstet Gynecol 1975;121:707–713.
61. Frantzen C, Schlosser HW. Microsurgery and postinfectious tubal infertility. Fertil Steril 1983;38:397–402.
62. Mulligan WJ. Results of salpingotomy. Int J Fertil 1966;11:424–430.
63. Rock JA, Katayama KP, Martin EJ, et al. Factors influencing the success of salpingostomy techniques for distal fimbrial obstruction. Obstet Gynecol 1978;52:591–596.
64. Clyman MJ. Silastic hoods in tuboplasty. A new approach to removal. Fertil Steril 1968;19:537–543.
65. Jessen H. 45 operations for sterility. Acta Obstet Gynecol Scand 1971;50:105–115.
66. Lamb EJ, Moscovitz W. Tuboplasty for infertility. Int J Fertil 1972;17:53–58.
67. Ozaras H. The value of plastic operations on the fallopian tubes in the treatment of infertility. Acta Obstet Gynecol Scand 1968;47:489–500.
68. Siegler AM. Salpingoplasty: classification and report of 115 operations. Obstet Gynecol 1969;34:339–344.
69. Foix A. Tratamiento quirugica de la esterilidad feminina. In: Esterilidad conjugal. Buenos Aires; Panamericana, 1974.
70. Young PE, Egan JE, Barlow JJ, et al. Reconstructive surgery for infertility at the Boston Hospital for Women. Am J Obstet Gynecol 1970;108:1092–1097.
71. Boyd IE, Holt EM. Tubal sterility. Patency tests and results of operation. J Obstet Gynaecol Br Commw 1973;80:142–151.
72. Mroueh A, Hajj SN. Tubal plastic surgery. Int J Fertil 1968;13:215–219.
73. Fjallbrant B. Tubal surgery. Report of 101 cases with special reference to the experience of the surgeon. Acta Obstet Gynecol Scand 1975;54:463–467.
74. Hanton EM, Pratt JH, Banner EA. Tubal plastic surgery at the Mayo Clinic. Am J Obstet Gynecol 1964;89:934–939.
75. Crane M, Woodruff JD. Factors influencing the success of tuboplastic procedures. Fertil Steril 1968;19:810–820.
76. Winston RML. Is microsurgery necessary for salpingostomy? The evaluation of results. Aust NZ J Obstet Gynaecol 1981;21:143–152.
77. Swolin K. Electromicrosurgery and salpingostomy. Long term results. Am J Obstet Gynecol 1975;121:418–419.
78. Gomel V. Microsurgery in female infertility. Boston: Little Brown & Co., 1983.
79. Betz G, Engel T, Penney LL. Tuboplasty—comparison of the methodology. Fertil Steril 1980;34:534–536.
80. Gomel V. The impact of microsurgery in gynecology. Clin Obstet Gynecol 1980;23:1301–1310.
81. Verhoeven H. Unpublished data.

Male Reproductive Physiology 10

Ronald S. Swerdloff and Shalender Bhasin

The human testis is an organ consisting of 2 related functional compartments: (1) the endocrine cells (Leydig or interstitial cells, and Sertoli cells), and (2) the germ cells (spermatozoa and sperm precursors). The Leydig, Sertoli, and germ cells are an anatomically and functionally integrated unit that affects normal reproductive function.

The Leydig cells, located between seminiferous tubules, are the source of most of the circulating testosterone and its metabolites. Testosterone and dihydrotestosterone are responsible for male sexual differentiation and maturation, normal sexual potency and ejaculatory capability, maturation of germ cells, and seminal fluid production. The Sertoli cells and germ cells are located within the seminiferous tubules and are separated from the Leydig cells by the tubular basement membrane. The Sertoli cells lie close to the germ cells and are believed to mediate the hormonal regulation of spermatogenesis. The Sertoli cells are also the source of androgen binding protein (ABP), the tubular contribution to the seminal fluid, müllerian inhibiting hormone, and inhibin. Spermatogonia, under the influence of these and other factors, differentiate into spermatozoa. Testicular function is regulated by a series of closed loop feedback systems involving the higher centers in the central nervous tissue, the hypothalamus, the pituitary, and testicular endocrine and germinal compartments (Fig. 10–1).

It is our purpose to describe the mechanisms that result in normal reproduction. An understanding of male reproductive function provides a basis for understanding derangements that may result in defective spermatogenesis and male infertility.

Regulation of the Testicular Endocrine Environment

GONADOTROPIN RELEASING HORMONE (GnRH). The hypothalamus is the integrating center of stimuli from the central nervous system and testes that influence the synthesis and secretion of gonadotropin-releasing hormone. The extrahypothalamic central nervous system inhibits and stimulates GnRH secretion. Neurotransmitters such as norepinephrine, dopamine, endorphins, and melatonin serve as regulators of GnRH synthesis and pulsatile release into the hypophyseal portal veins. Norepinephrine stimulates and dopamine and endorphins inhibit GnRH release from the hypothalamus (1). The hypothalamus, especially the supraoptic and arcuate nuclei, has androgen and estrogen receptors and responds to differences in circulating concentrations of sex steroid hormones by changing its rate of synthesis and/or release of GnRH.

GnRH is released into the portal circulation in pulses at a frequency of approximately 1 pulse every 70 to 90 minutes (2). The pulsatile nature of GnRH release appears to be essential for stimulating the synthesis and release of LH and FSH (3). Although GnRH stimulates the pituitary secretion of both LH and FSH, the pulse frequency of GnRH release may be important in determining the relative ratio of LH

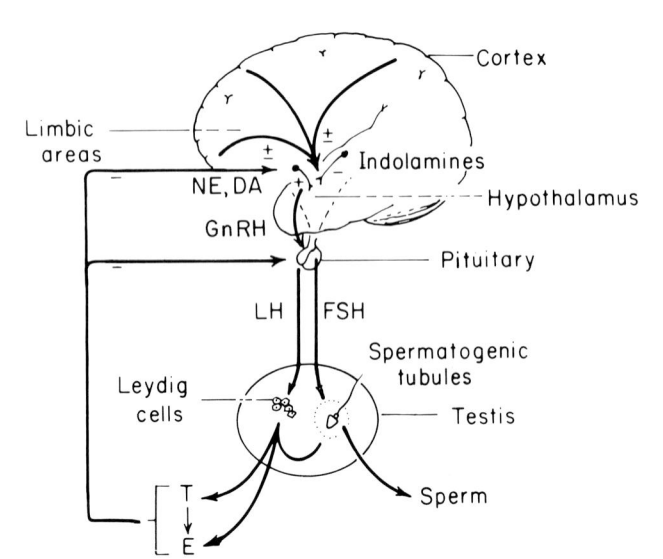

Fig. 10-1. The hypothalamic-pituitary-gonadal axis in the male. The hypothalamus is the integrating center for central nervous system (CNS) regulation of gonadotropin-releasing hormone. Extrahypothalamic CNS input has both inhibitory and stimulatory influences on GnRH secretion. Neurotransmitters such as norepinephrine (NE) and dopamine (DA), endorphins, and melatonin serve as regulators of GnRH synthesis and release from the hypothalamus. The human testis is a dual organ with endocrine and reproductive functions. Testicular function is regulated by a series of closed loop feedback systems involving the higher centers in the CNS, the hypothalamus, the pituitary, and the testicular endocrine and germinal compartments. T = testosterone; E = estrogen.

and FSH secreted into the peripheral circulation. Sex steroids, neurotransmitters, and pituitary gonadotropins modulate the pulse frequency and amplitude of GnRH secretion. Through an ultrashort feedback loop operating within the pituitary, gonadotropins may also regulate their own secretion (4).

LUTEINIZING HORMONE (LH). LH is a glycoprotein hormone that binds to Leydig cells and stimulates steroidogenesis. LH action is mediated by specific, high-affinity receptors on the cell membrane (5). Binding of LH to its receptors increases adenylate cyclase activity, which causes a rise in intracellular cyclic AMP (6); cAMP binding to protein kinase leads to dissociation of this holoenzyme, release of its regulatory unit, and RNA and protein synthesis. Four asparagine and 4 serine-linked carbohydrate units appear to be essential for biologic activity (7).

LH exerts its stimulatory effect upon steroidogenesis by accelerating the metabolism of cholesterol (8). Cholesterol entry into the mitochondria is proportionate to the quantity of cholesterol available to the Leydig cells. There, LH also stimulates the conversion of 20- and 22-alpha hydroxycholesterol to pregnenolone through the action of cholesterol esterase and cholesterol side chain cleavage enzymes (9). There is no evidence that LH directly affects any of the components of the seminiferous tubules.

FOLLICLE STIMULATING HORMONE (FSH). FSH receptors are present on Sertoli cell membranes. FSH binds to these receptors, stimulates adenylate-cyclase-mediated production of cAMP, and, finally, activation of the regulatory subunit of protein kinase (10).

One of the major actions of FSH is the stimulation of protein synthesis. FSH enhances testicular incorporation of amino acids into protein (10). FSH promotes the testicular production of at least 5 specific proteins: androgen-binding protein (ABP), inhibin, the plasminogen activator, gamma glutamyl transpeptidase, and a protein kinase inhibitor. The first 3 are secreted into the rete testis fluid (11–14).

FSH stimulates protein synthesis in the testes of immature rats, but not in the testes of rats older than 25 days. The responsiveness to FSH in mature rats returns following hypophysectomy (10). The loss of Sertoli cell response to FSH in the adult rat is caused by increased phosphodiesterase activity, which diminishes cAMP production. The number of FSH receptors, however, does not decrease with age, but actually increases (10).

FSH also stimulates aromatase activity in Sertoli cells cultured from testes of 5- to 20-day-old rats (15). Aromatase is the term for a group of enzymes that convert certain androgens (e.g., testosterone) to estrogens (e.g., 17-beta-estradiol). FSH also stimulates 5-alpha-reductase activity in Sertoli cells of 10-day-old rats.

The action of this enzyme results in the formation of dihydrotestosterone from testosterone. Finally, FSH stimulates a calcium-dependent regulatory protein that influences the distribution of intracellular calcium and the Sertoli cell cytoskeleton by microfilament realignment (11).

Hormonal Control of Spermatogenesis

Spermatogenesis is a complex process whereby primitive stem cells, type A spermatogonia, undergo a complex series of transformations to become mature spermatozoa. The development of germ cells in the seminiferous tubules occurs in 3 phases: spermatogonial multiplication, meiosis, and spermiogenesis. In the seminiferous epithelium, cells in these developmental phases are arranged in defined associations or stages. In most mammals these stages follow one another in a regular fashion and give rise to a wave of germ cell maturation along the seminiferous epithelium. The time interval between the successive appearance of the same cell association at a given point in the tubule is called the cycle of the seminiferous epithelium (16). In man, the average length of this cycle is 73 days (17) and includes all 3 phases. Subsequent sperm transport in the epididymis and vas deferens requires an additional 21 days.

FSH and androgens cause changes during different stages in the cycle of the seminiferous epithelium. Maximal binding of FSH in Sertoli cells occurs in those stages of spermatogenesis in which activity of adenylate cyclase in the haploid germ cells is greatest and when the secretion of cAMP by the seminiferous tubules is maximal (18). The other stages are found when secretion rates of androgen-binding protein and local concentrations of testosterone are highest (19). The stages of spermatogenesis that appear to be androgen dependent are also found when secretion of plasminogen activator and a meiosis-inducing substance is highest (20).

Steinberger et al. demonstrated that testosterone alone could initiate spermatogenesis in hypophysectomized immature rats, and that FSH was required only for maturation of spermatids to form spermatozoa (21,22). However, exogenous administration of testosterone to hypogonadotropic men does not induce spermatogenesis (23). This failure in the human is most likely owing to the practical limits of the dose that can be administered. Such doses increase circulating testosterone concentrations, but do not provide adequate intratesticular testosterone concentrations. By contrast, hCG administration stimulates an increase in intratesticular testosterone concentrations and promptly initiates spermatogenesis. Furthermore, precocious puberty may occur in boys with a localized Leydig cell tumor. The germ cells in tubules adjacent to this androgen-producing tumor undergo maturation while the germs cells distant from the tumor or in the contralateral testis remain unstimulated, despite virilizing peripheral serum concentrations of testosterone. In hypogonadal men treated with hCG alone, maturation of the seminiferous epithelium does not progress beyond the spermatid stage. FSH alone does not initiate spermatogenesis, but its administration to hCG-primed hypogonadal men results in completion of spermatogenesis and production of an adequate number of sperm to restore fertility (24). Thus, FSH appears to be essential for spermiogenesis (transformation of spermatids into mature spermatozoa). In hypogonadotropic men primed with hCG and FSH, spermatogenesis can be maintained by hCG alone.

In addition to androgens and FSH, many other proteins are secreted locally in the tubule in a cyclic fashion during the cycle of the seminiferous epithelium (25). These proteins probably mediate the interaction of Sertoli and germ cells—important for the intratesticular control of spermatogenesis.

Testicular Steroid Hormone Production

TESTOSTERONE AND ESTRADIOL. Testosterone is the major steroid hormone produced by the testis and cholesterol appears to be the obligatory precursor (25). The Leydig cells are the main source of the 4 mg to 7 mg of testosterone produced daily. Cholesterol is converted within the mitochondria of Leydig cells to pregnenolone, which is further metabolized outside the mitochondria to several other steroids, including testosterone (26,27). Pregnenolone can be converted to testosterone either via a delta-4 or a delta-5 pathway. With *in vitro* incubation of human testicular tissue, the delta-5 pathway appears to predominate, while in other species the delta-4 pathway via progesterone predominates (28,29).

About 40 mcg of estradiol are produced daily in an adult male. Three fourths of it is derived from peripheral aromatization of testosterone and androstenedione, while the rest is secreted directly from the testes. Virtually all of the dihydrotestosterone produced (300 mcg/day) is derived from peripheral conversion of testosterone, much in the prostate gland. Thus, testosterone also functions as a prohormone for both 17-beta-estradiol and dihydrotestosterone formation (25). Sertoli cells appear to be the intratesticular site of estradiol synthesis and the production of estradiol within the human testis may be important in the regulation of Leydig cell function. The role of dihydrotestosterone in spermatogenesis is probably minimal since little of this androgen is produced within the testes and is not required for spermatogenesis. Males with 5-alpha-reductase deficiency cannot produce normal quantities of dihydrotestosterone, yet spermatogenesis occurs (30).

Most of the circulating testosterone is bound to a high-affinity beta globulin, testosterone-estradiol binding globulin (TEBG), but only free, or unbound, testosterone is available for entry into testosterone-responsive cells. The hepatic production of TEBG is affected by a number of physiologic and metabolic factors. Estrogens stimulate and testosterone inhibits its production and the ratio of estrogen to androgen may be the major determinant of the hepatic production of TEBG (31). In men with hepatic cirrhosis, estrogen levels are normal or increased and TEBG synthesis is increased. While total testosterone concentrations are normal, free (unbound) concentrations diminish. This results in primary testicular failure, oligospermia, and, frequently, gynecomastia.

Thyroid hormones also influence TEBG levels: TEBG synthesis is less when thyroxine (T_4) or triiodothyronine (T_3) are low, but increased when T_4 and T_3 production is increased. TEBG concentrations are low in obese men with acromegaly.

ANDROGEN-BINDING PROTEIN (ABP). Androgen-binding protein is a glycoprotein found in the testis and epididymis (32,33). Its secretion by Sertoli cells into the seminiferous tubules is stimulated by FSH. ABP may sequester testosterone inside the seminiferous tubules and indirectly regulate spermatogenesis (34).

Androgen Receptors

Androgen-responsive tissues contain a specific receptor protein that binds dihydrotestosterone (DHT) with very high affinity. The binding affinity of this intracellular receptor is less for testosterone, and less yet for 3-alpha-androstanediol. The receptor has been found in the cytosolic fraction of cells from many androgen-responsive tissues (34,35). Dihydrotestosterone and testosterone are bound to a single androgen receptor protein, although claims of separate receptors for each steroid and distinct receptors in different tissues have been presented (36,37). In the majority of androgen-sensitive cells, testosterone readily diffuses through the cell membranes and is converted to DHT by 5-alpha-reductase. DHT binds to its receptor and the DHT-receptor complex undergoes a temperature-sensitive transformation before translocation into the nucleus (Fig. 10–2). In cells in which 5-alpha-reduction of testosterone occurs to a limited extent (e.g., seminiferous tubules), testosterone binds to the receptor, undergoes transformation, and the testosterone-receptor complex is translocated to the nucleus. A portion of the androgen-receptor complex binds to intranuclear acceptor molecules. This permits a tight association of androgen-receptor complexes with nuclear chromatin. These events are followed by synthesis of androgen-dependent RNA and proteins. The gene for the intracellular androgen receptor protein is located on the X-chromosome (38).

Paracrine Control of Testicular Function

REGULATION BY PRODUCTS OF STEROIDOGENESIS. Expression of testosterone action is the net consequence of the quantity of testosterone produced and androgen receptor

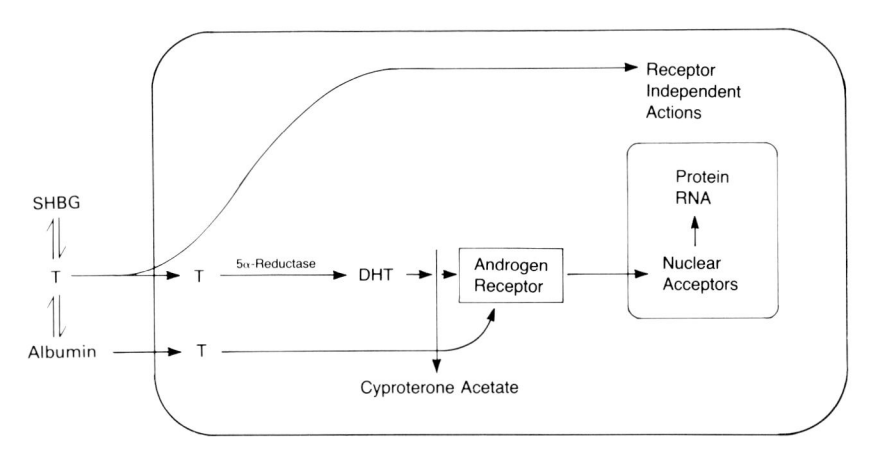

Fig. 10–2. Mechanism of androgen action at the cellular level. In a majority of androgen-sensitive cells, testosterone (T) penetrates the plasma membrane and is converted to dihydrotestosterone (DHT) by 5-alpha-reductase. DHT binds to a cytoplasmic androgen receptor and the DHT-receptor complex is translocated to the nucleus. In cells in which 5-alpha-reduction of testosterone occurs to a limited extent, testosterone binds to the receptor and the complex is translocated to the nucleus. Association of the androgen-receptor complex with nuclear acceptors is followed by synthesis of androgen-dependent messenger RNA and proteins. Antiandrogens such as cyproterone acetate inhibit androgen binding to the cytoplasmic receptor. Some actions of testosterone do not require receptor binding.

function. Testosterone formation is stimulated by LH, but its formation is modified by the presence of enzymes that promote the synthesis of steroids other than testosterone from cholesterol and progesterone. The conversion of 17-alpha-hydroxyprogesterone to androstenedione is catalyzed by C17–20 lyase and androstenedione is then converted to testosterone. 20-alpha-dehydrogenase diverts testosterone precursors from androgen synthesis and limits testosterone production (39).

Steroids with 21 carbon atoms that are reduced at the C-5 position (e.g., 5-alpha-pregnane-3,20 dione) inhibit C17–20 lyase. Thus, 5-alpha-reductase can be viewed as a potential inhibitor of testosterone and androstenedione synthesis (40).

The testes can also synthesize steroid sulfates and it has been proposed that these steroid sulfates serve as a reservoir to maintain intratesticular free testosterone concentrations at a constant level. Free steroids inhibit steroid sulfatase activity. When free steroid levels decline, inhibition of sulfatase activity diminishes and steroid sulfates are converted to free hormones (41).

SERTOLI-LEYDIG CELL INTERACTION. A large body of evidence suggests the existence of an intratesticular Leydig-Sertoli cell axis (42–45). Sertoli cell products regulate Leydig cell function and can inhibit testosterone synthesis. This is an example of a "short loop" feedback system, common in reproductive physiology. Sertoli cells appear to be the source of certain peptides that have a structure similar to that of GnRH. These peptides may bind to GnRH receptors on Leydig cells and modulate Leydig cell response to gonadotropins (46,47).

Sertoli cells can also convert androgens to estrogens. Estrogens reduce testosterone synthesis and do so independently of LH suppression (43,44). Furthermore, Leydig cells contain estradiol receptors (27). The net result of these functions is formation of estrogens from androgens secreted by the Leydig cells and modulation of Leydig cell function by the estrogens thus formed (43,45).

Testicular Regulation of Gonadotropin Secretion

FEEDBACK BY STEROID HORMONES. Androgens and estrogens regulate gonadotropin secretion differently. Administration of estradiol at physiologic levels results in decreases in FSH and LH concentrations. The decrease in circulating LH concentrations is associated with a decrease in LH pulse amplitude; LH pulse frequency remains unaltered (48).

The feedback effects of testosterone are complex in that it acts both as an androgen and as a precursor for estradiol. "Pure" androgens (i.e., nonaromatizable androgens, such as dihydrotestosterone), decrease the frequency of LH secretory pulses.

Aromatization of testosterone to form estradiol is also important in regulating gonadotropin secretion. In men pretreated with an antiestrogen such as clomiphene or with selective inhibitors of aromatization, testosterone fails to suppress LH and FSH (49). However, Swerdloff et al. showed that dihydrotestosterone, a nonaromatizable androgen, was more potent than testosterone in suppressing serum LH levels while equally potent to testosterone in suppressing FSH (50).

5-ALPHA-REDUCTASE. In a large number of mammalian species, the anterior pituitary, hypothalamus, hippocampus, and amygdala can convert testosterone to dihydrotestosterone, a 5-alpha-reduced androgen. Reduction of the keto group at C-3 of dihydrotestosterone also occurs to yield 5-alpha-androstane, 3-beta, 17-beta-diol (51). These conversions occur under the influence of an enzymatic complex that includes a 5-alpha-reductase and 2 hydroxysteroid dehydrogenases (3-alpha- and 3-beta-). These 5-alpha-reduced metabolites may act as intracellular mediators for the inhibitory control of LH secretion by testosterone (51).

INHIBIN. To explain the monotropic increase in FSH that follows seminiferous tubule injury, McCullagh proposed that the seminiferous tubules produced a factor capable of selective FSH suppression, a factor he termed inhibin (52). Inhibinlike activity has been reported in seminal plasma, rete testis fluid, aqueous extracts of testis, and Sertoli cell culture medium (53,54). Isolation of inhibin has not been successful to date. Sertoli cells are the likely source of inhibin.

Summary

Spermatogenesis is a continuous process occurring at all times in the seminiferous tubules of normal adult men. Formation of mature spermatozoa from spermatogonia requires 73 days in the human. Spermatogenesis is a testosterone-dependent process and intratesticular concentrations of testosterone are 100 times greater than peripheral serum concentrations. Such high local concentrations of testosterone appear to be necessary for spermatogenesis and subsequent transport of sperm in the epididymis and vas deferens. Hypothalamic GnRH and pituitary gonadotropins are important regulators of spermatogenesis by their role in modifying Leydig cell production of testosterone. Intratesticular testosterone production, and therefore spermatogenesis, are also modified by other secretory products of the testis, such as estradiol and androgen-binding protein. The testis also possesses the capacity to produce steroid sulfates. These appear to serve as a reservoir for free testosterone and, thereby, maintain a constant intratesticular testosterone concentration. Secretory products of the testis (e.g., testosterone and inhibin) also influence spermatogenesis by influencing hypothalamic and pituitary function.

Because the intratesticular mechanisms in the control of spermatogenesis are difficult to study and are not well understood, there are many gaps in our knowledge about the precise mechanisms of spermatogenesis and the pathophysiology of abnormal spermatogenesis. However, abnormalities of hypothalamic-pituitary function that result in altered secretion of FSH and LH will result in impaired reproductive capacity because of the resultant alteration in testosterone production by Leydig cells. Steroid enzyme defects that preclude normal production of testosterone and androgen receptor defects, which preclude normal expression of testosterone, also impair spermatogenesis.

By understanding the physiologic mechanisms of spermatogenesis, disorders of male reproduction become more understandable and treatment of these disorders more logical (Chapter 11).

REFERENCES

1. Barraclough CA, Wise PM. The role of catecholamines in the regulation of pituitary luteinizing hormone and follicle-stimulating hormone secretion. Endocr Rev 1982;3:91–120.
2. Carmel PW, Arakis S, Ferin M. Pituitary stalk portal blood collection in rhesus monkeys: evidence for pulsatile release of gonadotropin-re-

leasing hormone (GnRH). Endocrinology 1976;99:243–248.
3. Belchetz PE, Plant TM, Nakai Y, Keogh EJ, Knobil E. Hypophysial response to continuous and intermittent delivery of hypothalmic gonadotropin-releasing hormone. Science 1978;202:631–633.
4. LaBorde NP, Wolfsen AR, Odell WD. Short loop feedback system for the control of follicle-stimulating hormone in the rabbit. Endocrinology 1981;108:72–75.
5. Catt KJ, Tsuruhara T, Mendelson C, Ketelslegers MJ, Dufau ML. Gonadotropin binding and activation of the interstitial cells of the testis. In: Dufau ML, Means AR, eds. Hormone binding and target cell activation in the testes. New York: Plenum Press, 1974:1–30.
6. Tsuruhara T, Dufau ML, Cigurraga S, Catt KJ. Hormonal regulation of testicular LH receptors. Effects on cyclic AMP and testosterone responses in isolated Leydig cells. J Biol Chem 1977;252:9002–9009.
7. Dufau ML, Tsuruhara T, Horner KA, Podesta EJ, Catt KJ. Intermediate role of cyclic AMP and protein kinase during gonadotropin induced steroidogenesis in testicular interstitial cells. Proc Natl Acad Sci USA 1977;74:3419–3423.
8. Hall PF, Irby DC, deKretser DM. Conversion of cholesterol to androgens by rat testis. Comparison of interstitial cells and seminiferous tubules. Endocrinology 1967;84:488–496.
9. Hafiez A, Bartke A, Lloyd CW. The role of prolactin in the regulation of testis function: the synergistic effects or prolactin and LH on the incorporation of ^{14}C-acetate into testosterone and cholesterol by testis from hypophysectomized rats in vitro. J Endocrinol 1972;53:223–230.
10. Means AR, Fakunding JL, Huckins C, Tindall DJ, Vitale R. Follicle-stimulating hormone, the Sertoli cell, and spermatogenesis. Recent Prog Horm Res 1976;32:477–527.
11. Means AR, Dedman JR, Tindall DJ, Welsh MJ. Hormonal regulation of Sertoli cells. Int J Androl (Suppl 2) 1978;2:403–421.
12. Lacroix M, Smith FE, Fritz IB. Secretion of plasminogen activator by Sertoli cell enriched cultures. Mol Cell Endocrinol 1977;9:227–236.
13. Krueger PM, Hodgen GD, Sherins RJ. New evidence for the role of Sertoli cell and spermatogonia in the feedback control of FSH secretion in male rats. Endocrinology 1974;95:955–962.
14. Hansson VM, Ritzen EM, French FS, Nayfeh SN. Androgen transport and receptor mechanisms in the testis and epididymis. In: Greep RO, Astwood EB, Hamilton DW, eds. Handbook of Physiology. American Physiologic Society, Washington, D.C. 1975;7:173–201.
15. Van Damme MP, Robertson DM, Marana R, Ritzen EM, Diczfalusy E. A sensitive and specific in vitro bioassay method for the measurement of follicle-stimulating hormone activity. Acta Endocrinol 1979;91:224–237.
16. LeBlond CP, Clermont Y. Definition of the stages of the cycle of the seminiferous epithelium in the rat. Ann NY Acad Sci 1952;55:548–573.
17. Clermont Y. The cycle of the seminiferous epithelium in man. Am J Anat 1963;112:35–51.
18. Gordeladze JO, Parvinen VM, Clausen OP, Hansson V. Stage dependent variation in Mn 2^+-sensitive adenylyl cyclase (AC) activity in spermatids and FSH sensitive AC in Sertoli cells. Arch Androl 1982;8:43–51.
19. Ritzen EM, Boitani C, Parvinen M, French FC, Feldman M. Stage-dependent secretion of ABP by rat seminiferous tubules. Mol Cell Endocrinol 1982;25:25–33.
20. Lacroix M, Parvinen M, Fritz IB. Localization of testicular plasminogen activator in discrete portions (stages VII and VIII) of the seminiferous tubule. Biol Reprod 1982;25:143–146.
21. Steinberger E, Root A, Ficher M, Smith KD. The role of androgens in the initiation of spermatogenesis in man. J Clin Endocrinol Metab 1973;37:746–751.
22. Steinberger E. Hormonal control of mammalian spermatogenesis. Physiol Rev 1972;51:1–22.
23. Macleod J. The effects of urinary gonadotropin following hypophysectomy and in hypogonadotropic eunuchoidism. In: Rosemberg E, Paulsen CA, eds. The human testis. New York: Plenum Press, 1970:577–590.
24. Sherins RJ, Winters SJ, Wachslicht H. Studies of the role of hCG and low dose FSH in initiating spermatogenesis in hypogandotropic men. Endocrine Society 1977:(Abs. P312):212.
25. Parvinen M. Regulation of the seminiferous epithelium. Endocr Rev 1982;3:404–417.
26. Toren D, Menon KM, Forchielli E, Dorfman RI. In vitro enzymatic cleavage of the cholesterol side chain in rat testis preparations. Steroids 1974;3:381–390.
27. Van der Vusse GJ, Kalkman ML, Van der Molen HJ. Endogenous production of steroids by subcellular fractions from total rat testis and from isolated interstitial tissue and seminiferous tubules. Biochem Biophys Acta 193;297:179–185.
28. Yanaihara T, Troen P. Studies of the human testis I. Biosynthetic pathways for androgen formation in human testicular tissue in vitro. J Clin Endocrinol Metab 1972;34:783–792.
29. Samuels LT, Bussmann L, Matsumoto K, Huseby RA. Organization of androgen biosyn-

thesis in the testis. J Steroid Biochem 1975;6:291–296.
30. Peterson RE, Imperato-McGinley J, Gautier T, Sturla E. Male pseudohermaphroditism due to steroid 5 alpha-reductase deficiency. Am J Med 1977;62:170–191.
31. Chopra IJ, Tulchinsky D, Greenway FL. Estrogen-androgen imbalance in hepatic cirrhosis. Ann Intern Med 1973;79:198–203.
32. Hsu A-F, Troen P. An androgen-binding protein in the testicular cytosol of human testis. J Clin Invest 1978;61:1611–1619.
33. Rommerts FFG, Grootegold JA, Van der Molen HJ. Physiological role for androgen binding protein steroid complex in testis? Steroids 1976;28:43–49.
34. Rommerts FFG, Kruger-Sewnarain BC, Van Woerkom-Blik A., Grootegold JA, Van der Molen HJ. Secretion of proteins by Sertoli cell enriched cultures: effects of follicle stimulating hormone, dibutyryl cAMP and testosterone and correlation with secretion of estradiol and androgen binding protein. Mol Cell Endocrinol 1978;10:39–55.
35. Liao S. Cellular receptors and mechanisms of action of steroid hormones. Int Rev Cytol 1975;41:87–172.
36. Wilson J. Metabolism of testicular androgens. In: Hamilton DW, Greep RO, eds. Handbook of Endocrinology. American Physiological Society, Washington, D.C., 1975;5:491–508.
37. Verhoeven G, Heyns W, DeMoor P. Testosterone receptors in the prostate and other tissues. Vitam Horm 1975;33:265–281.
38. Ohno S. Major regulatory genes for mammalian sexual development. Cell 1976;7:315–321.
39. Inano H, Tamaoki B. Bioconversion of steroids in immature rat testes in vitro. Endocrinology 1966;79:579–590.
40. Brophy PJ, Gower DB. Studies on the inhibition by 5-alpha-pregnane 3,20-dione of the biosynthesis of 16-androstenes and dehydroepiandrosterone in boar testis preparations. Biochem Biophys Acta 1974;360:252–259.
41. Payne AH. Gonadal steroid sulfates and sulfatase V. Human testicular steroid sulfatase. Partial characterization and possible regulation by free steroid. Biochem Biophys Acta 1972;258:473–483.
42. Aoki A, Fawcett DW. Is there a local feedback from the seminiferous tubules affecting activity of the Leydig cell? Biol Reprod 1978;19:144–158.
43. Dufau ML, Hsueh AJ, Cigorraga S, Baukal AJ, Catt KL. Inhibition of Leydig cell function through hormonal regulatory mechanism. Int J Androl (Suppl 2) 1978;2:193–239.
44. Hsueh AJ, Dufau M, Catt KJ. Inhibitory effects of estrogen on Leydig cells function: studies of FSH treated hypophysectomized rat. Endocrinology 1978;103:1069–1102.
45. Mulder E, Van Beurden-Lamers WMO, DeBoer W, Brinkman AO, Van der Molen HJ. Testicular estradiol receptors in the rat. In: Dufau ML, Means AR, eds. Hormone binding and target cell activation in the testis. New York: Plenum Press, 1974:343–355.
46. Sharpe RM, Fraser HM, Cooper I, Rommerts FFG. Sertoli-Leydig cell communication via an LHRH-like factor. Nature 1982;290: 785–787.
47. Bhasin S, Heber D, Peterson M, et al. Partial isolation and characterization of testicular GnRH-like factors. Endocrinology 1983;112:1144–1146.
48. Winters SJ, Janick JJ, Loriaux DL, Sherins RJ. Studies on the role of sex steroids in the feedback control of gonadotropin concentrations in men. II. Use of the estrogen antagonist clomiphene citrate. J Clin Endocrinol Metab 1979;48:222–227.
49. Santen RJ. Is aromatization of testosterone to estradiol required for inhibition of LH secretion in men? J Clin Invest 1975;56:1555–1563.
50. Swerdloff RS, Walsh PC, Odell WD. Control of LH and FSH secretion in the male: evidence that aromatization of androgens to estradiol is not required for inhibition of gonadotropin secretion. Steroids 1972;20:13–18.
51. Martini L. The 5 alpha-reduction of testosterone in the neuroendocrine structures. Biochemical and physiological implications. Endocr Rev 1982;3:1–25.
52. McCullagh DR. Dual endocrine activity of the testis. Science 1932;76:19–21.
53. Baker HWG, Bremner WJ, Burger HG, et al. Testicular control of follicle-stimulating hormone secretion. Recent Prog Horm Res 1976;32:429–476.
54. Franchimont P, Chari S, Hagelstein MT, Duraiswami S. Existence of a follicle-stimulating hormone inhibiting factor "inhibin" in bull seminal plasma. Nature 1975;257:402–404.

Male Infertility: Diagnosis and Medical Management

11

Rebecca Z. Sokol and Ronald S. Swerdloff

The first and most important rule in the evaluation of infertility is to consider the couple as a unit in the evaluation and treatment of infertility. Too often a woman is investigated extensively only to discover later that her husband is azoospermic; likewise, a man may undergo lengthy treatment for oligospermia while his wife has an undiagnosed tubal obstruction or anovulatory cycles. The evaluation of both the man and woman should proceed in parallel until a significant problem is uncovered. Ideal management is best achieved when the couple is seen together by a team of physicians. When the man is under the care of either an endocrinologist or a urologist and the woman is under the care of a gynecologist, communication between physicians must be ongoing.

A prerequisite for a discussion of the evaluation and treatment of the male partner of an infertile couple is an understanding of the events responsible for the production and delivery of semen containing normal functioning spermatazoa into the vaginal canal. While the physiology of male reproduction was presented in depth in the previous chapter, several specific aspects will next be emphasized because of their clinical importance.

Reproductive Physiology

CONTROL OF SPERMATOGENESIS. Spermatogenesis results in the progressive maturation of germ cells from spermatogonia to mature spermatozoa. This process can be divided into 3 major phases: mitosis, meiosis, and spermiogenesis (1,2). The duration of spermatogenesis is constant for any given species and in man it takes approximately 72 days for an immature spermatogonium to evolve into a mature spermatozoa (2). Each phase in the process of spermatogenesis is also of fixed duration (3).

Testosterone stimulates spermatogenesis by direct action on germ cells or, possibly, by effecting changes in Sertoli cell function. Testosterone diffuses into the seminiferous tubules down a concentration gradient, and intratesticular testosterone concentrations are approximately 100 times greater than serum concentrations (4,5). Testosterone synthesis requires luteinizing hormone (LH) while follicle-stimulating hormone (FSH) is necessary for the terminal maturation of germ cells by its stimulation of Sertoli cell function (6,7). Sertoli cells also secrete inhibin, a peptide that selectively inhibits pituitary FSH secretion (8–10).

TRANSPORT OF SPERMATOZOA. Transport of sperm from the lumina of the seminiferous tubules to the ampulla of each vas deferens requires an additional 21 days. During their transit through the epididymis, spermatozoa become motile and acquire a greater capacity to fertilize an ovum. Fifteen percent to 30% of the human ejaculate volume is of prostatic origin, 50% to 80% is produced in the seminal vesicles, and the remainder is produced by the Sertoli cells (11,12).

CAPACITATION AND THE ACROSOME REACTION. Capacitation is a poorly understood process whereby ejaculated sperm undergo molecular changes during their transit through the female genital tract that enhance their ability to fertilize an ovum (13–15). There appears to be a "decapacitation factor" in seminal plasma that prevents premature capacitation of sperm (15). Separation of seminal plasma from sperm removes this factor, which is likely lost physiologically when sperm ascend through the cervix into the uterus and fallopian tubes (15). This factor has been identified in the rabbit and is a thermostable glycoprotein with an approximate molecular weight of 350 daltons (16,17).

Capacitation probably triggers the events leading to the acrosome reaction, the loss of the spermatozoa's outer acrosomal membrane, and the plasma membrane that occurs when spermatozoa are in the ampullary portion of the fallopian tubes. This results in the release of hyaluronidase, acrosin, and other enzymes needed for the fertilization process. Calcium, cAMP, and cellular shifts of sodium and potassium may be important in the acrosome reaction. Decapacitated spermatozoa are unable to undergo the acrosome reaction (16).

Spermatozoal penetration of the cumulus oophorus, corona radiata, and zona pellucida of the oocyte follows the acrosome reaction. The attachment and movement of spermatozoa through the zona pellucida in mammals appears to be facilitated by the various enzymes released during the acrosome reaction (18). Acrosin, a trypsinlike enzyme, is essential for sperm penetration of the zona pellucida (19,20). Hyaluronidase appears to be important for the dispersal of granulosa cells of the cumulus oophorus. Hyaluronidase may also modify the structure of the zona pellucida to make it more susceptible to acrosin activity (21).

Evaluation of the Male Partner

HISTORY AND PHYSICAL EXAMINATION. A thorough history and physical examination is the cornerstone of the evaluation of a potentially infertile man. Chronic illness, metabolic disease (e.g., diabetes mellitus), genital infection, certain hereditary diseases, certain drugs (22), and exposure to industrial or environmental toxins may impair spermatogenesis. Cryptorchidism, hypospadias, or other genital anomalies are also associated with male infertility. The presence of any of these should be sought and a sexual history that includes a description of sexual potency, ejaculation (premature or delayed), coital frequency, use of douches or lubricants, and technique (e.g., frequent extravaginal coitus) must also be obtained. Sexual impotency and frequent failure to ejaculate suggest inadequate testosterone effect; signs of this include a diminished rate of sexual hair growth, gynecomastia, and eunuchoid body proportions. Hypospadias may represent a mechanical cause of impaired sperm delivery or indicate deficient androgen effect during early fetal development. Scrotal examination will detect abnormal testes, a spermatocele, a varicocele, and absent vasa deferentia. Small testes (less than 4.0 cm in longest diameter or 15 cc by orchidometer) indicate impaired germinal tissue mass, either due to primary testicular failure or hypothalamic-pituitary insufficiency. Scrotal examination of a standing patient performing the Valsalva maneuver will assist in the diagnosis of smaller varicoceles. The presence of a nodular and thickened epididymis or vas deferens suggests a prior infection.

We have developed an algorithmic approach to the assessment of the potentially infertile male utilizing the findings from the history, physical examination, semen analysis, certain hormonal tests, and (when indicated) special ancillary tests (23).

LABORATORY ASSESSMENT OF THE INFERTILE COUPLE.

The Semen Analysis. The semen analysis has traditionally been the most important tool in the investigation of male infertility. The semen sample should be collected by masturbation after 2 to 4 days of sexual abstinence. The semen specimen should be kept at body temperature during transport and should be analyzed within 1 hour of collection. Three to 6 semen analyses should be performed before concluding that a man is infertile since there is considerable variation in semen quality. Samples collected at least 10 days apart is optimal, although longer intervals have been suggested to assess spermatogenesis through 1 full cycle (i.e., 90 days). The semen sample is evaluated for the following characteristics: appearance, volume, pH, and sperm motility, concentration, and morphology.

APPEARANCE. Freshly ejaculated semen is an opalescent, white, yellow, or gray fluid. Human semen coagulates at the time of ejaculation but liquefies 3 to 25 minutes later. The seminal coagulum is a dense network of long fibers, approximately 0.15 mm in diameter, that prevents free movement of spermatozoa. These fibers disappear as liquefaction occurs (24). Liquefaction occurs as a result of proteolytic activity by enzymes produced in the prostate. These are collagenaselike and chymotrypsinlike enzymes (25,26). Viscosity is a measure of liquefaction and a reflection of the enzymatic function of the prostate and seminal vesicles. Semen should flow freely when poured and viscosity is abnormal when it does not.

VOLUME. A normal semen volume is 2 ml to 6 ml. A volume less than 1 ml suggests incomplete collection, occlusion of the ejaculatory ducts, or congenital absence of the vasa deferentia and seminal vesicles.

pH. The normal range of pH is 7 to 8. A low pH suggests contamination of the specimen with urine or occlusion of the ejaculatory ducts.

SPERM MOTILITY. Within 2 hours of collection, more than 60% of the sperm should exhibit rapid forward motion. The percentage of sperm that are motile are estimated from a drop of semen examined at approximately 400 power magnification. Sperm velocity is estimated and graded on a scale of 0 to 4; 0 = no motility, 1 = tail movement but no forward progression, 2 = sluggish forward progression, 3 = more rapid forward progression, 4 = fast forward progression. More objective methods of measuring sperm velocity have been developed and the average velocity is approximately 30 micrometers per second (27–29).

SPERM CONCENTRATION. This is an extremely variable measurement and at least 3 semen samples must be analyzed before concluding that a man is azoospermic, oligospermic, or normal. On the basis of studies comparing sperm concentrations in men whose wives were pregnant with those men who, with their wives, were being evaluated for infertility, a sperm concentration greater than 20 million/ml is normally fertile (30,31). Eliasson could find no significant difference in fertility with concentrations as low as 5 million/ml (30).

SPERM MORPHOLOGY. The semen sample should contain more than 60% normal oval sperm, less than 6% tapering forms, less than 0.5% immature forms, and less than 8.6% amorphous forms. The remainder will be a variety of abnormal forms. The Papanicolaou stain is best for assessing sperm morphology. It is frequently difficult to distinguish immature spermatogenic cells from leukocytes, and special staining may be required. A recently published manual* by the World Health Organization is invaluable in the establishment of a standardized semen analysis laboratory.

ZONA-FREE HAMSTER *IN VITRO* FERTILIZATION ASSAY. The technique using hamster ova and guinea pig spermatozoa was originally described by Yanagimachi in 1972 (32), who later demonstrated that zona-free hamster eggs could be fertilized by human spermatozoa *in vitro* and thus serve as a substitute for human ova in the preliminary assessment of the fertilizing capacity of human spermatozoa (33). Essentially, the technique consists of collecting mature unfertilized ova from the oviducts of superovulated hamsters 15 to 17 days after an intraperitoneal injection of human chorionic gonadotropin. The ova are treated with hyaluronidase to remove the cumulus oophorus. The ova are then treated with trypsin to remove the zonae pellucida before mixing with human sperm (34–35). The test has now been characterized and standardized (35–38). An ovum has been penetrated when the sperm heads are swollen or sperm pronuclei are seen. Results are expressed as the percentage of ova penetrated, and at least 30 are examined. Fourteen percent to 100% of ova are penetrated by sperm from fertile men while fewer than 10% of ova are penetrated by sperm from infertile men (35,39). While not a substitute for a semen analysis, this test improves the identification of abnormal sperm and may be a reliable predictor of fertility potential.

IN VITRO CERVICAL MUCOUS PENETRATION TEST. This method provides a standardized, simple procedure for the measurement of sperm penetration in cervical mucus

---

* Laboratory Manual for the Examination of Human Semen and Semen-Cervical Mucus Interaction

(40) and serves as an alternative to the postcoital test. The ability to penetrate cervical mucus is one of the most important tests of human sperm function and the results of *in vitro* tests of sperm penetration are significantly correlated with pregnancy (40). The procedure is performed as follows:

a. One end of a flat capillary tube, prefilled with bovine cervical mucus, is placed in a reservoir of 1 ml of freshly collected semen for 90 minutes.
b. The tube is then removed from the semen reservoir, wiped clean of any residual semen, placed on a glass slide, and evaluated with a phase-contrast microscope at 400 power magnification. Each assay is run in duplicate. The distance traveled by the spermatozoa into the mucus is measured; a distance greater than 20 mm is considered adequate penetration.

HORMONAL TESTS. Once a man is determined to be either azoospermic or consistently oligospermic, serum concentrations of LH, FSH, and testosterone are measured. Because of the episodic nature of hormone secretion, we obtain 3 blood samples at least 20 minutes apart and pool equal volumes of serum from each for a single determination of these hormones. The results of these tests are essential for the characterization of the man's problem and determination of the therapeutic approach according to our algorithm.

Algorithmic Approach to Infertile Men

AZOOSPERMIA.

Low Serum Testosterone, Elevated LH and FSH (Algorithm 11–1). Such men have primary testicular failure involving both the Leydig cells (testosterone secretion) and germinal elements (sperm production). The elevated serum gonadotropin levels distinguish primary testicular insufficiency from hypothalamic-pituitary disease.

Normal Testosterone, Normal LH, Elevated FSH (Algorithm 11–1). These results may be seen in azoospermic or severely oligospermic men who have primary germinal tubular failure without associated Leydig cell damage. FSH concentrations may be high because inhibin production by the Sertoli cells is deficient (9,41).

Low Testosterone, LH and FSH (Algorithm 11–2). Such men have hypogonadotropic hypogonadism due to a congenital or an acquired abnormality. Anosmia is often found in men with congenital LH and FSH deficiency (Kallmann's syndrome). Men (and women) with hypogonadotropic hypogonadism should be tested for deficiencies of other pituitary hormones (TSH, ACTH, and growth hormone). Serum prolactin should be measured, as it is elevated in many with a pituitary tumor but is normal in men with hypogonadotropic hypogonadism. If a pituitary tumor is suspected, a careful neurologic examination, including visual field testing, should be performed to assess the possibility of impingement on the optic chiasm by an expanding pituitary tumor. Anorexia nervosa and severe malnutrition are suggested by physical examination. "Cone down" X-rays of the sella turcica should be performed on all hypogonadotropic men with a normal prolactin level to exclude the possibility of a nonsecreting pituitary adenoma. Men with elevated prolactin concentrations or an abnormal "cone down" X-ray of the sella turcica require polytomography or, preferably, a high-resolution CAT scan of the pituitary.

Normal Testosterone, LH, and FSH (Algorithm 11–3). Azoospermic men with this hormonal pattern have either retrograde ejaculation, congenital absence of the vasa deferentia, or an obstruction of the ejaculatory system. Azoospermia caused by impaired spermatogenesis is almost always associated with an elevated FSH concentration (42). The distinction between these disorders is important since some obstructive problems can be corrected surgically (see Chapter 12).

Ejaculate volumes less than 1 ml and absence of fructose in semen suggest either bilateral obstruction of the ejaculatory ducts or congenital absence of the vasa deferentia and seminal vesicles. Semen volumes and fructose concentrations will be normal in azoospermic men with obstruction of the epididymata or vasa deferentia since most of the volume and the fruc-

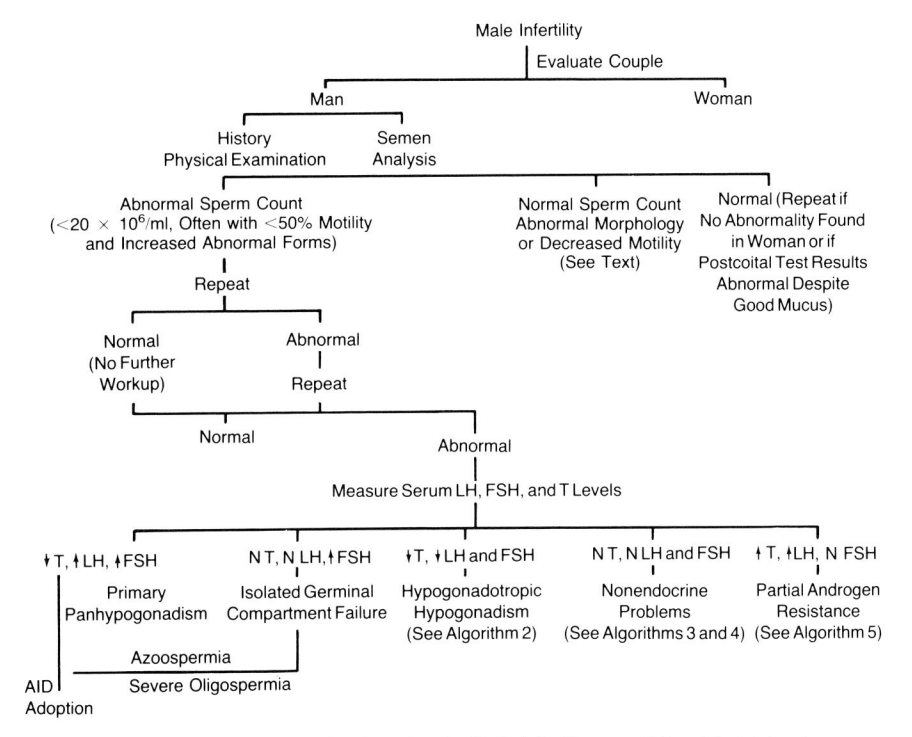

Algorithm 11–1. Diagnostic evaluation of potentially infertile men. LH = luteinizing hormone; FSH = follicle-stimulating hormone; T = testosterone; N = normal; AID = artificial insemination donor. (Reproduced with permission from Swerdloff RS, Boyers SP. JAMA 1982;247:2419. Copyright 1982, American Medical Association.)

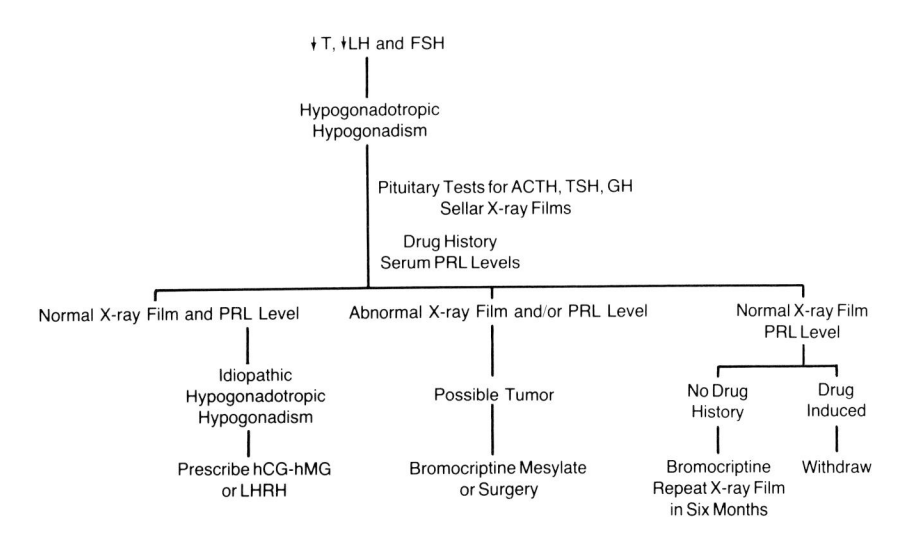

Algorithm 11–2. Evaluation and treatment of men with hypogonadotropic hypogonadism. T = testosterone; LH = luteinizing hormone; FSH = follicle-stimulating hormone; ACTH = adrenocorticotropic hormone; TSH = thyroid-stimulating hormone; GH = growth hormone; PRL = prolactin; hCG = human chorionic gonadotropin; hMG = menotropins (human menopausal gonadotropin); LHRH = gonadotropin releasing hormone (luteinizing hormone-releasing hormone). (Reproduced with permission from Swerdloff RS, Boyers SP. JAMA 1982;247:2419. Copyright 1982, American Medical Association.)

tose come from the seminal vesicles, which are not obstructed in this instance. Scrotal exploration, vasography, and biopsy of the testes may be necessary to define the location and extent of the obstruction.

Men with diabetes mellitus, previous genital surgery (e.g., prostatic resection) or certain neuropathies may not produce an ejaculate or may have retrograde ejaculation. The presence of many sperm in the urine after ejaculation confirms the latter.

OLIGOSPERMIA.

Low Testosterone, Elevated LH and FSH (Algorithm 11–1). These men have primary gonadal insufficiency.

Normal Testosterone and LH, Elevated FSH (Algorithm 11–1). These men usually have severe oligospermia secondary to damage of the germinal epithelium.

Low Testosterone, Low or Normal LH and FSH (Algorithm 11–2). These oligospermic men usually have partial deficiencies of gonadotropin secretion, usually brought on by acquired hypothalamic or pituitary disease. Serum prolactin should be measured in these men and a pituitary tumor suspected if the prolactin concentration is high.

Most very obese men and some lean men have normal serum LH and FSH concentrations but a low total testosterone concentration. The latter finding occurs as a result of decreased sex-hormone-binding protein synthesis (43). Such men have normal serum concentrations of free (unbound) testosterone.

Normal Testosterone, LH and FSH (Algorithm 11–4). This hormonal pattern is seen in the majority of oligospermic men and many have a varicocele. Men with this hormonal pattern who do not have a varicocele are categorized as having idiopathic oligospermia.

Elevated Testosterone and LH, Low FSH (Algorithm 11–5). These men may have partial androgen resistance (deficient response to testosterone in androgen target cells). Resistance to the action of testosterone in the hypothalamus and pituitary gland causes an increase in LH concentrations, which stimulate an increased testicular secretion of testosterone and estradiol. Profound degrees of androgen resistance during fetal life often result in genital ambiguity. However, lesser degrees of androgen resistance may cause only hypospadias (the Reifenstein syndrome) or gynecomastia. Since the germinal epithelium is a testosterone target tissue, oligospermia or azoospermia are invariably found in androgen-resistant subjects. Loss of germinal epithelium may also occur because of increased estradiol synthesis by the testes. Androgen resistance may be a frequent cause of idiopathic oligospermia or azoospermia in men without genital ambiguity or gynecomastia (44). Serum concentrations of testosterone, LH, and estradiol may be normal in androgen-resistant infertile men. At present, the most reliable means to make the diagnosis of androgen resistance is measurement of androgen receptor binding capacity in fibroblasts cultured from a scrotal skin biopsy.

ABNORMAL SPERM MORPHOLOGY OR MOTILITY. Dead sperm can be identified with supravital stains. Treatment of necrospermia may be possible in the future as the relationship between abnormal sperm metabolism and absent sperm motility is clarified. Genital infections may impair sperm motility and the presence of leukocytes in semen suggests this diagnosis. Men with evidence of a genital infection should receive antibiotics that reach therapeutic levels in the genital tract (e.g., trimethoprim).

Immotile or agglutinated sperm may indicate the presence of an autoantibody against sperm. Agglutinating antibodies are present in the sera of 2% to 13% of subfertile men, many of whom have a history of genital trauma or infection. However, as many as 2% of fertile men may have a circulating antibody against their own sperm. This agglutinating substance may not be an antibody but a steroid-beta-lipoprotein complex in some of these men. There is, at best, a poor correlation between the presence of serum and seminal antisperm antibodies. As a consequence, a causal relationship between sperm-agglutinating antibodies and male infertility is not established. Haas and Galle have discussed the role of antibodies in infertile couples (Chapter 7).

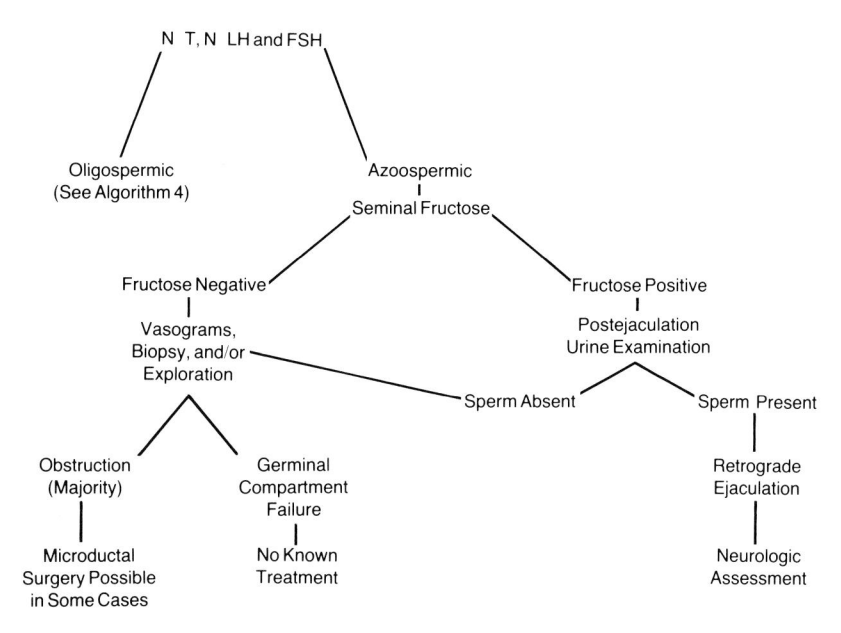

Algorithm 11–3. Diagnostic evaluation of azoospermic men. N = normal; T = testosterone; LH = luteinizing hormone; FSH = follicle-stimulating hormone. (Reproduced with permission from Swerdloff RS, Boyers SP. JAMA 1982;247:2419. Copyright 1982, American Medical Association.)

Treatment of the Infertile Male

AZOOSPERMIA.

Hypogonadotropic Hypogonadism (Algorithm 11–2). Since FSH and LH secretion is deficient in these men, fertility can often be restored with human chorionic gonadotropin (hCG) and human menopausal gonadotropin (Pergonal®) (45.) Gonadotropin-releasing hormone has stimulated spermatogenesis, but repetitive doses every several hours for several months were necessary (46). Treatment of men with a pituitary tumor is analogous to that

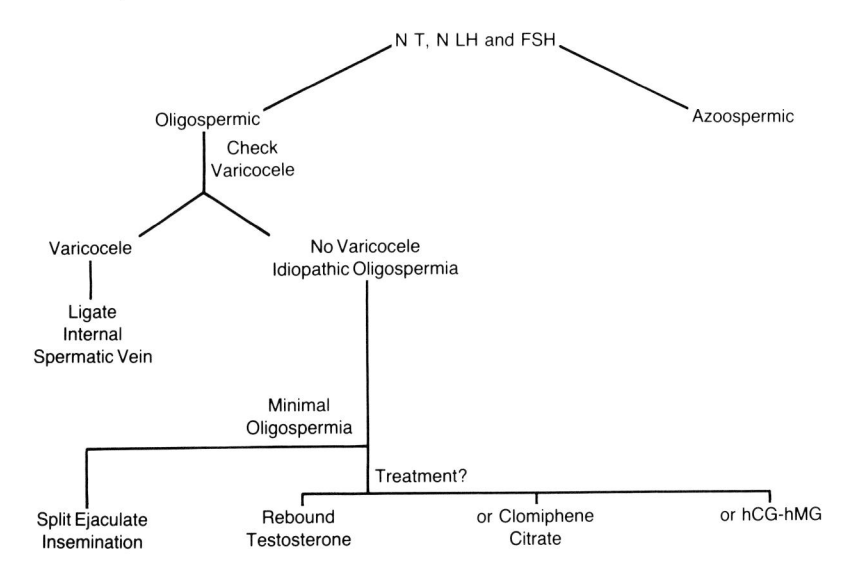

Algorithm 11–4. Diagnostic evaluation of oligospermic men. N = normal; T = testosterone; LH = luteinizing hormone; FSH = follicle-stimulating hormone; hCG = human chorionic gonadotropin; hMG = menotropins (human menopausal gonadotropin). (Reproduced with permission from Swerdloff RS, Boyers SP. JAMA 1982;247:2419. Copyright 1982, American Medical Association.)

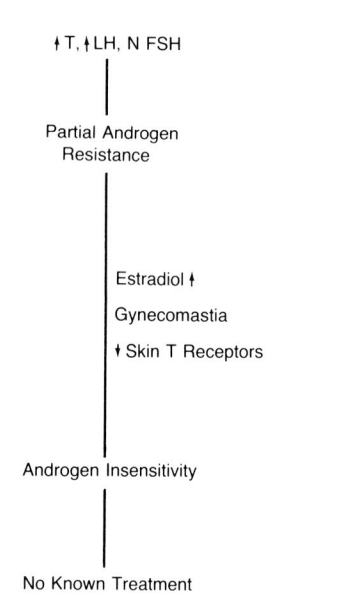

↑T, ↑LH, N FSH
|
Partial Androgen Resistance
|
Estradiol ↑
Gynecomastia
↑ Skin T Receptors
|
Androgen Insensitivity
|
No Known Treatment

Algorithm 11–5. Diagnostic evaluation of men with partial androgen resistance. T = testosterone; LH = luteinizing hormone; FSH = follicle-stimulating hormone; N = normal. (Reproduced with permission from Swerdloff RS, Boyers SP. JAMA 1982;247:2419. Copyright 1982, American Medical Association.)

of women and has been discussed in Chapter 4.

Ductal Obstruction (Algorithm 11–3). Surgical management of these men is discussed in Chapter 12.

Retrograde Ejaculation (Algorithm 11–3). Pregnancies have resulted from insemination of semen voided or recovered from the bladder after retrograde ejaculation. Occasionally, retrograde ejaculation is corrected by drugs such as ephedrine and brompheniramine (47). This is also discussed in Chapter 17.

Primary Testicular Spermatogenic Failure (Algorithm 11–4). Men with pantesticular insufficiency do not respond to any known therapy, and artificial insemination with donor semen (AID) or adoption are the only avenues available currently.

No known therapy exists for men with selective spermatogenic failure (elevated serum FSH with normal serum LH and testosterone) and AID or adoption are their only alternatives for having a child.

OLIGOSPERMIA.

Mild Primary Spermatogenic Deficiency (Algorithm 11–1). Men with incomplete damage to the germinal elements may be oligospermic, not azoospermic. Generally, men with elevations of serum FSH fail to respond to any of the treatments described below for idiopathic oligospermia.

Artificial insemination with the first portion of the husband's ejaculate (AIH) may be beneficial when the sperm concentration is low, but greater than 5 million/ml. The pregnancy rate with split ejaculate AIH is about 23% (with a reported range of 13% to 56%). When the whole ejaculate is inseminated, the pregnancy rate is slightly lower, approximately 15% (range of 0% to 55%) (48). The slight improvement when the first portion of a split ejaculate is inseminated is probably a result of the fact that 80% or more of the sperm are in this first portion (49,50). Sperm morphology and motility are similar in the 2 fractions (51). We have found no differences in sperm penetration of hamster ova in the 2 portions of a split ejaculate. This suggests that the fertilizing capacity of the more concentrated portion of the ejaculate is not enhanced and the greater pregnancy rate with split ejaculate insemination is not significant.

Pregnancy rates are not increased in the wives of oligospermic men in whom successive whole ejaculates are frozen, pooled, and then used for artificial insemination (52). This is understandable since the ejaculate has a lower sperm concentration and cryopreservation further reduces the concentration and percentage of motile sperm.

Partial Hypogonadotropic Hypogonadism (Algorithm 11–2). These men are treated in a similar fashion to those with low gonadotropins and azoospermia.

Treatment of men with hyperprolactinemia is dictated by the nature of the pathologic findings. Lowering the serum prolactin concentration frequently returns gonadal function to normal.

Idiopathic Oligospermia (Algorithm 11–4). There is no standard treatment of idiopathic oligospermia that is especially effective. Few studies testing the value of a drug have been done in a controlled fashion using a placebo as a basis of comparison. Idiopathic oligospermia is not a specific entity, but is the result of a variety of abnormalities that each cause a reduction in sperm concentration. The use of any of the following drugs is, therefore, largely empiric. For these reasons, it should not be a surprise that pregnancy rates are disappointingly low when any of these are used.

ANTIESTROGENS. Clomiphene and tamoxifen act as competitive inhibitors of estrogen action by occupying estrogen receptors. Testolactone (Teslac®), an aromatase inhibitor, prevents the conversion of testosterone to estradiol. These drugs exert their effects in at least 2 ways. Androgens and estrogens modulate hypothalamic and pituitary function to regulate gonadotropin production. Androgens affect hypothalamic function directly, but also influence the hypothalamus and pituitary by acting as substrates for aromatization to estradiol. Antiestrogens displace estrogens from their receptors and interfere with the normal feedback by circulating or locally produced estrogens. As a result, secretion of GnRH increases and stimulates increased gonadotropin secretion. This, in turn, stimulates an increased rate of testosterone production, which, in theory, induces germinal cell maturation. Antiestrogens also may have a direct effect on the testes by blocking the inhibitory action of estradiol on Leydig cell function. Decreasing the effective levels of estradiol by administering an estrogen inhibitor or an aromatase inhibitor should lead to an increase in sperm production by the testes of oligospermic men.

Clomiphene has been one of the most commonly used drugs in the treatment of male infertility. Yet, no study has been published that is a well-controlled, double-blind, longitudinal experiment designed to assess its true effectiveness. Three studies using clomiphene in male infertility have attempted to include controls. Weiland et al. (53) administered 5 mg or 10 mg of clomiphene per day for 12 weeks, then a placebo for 12 weeks. Although sperm concentrations were increased with clomiphene, the increase was erratic and there were no pregnancies. Masala et al. administered clomiphene, 50 mg, twice daily for 5 days to 10 oligospermic men and 10 control subjects (54). They found no statistical differences in hormonal response between the 2 groups. Foss et al. gave either clomiphene (100 mg/day) or a placebo for 10 days in each of 3 months (55). Although 19 pregnancies occurred, they were unable to implicate clomiphene as the effective agent. Unfortunately, the duration of the treatment course in each of these experiments may have been too short if one recalls that a sperm cycle is 72 days.

Tamoxifen citrate is also an antiestrogen, but with weaker intrinsic estrogenic activity than clomiphene. Few studies have been published that evaluate its effectiveness in restoring male fertility. Tamoxifen increases serum concentrations of LH, FSH, testosterone, and estradiol. The sperm concentration or motility improved in 12 men with idiopathic oligospermia (56). Although Willis et al. reported no statistically significant improvement in the sperm concentration of oligospermic men, 1 of the wives conceived (57). Comhaire reported an increase in sperm concentration and 3 pregnancies (58). Recently, Buvat et al. treated 25 normogonadotropic oligospermic infertile men with tamoxifen (20 mg/day) for 4 to 12 months (59). The mean sperm concentration was significantly increased ($P < 0.001$) and 10 pregnancies were reported during the treatment period. Comhaire has reviewed the biochemical and spermatogenic effects of tamoxifen (60).

Testolactone, an aromatase inhibitor, may also stimulate spermatogenesis. One gram orally each day for 6 to 12 months resulted in a significant increase in sperm concentration in 8 of 9 men with idiopathic oligospermia (61). Three pregnancies occurred in their partners. There were no significant changes in motility or semen volume, or in the results of GnRH stimulation at the end of the treatment period. Estradiol levels decreased, testosterone levels increased, and LH, FSH, and prolactin levels did not change. No other clinical trials using this drug have yet been reported.

ANDROGEN THERAPY. Testosterone enanthate or other testosterone esters suppress LH and possibly FSH secretion when given intramuscularly in doses of 200 mg to 250 mg every 2 weeks (62–67). Spermatogenesis is inhibited secondarily. Three months after therapy, gonadotropin secretion will return and sperm concentrations may rebound to a higher level. This is the premise for what is called "testosterone rebound therapy." However, only 28% of the wives of treated men conceive (68) and pregnancy did not occur more frequently than in an untreated infertile group (69).

Androgens in low doses have also been used to stimulate spermatogenesis. Methyltestosterone (10 mg to 50 mg/day), mesterolone (50 mg to 75 mg/day), fluoxymesterone (5 mg to 20 mg/day), and others have been administered for 3 months or more in an effort to increase sperm concentration or motility. Direct stimulation of the germinal epithelium and epididymis has been proposed, but results have been variable (70–72). These studies have not always excluded a female factor or compared the results of testosterone against the effect of a placebo.

GONADOTROPINS. Receptors for follicle-stimulating hormone (FSH) and luteinizing hormone (LH) are present on Leydig cells (73) and on cells in the seminiferous tubules (74). Based on these observations and the stimulation of spermatogenesis by gonadotropins in hypogonadotropic hypogonadal men, chorionic gonadotropin (hCG), and/or menopausal gonadotropins (e.g., Pergonal®) have been given to men with idiopathic oligospermia in an attempt to stimulate spermatogenesis. Unfortunately, their use has not improved the fertility of men with idiopathic oligospermia (75–79).

SPERM ANTIBODIES. Haas and Galle have reviewed the diagnosis and therapy of sperm antibodies in the female (Chapter 7). The same diagnostic limitations exist in ascribing the presence of such an antibody in a man as the cause of infertility. Although glucocorticoids have been recommended for men with an antibody against his own sperm (80), Hendry and colleagues found no significant improvement in fertility after 5-day courses of 96 mg methylprednisolone each day repeated at 2 to 3 month intervals (81). There may be significant side effects with glucocorticoid therapy. For these reasons, glucocorticoids should be used only when other causes of infertility have been excluded and the presence of an antisperm antibody is certain.

SEMINAL INFECTION OR INFLAMMATION. Because nonspecific infections of the male genital urinary tract have been implicated as a cause of infertility, antibacterial agents have been prescribed for men with normal or low sperm concentrations who have leukocytes in their semen or other findings to suggest an infection. Recommended treatment regimens have included doxycycline, 100 mg orally 2 times per day, tetracycline, 250 mg to 500 mg 3 to 4 times per day, and sulfamethoxazole, 160 mg to 800 mg per day for 1 to 3 months. Eighteen of 32 oligospermic men had an improvement in the percentage of hamster eggs penetrated by their sperm after receiving doxycycline (100 mg twice daily for 10 days, then 100 mg daily for 10 days) (82). Improvement in hamster egg penetration correlated with a decrease in the number of leukocytes in semen and 6 of the wives conceived during or within 1 month after their husband's treatment. The role of these infections in male infertility and the success with antibiotics is, nonetheless, unsettled at present. The relationship of infertility and genital infections in men and women has been reviewed recently (83).

Conclusion

The algorithmic approach that we have described to evaluate the male partner of an infertile couple uses the combination of a thorough history and physical examination, 1 or more semen analyses, and measurement of specific hormones. By categorizing each infertile male in this manner, a rational and effective therapy can be selected for many causes of impaired fertility. Unfortunately, many infertile men have no apparent cause of impaired spermatogenesis because our understanding of male reproductive physiology is incomplete. For these men, therapy is empiric and often unsuccessful. Circumventing the problem by artificial insemination, adoption, or perhaps *in vitro* fertilization may be these couples' only hope of having children.

REFERENCES

1. Heller CG, Clermont Y. Kinetics of the germinal epithelium in man. Recent Prog Horm Res 1964;20:545–575.
2. Mann T. Biochemistry of semen in the male reproductive tract. London: Methuen, 1964:1–493.

3. Monesi V. Spermatogenesis and the spermatozoa. In: Austin CR, Short RV, eds. Reproduction in mammals. Cambridge: University Press, 1972:46–84.
4. Ruokonen A, Laatikainen T, Laitinen EA, Vihko R. Free and sulfate-conjugated neutral steroids in human testis tissue. Biochemistry 1972;11:1411–1416.
5. Morse HC, Horike N, Rowley MJ, Heller CG. Testosterone concentrations in testes of normal men: effects of testosterone proprionate administration. J Clin Endocrinol Metab 1973;37:882–886.
6. Bardin CW, Paulsen CA. The testes. In: Williams RH, ed. Textbook of endocrinology, 6th. ed. Philadelphia: WB Saunders Co., 1981:293–354.
7. Swerdloff RS. Physiology of male reproduction. Hypothalamic-pituitary function and the hypothalamic-pituitary-gonadal axis. In: Harrison JH, ed. Campbell's urology, 4th ed. Philadelphia: WB Saunders Co., 1978:125–133.
8. Baker HWG, Bremner WJ, Burger HG, et al. Testicular control of follicle stimulating hormone secretion. Recent Prog Horm Res 1976;32:429–476.
9. Van Thiel DH, Sherins RJ, Meyers GH Jr, De Vita VT Jr. Evidence for a specific seminiferous tubular factor affecting FSH secretion in man. J Clin Invest 1971;51:1009–1019.
10. Ward DN, Glenn SD, Wan-Kyng L, Gordon WL. Chemistry of gonadal peptides. In: Greenwald GW, Teranova PF, eds. Factors regulating ovarian function. New York: Raven Press, 1983:151–156.
11. Mann T, Lutwak-Mann C. Epididymis and epididymal semen. In: Male reproductive function and semen. Berlin: Springer-Verlag, 1981:147–148.
12. Mann T. Secretory function of the prostate, seminal vesicle and other male accessory organs of reproduction. J Reprod Fertil 1974;37:179–188.
13. Rogers G. Mammalian sperm capacitation and fertilization in vitro: a critique of methodology. Gamete Research 1978;1:165–223.
14. Shapiro BM, Eddy EM. When sperm meets egg: biochemical mechanisms of gamete interaction. Int Rev Cytol 1980;66:257–302.
15. Chang MC. A detrimental effect of seminal plasma on the fertilizing capacity of sperm. Nature 1957;179:258–259.
16. Eng LA, Oliphant G. Rabbit sperm reversible decapacitation by membrane stabilization with a highly purified glycoprotein from seminal plasma. Biol Reprod 1978;19:1083–1094.
17. Reyes A, Oliphant G, Brackett BG. Partial purification and identification of a reversible decapacitation factor from rabbit seminal plasma. Fertil Steril 1975;26:148–157.
18. Edwards RG. "Fertilization" in the human female. New York: Academic Press, 1980:586–592.
19. Hartree EF, Srivastava PN. The chemical composition of the acrosomes of ram spermatozoa. J Reprod Fertil 1965;9:47–60.
20. Zaneveld LJD, Williams WL. A sperm enzyme that disperses the corona radiata and its inhibition by decapacitation factor. Biol Reprod 1970;2:363–368.
21. Reddy JM, Joyce C, Zaneveld LJD. Role of hyaluronidase in fertilization; the antifertility activity of myocrisin, a nontoxic hyaluronidase inhibitor. J Androl 1980;1:28–32.
22. Aiman J. Infertility. In: Duenhoelter J, ed. Greenhill's office gynecology. Chicago: Yearbook Medical Publishers, 1983:188–223.
23. Swerdloff RS, Boyers SP. Evaluation of the male partner in an infertile couple. JAMA 1982;247:2418–2422.
24. Zaneveld LJD, Tauber PF, Port C, Propping D, Schumacher GFB. Scanning election microscopy of the human, guinea-pig and rhesus monkey seminal coagulum. J Reprod Fertil 1974;40:223–225.
25. Lukac J, Koren E. Mechanism of liquefaction of the human ejaculate. II. Role of collagenase-like peptidase in seminal proteinase. J Reprod Fertil 1979;56:501–506.
26. Koren E, Milkovic S. "Collagenase-like" peptidase in human rat and bull spermatozoa. J Reprod Fertil 1973;32:349–356.
27. Jouannet P, Volocnine B, Deguent P, et al. Light scattering determination of various characteristic parameters of spermatozoa motility in a series of human sperm. Andrologia 1977;9:36–49.
28. Sokolowski JE, Blasco L, Storey BP. Turbidimetric analysis of human sperm motility. Fertil Steril 1977;28:1337–1341.
29. Overstreet JW, Jatv BF, Hanson FW, et al. A simple, inexpensive method for objective assessment of human sperm movement characteristics. Fertil Steril 1979;31:162–172.
30. Eliasson R. Analysis of semen. In: Behrman SJ, Kistner RW, eds. Progress in infertility. Boston: Little, Brown & Co., 1975:691–714.
31. Sherins RJ, Brightwell D, Sternphal PM. Longitudinal analysis of semen of fertile and infertile men. In: Troen P, Nankin H, eds. The testis in normal and infertile men. New York: Raven Press, 1977:473–478.
32. Yanagimachi R. Penetration of guinea pig spermatozoa into hamster eggs in vitro. J Reprod Fertil 1972;28:477–480.
33. Yanagimachi R, Yanagimachi H, Rogers BJ.

The use of zona-free animal ova as a test system for the assessment of the fertilizing capacity of human spermatozoa. Biol Reprod 1976; 15:471–476.
34. Hanada A, Chang MC. Penetration of zona-free eggs by spermatozoa of different species. Biol Reprod 1972;6:300–309.
35. Rogers BJ, Van Campen H, Ueno M, Lambert H, Bronson R, Hale R. Analysis of human spermatozoal fertilizing ability using zona-free ova. Fertil Steril 1979;32:664–670.
36. Hall JL. Relationship between semen quality and human sperm penetration of zona-free hamster ova. Fertil Steril 1981;35:457–463.
37. Blazak WF, Overstreet JW. Competitive penetration of zona-free hamster eggs by spermatozoa from fertile donors. Fertil Steril 1981;35:246–247 (Abs).
38. Gudman BA, Sokolowski JE, Blasco L, Wolf DP. The "Humster Test": its use and variability in analyzing human sperm fertilizing ability. Fertil Steril 1981;35:251–252 (Abs).
39. Rudak E. Interspecific fertilization. In: Jagillo G, Vogel HJ, eds. Bioregulators of reproduction. New York: Academic Press, 1981:168–186.
40. Alexander NJ. Evaluation of male infertility with an in vitro cervical mucous penetration test. Fertil Steril 1981;36:201–208.
41. Chappel SC, Ulloa-Aguirre A, Coutifaris C. Biosynthesis and secretion of follicle-stimulating hormone. Endocr Rev 1983;4:179–211.
42. de Kretser DM. The endocrinology of male infertility. Br Med Bull 1979;35:187–192.
43. Glass AR, Swerdloff RS, Bray GA, et al. Low serum testosterone and sex-hormone-binding-globulin in massively obese men. J Clin Endocrinol Metab 1977;45:1211–1219.
44. Aiman J, Griffin JE. The frequency of androgen receptor deficiency in infertile men. J Clin Endocrinol Metab 1982;54:725–732.
45. Rosemberg E. Gonadotropin therapy of male infertility. In: Hafez ESE, ed. Human semen and fertility regulation in men. St. Louis: CV Mosby Co., 1976:464–475.
46. Hoffman AF, Crowley WF. Induction of puberty in men by long-term pulsatile administration of low-dose gonadotropin-releasing hormone. N Eng J Med 1982;307:1237–1241.
47. Andaloro UA and Duke A. Treatment of retrograde ejaculation with brompheniramine. Urology 1975;5:520–522.
48. Moghissi KS, Gruber JS, Evans S, Yanez J. Homologous artificial insemination. Am J Obstet Gynecol 1977;129:909–915.
49. MacLeod J, Hotchkiss RS. The distribution of spermatozoa and of certain chemical constituents in human ejaculate. J Urol 1942:48:225–229.
50. Amelar RD, Hotchkiss RS. The split ejaculate. Fertil Steril 1965;16:46–60.
51. Eliasson P, Lindholmer C. Distribution and properties of spermatozoa in different fractions of split ejaculates. Fertil Steril 1972;23:252–256.
52. Dixon RE, Buttram VC, Schum CW. Artificial insemination using homologous semen: a review of 158 cases. Fertil Steril 1976;27:647–654.
53. Weiland RG, Amari AH, Klein DE, Doshi NS, Hallberg MC, Chen JC. Idiopathic oligospermia: control observations and response to cisclomiphene. Fertil Steril 1972:23:471–474.
54. Masala A, Delitala G, Alagna S, Devilla L, Lotti G. Effect of clomiphene citrate on plasma levels of immunoreactive luteinizing hormone releasing hormone, gonadotropin and testosterone in normal subjects and in patients with idiopathic oligospermia. Fertil Steril 1978;29:424–427.
55. Foss GL, Tindall VR, Birkett JP. The treatment of subfertile men with clomiphene citrate. J Reprod Fertil 1973;32:167–170.
56. Vermeulen A, Comhaire F. Hormonal effects of an antiestrogen, tamoxifen, in normal and oligospermic men. Fertil Steril 1978;29:320–327.
57. Willis KJ, London DR, Bevis MA, Butt WR, Lynch SS, Holder G. Hormonal effects of tamoxifen in oligospermic men. J Endocrinol 1977;73:171–178.
58. Comhaire F. Treatment of oligospermia with tamoxiphen. Int J Fertil 1976;21:232–238.
59. Buvat J, Ardaens K, Lemaire A, Gauthier A, Gasnault JP, Buvat-Herbaret M. Increased sperm count in 25 cases of idiopathic normogonadotropic oligospermia following treatment with tamoxifen. Fertil Steril 1983;39:700–703.
60. Comhaire FH, Tamoxifen. In: Bain J, Schill W-B, Schwarzstein L, eds. Treatment of male infertility. New York: Springer-Verlag, 1982:45–53.
61. Vigersky RA, Glass AR. Effects of delta-1-testolactone on the pituitary-testicular axis in oligospermic men. J Clin Endocrinol Metab 1981;52:897–902.
62. Lacroix A, McKenna TJ, Rabinowitz D. Sex steroid modulation of gonadotropins in normal men and in androgen insensitivity syndrome. J Clin Endocrinol Metab 1979;48:235–240.
63. Franchimont P, Chari S, Demoulin A. Hypothalamic-pituitary testis interaction. J Reprod Fertil 1975;44:335–350.
64. Peterson NT Jr, Midgley AR, Jaffe RB. Regulation of human gonadotropins. III. Luteinizing

hormone and follicle stimulating hormone in sera from adult males. J Clin Endocrinol Metab 1968;28:1473–1478.
65. Sherins RJ, Loriaux DL. Studies on the role of sex steroids in the feedback control of FSH concentrations in man. J Clin Endocrinol Metab 1973;36:886–893.
66. Stewart-Bentley M, Odell W, Horton R. The feedback control of luteinizing hormone in normal adult men. J Clin Endocrinol Metab 1974;38:545–553.
67. Swerdloff RS, Odell WD. Some aspects of the control of secretion in LH and FSH in humans. In: Rosemberg E, ed. Gonadotropins. Los Altos: Geron-X, 1968:155–166.
68. Schill WB. Recent progress in pharmacological therapy of male subfertility—a review. Andrologia 1979;11:77–107.
69. Baker HWG. Male infertility of undetermined etiology. In: Krieger PT, Bardin W, eds. Current therapy in endocrinology. Philadelphia: BC Decker Inc., 1983:366–371.
70. Giarola A. Effect of mesterolone in the spermatogenesis of infertile patients. In: Mancini RE, Martini E, eds. Male fertility and sterility. Proceedings of the Serono Symposia. New York: Academic Press, 1974:479–495.
71. Brown JS. The effect of orally administered androgens on sperm motility. Fertil Steril 1975;26:305–308.
72. Keough EJ, Burger HG, De Kretser DM, Hudson B. Nonsurgical management of male infertility. In: Hafez ESE, ed. Human semen and fertility regulation in men. St. Louis: CV Mosby Co., 1976:452–463.
73. de Kretser DM, Burger HG, Hudson B. Relationship between serum FSH levels and germinal cells in males with infertility. J Clin Endocrinol Metab 1974;38:787–793.
74. Means AR, Fakunding JL, Huckins C, Tindall DJ, Vitale R. Follicle-stimulating hormone, the Sertoli cell and spermatogenesis. Recent Prog Horm Res 1976;32:477–525.
75. Rosemberg E. Medical treatment of male infertility. Andrologia 1976;8:95–107.
76. Sherins RJ. Clinical aspects of treatment of male infertility with gonadotropins: testicular response of some men given hCG with and without pergonal. In: Mancini RE, Martini L, eds. Male fertility and sterility. New York: Academic Press, 1974:545–565.
77. Troen P, Yanaihara T, Nankin H, Tominaga T, Lever H. Assessment of gonadotropin therapy in infertile males. In: Rosemberg E, Paulsen CA, eds. The human testis. New York: Plenum Press, 1970:591.
78. Lunenfeld B, Mor A, Mani M. Treatment of male infertility: I. human gonadotropins. Fertil Steril 1967;18:581–592.
79. Margolieth EJ, Laufer N, Persistz E, Gaulayere B, Shemesh A, Schenker JG. Treatment of oligoasthenospermia with human chorionic gonadotropin: hormonal profiles and results. Fertil Steril 1983;39:841–844.
80. Shulman S, Harlin B, Daries P, Reyniak JV. Immune infertility and new approaches to treatment. Fertil Steril 1978;29:309–313.
81. Hendry WF, Stedronska J, Parslow J, Hughs L. The results of intermittent high dose steroid therapy for male infertility due to antisperm antibodies. Fertil Steril 1981;36:351–355.
82. Berger RE, Smith WD, Critchlow CW, et al. Improvement in the sperm penetration (hamster ova) assay (SPA) results after doxycycline treatment of infertile men. J Androl 1983;4:126–130.
83. Sherris JD, Fox G. Infertility and sexually transmitted disease: a public health challenge. Population Reports, Series L, July 1983, No. 4.

The Surgical Management of Male Infertility

Howard Frey and Jacob Rajfer

Fifteen percent of all marriages are involuntarily childless and men are directly responsible in 30% and contributory in another 20% of these (1). The most common category of male infertility is idiopathic oligospermia for which surgery is not appropriate. The urologist nevertheless plays an important role in the treatment of a number of other causes of infertility. A prime example is the improvement in sperm concentration, motility, and morphology that often results in pregnancy following varicocelectomy.

The introduction of the operating microscope has also created new opportunities for the urologist to help restore fertility in some men. Surgical reconstruction of certain abnormalities of the male genital tract was once considered impossible, but now fertility is restored frequently enough to offer hope to these men. It is our purpose in this chapter to provide current information about those surgically reversible conditions that cause or contribute to infertility in the male partner.

Anatomy of the Male Genital System

TUBULAR SYSTEM. The testis is divided into 200 to 300 lobules, each of which contains 1 to 3 seminiferous tubules (Fig. 12–1). The uncoiled length of each tubule is 70 cm to 80 cm and each has a diameter of 0.12 mm to 0.3 mm. Spermatogenesis occurs in the highly coiled portion of the seminiferous tubules, which assume a straight course near the apex of the lobule. These unite to form a network of 20 to 30 ducts, 0.5 mm in diameter, known as the rete testis. At the superior portion of the rete testis, 12 to 20 efferent ductules emerge from each testis after perforating the tunica albuginea. Each ductule, uncoiled, measures 15 cm to 20 cm in length. The efferent ductules become convoluted and condense into a number of cortical masses called the lobule of the epididymis. Together, these lobules constitute the head of the epididymis. The ductules converge into the epididymal duct, which is also highly convoluted. The epididymal duct, which measures 6 m (19.7 feet) in length, continues from the tail of the epididymis as the convoluted portion of the vas deferens, which becomes straight as it leaves the epididymis. The vas deferens is unique in possessing a very thick muscular wall and an extremely narrow lumen (0.3 mm to 0.5 mm). It passes through the inguinal ring, around the inferior epigastric vessels, then medially across the ureter. It dilates to form the ampulla behind the prostate, narrows again, then joins the duct of the seminal vesicle to form the ejaculatory duct (Fig. 12–2).

Each seminal vesicle is a tubular structure that is coiled on itself and contains several diverticula. Its diameter is 3 mm to 4 mm and, when uncoiled, is 10 cm to 15 cm in length. The seminal vesicles are separated from the rectum by Denonvilliers' fascia, which is a double leaf of peritoneum that extends into the deep pelvis. Goblet cells in the seminal vesicle secrete fructose and an anticoagulating enzyme. Seminal vesicular secretion accounts for the greatest portion of the ejaculate volume.

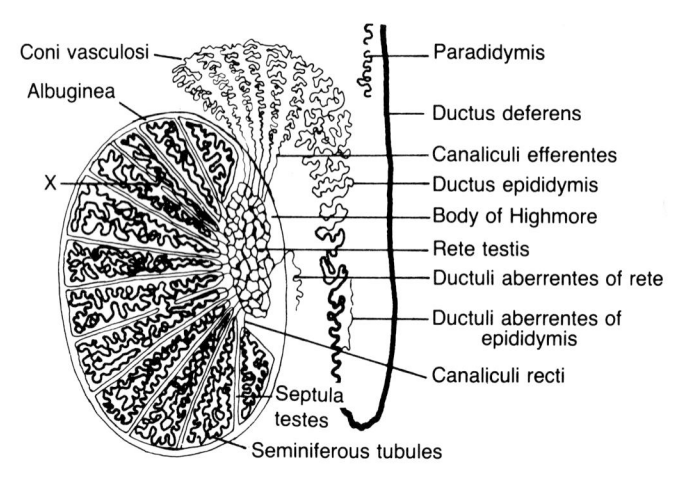

Fig. 12–1. Anatomy of the testis, epididymis, and vas (ductus) deferens. Spermatozoa are manufactured in the seminiferous tubules and transported by physical forces into the epididymis and vas deferens. The entire process of spermatogenesis and sperm transport takes approximately 90 days. (Reproduced with permission. Bloom W, Fawcett DW. A textbook of histology, 10th ed. Philadelphia: WB Saunders, 1975.)

Sperm are not stored in the seminal vesicles but in the cauda epididymis and vas deferens.

The ejaculatory ducts pass obliquely through the prostate gland and terminate along the verumontanum in the prostatic urethra. The bladder neck is situated proximal to the urethral entrance of the ejaculatory ducts, while the external urinary sphincter lies just distal to it (Fig. 12–2).

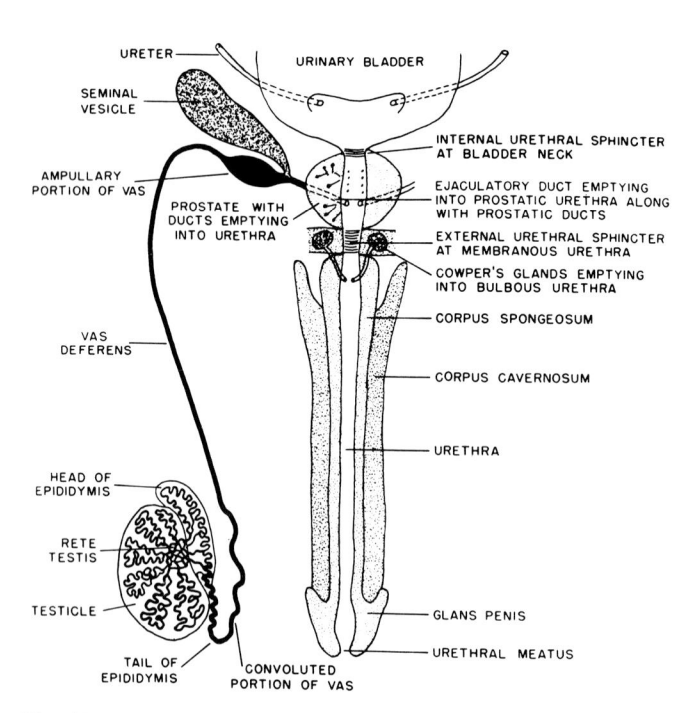

Fig. 12–2. Anatomy of the vas deferens and its relationship to the seminal vesicle, prostate, bladder, and urethra. (Reproduced with permission. Amelar RD. Infertility in men. Philadelphia: FA Davis Co., 1966.)

ARTERIAL SUPPLY. The testis receives its blood supply primarily from 3 anastomosing vessels: the spermatic, vasal (deferential), and cremasteric arteries (Fig. 12–3). The main supply is from the spermatic artery, which arises from the aorta, just beneath the renal arteries. The artery courses obliquely downward, crosses and then lies lateral to the ureter, and passes through the internal inguinal ring. The artery travels with the spermatic cord; it enters the testis via 1 or 2 superficial vessels that lie just beneath the tunica albuginea and forms the tunica vasculosa. Septal branches that emerge from the tunica vasculosa travel along the tubules. The vasal artery, the larger of the collateral vessels, and the cremasteric artery do not enter the testis directly but anastomose with the spermatic artery close to the testis (2).

VENOUS DRAINAGE. The venous drainage of the testis unites with veins draining the epididymis to form an anastomosing venous system, the pampiniform plexus, which runs along the spermatic cord. After emerging from the internal ring, these veins usually coalesce to form at least 2 major veins situated on either side of the spermatic artery. These unite to form a single vein, which drains into the vena cava on the right and the renal vein on the left. The spermatic vein, like most veins, contains valves that prevent retrograde flow. The left renal vein is anterior to the aorta and posterior to the superior mesenteric artery. With each arterial pulse, an intermittent obstruction to flow in the left renal vein may occur (3) and result in intermittent obstruction of flow in the left spermatic vein. Unlike the arteries, the veins of the testis anastomose freely with collateral vessels from the contralateral side (4,5).

THE NERVOUS SYSTEM. The bladder neck and the muscularis of the vasa deferentia and seminal vesicles are innervated by the sympathetic aspect of the autonomic nervous system. This sympathetic outflow arises from T11 to T12 and coalesces into the hypogastric nerve plexus. These sympathetic plexi lie anterior to the aortic bifurcation (presacral nerve) and along the medial borders of the psoas muscles; they lie under the vena cava on the right and the aorta on the left. Stimulation of these ganglia causes contraction of the vasa deferentia and seminal vesicles, and closure of the bladder neck. This results in seminal emission and the deposition of sperm and seminal fluid into the prostatic urethra (Table 12–1), and prevents retrograde flow of sperm into the bladder.

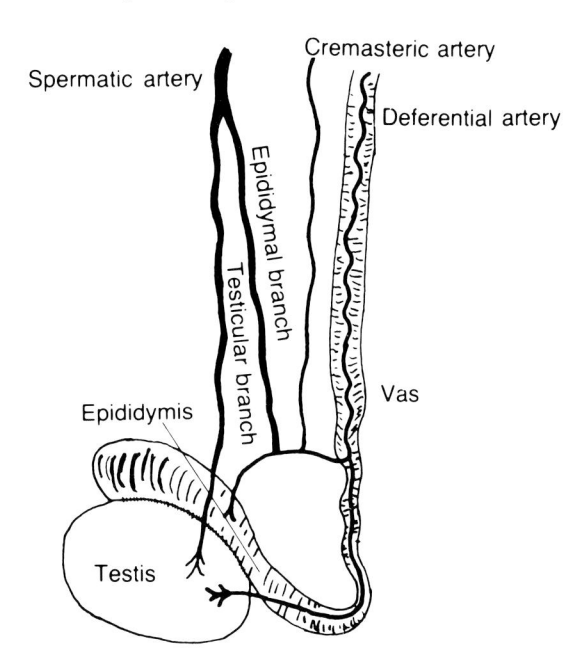

Fig. 12–3. Arterial blood supply of the testis. Anastomoses exist between the arteries of the testis.

Preventive Surgery

There are a number of clinical disorders that may subsequently lead to infertility. Appropri-

TABLE 12–1. Autonomic Nervous System in Male Sexual Function

FUNCTION	SPINAL ORIGIN	AUTONOMIC SYSTEM	PATHWAY
Erection	S2-S4	Parasympathetic	Pelvic nerve
Seminal emission	T12-L3	Sympathetic	Pudendal nerve
Ejaculation	S2-S4	Parasympathetic	Pudendal nerve

ate surgical intervention when these disorders manifest themselves may prevent infertility in these men.

CRYPTORCHIDISM. To produce viable and mature spermatozoa, the human testis must descend from the warmer intraabdominal cavity to the cooler scrotum (6). The slight temperature elevation of 1.5°C to 2.0°C of the testis out of the scrotum inhibits spermatogenesis but does not interfere with testosterone production by the Leydig cells.

Ultrastructural changes in the cryptorchid testis have been described as early as the second year of life (7–9). These changes includes degeneration of the mitochondria, loss of ribosomes, and an increase in collagen fibers in the seminiferous tubules and interstitium. The longer the testis is out of the scrotum, the greater the likelihood of damage to the seminiferous tubules. Conversely, the earlier a testis is brought into the scrotum, the greater the potential for normal spermatogenesis. However, Silber has observed sperm production in a testis that was cryptorchid for 17 years before it was autotransplanted into the scrotum (10).

Although it is not surprising that sperm production and the resultant fertility of men with bilateral cryptorchid testes is often negligible, the sperm density in men with unilateral cryptorchidism is only 40% of normal (11–13). This suggests that a defect in spermatogenesis also exists in the normally descended testis. Orchiopexy should be performed before degeneration of the seminiferous epithelium, which is often by the second year of life (14).

TORSION. Torsion of the testis and/or spermatic cord is another common problem that can alter fertility through loss of spermatogenesis. Torsion is caused by an anatomic abnormality between the testis and the mesentery from which it is suspended (Fig. 12–4) (15). Normally, the mesentery of the testis holds the testis in an almost upright position. If the testis is much broader than its mesentery, it will have a tendency to twist and torsion may occur. This occurs most often at puberty when the testis grows rapidly while the mesenteric insertion of the testis remains unchanged. Because this abnormality between the testis and its mesentery is often bilateral, simultaneous exploration and orchiopexy of the contralateral testis is mandatory when torsion of 1 testis occurs. Torsion of the contralateral testis may occur in 40% of men who had only a unilateral orchiopexy (16).

Torsion causes testicular ischemia and this

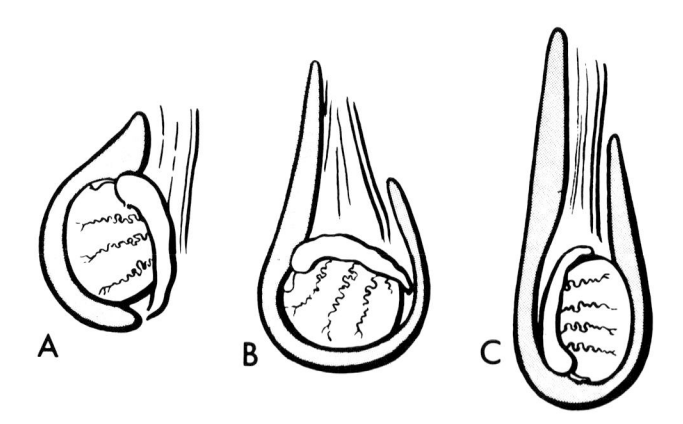

Fig. 12–4. Relationship between the mesentery of the testis (shaded area), the tunica vaginalis around the testis, and the testis itself. **A** Normal anatomic relationship, **B** Horizontal lie of testis (bell clapper deformity), **C** Inversion of the testis. **B** and **C** predispose to testicular torsion. (Reproduced with permission. Scorer CG, Farrington GH. Congenital anomalies of the testes: cryptorchidism, testicular torsion, and inguinal hernia and hydrocele. In Harrison JH, Gittes RF, Perlmutter AD, Stamey TA, Walsh PC, eds. Campbell's urology. Philadelphia: WB Saunders, 1979:1549–1565.)

results in a progressive loss of both the germinal epithelium and Sertoli cells (17,18). These degenerative changes begin 4 to 6 hours after total ischemia; Leydig cell function becomes impaired after only 10 hours of ischemia. Cellular damage is delayed with lesser degrees of torsion. However, immediate surgical exploration is mandatory, regardless of the time interval of ischemia, since salvage of the testis depends upon the early recognition and treatment of the condition (19,20).

In some studies a decreased fertility potential was found in both humans and animals who had an orchiopexy for unilateral torsion (21,22). When an orchiectomy rather than an orchiopexy was performed, fertility was normal, which suggests that a testis, after it has undergone torsion, may induce damage to the contralateral testis. However, the mechanism is unknown and these observations are preliminary. Further studies are required before orchiectomy becomes the treatment of choice for testicular torsion.

TRAUMA. Testicular trauma requires prompt surgical intervention if potential loss of testicular tissue is to be avoided. The scrotum and its contents often avoid injury because they are mobile; however, blunt or penetrating trauma directly to the scrotum may cause testicular injury. Surgical exploration is indicated if marked swelling and pain are present to suggest damage of the testis. A testicular scan may demonstrate a viable and intact testis in the presence of a large scrotal hematoma. If necessary, a hematoma can be drained and testicular rupture treated by debridement of necrotic seminiferous tubules and repair of the tunica albuginea. Minor trauma that causes marked testicular pain, tenderness, and swelling suggests the presence of testicular torsion, epididymitis, or a bleeding testicular tumor, since these may present with the signs and symptoms of trauma. An ultrasound may reveal a testicular tumor in such situations. Penetrating injuries of the scrotum that pierce the dartos muscle require surgical exploration and debridement with drainage.

RETROPERITONEAL SURGERY AND SYMPATHECTOMY. As described earlier, the sympathetic nervous system causes contraction of the vasa deferentia, seminal vesicles, and bladder neck such that seminal emission results. Interruption of these sympathetic nerves may result in the loss of seminal emission and/or retrograde ejaculation. This may occur as a result of a bilateral retroperitoneal node dissection for a testicular tumor or a sympathectomy for vascular disease.

Because of the potential loss of fertility, the sympathetic chain should be preserved, if possible, during a retroperitoneal lymph node dissection. A modified retroperitoneal node dissection is used in some centers to spare one of the paired sympathetic ganglia near the aortic bifurcation (23).

The treatment for loss of seminal emission is medical and not surgical. Pharmacologic stimulation by alpha-adrenegic agents may be used (24) but, in our experience, the results are poor. It is possible to retrieve sperm from the bladder of men with retrograde ejaculation for artificial insemination. Sodium bicarbonate (1 teaspoon in a glass of water every 4 hours) beginning the day before retrieval of sperm will alkalinize the urine and enhance sperm survival. Within 30 minutes after voiding and then ejaculation, the bladder is catheterized and the urine is centrifuged. After decanting the urine, the pellet containing the sperm is suspended in a physiologic buffer (e.g., Baker's solution) and inseminated. There is no large series of men so treated and only isolated instances of pregnancy have been reported.

Surgery for Infertility

VARICOCELE. A varicocele is a varicosity or dilatation of the veins of the pampiniform plexus that is caused by reverse blood flow in the affected spermatic vein. To accommodate the increased volume of blood, the veins of the pampiniform plexus engorge and dilate. A varicocele is present in as many as 39% of infertile men (25), but is also present in 8% to 13% of fertile men (26). Classically, a varicocele feels like a "bag of worms" in the scrotum. However, a pulsation along the spermatic vein with increased intraabdominal pressure (a Valsalva maneuver) may be the only clinical manifestation of a varicocele. Each hemiscrotum must be examined carefully since a varicocele may be present on the left (most common), only on the right, or on both sides. To detect a varicocele the man must be examined in both the standing and supine positions, and with and without the Valsalva maneuver. A varicocele may be missed if the man is examined only in the supine position. Since testicular size may be reduced in the presence of a varicocele, measurement of testicular volume or linear dimensions is important. If there is any doubt about the presence of a varicocele, a venogram should be performed (Fig. 12–5). We have no faith in thermography or Doppler studies to detect the presence of a varicocele.

Ample evidence exists that a varicocele is not merely an associated finding in infertile men, but may be the cause of the infertility as well. Not only do varicoceles occur more commonly in the male partner of infertile couples, but they are also associated with reduced sperm concentrations (26,27). Two thirds of infertile men with a varicocele will have an abnormality in sperm morphology; primarily tapered forms are found, but immature spermatids may also be present. A marked depression in sperm motility is also a common finding. Germinal cell hypoplasia with premature sloughing of immature cells into the seminiferous tubules is the most common finding in a testicular biopsy from these men (28).

Varicocelectomy results in improved semen quality in 70% of men and 50% of their wives subsequently conceive (26,29,30). The most impressive response following varicocelectomy is an improvement of sperm motility; pregnancies have resulted even when the sperm concentration remains low (27). While chorionic gonadotropin (hCG) has been used as an adjunct to varicocelectomy, only Amelar and Dubin have demonstrated a therapeutic benefit (1). Dubin and Amelar have demonstrated that the size of a varicocele bears no relationship to the probability of fertility after varicocelectomy (31).

Despite its strong association with infertility, the mechanism by which a varicocele causes infertility is still unknown. An abnormally high scrotal temperature secondary to increased venous blood flow (32,33), and retrograde venous flow into the scrotal circulation of adrenal substances toxic to spermatogenesis have been proposed, although evidence for an excess concentration of such substances is generally lacking (27,33). Peripheral plasma concentrations of LH, FSH, testosterone, and estradiol are normal in men with a varicocele (34).

The rationale for surgical ligation of a varicocele is that retrograde venous flow into the spermatic vein is prevented. Reverse flow may occur with total absence or incompetence of valves in the spermatic vein (35). Since the left spermatic vein joins the left renal vein at an angle of approximately 90°, it may become intermittently and partially obstructed by compression of the renal vein between the aorta and superior mesenteric artery (3). When a varicocele is present on both sides, not an uncommon occurrence (3), each should be ligated.

There are various surgical techniques to correct a varicocele. Ligation of the pampiniform plexus via a scrotal incision should not be done because the recurrence rate (due to the presence of unligated collateral vessels) is high and postoperative hydrocele formation is common (36). In addition, the testicular artery, which is difficult to identify in the scrotal area, may be ligated; this may result in testicular atrophy. Most surgeons perform a "high ligation" of the spermatic vein through an incision in the in-

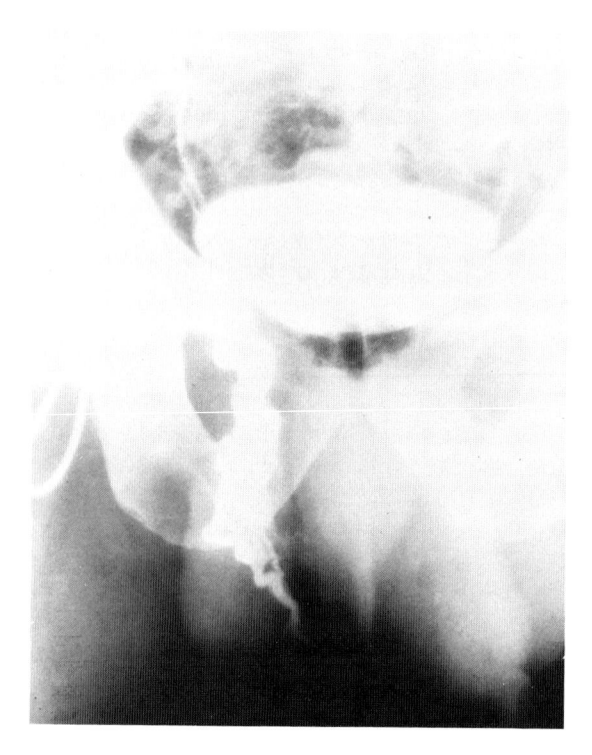

Fig. 12–5. Venogram demonstrating a large right varicocele in a man with oligospermia. This man's vena cava was on the left and his right spermatic vein drained into the right renal vein.

guinal canal or flank. With either incision, a hydrocele is rare, as is ligation of the testicular artery. Of 504 varicocelectomies done with a high ligation technique, a recurrence occurred in only 1 man and none developed testicular atrophy (30). We prefer the inguinal approach because large perforating vessels to the abdominal wall are best seen with this approach.

In the past few years, nonoperative correction of a varicocele has been used successfully (37,38). A removable balloon is inserted into the main branches of the internal spermatic vein at the time of venography (Fig. 12–6). The principal drawback of this technique is the possibility that the balloon will embolize into the pulmonary vasculature.

DUCTAL OBSTRUCTION. The surgical correction of a congenital or acquired ductal (vas deferens and epididymis) obstruction is difficult because of the narrow lumina of these structures. Obstruction may result from inflammatory conditions (e.g., tuberculous, gonorrheal, or chlamydial epididymitis), iatrogenic injury during herniorrhaphy, traumatic injuries, or, most commonly, a vasectomy for sterilization. Congenital abnormalities account for approximately 2% of male infertility (25) and are more difficult to overcome since large segments of the ductal system may be absent.

Men with acquired ductal obstruction present with azoospermia, fructose in their seminal fluid, and normal FSH concentrations. Prior to definitive surgery or when the diagnosis of obstruction is uncertain, a testicular biopsy should be done to document the presence of normal spermatogenesis. Some men with the Sertoli cell only syndrome may have normal FSH levels (39) and the other findings of ductal obstruction. A testicular biopsy is the only way to identify these men. Generally, a testicular biopsy is useful in all azoospermic men to differentiate those with primary testicular failure from those with a potentially correctable ductal obstruction. Spermatogenesis will be abnormal if the problem is primary testicular failure. Conversely, spermatogenesis is normal in men with ductal obstruction. Absence of fructose in the seminal fluid is most often the result of congenital absence of the vasa deferentia and seminal vesicles (from which the fructose is derived), or, rarely, an obstruction of the ejaculatory ducts.

Men with oligospermia rarely need a testicular biopsy since the presence of ejaculated sperm excludes the diagnosis of complete bilateral ductal obstruction. An exception to this is the rare individual with a normal testis but obstructed or absent ducts on one side and an atrophic testis on the opposite side. Also, a man with fewer than 1 million sperm per milliliter of ejaculate but normal-sized testes may have a partial obstruction.

Proper technique in obtaining a testicular biopsy is essential for optimal interpretation. Several points should be emphasized. The tunica albuginea should be incised transversely to avoid injury to the tunica vasculosa. A small portion of the testis will then protrude through the incision in the tunica albuginea and this should be excised with a scalpel, without otherwise grasping the tissue (Fig. 12–7). Bouin's, Zenker's, or Carnoy's solution can be used for fixation. Formalin or formaldehyde should never be used since they will greatly distort the histology and make interpretation impossible. For electron microscopic studies, 2.5% glutaraldehyde should be used. We believe that a biopsy should be obtained from each testis since results may, rarely, differ. This procedure is performed on an outpatient basis using local anesthesia.

VASOGRAPHY. As with a testicular biopsy, a vasogram is rarely indicated for the investigation of oligospermia, but may be useful in an azoospermic man to diagnose ductal obstruction. It is our feeling that testicular biopsies should be performed first to determine whether primary testicular failure is present. If spermatogenesis appears normal, then the site of ductal obstruction may be identified by vasography. If warranted, repair of the ductal obstruction should be performed at the same time as the vasogram and closure of the vasotomy. To perform vasography, we incise the vas under magnification and inject X-ray contrast material after inserting a blunt 25-gauge needle into the lumen of the vas deferens (Fig. 12–8). We close the vas in 1 or 2 layers with 9–0 Nylon. Blind injection into the vas should be avoided because there is a risk of submucosal extravasation of contrast material and subsequent obstruction of the lumen.

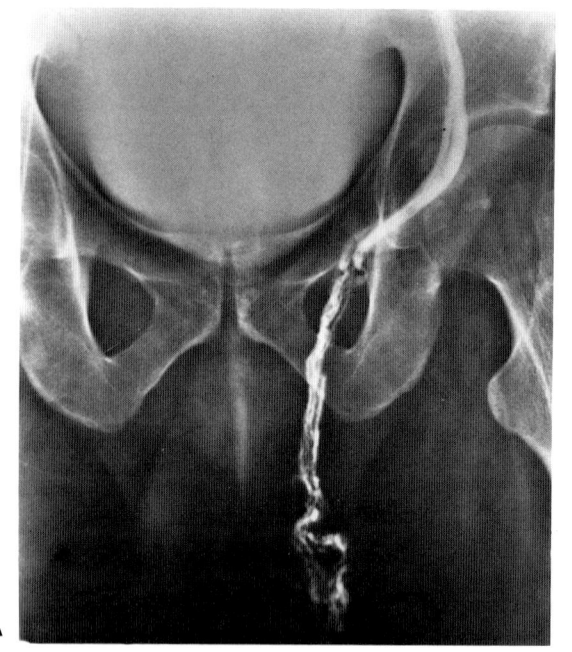

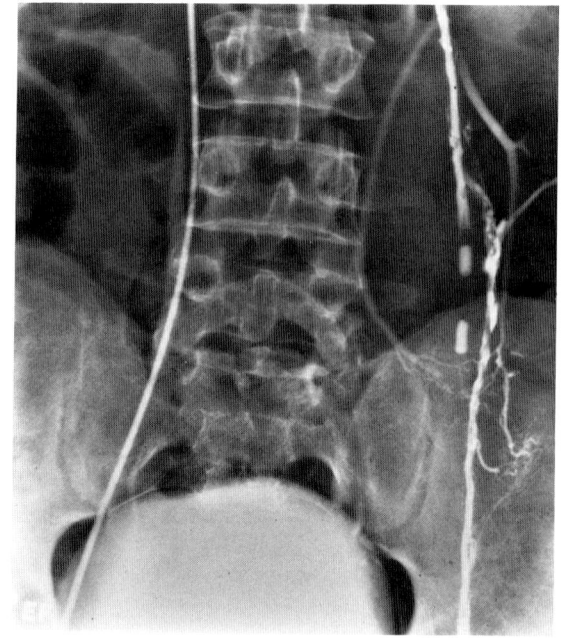

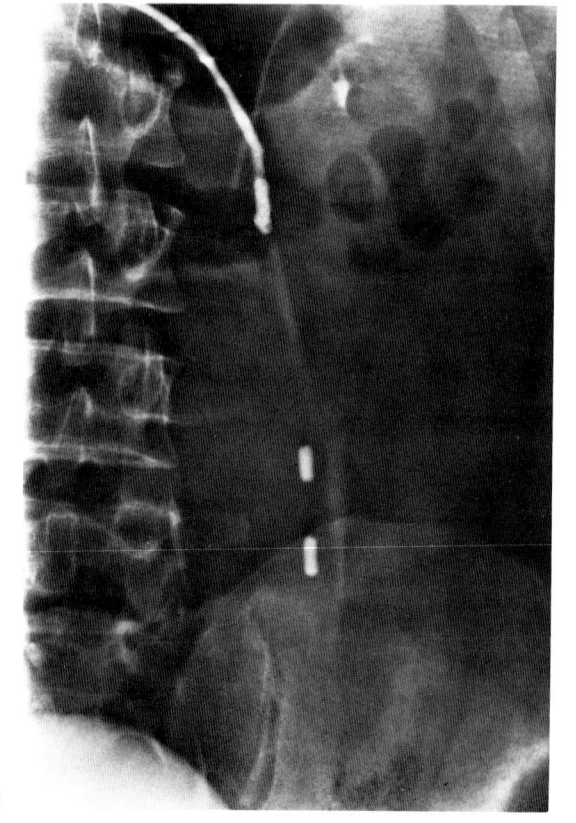

Fig. 12-6. Percutaneous embolization of a left varicocele. **A** Identification of the varicocele, **B** Demonstration of additional perforatoring veins proximal to the occlusive detachable balloons, **C** Total occlusion of the spermatic vein with additional balloons.

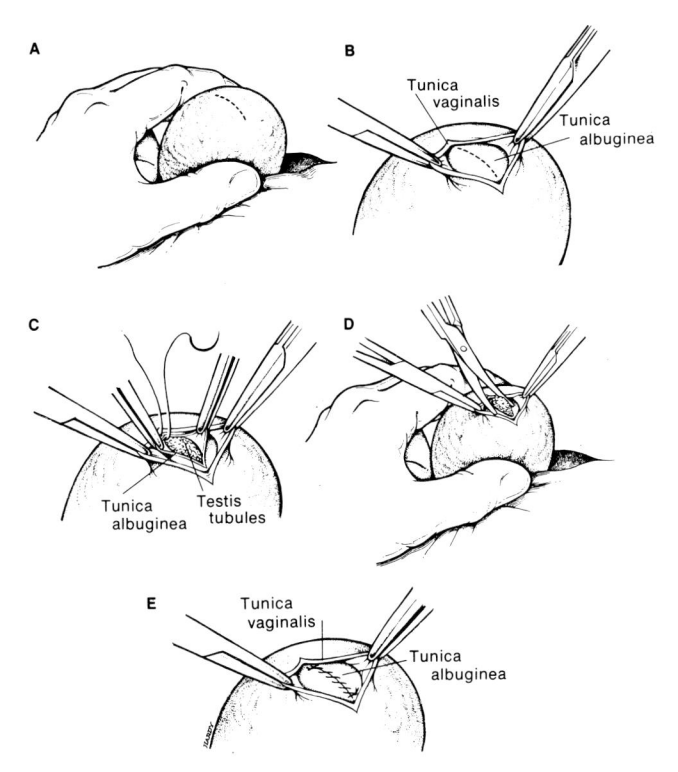

Fig. 12–7. "No touch" technique of testicular biopsy (**A** to **E**) that may be performed as an outpatient under local anesthesia. (Reproduced with permission. Amelar RD, Dubin L, Walsh PC. Male infertility. Philadelphia: WB Saunders, 1977.)

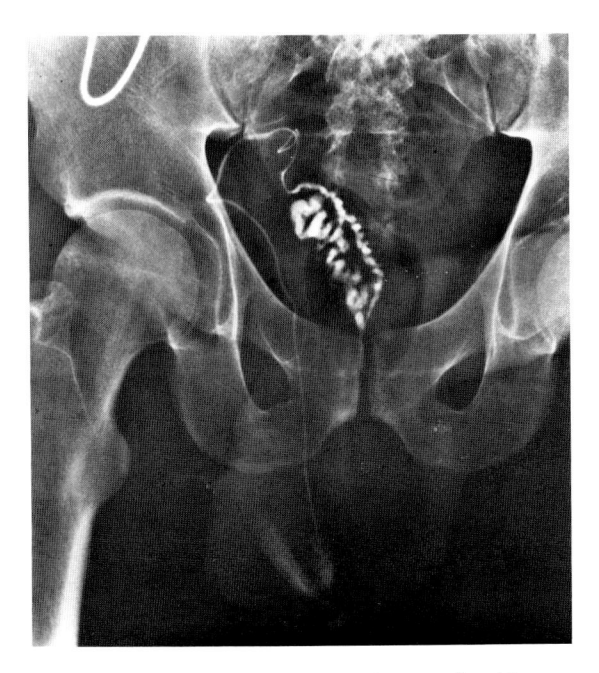

Fig. 12–8. Vasogram demonstrating the ampulla of the vas deferens and retrograde filling of the more lateral portion of the seminal vesicle.

VASECTOMY. Besides circumcision, vasectomy is the most common operation performed in the male (40). Since requests to reverse a vasectomy are common, the vasectomy should be done in a way that allows the greatest chance for reversal in those men most likely to request it. Obviously, the technique must also be effective in preventing unwanted pregnancies. Pregnancy after vasectomy has been related to the technique of the procedure. Ligation of the terminal part of the vas may be followed by necrosis and sloughing of the segment distal to the ligature (40). This may result in formation of a sperm granuloma, which may canalize and provide an alternate pathway for transport of viable sperm (41,42). Fulguration instead of ligation of the proximal vas may prevent such necrosis and reduce the incidence of sperm granuloma (40). Of interest, however, is the observation that the presence of a sperm granuloma at the vasectomy site is associated with a greater chance for successful vasovasostomy (43). A sperm granuloma may reduce intraluminal pressure in the epididymis and reduce the frequency of "epididymal blowouts" after a proximal vasectomy (44). The epididymal "blowout" will result in secondary epididymal obstruction and failure of sperm to traverse the length of the epididymis, which is necessary for spermatozoal maturation and normal sperm transport (43).

Shapiro and Silber performed open-ended vasectomies (the testicular end of the vas was neither cauterized nor ligated) on a group of men to encourage sperm granuloma formation at the vasectomy site (42). While it is too soon to assess the value of this technique in improving the chance of successful vasovasostomy, there was a high incidence of recanalization. Few urologists utilize this technique today.

In performing a vasectomy, other factors are also important for enhancing the chance of successful vasovasostomy. The vasectomy should not include the convoluted portion of the vas, a location in which vasovasostomy is more difficult to perform. Only a short length of vas (less than 2 cm) should be removed. Removal of a longer segment reduces the likelihood of a successful reanastomosis at a later date.

VASECTOMY REVERSAL. Vasovasostomy is a rather unique procedure since it is complicated by the fact that the vas deferens has a thick, tough muscular wall but a minute lumen of 0.3 mm to 0.7 mm diameter. In addition, the testicular end of the ligated vas usually has a dilated lumen from chronic obstruction, whereas the portion of the vas distal to the ligation still has a narrow lumen. Anastomosis of structures with disproportionate lumina is difficult. Vasovasostomy with optical loupes (2.5× to 6×) is usually done with a 1-layer anastomosis using a 7–0 suture. Thus, the muscularis and mucosa are approximated with the same suture. A splint of Nylon or absorbable chromic catgut suture, which is brought out through a separate vasotomy, is sometimes employed. We do not recommend the use of a splint because it may cause additional scarring, inflammation, and sperm leakage (Fig. 12–9) (45). Because of the disproportionate diameters of the lumina, a 1-layer closure may not result in a patent, sperm-tight vas. Nevertheless, various authors have reported good

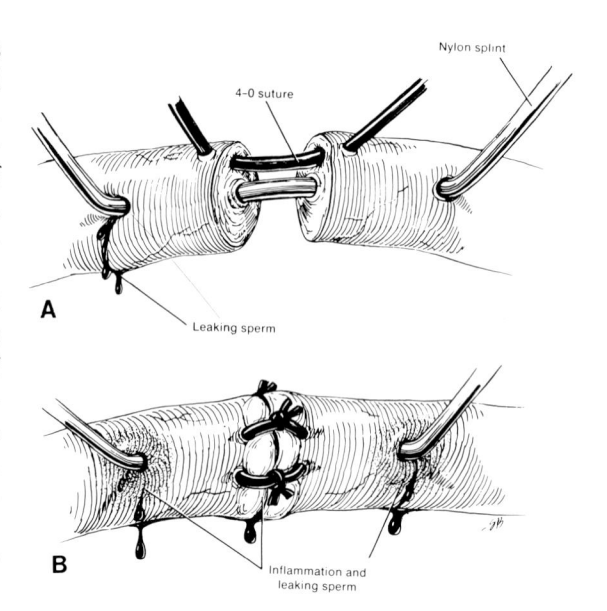

Fig. 12–9. Macroscopic 1-layer vasovasostomy using a Nylon stent in the vasal lumen **(A).** Sutures are large with respect to the size of the vas and this may result in leakage of sperm at the anastomotic site and the exit sites of the stent **(B).** (Reproduced with permission. Silber SJ. Microsurgery. Baltimore: Williams & Wilkins, 1979. Figs. 12–9, 12–10, 12–12 to 12–14 copyright 1979, The Williams & Wilkins Co., Baltimore.)

results with this macroscopic technique (46–49) and a subsequent pregnancy rate as high as 55% (50).

It is our opinion that a more precise anastomosis is best accomplished by microscopic vasovasostomy. This precision seems to be the consequence of a 2-layer closure in which the luminal mucosa is first approximated and followed by anastomosis of the muscularis (51). The problem of disproportionate luminal diameters can be managed more effectively and the chances for a sperm-tight, patent lumen are increased. Gentle dilatation of the lumen proximal to the vasectomy may reduce the disproportion. Lacrimal duct or coronary artery dilators are effective for this. While the operating microscope is cumbersome, the resulting visualization enables the surgeon to place the sutures more precisely. We use 10–0 Nylon for the mucosal layer and 9–0 Nylon on a cutting needle for the tough muscular wall of the vas (Fig. 12–10).

Results of microscopic vasovasostomy have, in general, been better than for macroscopic techniques (49,51,52). Silber reported a 95% patency rate in 42 consecutive men undergo-

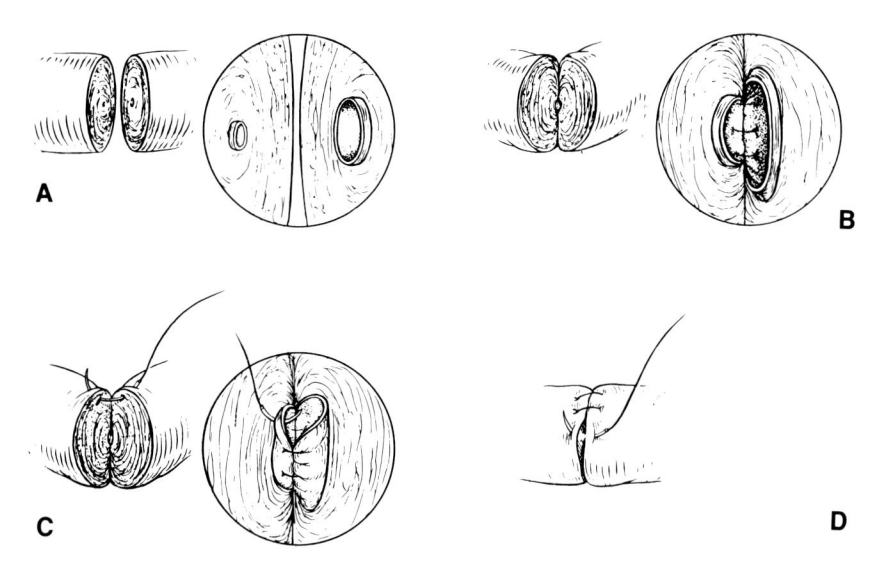

Fig. 12–10. Microscopic 2-layer vasovasostomy as described by Silber **(A to D):** 10–0 Nylon is used for the inner mucosal layer and 9–0 Nylon is used for the outer muscularis and adventitial layers. (Reproduced with permission. Silber SJ. Microsurgery. Baltimore: Williams & Wilkins, 1979.)

ing microscopic vasovasostomy (53). Seventy-one percent of their wives conceived within 1.5 years of their husband's surgery. Owen obtained a 70% pregnancy rate with a 2-layer microscopic anastomosis (52). However, Lee and McLoughlin obtained comparable pregnancy rates with macroscopic (loupes) and microscopic techniques—46% and 54%, respectively (49).

There is a discrepancy between patency rates (determined by the presence of sperm in the ejaculate following vasectomy reversal) and pregnancy rates. This discrepancy suggests that factors other than surgical technique are important. An interval between vasectomy and vasovasostomy of greater than 10 years is associated with a lesser chance of pregnancy (51,53). This may be a result of long-term increases in intraluminal pressure, atrophy of seminiferous epithelium within the testis (54), secondary ductal changes (53,55,56), or other, undetermined factors. Antisperm antibodies are commonly present following vasectomy (57), but their presence does not correlate with fertility following vasovasostomy (46,50). The presence of sperm in the fluid emanating from the testicular side of the vas lumen at the time of reversal denotes a good prognosis for fertility. Normal sperm concentrations were obtained in 75% of 121 men after vasovasostomy if sperm were seen in the vas fluid at the time of reanastomosis (53).

VASOEPIDIDYMOSTOMY. Men with azoospermia and normal serum FSH levels will frequently have an epididymal obstruction and require vasoepididymostomy. Dubin and Amelar observed a 25% prevalence of ductal obstruction in azoospermic men (25). Some men undergoing vasectomy reversal will have no sperm present in the lumen of the vas and will require a more proximal anastomosis to the cauda epididymis (Fig. 12–11) (53). In performing a macroscopic vasoepididymostomy, a longitudinal incision is made through the tunic of the epididymis into the convoluted epididymal duct. In so doing, the epididymis is transected in numerous locations (Fig. 12–12). A longitudinal incision is also made in the vas and a side-to-side anastomosis to the epididymal tunic is performed. A successful operation depends on the creation of a permanent fistula between the epididymal duct and the vas. Macroscopic vasoepididymostomy is infrequently successful (58).

With a microscopic technique, the one draining epididymal duct is anastomosed directly to the vas (Fig. 12–13) (59). The appropriate duct must be identified by observing seminal fluid draining from the horizontally transected epi-

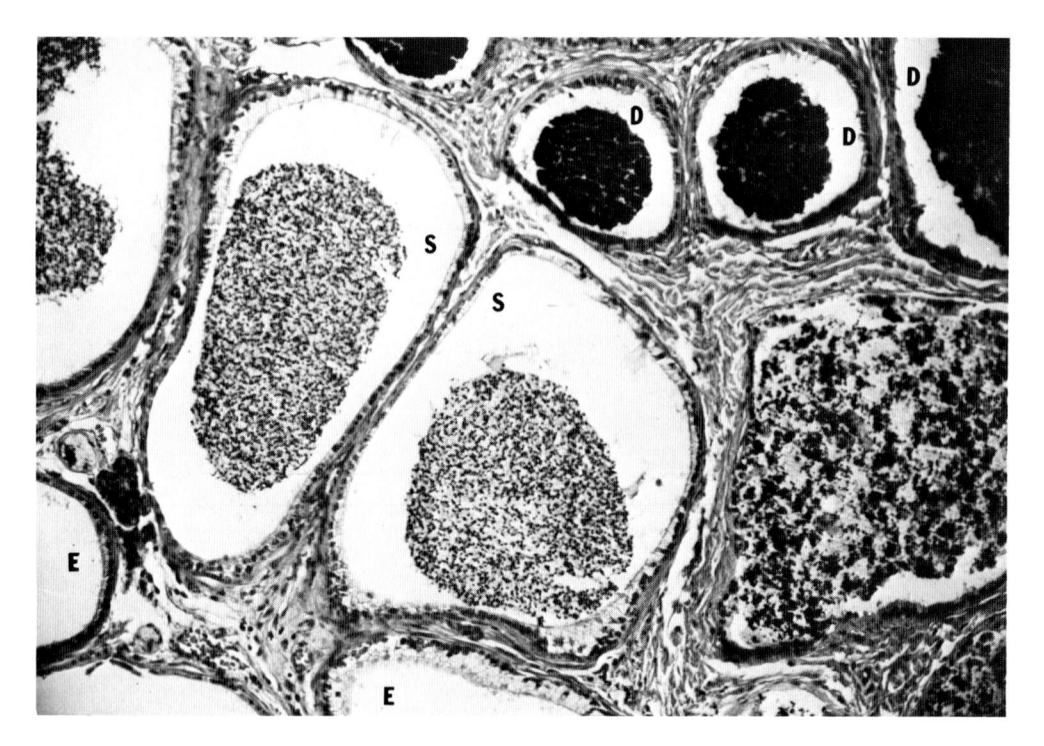

Fig. 12–11. Histology of the epididymis in a man with azoospermia whose ejaculate contained fructose. His FSH concentrations were normal. These findings suggested a ductal obstruction. At surgery, an obstruction was found in the epididymis. In this area some of the epididymal tubules are filled with sperm (S), some are filled with necrotic debris and degenerating sperm (D), while other tubules are empty of any contents (E). It appears as if the sperm are being digested and reabsorbed proximal to the obstruction in the epididymis.

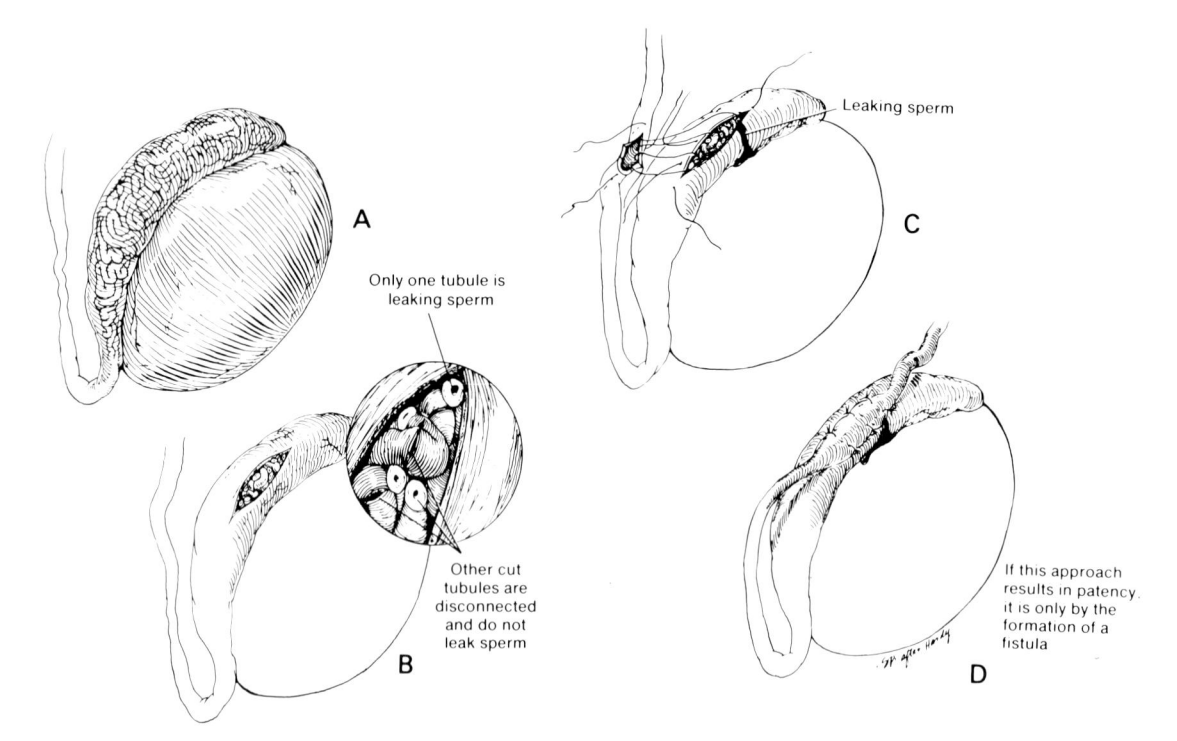

Fig. 12–12. Vasoepididymostomy performed by incising the epididymis blindly **(B)** and anastamosing the vasal lumen, which has been also incised longitudinally **(C)** in hopes of creating a patent fistula between the epididymal tubule and the vas. (Reproduced with permission. Silber SJ. Microsurgery. Baltimore: Williams & Wilkins, 1979.)

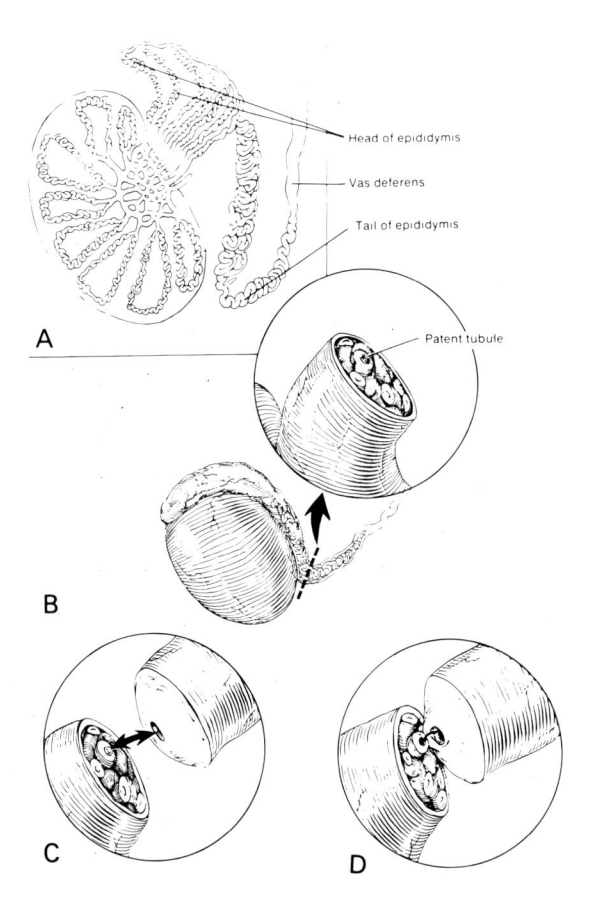

Fig. 12-13. Microscopic vasoepididymostomy performed by anastomosing the 1 patent tubule end to end with mucosa of the vas using 10-0 Nylon. (Reproduced with permission. Silber SJ. Microsurgery. Baltimore: Williams & Wilkins, 1979.)

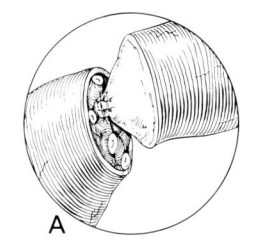

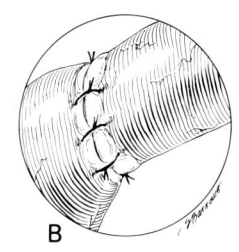

Fig. 12-14. Completion of a microscopic vasoepididymostomy by anastomosing the muscularis of the vas deferens to the adventitia of the epididymis. (Reproduced with permission. Silber SJ. Microsurgery. Baltimore: Williams & Wilkins, 1979.)

didymis. The fluid is examined for the presence of sperm. If none is present, a more proximal part of the epididymis is incised. A patent epididymal duct has a diameter of 0.1 mm to 0.3 mm and an extremely thin wall (53). The anastomosis between the epididymal duct and vas lumen is made with approximately 3 interrupted sutures of 9-0 or 10-0 Nylon. The muscularis of the vas is then sutured to the epididymal edge to secure the anastomosis (Fig. 12-14). Microscopic vasoepididymostomy is technically demanding but affords greater chance for success than previous macroscopic procedures. Eleven of 14 men had normal sperm concentrations in their ejaculates after this procedure (53).

CREATION OF A SPERMATOCELE. When the vasa deferentia are scarred and occluded over a long segment or when the vasa are congenitally absent, neither a vasovasostomy or vasoepididymostomy is possible. A history of genital trauma or infection in an azoospermic man with a normal ejaculate volume and fructose in the semen suggests the diagnosis of ductal obstruction. Scrotal exploration and a vasogram are the only means to confirm the diagnosis and ascertain the location and length of ductal obstruction. Men with congenital absence of the vasa deferentia (and seminal vesicles) will have no palpable vasa or seminal vesicles (Fig. 12-15). The ejaculates of these men

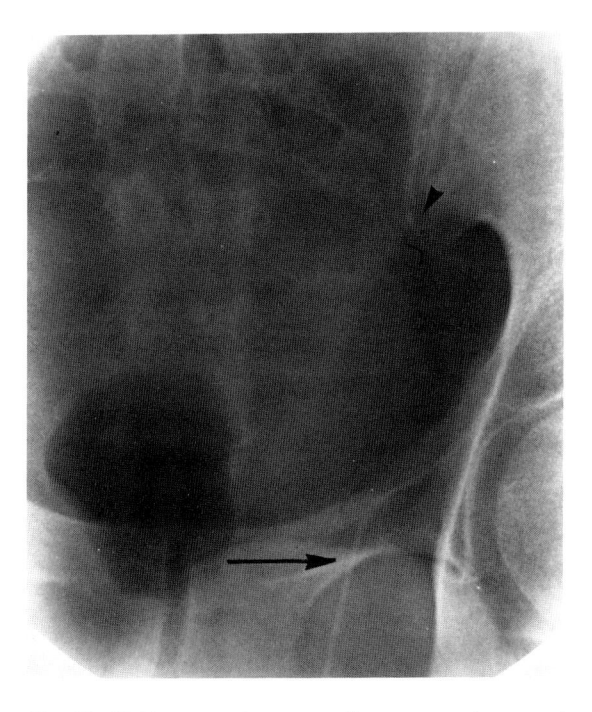

Fig. 12-15. Vasogram in a man with azoospermia, normal ejaculatory volume, positive seminal fructose and a normal testicular biopsy. Vas (arrowhead) ends blindly in the deep pelvis (arrow).

are 1 cc or less, contain no fructose, do not coagulate, and have an acidic pH. The epididymides may also be partially absent. Spermatogenesis is normal in these men.

By creating a spermatocele, semen can be aspirated percutaneously and inseminated into the cervix of the spouse. Schoysman recovered sperm in 33% of men and achieved a pregnancy in 10.8% of their wives after using a segment of saphenous vein to create a spermatocele (60). Others have been unable to achieve this rate of success (61). Use of a tunica vaginalis graft has been recommended to circumvent some of the problems of using a saphenous vein graft (44). In our experience, the results of this are as dismal as those with a saphenous vein graft (Fig. 12–16).

A silicone reservoir has recently been developed expressly for the purpose of creating a spermatocele (62). It may be anastomosed to the epididymis and may be easier to work with than a saphenous vein or tunica vaginalis. In animal experiments, sperm were recovered more frequently when the silicone prosthesis was implanted closer to the tail of the epididymis. However, use of this prosthesis for creation of a spermatocele is currently not approved in the United States.

Summary

While the internist, endocrinologist, and gynecologist may be able to evaluate the male partner of an infertile couple, it is the urologist whose skills are ultimately called upon once the physical exam, semen analysis, and other diagnostic procedures suggest the presence of a varicocele, ductal obstruction, or other abnormality.

Caring for an infertile couple as a couple has been suggested or emphasized many times in

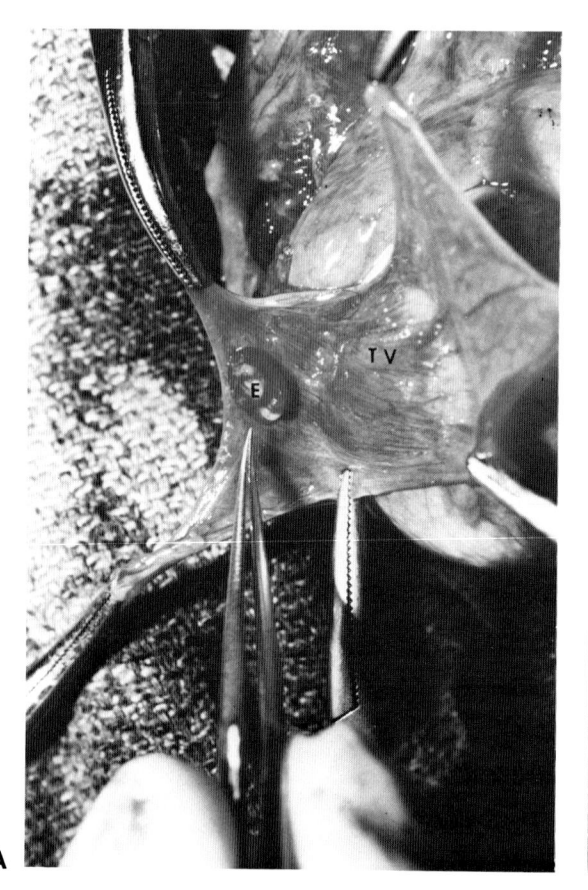

Fig. 12–16. Creation of an artificial spermatocele with tunica vaginalis. **A** Transected cauda epididymis (*E*) being anastomosed to the tunica vaginalis (*TV*) so that the epididymal contents would drain into it. **B** Completion of the closure of the tunica vaginalis around the epididymis.

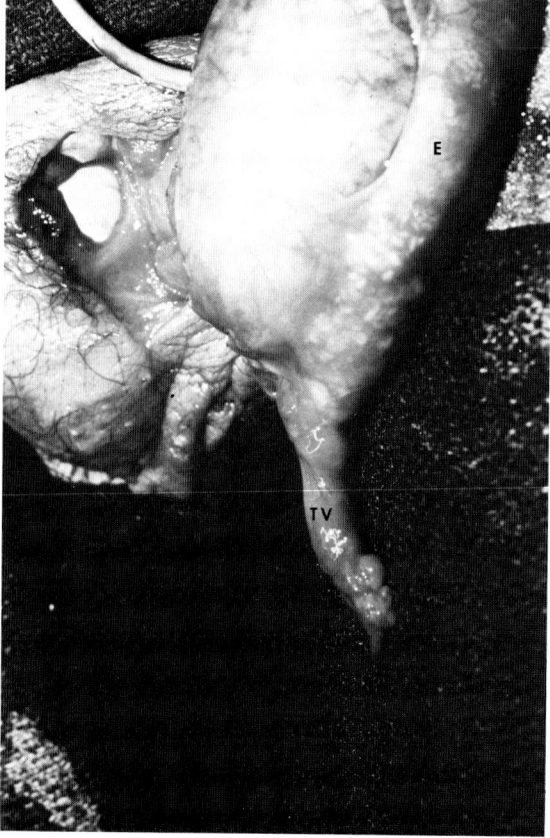

this text and the urologist is essential in the care of many of these couples because of his or her knowledge of surgical anatomy, testicular and adnexal pathology, and surgical skills. Improvement in microsurgical instruments, advances in surgical techniques, and the acquisition of new knowledge of the function of the male reproductive organs will lead to improved results in the surgical restoration of fertility in men.

REFERENCES

1. Amelar RD, Dubin L, Walsh PC. Male infertility. Philadelphia: WB Saunders, 1977.
2. Fowler R and Stephens FD. The role of testicular vascular anatomy in the salvage of high undescended testes. Aust NZ J Surg 1959;29:92–106.
3. Brown JS, Dubin L, Becker M, Hotchkiss RS. Venography in the subfertile man with varicocele. J Urol 1967;98:388–392.
4. Brown JS, Dubin L, Hotchkiss RS. The varicocele as related to fertility. Fertil Steril 1967;18:46–56.
5. Ed-Sadr AR, Mina E. Anatomical and surgical aspects in the operative management of varicocele. Urol Cut Rev 1950;54:257–262.
6. Moore CR, Quick WJ. The scrotum as a temperature regulator for the testes. Am J Physiol 1924;68:70–79.
7. Mengel W, Heinz HA, Sippe WG, Hecker WC. Studies on cryptorchidism: a comparison of histological findings in the germinative epithelium before and after the second year of life. J Pediatr Surg 1974;9:445–450.
8. Hadziselimovic F, Herzog B, Seguchi H. Surgical correction of cryptorchidism at 2 years: electron microscopic and morphometric investigations. J Pediatr Surg 1975;10:19–26.
9. Wronecki K, Czernik J. Electron microscopic studies of the undescended testicle in boys under 5 years. Z Kinderchir 1980;30:167–171.
10. Silber SJ. Microsurgery for the undescended testicle. Urol Clin North Am 1982;9:429–438.
11. Hecker W, Heinz HA. Cryptorchidism and fertility. J Pediatr Surg 1967;2:513–517.
12. Woodhead DM, Pohl DR, Johnson DE. Fertility of patients with solitary testis. J Urol 1973;109:66–67.
13. Lipshultz LI, Caminos-Torres R, Greenspan CS, Snyder PJ. Testicular function after orchiopexy for unilaterally undescended testis. N Engl J Med 1976;295:15–18.
14. Scorer CG. Early operation for the undescended testis. Br J Surg 1967;54:694–698.
15. Scorer CG, Farrington GH. Congenital deformities of the testicle and epididymis. New York: Appleton-Century-Crofts, 1971.
16. Skoglund RW, McRoberts JW, Ragde H. Torsion of the spermatic cord: a review of the literature and an analysis of 70 new cases. J Urol 1970;104:604–607.
17. Smith GI. Cellular changes from graded testicular ischemia. J Urol 1955;73:355–362.
18. Sonda LP, Lapides J. Experimental torsion of the spermatic cord. Surg Forum 1961;12:502–504.
19. Cass AS, Cass BP, Veeraraghavan K. Immediate exploration of the unilateral acute scrotum in young male subjects. J Urol 1980;124:829–832.
20. Ransler CW, Allen TD. Torsion of the spermatic cord. Urol Clin North Am 1982;9:245–250.
21. Bartsch G, Marberger FH, Mikuz G. Testicular torsion: late results with special regard to fertility and endocrine function. J Urol 1980;124:375–378.
22. Nagler HM, deVere White R. Long-term effects of testicular torsion on reproductive capacity in the adult male rat. Surg Forum 1982;33:619–620.
23. Leiter E, Brendler H. Loss of ejaculation following bilateral retroperitoneal lymphadenectomy. J Urol 1967;98:375–378.
24. Kedia KR, Markland C, Fraley EE. Sexual function after high retroperitoneal lymphoadenectomy. Urol Clin North Am 1977;4:523–527.
25. Dubin L, Amelar RD. Etiologic factors in 1294 consecutive cases of male infertility. Fertil Steril 1971;22:469–474.
26. Verstoppen GR, Steeno OP. Varicocele and the pathogenesis of the associated subfertility: a review of the various theories. II. Results of Surgery. Andrologia 1977;9:293–305.
27. MacLeod J. Seminal cytology in the presence of varicocoele. Fertil Steril 1965;16:735–757.
28. Dubin L, Hotchkiss RS. Testis biopsy in subfertile men with varicocele. Fertil Steril 1969;20:50–57.
29. Tulloch WS. A consideration of sterility factors in the light of subsequent pregnancies. II. Subfertility in the male. Edinburgh Obstet Soc 1952;104:29–34.
30. Dubin L, Amelar RD. Varicocelectomy as therapy in male infertility: a study of 504 cases. J Urol 1975;113:640–641.
31. Dubin L, Amelar RD. Varicocele size and results of varicocelectomy in selected subfertile men with varicocele. Fertil Steril 1970;21:606–609.
32. Zorgniotti AW, MacLeod J. Studies in tempera-

ture, human semen quality, and varicocele. Fertil Steril 1973;24:854–863.
33. Verstoppen GR, Steeno OP. Varicocele and the pathogenesis of the associated subfertility: a review of the various theories. III. Theories concerning the deleterious effects of varicocele on fertility. Andrologia 1978;10:85–102.
34. Swerdloff RS, Walsh PC. Pituitary and gonadal hormones in patients with varicocele. Fertil Steril 1975;26:1006–1012.
35. Ahlberg NE, Bartley O, Chidekel N, Fritjofsson A. Phlebography in varicocele scroti. Acta Radiol [Diagn] (Stockh) 1966;4:517–528.
36. Scott LS, Young D. Varicocele: a study of its effects on human spermatogenesis and of the results produced by spermatic vein ligation. Fertil Steril 1962;13:325–334.
37. Walsh PC, White RI. Balloon occlusion of the internal spermatic vein for the treatment of varicoceles. JAMA 1981;246:1701–1702.
38. White RI, Kaufman SL, Barth KH, DeCaprio V, Strandbert JD. Therapeutic embolization with detachable balloons, technique and clinical results. Radiology 1979;131:619–627.
39. Baker HWG, Bremner WJ, Burger HG, et al. Testicular control of follicle stimulating hormone secretion. Recent Prog Horm Res 1976;32:429–476.
40. Schmidt SS, Morris RR. Spermatic granuloma: the complication of vasectomy. Fertil Steril 1973;24:941–947.
41. Schmidt SS. Techniques and complications of elective vasectomy. The role of spermatic granuloma in spontaneous recanalization. Fertil Steril 1966;17:467–482.
42. Shapiro EI, Silber SJ. Open-ended vasectomy, sperm granuloma and post-vasectomy orchialgia. Fertil Steril 1979;32:546–550.
43. Silber SJ. Sperm granuloma and reversibility of vasectomy. Lancet 1977;2:588–589.
44. Silber SJ. Epididymal extravasation following vasectomy as a cause for failure of vasectomy reversal. Fertil Steril 1979;31:309–315.
45. Fernandes M, Shah KN, Draper JW. Vasovasostomy: improved microsurgical technique. J Urol 1968;100:763–766.
46. Fallon B, Jacobo E, Bunge RG. Restoration of fertility by vasovasostomy. J Urol 1978;119:85–86.
47. Middleton RG, Henderson D. Vas deferens reanastomosis without splints and without magnification. J Urol 1978;119:763–764.
48. Amelar RD, Dubin L. Vasectomy reversal. J Urol 1979;121:547–550.
49. Lee L, McLoughlin MG. Vasovasostomy: a comparison of macroscopic and microscopic techniques at one institution. Fertil Steril 1980;33:54–55.
50. Phadke GM, Phadke AG. Experiences in the reanastomosis of the vas deferens. J Urol 1967;97:888–890.
51. Yong Lee H. Observations of the results of 300 vasovasostomies. J Androl 1980;1:11–15.
52. Owen ER. Microsurgical vasovasostomy: a reliable vasectomy reversal. Aust NZ J Surg 1977;47:305–309.
53. Silber SJ. Microsurgery of male genitalia: nonvascular. In: Silber SJ, ed. Microsurgery. Baltimore: Williams & Wilkins, 1979:307–375.
54. Derrick FC Jr, Glover WL, Kanjuparamban Z, et al. Histologic changes in the seminiferous tubules after vasectomy. Fertil Steril 1974;25:649–658.
55. Howards SS, Jesse S, Johnson A. Micropuncture and microanalytic studies of the effect of vasectomy on the rat testis and epididymis. Fertil Steril 1975;26:20–28.
56. Pardanani DS, Patil NG, Pawar HN. Some gross observations of the epididymis following vasectomy: a clinical study. Fertil Steril 1976;27:267–270.
57. Alexander NJ. Vasectomy and vasovasostomy in rhesus monkeys: the effect of circulating antisperm antibodies on fertility. Fertil Steril 1977;28:562–569.
58. Hanley HG. The surgery of male infertility. Ann R Coll Surg Engl 1955;17:159–183.
59. Silber SJ. Microscopic vasoepididymostomy: specific microanastomosis to the epididymal tubule. Fertil Steril 1978;30:565–571.
60. Schoysman R, Drouart JM. Progrès recent dans la chirurgie de la stèrilitè masculine et feminine. Acta Chirurg Belgica 1972;71:261–280.
61. Vickers MA. Creation and use of a scrotal sperm bank in aplasia of the vas deferens. J Urol 1975;114:242–245.
62. Wagenknecht LV, Holstein AF, Schirrin C. Alloplastic spermatocele for the treatment of male infertility. Urol Res 1976;4:177.

Extracorporeal Fertilization and Embryo Transfer

Anibal A. Acosta and Jairo E. Garcia

The process of fertilization and embryo transfer can be accomplished in different ways: *in vivo* fertilization of spontaneously ovulated oocytes or *in vivo* fertilization of superovulated females followed by embryo retrieval from the tube or the uterine cavity. Subsequently, those embryos can be transferred to some other recipient(s) whose reproductive cycles have been synchronized with the donor's cycle. These procedures have been used extensively in veterinary medicine.

In the human with reproductive problems, oocytes retrieved from the ovary close to the time of spontaneous or induced ovulation have been fertilized in the laboratory after retrieval (extracorporeal fertilization *in vitro*) and then transferred into the uterus of the donor in an effort to achieve implantation and pregnancy (embryo transfer).

Another possibility is to place the retrieved oocyte or oocytes into the uterine cavity immediately after recovery and inseminate (naturally or artificially) the woman just before or after the oocyte transfer. We will refer to this procedure as *in vivo* intrauterine fertilization, which obviously does not require subsequent embryo transfer.

In this chapter, we will refer primarily to extracorporeal fertilization and embryo transfer to the oocyte's donor. This is the procedure that is most commonly used in humans. *In vivo* intrauterine fertilization has not been very successful in humans or other primates (1,2).

We will also describe, for the most part, the program at Norfolk, Virginia, which has been in existence since 1980, and use our data as a basis for discussion.

Historical Review

Physiologists have long been interested in the process of fertilization and embryo transfer. The first paper reporting success was published on April 27, 1890 after more than a half-century of unsuccessful and apparently unpublished trials (3). In the United States, McLaren and Biggers in 1958 and Chang in 1959 were the first to accomplish *in vivo* fertilization and embryo transfer successfully in mice and rabbits, respectively (4,5). In the following years, several different centers published their experience on *in vitro* fertilization of ovulated oocytes in rabbits, mice, and rats.

Veterinarians quickly saw the economic advantages of these techniques in improving the quantity and quality of cattle. They adopted the techniques of superovulation, *in vivo* fertilization, and surgical or nonsurgical embryo transfer.

In 1965 and 1966, Edwards was the first to try to fertilize human oocytes in the laboratory (6,7). He published the first success in 1970 (8) and other reports soon followed (9,10). Immediately thereafter, embryo transfer was begun and the first successful term infant was born in England on July 25, 1978 (11). A second child was born January 14, 1979. In Australia, the first baby conceived with this procedure was born June 23, 1980 (12). The department of obstetrics and gynecology at Eastern Virginia Medical School was the first to start such a program in the United States and planning was begun in September 1978. By January 1980 the protocol was approved and the certificate of need granted. Our clinical efforts began in

March 1980 and the first pregnancy was announced May 11, 1981. Several months later, a second pregnancy was achieved. The first baby was born at Norfolk General Hospital by Cesarean section on December 28, 1981.

Several other groups in the United States, Europe, Australia, and, most recently, South America have established programs of *in vitro* fertilization.

In addition to surmounting intractable problems of infertility, programs of *in vitro* fertilization have contributed much to our knowledge of reproductive physiology. Our understanding of the process of oocyte maturation, function of the ovarian follicle, the follicular microenvironment, fertilization, sperm physiology, oocyte-sperm interaction, and early embryo development have all been enhanced.

Indications

Women with gamete transport problems are the first and most common group for whom *in vitro* fertilization is indicated. Initially, *in vitro* fertilization was considered to be complementary to reconstructive surgery of the fallopian tube. However, the results of certain types of tubal procedures have not improved. For example, term pregnancy rates are only 14.1% (13) to 36% (14) in women who undergo a salpingostomy. Second attempts at tubal surgery seldom result in a pregnancy rate greater than 10% (15). *In vitro* fertilization may, therefore, supplant tubal surgery provided success rates continue to improve and exceed those of reconstructive surgery (see Results). *In vitro* fertilization offers the only chance of pregnancy when both tubes have been removed.

The presence of a male factor is the second indication. *In vitro* fertilization offers hope of pregnancy when women are married to men with severe oligospermia, azoospermia, or nonmotile sperm for which no medical or surgical therapy is available. Although the number of sperm necessary for *in vitro* fertilization of the human oocyte is unknown, most groups are achieving success with progressively fewer sperm. Fewer than 100,000 sperm per oocyte may be sufficient and conception has occurred with even fewer sperm. Factors that control the fertilizing capacity of sperm from oligospermic men are being identified and knowledge of these should improve the results of *in vitro* fertilization. It may be possible to correlate sperm attachment to the oocyte and tests of sperm penetration capacity (e.g., zona-free hamster test, human nonviable oocyte penetration test) with the results of *in vitro* fertilization using human gametes.

Unexplained infertility, which occurs in 10% to 20% of all infertile couples (16), is the third indication for extracorporeal fertilization and embryo transfer. In some of these couples, egg-sperm interaction or embryo development and cell division may be impaired (17). In others, there may be an immunologic impediment that results in interference of egg-sperm interaction and fertilization. *In vitro* fertilization may not only be a diagnostic tool in these couples, but may be therapeutic as well.

Women with an intractable cervical factor or an antibody to sperm in the cervical mucus (see Chapter 7), endometriosis with distortion and impairment of the pelvic peritoneum and cul-de-sac, mild endometriosis that has not responded to conventional medical or surgical therapy, or those who failed to conceive with artificial insemination may also benefit from extracorporeal fertilization and embryo transfer.

Patient Selection and Preparation

All previous medical records of the couple are reviewed and they are then assigned to 1 of 3 groups: infertility of tubal, male, or undetermined origin. Each couple is then given a brochure specific for each group. The brochure gives the couple a detailed description of the procedure, techniques, diagnostic tests to be performed, and costs.

The couple is then interviewed. A complete medical history is obtained from each, previous records are again reviewed, and their questions are answered.

A "screening" laparoscopy is performed when the indication for *in vitro* fertilization is the presence of a tubal factor. We do this to assess the actual anatomic conditions of the pelvic cavity and the availability of at least 1 ovary for oocyte retrieval. Only if the results of this laparoscopy suggest a reasonable chance of success is this couple accepted into the program.

We do not perform a screening laparoscopy when a male factor is present and the wife has no history of pelvic pathology or prior abdominal or pelvic surgery. We do obtain a semen analysis, search for an immunologic factor, obtain bacteriologic cultures of the seminal plasma, separate and recover the motile sperm fraction, artificially stimulate sperm motility, and perform a zona-free hamster egg and a human nonviable oocyte penetration test.

Evaluation of the woman includes a general physical and pelvic examination. The uterus is sounded and the results recorded as this information is extremely useful at the time of embryo transfer. Routine laboratory screening tests are also performed. Special laboratory tests are obtained only if indicated from the medical history.

Until the present we have accepted only couples when the woman was younger than 35 years. However, some women up to the age of 40 years may benefit from extracorporeal fertilization. Only stable, married couples in whom conventional methods of treatment have failed are accepted. After a couple is accepted, we again discuss all aspects of the program with them and obtain a written consent to proceed.

Human Menstrual Cycle (Natural Cycle for Oocyte Retrieval)

After several years of pioneering work, Steptoe and Edwards concluded that the natural menstrual cycle afforded the best opportunity to achieve a successful pregnancy since the first baby was born from an oocyte recovered several minutes before spontaneous ovulation in an unstimulated menstrual cycle (18). The group in Australia reached the same conclusion. Detection of impending ovulation depends upon detection of the LH (luteinizing hormone) surge with an assay of urinary LH excretion or serum LH concentration. We monitor the 2 menstrual cycles immediately preceding the one in which oocyte retrieval will be attempted (19). To pinpoint the time of ovulation, we obtain the following each day of the cycle:

1. A maturation index from the lateral vaginal walls (to measure the percent of pyknotic cells).
2. Cervical mucus to identify the day on which the volume is greater than 0.2 cc, the spinnbarkeit is more than 10 cm, and ferning is 4+.
3. Pelvic ultrasound to measure follicular diameter.
4. Serum concentrations of estradiol and LH.

When the results of these suggest that ovulation is close, we then measure serum LH concentrations every 4 hours to detect the LH surge. The peak in serum estradiol concentration is not a good predictor since it may occur just prior to the LH surge or as early as 72 hours before.

Laparoscopy and oocyte retrieval are performed 28.5 hours after the woman's LH concentration enters the ascending limb of the midcycle surge (Fig. 13–1). The ascending limb of her LH surge is defined as a continuously increasing concentration over 60 mIU/ml. Measurement of follicular diameter is a useful, though not infallible, adjunct to serial LH determinations. Oocytes can be obtained from follicles with a diameter of 18 mm to 25 mm (Fig. 13–2).

Based on the results of these clinical, hormonal, and ultrasonic studies, we performed 41 timed laparoscopies. Twenty-one preovulatory oocytes were recovered, but in 9 a fresh corpus luteum was found. Two women had ovarian cysts that were mistaken for dominant follicles. There were 9 technical failures. The finding of a corpus luteum was the consequence, in part, of not monitoring the 2 previous menstrual cycles and of estimating the time of ovulation from the peak concentration of LH rather than from the ascending limb of the LH surge.

Serum progesterone concentrations were important for retrospective analysis of the cycles of women in whom a corpus luteum was found or to reassure ourselves that the aspiration failure resulted from technical problems rather than from improper monitoring of the spontaneous menstrual cycle. Unfortunately, the progesterone radioimmunoassay is not rapid enough to allow the results to be used to predict ovulation. Stress caused some women to have a delay of ovulation and some women failed to ovulate in the cycle of oocyte retrieval. The presence of only 1 available follicle reduced the chances of obtaining a preovulatory oocyte. This was a special problem in those

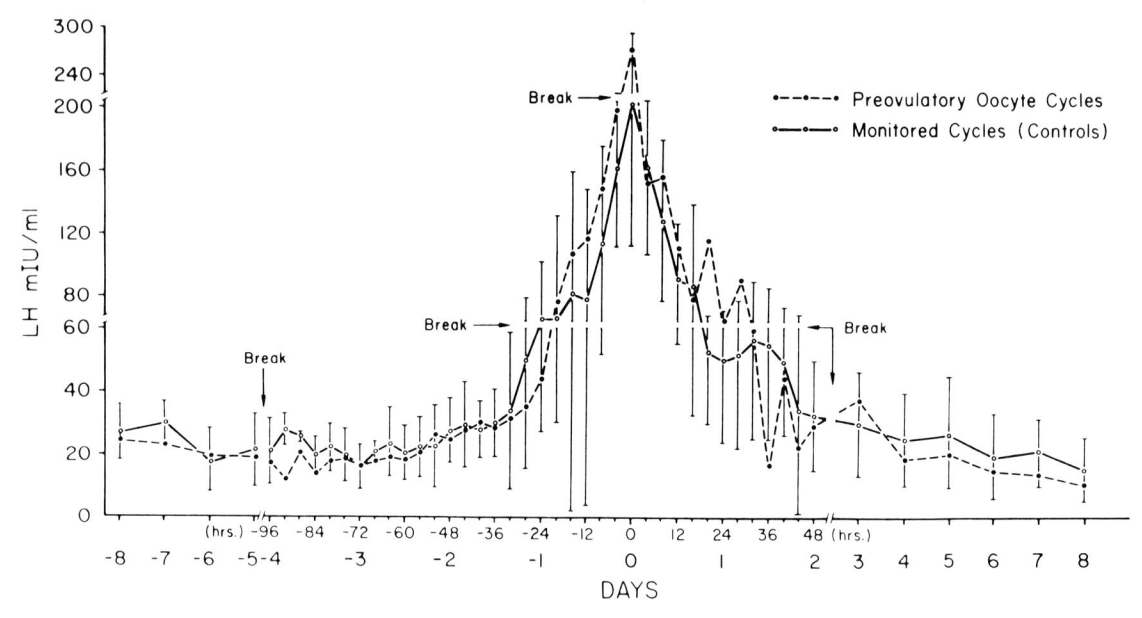

Daily Serum LH Values in 50 Menstrual Cycles from 28 Normal Women

Fig. 13–1. Daily and every 4-hour serum LH levels from day −8 to day +8 from the LH peak in 50 natural menstrual cycles. Solid line = control subjects (mean and SD); broken line = preovulatory oocyte group. Notice the true ascending limb of LH above 60 mIU/ml.

women who had already ovulated and had a corpus luteum. The need to monitor 2 previous menstrual cycles to provide a baseline is cumbersome and expensive. As noted above, we were able to retrieve an oocyte in only 50% of women during a spontaneous menstrual cycle. All of these make the spontaneous menstrual cycle less than ideal for *in vitro* fertilization.

Ovulation Induction

Since January 1981, we have induced ovulation with human menopausal gonadotropin

- ⓐ Preovulatory Oocyte : 17
- ↓ Corpus Luteum : 9
- ⓐ↓ Corpus Luteum & Preovulatory Oocyte : 4
- ⊗ Oocyte Retrieval Failure : 8
- ○ Immature Oocyte : 1
- ⓘ Cyst : 2

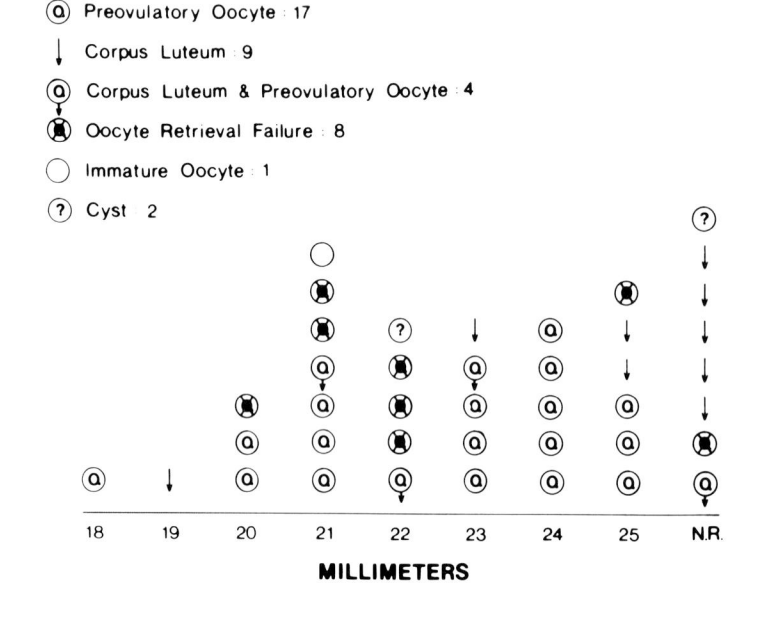

Fig. 13–2. Follicle diameter determined by ultrasound in 41 cycles in which oocyte aspiration was attempted. Preovulatory oocytes could be obtained from 18-mm to 25-mm follicles. Small ovarian cysts can be misinterpreted as a follicle. Preovulatory oocytes have been recovered from the cul-de-sac if ovulation had already occurred. N.R. = not reliable.

(hMG) and chorionic gonadotropin (hCG). HMG injections are begun on the third or fifth day of a 28- or 35-day menstrual cycle (20,21). Serum concentrations of estradiol are determined daily from the start of hMG therapy. The maturation index, characteristics of cervical mucus, dilatation of the external cervical os, and follicular diameter measured by ultrasound are observed beginning on the sixth day of the menstrual cycle. In general, hMG is continued until the clinical indices suggest impending ovulation and the serum estradiol concentration is 300 to 600 pg/ml. Clinical indices for impending ovulation were described in the discussion of the spontaneous menstrual cycle. Ultrasound was helpful in determining the number and size of preovulatory follicles, to ensure that the follicle(s) were developing on the side of an accessible ovary, and to ascertain that no ovarian cysts were developing.

The estradiol concentration in response to hMG differed in these women and we were able to define 3 groups based on the response. One group of women had a diminished response to hMG and we continued gonadotropin therapy until their serum estradiol concentrations reached 300 pg/ml and their clinical indices suggested an adequate estrogenic response. The second group of women responded to hMG with an increase in estradiol to concentrations between 300 pg/ml and 600 pg/ml, but their clinical indices lagged. In this group, hMG was decreased to 1 ampule per day and continued until their clinical indices suggested an adequate estrogenic response. The third group of women was defined by the presence of a serum estradiol concentration of 600 pg/ml and hMG was stopped once these women reached this level unless a reliable ultrasound revealed no follicles greater than 1 cm in diameter. Each woman tended to respond to hMG in a similar fashion in subsequent cycles. This made it somewhat easier to adjust the dosage of hMG since the response was more predictable.

HCG (10,000 units) is administered about 50 hours after the last injection of hMG. Laparoscopy and oocyte retrieval is then performed 34 hours after the injection of hCG.

Immature or degenerated oocytes are often recovered with preovulatory oocytes. Usually, smaller follicles yield an abnormal oocyte, while larger follicles more often yield healthy oocytes. Follicular diameter is frequently less in hMG-stimulated cycles than in spontaneous or clomiphene-induced cycles (19,22). The mean diameter of preovulatory follicles after hMG stimulation is 16.3 mm (23). Because smaller follicles may yield a healthy, preovulatory oocyte and a larger follicle produce a degenerated oocyte, all follicles visualized at laparoscopy are aspirated. An average of 2.85 oocytes are recovered from each woman after hMG and hCG stimulation. In 80% of women, follicles develop in both ovaries, although 1 ovary always contains a dominant follicle. Thus far, no woman has developed the hyperstimulation syndrome (see Chapter 6).

Other groups performing *in vitro* fertilization induce ovulation with clomiphene and their success rates are comparable to ours. However, the rate of spontaneous abortion appears to be higher in clomiphene-induced cycles. This may be due to a higher frequency of luteal phase defects in these cycles.

Oocyte Retrieval and Aspiration Device

Laparoscopy is done as outpatient surgery at the determined time under balanced general endotracheal anesthesia. The ideal anesthetic for oocyte retrieval should accomplish the following (24):

1. Cause no oocyte toxicity.
2. Have no effect on gonadotropic hormone concentrations.
3. Minimize the stress of the laparoscopy.
4. Provide abdominal muscle relaxation.
5. Allow a rapid recovery.
6. Have no effects that may develop with repeated administration.
7. Be comfortable for the woman and cause minimal side effects.
8. Be a standardized technique that is easy to administer.

Balanced general endotracheal anaesthesia fulfills most of these criteria and we use an anticholinergic, fentanyl, sodium pentothal, succinylcholine for intubation, nitrous oxide and oxygen, and a succinylcholine drip for intraoperative muscle relaxation.

The laparoscopy is performed in a routine fashion except that no vaginal, cervical, or uterine instruments to manipulate the uterus are used. Visualization and follicular aspiration are performed using a standard 10-mm Wolff operating laparoscope with a 5-mm probe channel and 180° viewing angle. A 6-mm plastic sleeve with trocar is inserted through a second incision in the suprapubic area. A Semm-type atraumatic grasping forceps is used for intraabdominal maneuvers. Other centers use a third trocar to pass the needle for oocyte retrieval.

Carbon dioxide (CO_2) is instilled into the peritoneal cavity until the intraabdominal pressure is 12 mm of mercury. Three liters are usually sufficient. Although CO_2 may change the pH of the aspirated follicular fluid, little or none enters the fluid and no changes in pH have occurred. If ovulation has already occurred and it is necessary to retrieve the oocyte(s) from the cul-de-sac, it should be done at the beginning of the procedure to minimize CO_2-induced changes in peritoneal fluid pH.

Once the laparoscope is in place, inspection of the pelvic cavity is rapid since the women have either had a screening laparoscopy or have no pelvic pathology to delay oocyte retrieval. Also, inspection is rapid because the size, location, and number of follicles are known from the ultrasound exams performed during hMG stimulation.

The procedure is viewed on a television monitor and videotaped with a Circon® color microvideo camera. The camera attaches easily to the laparoscope and all is ready for oocyte retrieval very quickly.

After placing the woman in the Trendelenburg position (20° to 25°), the ovary containing the dominant follicle is inspected first and stabilized with the grasping forceps. All instruments, containers, and fluids that will be used during the procedure have been kept at 37°C in an incubator and are transferred to the surgical instrument table and maintained at the same temperature with a heating pad. The aspiration now begins.

The aspiration device is illustrated in Fig. 13–3 (25). A 12-gauge (2.16 mm, internal diameter) stainless steel needle (43 cm long) is passed through the operating channel of the laparoscope. The tip of the needle has a 45° bevel and a relatively blunt end. These features help to minimize damage to the oocyte-cumulus oophorous complex at the time of aspiration. A raised sleeve is present 5 mm behind the tip of the needle. This is useful to indicate the depth of penetration into the follicle and to seal the puncture site at the time of aspiration and irrigation. The hub of the needle has one flat surface to indicate the direction of the bevel. Each needle is identified by num-

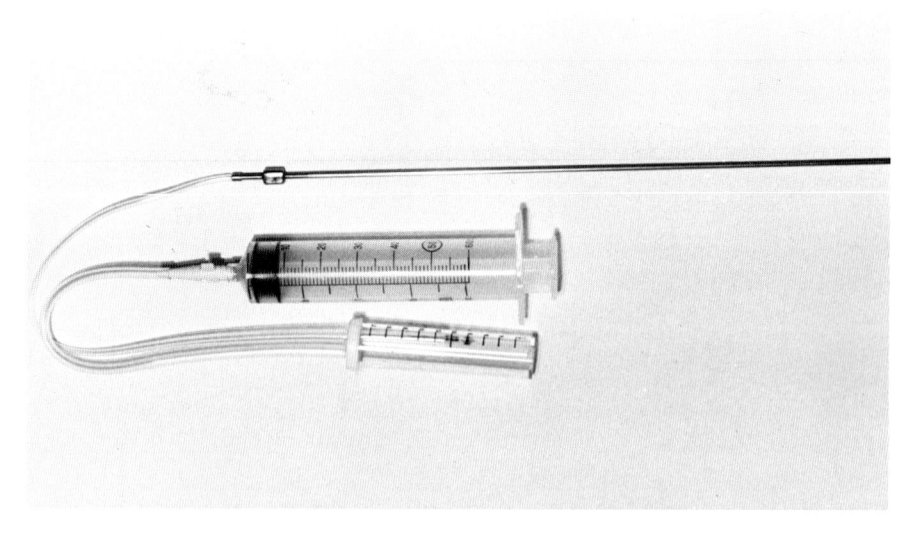

Fig. 13–3. Aspiration device. This equipment is commercially available. Only the needle has been specially designed and made. Manual aspiration provides suitable suction pressure at the proper time, thus preventing CO_2 from entering the system.

ber. A 16-gauge needle is also available when a smaller needle is required. The needle is attached to plastic tubing (No. 10 French, 37.5 mm long) and the plastic tubing to a DeLee suction catheter with a mucous trap. There are no other connections that, if present, might trap the oocyte. The DeLee trap, with a 20-cc capacity, is connected to a 60-cc syringe via a second plastic tube, 25.5 cm long. The total dead space of the system is 4 cc from the tip of the needle to the trap.

Two milliliters of Dulbecco's phosphate buffer are aspirated into the trap. This washes the needle and tubing and assures an appropriate pH for the follicular fluid and oocyte-cumulus complex. The needle is then inserted into the selected follicle (Fig. 13–4). Negative pressure is applied to the syringe (190 mm Hg) and the follicular fluid is aspirated into the DeLee trap. After the follicle collapses, the needle is withdrawn and another 2 cc of buffer are aspirated into the trap. The appearance of the punctured follicle and the follicular fluid is recorded and the trap containing the fluid is taken to the adjacent laboratory. The follicle is then irrigated with 4 cc or 8 cc of buffer that contains a heparin concentration of 10 units per cc buffer. The volume of buffer used depends on the size of the follicle and the amount of fluid obtained. The irrigation system consists of an identical needle that is, however, attached to a 60-cc syringe and tubing without a trap. Through the initial puncture site the follicle is distended and irrigated once or twice with 4 cc of buffer, which is then aspirated into the syringe. Another 4 cc of Dulbecco's buffer are then used to wash the needle and tubing. This fluid is also sent to the laboratory.

In the laboratory, the appearance of the fluid and the granulosa cells is assessed and the results reported immediately to the surgeons. If an adequate number of preovulatory oocytes has been recovered, the laparoscopy is ended. If not, additional follicles are punctured—even those that appear as immature oocytes since they can mature and be fertilized *in vitro*.

Other centers use different procedures. Some use a 2-channel needle and the diameter of the needle varies from 0.9 mm to 2.2 mm. Some prefer needles coated with Teflon on the inner surface. Suction varies from 20 mm Hg to 200 mm Hg and is applied by hand or with wall suction. Some prefer a mixture of nitrous oxide, oxygen, and carbon dioxide for the pneumoperitoneum. Thus, the procedure is not standardized and optimal conditions have not been determined in a systematic fashion.

The rate of recovery of preovulatory oocytes is 50% to 100% per follicle and 58% to 91% per cycle for most groups.

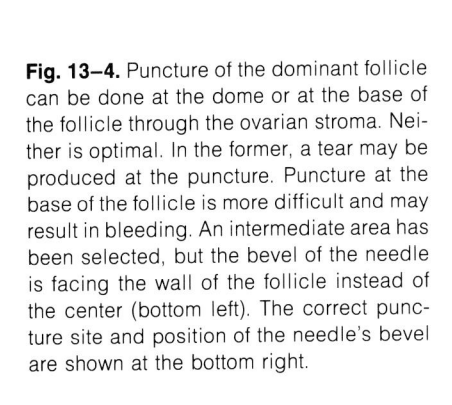

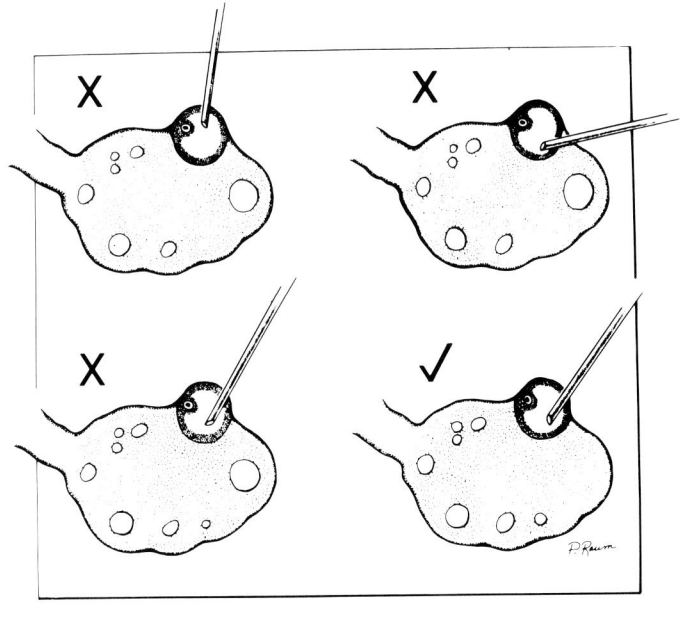

Fig. 13–4. Puncture of the dominant follicle can be done at the dome or at the base of the follicle through the ovarian stroma. Neither is optimal. In the former, a tear may be produced at the puncture. Puncture at the base of the follicle is more difficult and may result in bleeding. An intermediate area has been selected, but the bevel of the needle is facing the wall of the follicle instead of the center (bottom left). The correct puncture site and position of the needle's bevel are shown at the bottom right.

Evaluation of Follicular Fluid, Granulosa Cells, and Oocytes at the Time of Retrieval

Pure follicular fluid is straw-colored. Occasionally it has an amber appearance and is blood tinged; this may be an early sign of postmaturity. The volume of follicular fluid increases as the size of the follicle increases, although the pH of the fluid is always between 7.2 and 7.4.

To facilitate rapid identification of any oocyte, the follicular fluid in buffer is poured into several Petri dishes and the contents of each is inspected with a dissecting or inverted microscope. The stage of oocyte maturation is based upon the presence of the extracoronal mass of cumulus cells, morphology of the coronal cells, the appearance of the ooplasm, and the morphology of the granulosa cells. If all these are present and appear normal, the oocyte is mature and preovulatory (Fig. 13–5). The presence of a polar body is a good indicator of a mature oocyte but it is often difficult to find. If the cumulus has not developed and consists only of a compact layer of cells adherent to the zona pellucida and immature granulosa cells are present, the oocyte-cumulus complex is immature (Fig. 13–6). The oocyte may be so immature that a germinal vesicle is present. Atretic or degenerated oocytes have a contracted, misshapen, and dark ooplasm and the cumulus is absent (Fig. 13–7).

Many granulosa cells are obtained with the oocyte. The number varies with the vigor of the aspiration and the number of follicular irrigations. Immature granulosa cells from small follicles are small, compact, have a scant cytoplasm, and a tendency to be shed in sheets or clumps. In contrast, mature granulosa cells are not clumped and are larger because of the increased quantity of glycosaminoglycans induced by the midcycle surge of FSH. Mature granulosa cells also exhibit some degree of luteinization, which is identified by the presence of an increased amount of cytoplasm.

The hormonal milieu of the follicular fluid depends on the extent of granulosa cell maturation and follicular size. Mature follicles have

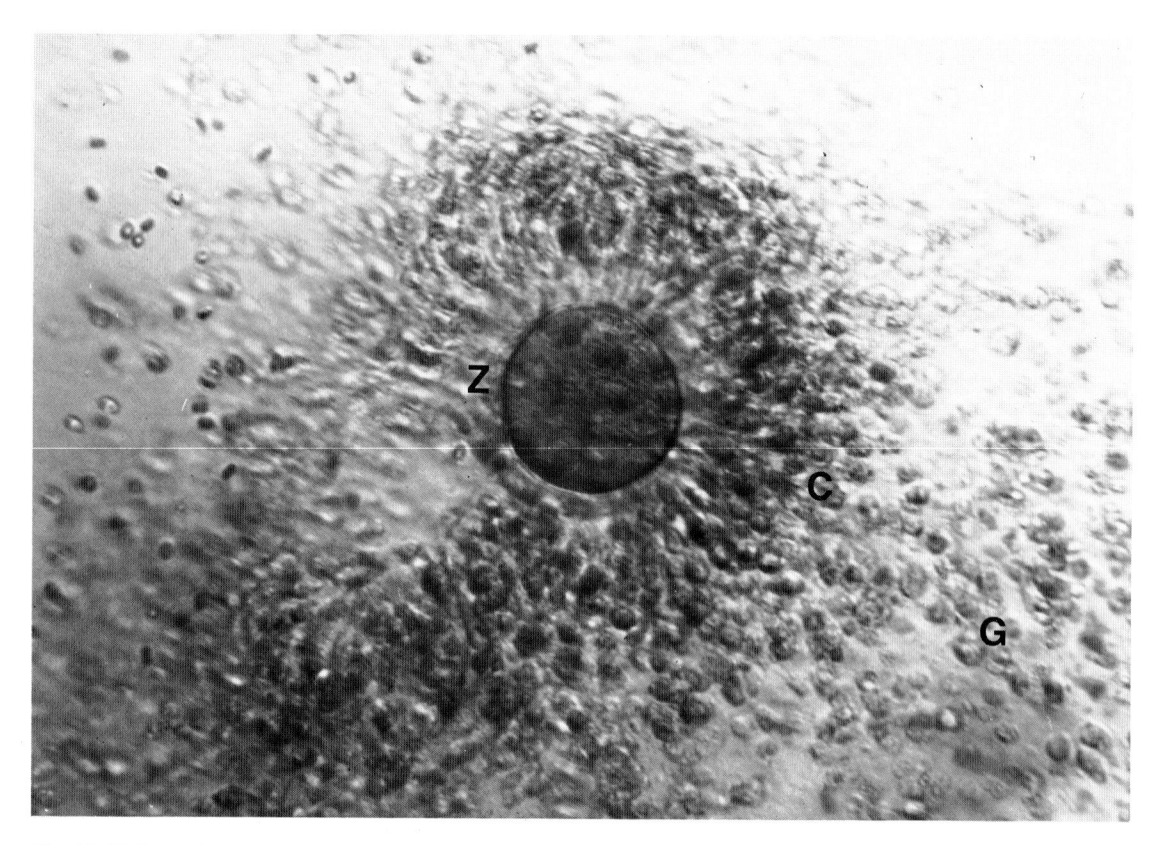

Fig. 13–5. Preovulatory oocyte. Photomicrograph (100×) that also shows the corona radiata (C), granulosa cells (G), the vitelline membrane and the zona pellucida (Z). The polar body is not seen.

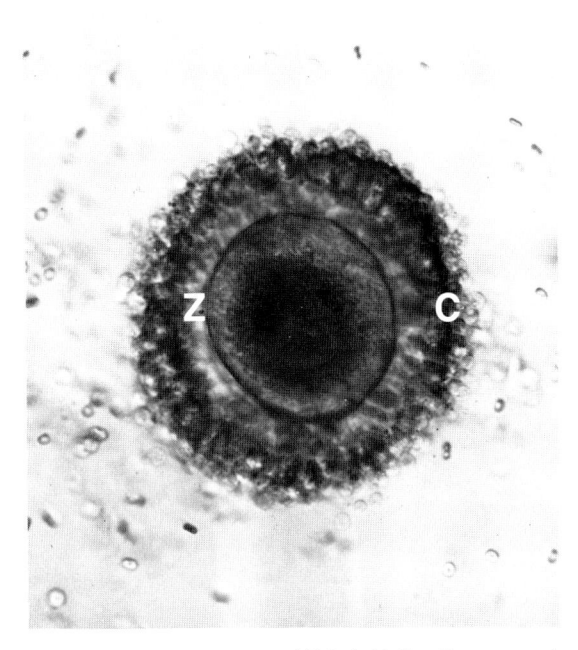

Fig. 13-6. Immature oocyte (100×). Notice the compactness of the cumulus around the zona pellucida.

high concentrations of estradiol, FSH, LH, and progesterone but a low concentration of androstenedione. Androstenedione is the predominant steroid in follicular fluid of imma-

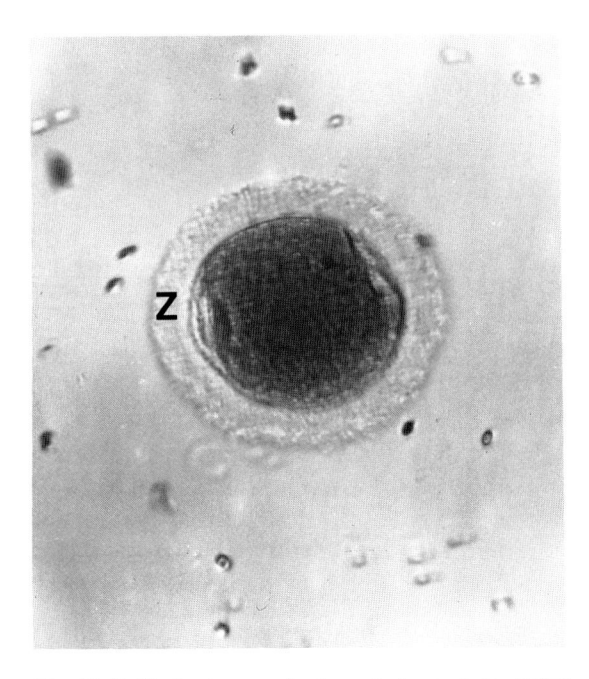

Fig. 13-7. Photomicrograph of an atretic or degenerated oocyte (100×). The zona pellucida has no surrounding cumulus cells.

ture or degenerated follicles (26). Thus, an estrogenic environment correlates with the presence of a mature follicle and such an environment may be necessary for follicular maturation.

In Vitro Fertilization

In vitro fertilization and cleavage is carried out in Ham's F-10 culture medium supplemented with human fetal cord serum. The technique involves (a) preincubation of the oocyte, (b) preparation of the sperm, (c) fertilization, and (d) cleavage (27).

PREINCUBATION OF THE OOCYTE. Once the oocyte has been identified and isolated from the follicular fluid, it is placed in a Falcon No. 3037 organ culture dish containing 3 ml of culture (insemination) medium. This medium is supplemented with 7.5% fetal serum. The preincubation is carried out in an incubator in an atmosphere of 5% CO_2 in air. The humidity of the incubator is 97% to 98% and the temperature is 37°C. As indicated by the extrusion of the first polar body, a preincubation time of 6 to 8 hours (preovulatory oocyte), or about 26 hours (immature oocyte), seems to be optimal.

PREPARATION OF SPERM. A semen sample is obtained 2 hours before the insemination. The husband is requested to observe a 3- to 5-day period of sexual abstinence. The semen sample is collected by masturbation into a sterile polypropylene container. After liquefying at room temperature, a semen analysis is done. Two milliliters of semen are diluted with 2 ml of insemination medium, mixed, and centrifuged (427 × g for 10 minutes). The supernatant is discarded and the pellet containing the sperm is mixed, diluted in medium, and centrifuged twice more. The pellet containing the sperm is then resuspended in 1 ml of insemination medium. The sperm are incubated for 30 minutes in an atmosphere of 5% CO_2. The supernatant containing the motile fraction of sperm is removed and the sperm concentration and motility determined. The oocyte is then inseminated with 1.5 million sperm in 3 ml of insemination medium.

FERTILIZATION. After 12 to 16 hours the oocyte is transferred to growth medium (Ham's F-10 supplemented with 15% fetal cord serum). This medium was prepared at the same time as the insemination medium and incubated overnight. The oocyte is examined for evidence of pronuclear formation after it is transferred to this medium. Occasionally, the oocyte is surrounded by cells that should have been removed or dispersed by the sperm. These cells are mechanically removed at this stage to ensure that fertilization has occurred and polyspermia has not.

CLEAVAGE. After the pronuclear stage has been confirmed, the fertilized oocyte is returned to the incubator to allow cleavage to occur. Forty to 44 hours after insemination, the zygote is inspected. If cell division has occurred normally and the conceptus is 2 to 6 cells (Fig. 13–8), it is now transferred to the woman's endometrial cavity.

Embryo Transfer

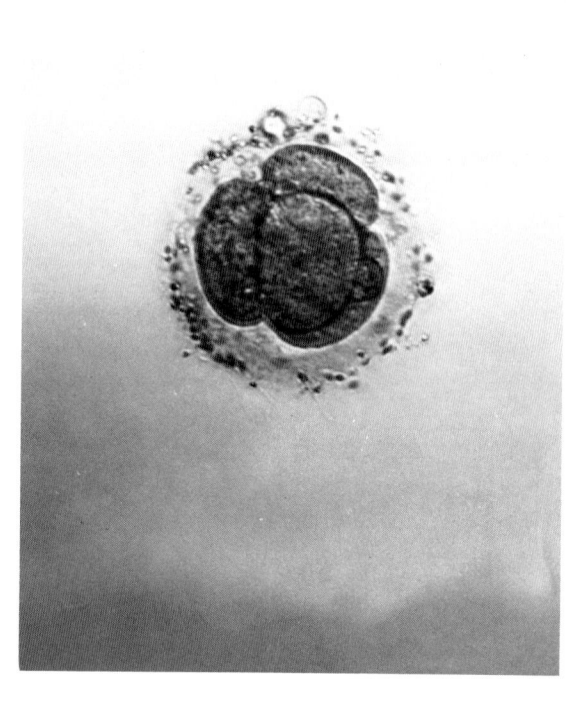

Fig. 13–8. Four-cell embryo prior to transfer. The cumulus mass has been dispersed. There are still some spermatozoa attached to the zona pellucida.

Embryo transfer after *in vivo* fertilization of livestock is very successful. With human extracorporeal fertilization, embryo transfer is the least successful step of the entire procedure.

Implantation depends on 2 factors: the quality of the conceptus and the adequacy of the endometrial environment. Both of these are extremely difficult to evaluate. Morphologic appearance of the conceptus is not a good criterion since healthy-looking embryos may not implant and those that appear less healthy may result in a normal pregnancy and fetus. The uterine environment cannot be investigated directly in the cycle of transfer since damage to the endometrium may otherwise occur. It is necessary to rely on indirect evidence that the endometrial environment is normal (e.g., progesterone and estradiol concentrations).

Embryo transfer can be done very early in development: shortly after fertilization and pronuclear formation, in the 2-cell stage, or even in the 4- to 8-cell stage. The last is the most frequently used stage for transfer by the existing programs.

A very early transfer has the theoretical advantage of shortening the culture period and of returning the embryo to a more natural environment (the uterine cavity) much earlier. However, there is no way to judge subsequent development when a very young embryo is transferred and the quality of the laboratory technique cannot be assessed by observing division into later stages.

Late transfer allows more active control of embryo development and cleavage, and the embryo is transferred to the endometrial cavity closer to the time when a conceptus normally reaches it. Late transfer is more successful.

The time of transfer is determined by the characteristics of the oocytes obtained. Transfer is done 44 to 46 hours after insemination (4- to 6-cell stage) when only preovulatory oocytes are obtained. A longer incubation period before transfer is necessary when only immature oocytes are obtained. When a combination of immature and preovulatory oocytes are obtained, the transfer time has to be delayed to allow the immature ones to be fertilized and start cell division without delaying so long that the more developed concepti are jeopardized.

At the chosen time, the woman returns to the operating room (adjacent to the laboratory). Knowledge of the size and position of her uterus and cervical canal (from the uterine sounding done at the first visit) is extremely helpful at the time of transfer. Discomfort to the woman and damage to her endocervix or endometrium are lessened.

The transfer apparatus (Fig. 13–9) consists of a 31-cm metal cannula with an internal and external diameter of 1.6 mm and 1.9 mm, respectively. The cannula curves gently to follow the curvature of the endocervical canal and endometrial cavity. A 46-cm Teflon catheter with an internal diameter of 1.2 mm has been designed to pass through the metal cannula. A piece of tape is put on the catheter 39 cm from its distal end. When the tape on the catheter reaches the proximal end of the metal cannula, there is 7 cm of catheter protruding from the other end of the cannula. If the catheter is advanced slowly and gently into the uterine cavity, resistance is encountered when the tip reaches the uterine fundus. The tip of the catheter is solid, round, and slightly narrower than the proximal end; this facilitates passage through the cervix. Four millimeters proximal to the tip there is a 1.2-mm notch in the side of the catheter through which the embryo(s) are first aspirated and then ejected into the uterine cavity.

A tuberculin syringe attached to the proximal end of the catheter is used to draw the embryo(s) into the catheter. Drawn into the catheter in succession are:

1. 0.03 ml of culture medium.
2. 0.02 ml of air.
3. 0.03 ml of culture medium containing the embryo(s).
4. 0.02 ml of air.
5. 0.03 ml of culture medium.

The embryo lies between layers of air and culture medium. If there is a change in surface tension when the catheter is inserted through the cervical mucus, the first drop of medium and the air space protect the embryo. If several embryos are being transferred, they are loaded and transferred together in the manner described, without an increase in media volume.

The woman is put in the knee-chest position if her uterus is anteverted or the dorsal lithotomy position if her uterus is retroverted. The cervix is visualized by placing a speculum into the vagina, then cleansed with a dry cotton applicator and grasped with a tenaculum. A tenaculum is used only if the cervical canal is difficult to sound.

The loaded transfer apparatus, protected by a sterile cover, is brought to the operating room from the adjacent laboratory. The tip of the metal cannula is placed at the lower one third of the cervical canal and the catheter is

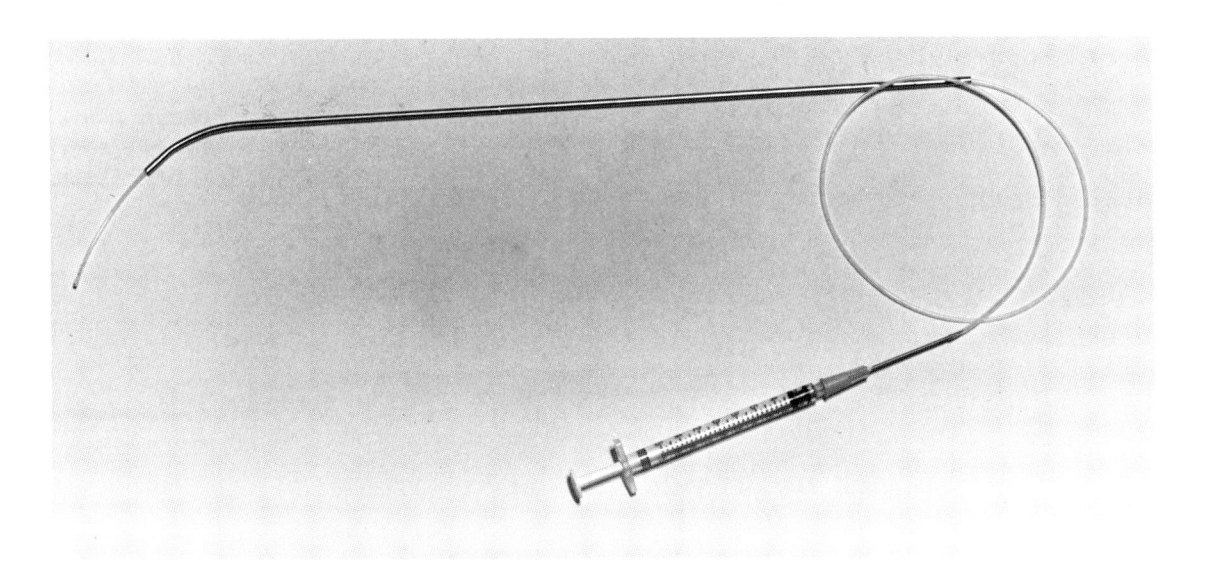

Fig. 13–9. Transfer device. The metal cannula (guide) and the Teflon catheter used in embryo transfers are shown. The tuberculin syringe attached to the proximal end of the Teflon catheter is used for both loading and ejecting the conceptus.

then passed through the cannula and the internal os into the uterine cavity until it reaches the fundus. The catheter is then withdrawn 2 mm to 3 mm and the contents of the catheter are injected. A small volume of air is used to flush the catheter, which is then rotated gently to ensure disengagement of the embryo. The catheter is then withdrawn, taken to the laboratory, and flushed with fluid. This fluid and the catheter are examined microscopically to be certain that the embryo has been expelled into the uterus.

After removing the cannula and speculum, the woman is put into the prone or supine position (depending upon the position used for embryo transfer) and kept in that position for 4 hours. She is then allowed to go home and is advised to remain in the same position until the next morning. During the 24 hours preceding and following the transfer, the woman receives 250 mg of tetracycline every 4 hours.

With this technique, the transfer proceeds smoothly and has never had to be stopped because of complications or inability to pass the catheter into the uterine cavity.

Results

Human reproduction is rather ineffective. Only 25% of women conceive each cycle and 50% of these conceptions eventuate in expulsion of the embryo by the expected time of menses. A positive radioimmunoassay of hCG is the only evidence of pregnancy (28). Such inefficiency may result from problems related to the oocyte, the sperm, the embryo, or the endometrium. Only 84% of all ovulated oocytes will be fertilized and only one third of these will result in a term pregnancy.

In vitro fertilization magnifies the inefficiency of human reproduction. The ultimate success rate with this procedure is 11% to 26% in the established programs. In our program, no pregnancies occurred in 41 women when oocytes were obtained from natural cycles, despite proper monitoring and retrieval of normal-appearing oocytes (19). From January 1981 until September 1982, ovulation has been induced with hMG and hCG. Laparoscopies have been performed in 221 cycles. Fertilizable oocytes were recovered in 184 of these cycles (83%). Fertilization occurred with 164 oocytes (89%) and transfer of an embryo was accomplished in 152 cycles (69%). A pregnancy occurred in 38 cycles, or 17% of the number of laparoscopies, and 25% of the women who had an embryo transferred (Table 13–1).

Pregnancy has occurred after fertilization of either preovulatory or immature oocytes that were allowed to mature *in vitro*.

The success rate is directly related to the number of embryos transferred into the endometrial cavity (Table 13–2). The 38 pregnancies resulted from the transfer of a single embryo in 13 of 73 cycles (17.8%). In 55 cycles, 2 embryos were transferred and 15 conceptions resulted (27.2%). Conception occurred in 8 of 18 cycles when 3 embryos were transferred (44.2%), and in 2 of 6 cycles when 4 or more embryos were transferred. Although the transfer of multiple embryos appears to be more successful, only 2 sets of twins have been identified. Multiple pregnancy has not been a frequent occurrence in the other programs.

There are several factors that could account for the low pregnancy rate. The embryo might flow out of the uterus through a track in the endometrium made by the catheter. The transfer procedure might elicit uterine contractions. Mucus or blood carried into the uterus at the time of transfer might prevent implantation. The absence of a putative physiologic signal from the conceptus or endometrium may result in failure of implantation. Such a signal is hypothetical. Asynchrony between embry-

TABLE 13–1. Results of *In Vitro* Fertilization and Embryo Transfer*

	NUMBER	% OF A	% OF B	% OF C	% OF D
A. Laparoscopies	221	—	—	—	—
B. Fertilizable eggs	184	83	—	—	—
C. Eggs fertilized	164	74	89	—	—
D. Transfer	152	69	83	93	—
E. Pregnancies	38	17	21	23	25

* Norfolk, Virginia: 1/1/81 to 10/15/82 (series 1 to 6).

TABLE 13-2. Effect of the Number of Embryos Transferred on the Pregnancy Rate*

NUMBER OF EMBRYOS TRANSFERRED	NUMBER OF CYCLES	NUMBER OF PREGNANCIES	PERCENT PREGNANCIES
1	73	13	17.8†
2	55	15	27.2
3	18	8	44.8
4 or more	6	2	33.3
Total	152	38	

* Norfolk, Virginia: 1/1/81 to 10/15/82.
† Percent of cycles.

onic development and endometrial maturation impedes implantation in several species of mammals, although the importance of this has not been documented in humans. Successful pregnancy after transfer of embryos from 2 to 8 cells argues against the importance of embryo-endometrial synchrony.

Initially, the risk of ectopic pregnancy was considered to be nonexistent. However, 3 ectopic pregnancies have occurred in women conceiving with *in vitro* fertilization. These occurred in women who still had fallopian tubes.

Luteal Phase after Oocyte Retrieval

Although the quality of the embryo transferred is important in determining the success of *in vitro* fertilization, the environment in which it implants and develops must be equal in importance. It is unfortunate that Edwards and Steptoe attributed part of their early failure to delayed or suboptimal luteinization of a follicle as a result of gonadotropin induction of ovulation (18). Because of their early lack of success, they recommended the use of natural cycles for oocyte retrieval. Subsequent experience has yielded contrary results: gonadotropin-stimulated cycles are more successful.

The effect of oocyte aspiration on the subsequent luteal phase of natural or stimulated cycles is scant and, occasionally, contradictory (29). Kreitmenn has reported 2 types of luteal phase deficiency following aspiration of the dominant follicle of monkeys (30). The first was an early postaspiration deficiency of progesterone secretion and the second was a persistent deficiency of progesterone secretion throughout the entire luteal phase. Administration of hCG late in the luteal phase did not always correct the deficiency. The degree of corpus luteum deficiency seems to correlate with the number of granulosa cells aspirated with the oocyte. We have reported significant decreases in peripheral concentrations of progesterone and estrogen after follicular puncture and aspiration (29). This occurred primarily in the cycles in which the most vigorous aspiration of a follicle was performed. Progesterone supplementation can overcome this deficiency in steroid secretion, at least in natural cycles.

Krein and co-workers found no difference in peripheral venous steroid concentrations when they compared natural cycles of women undergoing oocyte aspiration with those who did not undergo aspiration (31). They did find that prolactin concentrations were increased significantly 30 minutes after induction of anesthesia and the increase persisted for 8 hours after laparoscopy. However, the stress of any surgical procedure causes similar increases in prolactin concentration. Increased prolactin concentrations may still be important in these women since hyperprolactinemia is a recognized cause of luteal phase deficiency. Others have also reported increased concentrations of prolactin on isolated days of the luteal phase, as well as a transient decrease in progesterone concentrations (32).

Feichtinger, however, found evidence of a luteal phase deficiency in only 2 of 32 women after laparoscopic retrieval of oocytes in natural cycles (33). The importance of a luteal phase deficiency and hyperprolactinemia in natural cycles after oocyte retrieval is arguable. Nontheless, it is clear that pregnancy rates after oocyte retrieval in natural cycles are low.

There is no evidence of a luteal phase deficiency in cycles stimulated with gonadotropins.

Rather, the corpora lutea from these cycles produce quantities of progesterone higher than normal (Fig. 13–10). Estradiol concentrations are also higher in these cycles (Fig. 13–11) (34). An occasional patient may still have a corpus luteum deficiency (35). Clomiphene also stimulates the secretion of estradiol and androstenedione (32). When hCG was also used, the increased concentrations of androstenedione were sustained longer. When studied, progesterone concentrations were also increased. Luteal phase deficiency is generally not observed in stimulated cycles. However, we routinely supplement the luteal phase with progesterone because of the occasional cycle with evidence of luteal phase deficiency.

Follow-up of Pregnancies

All women who have had an embryo transfer in our program receive 12.5 mg of progesterone in oil daily. The occurrence of a pregnancy is confirmed by a positive radioimmunoassay of the hCG beta subunit as early as the twelfth day after aspiration of the follicle. Once pregnancy is confirmed, the progesterone is stopped and 17-hydroxyprogesterone caproate (Delalutin®), 250 mg, is given intramuscularly each week. This is continued until the eighteenth week of pregnancy.

Prenatal care is given by the woman's own obstetrician. Estradiol, progesterone, and hCG concentrations were measured throughout pregnancy in the first few women to conceive. These were normal. Currently, we obtain the concentration of these 1 week after confirming the pregnancy and every 4 weeks until the eighteenth week. Realtime ultrasound is obtained by the tenth week of pregnancy to confirm the presence of a fetus.

One fetus conceived by *in vitro* fertilization had a trisomy and was aborted. One twin was born with a congenital cardiac malformation. No other chromosomal or congenital abnormalities have been reported. Unless subsequent experience discloses a higher rate of such abnormalities, we do not recommend am-

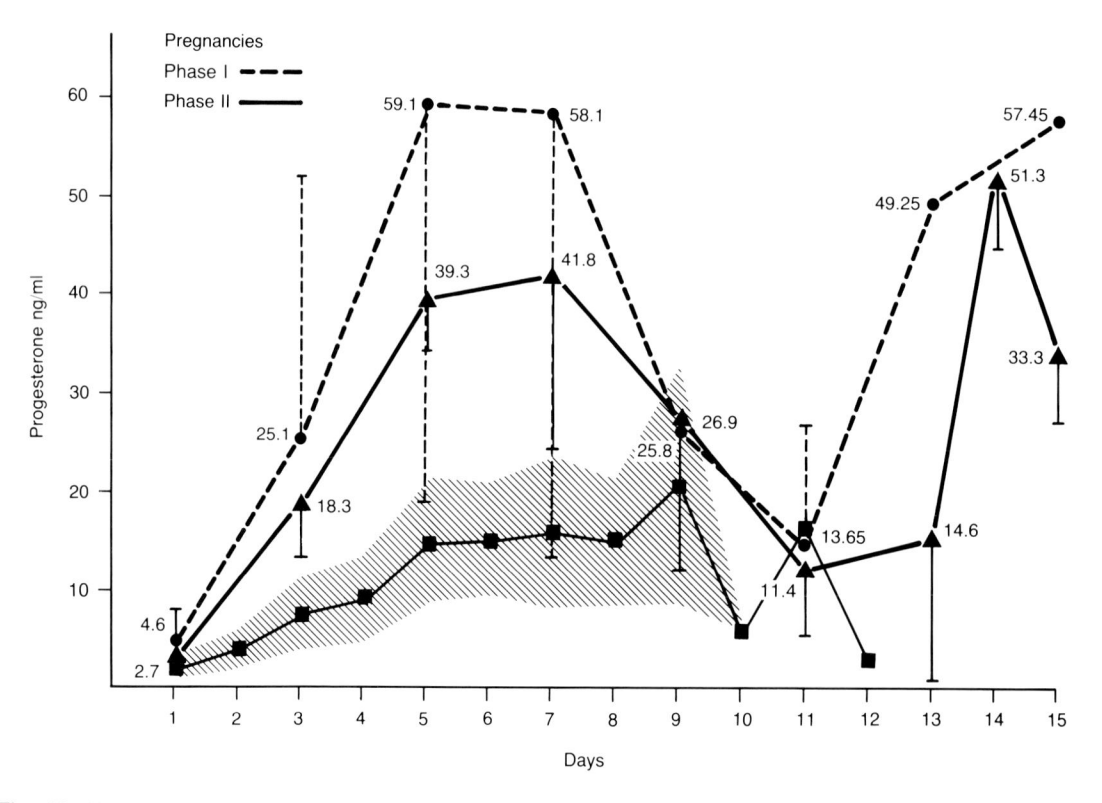

Fig. 13–10. Normal progesterone values in the luteal phase (mean and SD shaded area) are compared with progesterone values (mean and SD) in 2 different groups of women who had oocyte retrieval after ovulation induction using hMG and hCG. In the latter 2 groups, significantly increased progesterone values were found almost every day.

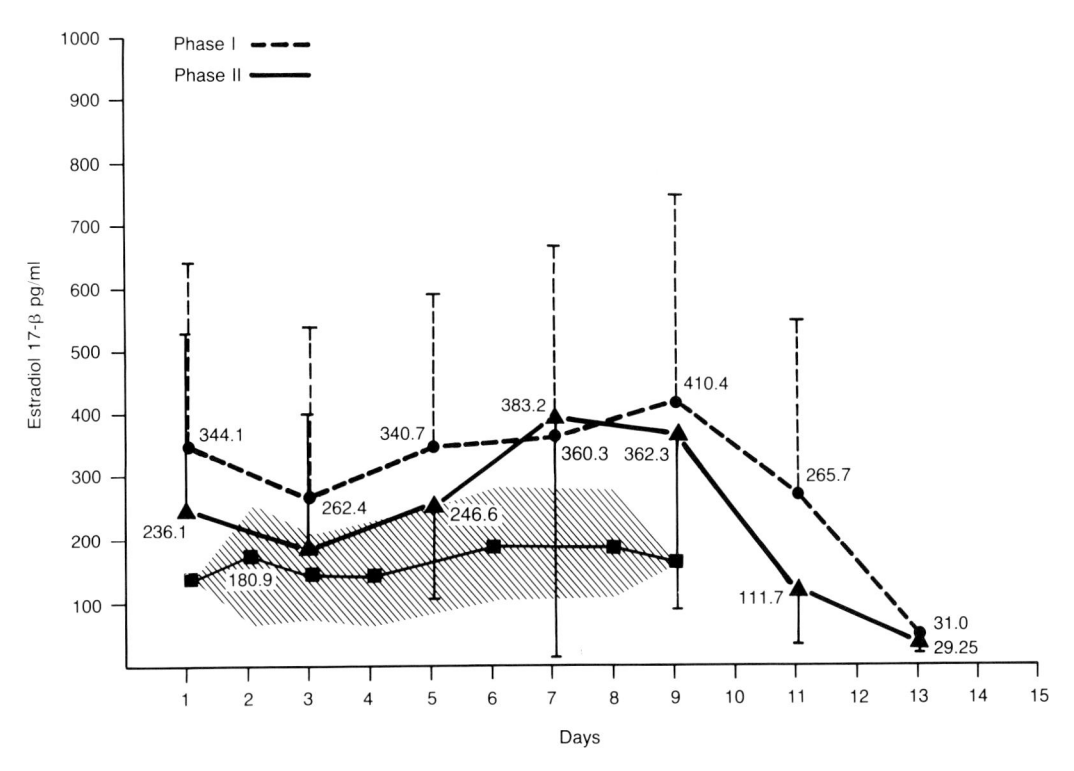

Fig. 13–11. Normal estrogen values in the luteal phase (mean and SD, shaded area) are compared with the same 2 groups shown in Figure 13–10. In neither group was there evidence of estradiol deficiency.

niocentesis if no other indication (e.g., maternal age) exists.

While the members of some programs recommend that delivery be by Cesarean section, we believe that a vaginal delivery should be attempted unless there is an obstetric contraindication. Ten infants have been born that were conceived in our program. Two have delivered vaginally. The other 8 were delivered by Cesarean section because of prematurity and severe preeclampsia (n = 1), advanced maternal age (n = 3), cephalopelvic disproportion (n = 2), or the presence of a uterine scar (n = 2). The cumulative experience is still insufficient to judge if pregnancy complications occur more frequently after *in vitro* fertilization. Since the oldest child was born in July 1978, it is too early to know if growth and development of these children will be normal.

REFERENCES

1. Craft I, McLeod F, Green S, et al. Human pregnancy following oocyte and sperm transfer to the uterus. Lancet 1982;1:1031–1033.
2. Hodgen G. Personal communication.
3. Heape W. Preliminary note on the transplantation and growth of mammalian ova within a uterine foster-mother. Proc R Soc 1890; 48:457–458.
4. McLaren A, Biggers JD. Successful development and birth of mice cultivated *in vitro* as early embryos. Nature 1959;182:877–878.
5. Chang MC. Fertilization of rabbit ova *in vitro*. Nature 1959;184:466–467.
6. Edwards RG. Maturation *in vitro* of human ovarian oocytes. Lancet 1965;2:926–929.
7. Edwards RG, Donahue RP, Baramki TA, Jones HW. Preliminary attempts to fertilize human oocytes matured *in vitro*. Am J Obstet Gynecol 1966;96:192–200.
8. Edwards RG, Steptoe PC, Purdy JM. Fertilization and cleavage *in vitro* of preovulatory human oocytes. Nature 1970;227:1307–1309.
9. DeKretzer D, Dennis P, Hudson B, et al. Transfer of a human zygote. Lancet 1973;2:728–729.
10. Soupart P, Strong PA. Ultrastructural observations on human oocytes fertilized *in vitro*. Fertil Steril 1974;25:11–44.
11. Steptoe PC, Edwards RG, Purdy JM. Clinical aspects of pregnancies established with cleaving embryos grown *in vitro*. Br J Obstet Gynaecol 1980;87:757–768.
12. Lopata A, Johnston IWH, Hoult IJ, Speirs AI.

Pregnancy following intrauterine implantation of an embryo obtained by in vitro fertilization of a preovulatory egg. Fertil Steril 1980;33:117–121.
13. Frantzen C, Schlosser HW. Microsurgery and postinfectious tubal infertility. Fertil Steril 1982;38:397–402.
14. Swolin K. Electromicrosurgery and salpingostomy: long term results. Am J Obstet Gynecol 1975;121:418–419.
15. Lauritsen JG, Pagel JD, Vangsted P, Starup J. Results of repeated tuboplasties. Fertil Steril 1982;37:68–72.
16. Drake T, Tredway D, Buchanan G, Takaki N, Daane T. Unexplained infertility. Obstet Gynecol 1977;50:644–646.
17. Trounson AO, Leeton J, Wood CK, Webb J, Kovacs G. The investigation of idiopathic infertility by *in vitro* fertilization. Fertil Steril 1980;34:431–438.
18. Edwards RG, Steptoe PC, Purdy JM. Establishing full-term human pregnancies using cleaving embryos grown *in vitro*. Br J Obstet Gynaecol 1980;87:737–756.
19. Garcia JE, Jones GS, Wright GL Jr. Prediction of the time of ovulation. Fertil Steril 1981;36:308–315.
20. Garcia JE, Jones GS, Acosta AA, Wright G Jr. Human menopausal gonadotropin/human chorionic gonadotropin follicular maturation for oocyte aspiration: phase 1, 1981. Fertil Steril 1983;39:167–173.
21. Garcia JE, Jones GS, Acosta AA, Wright G Jr. Human menopausal gonadotropin for oocyte aspiration: phase II, 1981. Fertil Steril 1983;39:174–179.
22. Vargyas JM, Marrs RP, Kletzky OA, Mishell DR. Correlation of ultrasonic measurement of ovarian follicle size and serum estradiol levels in ovulatory patients following clomiphene citrate for *in vitro* fertilization. Am J Obstet Gynecol 1982;144:569–573.
23. Mantzavinos T, Garcia JE, Jones HW Jr. Ultrasound measurements of ovarian follicles stimulated by human gonadotropins for oocyte recovery and *in vitro* fertilization. Fertil Steril 1983;40:461–465.
24. Evans J. Anesthesia in a program of *in vitro* fertilization. First *In Vitro* Workshop, Norfolk, Virginia, September 12, 1982.
25. Jones HW Jr, Acosta AA, Garcia JE. A technique for the aspiration of oocytes from human ovarian follicles. Fertil Steril 1982;37:26–29.
26. McNatty KP, Moore-Smith D, Makris A, Osanthanondh R, Ryan KJ. The micro environement of the human antral follicle: interrelationships among the steroid levels in antral fluid, the population of granulosa cells, and the status of the oocyte *in vivo* and *in vitro*. J Clin Endocrinol Metab 1979;49:851–859.
27. Veeck LL. Laboratory procedures. First *In Vitro* Workshop. Norfolk, Virginia, September 12, 1982.
28. Miller JF, Williamson E, Glue I. Fetal loss after implantation. Lancet 1980;13:554.
29. Garcia J, Jones GS, Acosta AA, Wright GL Jr. Corpus luteum function after follicle aspiration for oocyte retrieval. Fertil Steril 1981;36:565–572.
30. Kreitmenn O, Nixon WE, Hodgen GD. Induced corpus luteum dysfunction after aspiration of the preovulatory follicle in monkeys. Fertil Steril 1981;35:671–675.
31. Krein JF, Broom TJ, Ralph NM, et al. Human luteal phase function following oocyte aspiration from the immediately preovular graafian follicle of spontaneous ovular cycles. Br J Obstet Gynaecol 1981;88:1021–1028.
32. Frydman R, Testart J, Giacomini P, Imbert MC, Martin E, Nahoul K. Hormonal and histological study of the luteal phase in women following aspiration of the preovulatory follicle. Fertil Steril 1982;38:312–317.
33. Feichtinger W, Kemeter P, Szalay S, Beck A, Janisch H. Could aspiration of the graafian follicle cause luteal phase deficiency? Fertil Steril 1982;37:205–208.
34. Acosta AA, Garcia JE, Jones GS, Wright GL Jr. Corpus luteum function in patients with hMG/hCG induced ovulation for *in vitro* fertilization. Submitted.
35. Jones GS, Garcia JE, Acosta AA, et al. The occurrence of luteal phase defects during a program for *in vitro* fertilization. In: Van de Molen HJ, Klopper A, Lunenfeld B, Neves de Castro M, Sciarra F, Vermeulen A, eds. Fertility, infertility, and contraception. Amsterdam: Excerpta Medica, 1982:244–255.

Environmental Factors in Infertility

A. F. Haney

Human reproduction increasingly occurs in an environment contaminated by a diverse group of xenobiotics (pharmaceutical drugs, pesticides, herbicides, plastics, heavy metals, etc.), reflecting our dependence on sophisticated modern chemicals. As a result, there are a myriad of opportunities for environmental agents to influence our procreation adversely. A list of potential areas for environmental interaction with reproduction is presented in Table 14–1. Heightened awareness by both physicians and the public of occupational and environmental hazards resulted in passage of the Occupational Safety and Health Act. This concern is amplified by the rising numbers of women in the workplace, with greater than 40% of pregnancies occurring in working women (1). Smaller family sizes and the trend toward delayed childbearing to attain socioeconomic and educational goals intensifies the concern for a safe pregnancy.

Environmental agents are potentially hazardous to reproduction anywhere from gametogenesis to sexual maturation of the offspring, including such diverse areas as gamete transport, sexual behavior, and genital tract differentiation. Excluding gross teratology, the endpoints of functional reproductive toxicity, i.e., infertility, oligomenorrhea, oligospermia, etc., are poorly characterized even in normal populations. Subtle changes in these parameters are likely to be overlooked unless they draw immediate attention by their uniqueness, such as the genital abnormalities induced by prenatal diethylstilbestrol (DES) exposure (Fig. 14–1) (2), or by an overwhelmingly apparent increase in the frequency of a rare defect as illustrated by the phocomelia induced by thalidomide (3). The implications of these reproductive hazards have been apparent to industry even to the point of employers allegedly requiring women to "prove" they are infertile and to take less attractive job alternatives away from putative reproductive toxicants (4).

Vital to reducing the hazard is the identification of environmental chemicals posing a threat to reproduction prior to large-scale manufacture and widespread human exposure. With several thousand commercial chemicals being introduced each year, this is a monumental task. The magnitude of the contamination of the environment by xenobiotics has been generally underestimated; this was dramatized by the recent report that 8.5 kg per day of salicylic acid was found in the wastewater effluent of Kansas City, Missouri (5). Similarly, o,p'DDT is a ubiquitous contaminant in our environment, with an estimated cumulative utilization of 200 million pounds (6). As much as 1.9 million kg of DDT may have been discharged by the Los Angeles sewer system alone, resulting in a massive contamination of the southern California seashore (7). The most significant environmental contaminant may be estrogen, considering the millions of women taking oral contraceptive tablets and the quantity of diethylstilbestrol (DES) used as a growth-promoting agent for poultry, cattle, and sheep—27,000 kg of DES were used in 1970 by the livestock industry (8). Despite a withdrawal of official approval, its use continues. The impact of these and other envi-

TABLE 14–1. Sites and Functions of the Reproductive Tract Susceptible to Alteration by Environmental Influences

SITE	FUNCTION
Reproductive tract	
Central nervous system	Sexual behavior
Hypothalamus	Synthesis or release of neurotransmitters, neuromodulators, or neurohormones
Pituitary	Synthesis or release of trophic hormones
Testis	Steroidogenesis
	Production of regulatory factors (e.g., inhibin)
	Gametogenesis
Male accessory glands	Secretory function
Ovary	Gametogenesis
	Follicular/luteal function: steroidogenesis, oocyte maturation, production of intrafollicular regulatory factors (e.g., inhibin)
Oviduct	Oviduct secretions
	Gamete transport
Uterus	Uterine-tubal junction structure/function
	Uterine structure/function
	Uterine luminal secretions
	Endometrial decidualization
Cervix	Structural changes
	Endocervical mucous production
Vagina, vulva	Structural changes
	Adenosis
Nonreproductive tract	
Liver	Metabolism of reproductive hormones
	Synthesis/degradation of proteins related to reproductive function
Adrenal	Steroidogenesis

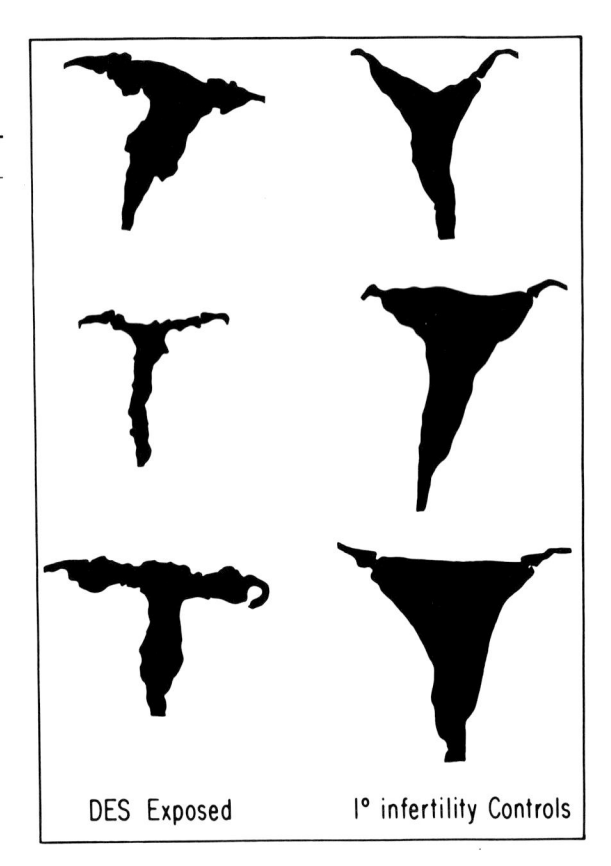

Fig. 14–1. Uterine contours in women exposed to diethylstilbestrol prenatally. Tracings of hysterosalpingograms of DES-exposed women and control subjects with primary infertility are compared to illustrate differences. The DES-exposed women have a characteristic T-shaped endometrial cavity and, occasionally, a dilated lower uterine segment and marked irregularity of the endometrial cavity. (Reproduced with permission. Haney AF et al. Diethylstilbestrol-induced upper genital tract abnormalities. Fertil Steril 1979;31:142.)

ronmental agents on human reproduction remains unclear at the present, but the potential problems are of such magnitude that closer scrutiny is urgently needed.

Environmental Agents Affecting Human Reproduction

Physicians caring for infertile couples have generally focused on treating pathologic conditions such as anovulation, oligospermia, and inadequate luteal function, frequently without being able to discern the etiology of these problems. The possibility that an environmental agent may be responsible for a portion of these conditions has received surprisingly little attention despite the knowledge that several chemicals have effects at extremely low levels of exposure. For example, the Occupational Safety and Health Administration of the Department of Labor has set the permissable exposure limit to dibromochloropropane (DBCP) at 1 part per billion (9). Dioxin has caused teratogenic effects in monkeys in concentrations as low as 50 parts per trillion (10).

It has been proposed that environmental agents may be responsible for a decrease in the average sperm concentration observed over the past 25 years (11). The percentage of men with a concentration greater than 100 million sperm per milliliter has declined from 44% to 22%, while the percentage of men with a concentration of 20 to 40 million sperm per milliliter has increased from 12% to 22%. Similarly, it has been suggested that ovulatory dysfunction may be related to the seasonal use of DDT (12). Whether these represent real environmental effects is controversial, but a large number of agents have altered human reproductive physiology, and selected examples are described below.

ESTROGENS. Occupational exposures resulting in hyperestrogenism have been reported with the manufacture and use of diethylstilbestrol as well as natural estrogens (13,14). Similar effects have also been noted in the manufacture of progestogens in combination with estrogens in oral contraceptive tablets (15). In a report by company physicians in the pharmaceutical industry, 181 cases of clinical hyperestrogenism were noted in workers from 1941 through 1978 (Table 14–2). The clinical manifestations of hyperestrogenism may even extend to the workers' children as a result of contaminated clothing brought home from the workplace (16). Symptoms include loss of libido and gynecomastia in men and irregular menses, nausea, headaches, breast pain, leukorrhea, and ankle edema in women. Comparable findings have been noted in workers involved with the manufacture of conjugated estrogens, hexestrol, and ethinyl estradiol.

Inadvertent pharmaceutical exposure to estrogens has also occurred as a result of vitamin tablet production with stilbestrol-contaminated equipment. This has caused gynecomastia in children (17). A similar phenomenon was observed during the treatment of tuberculosis with isoniazid tablets contaminated with stilbestrol (18). Even hair lotion tainted with diethylstilbestrol has been absorbed through the scalp with clinical effect (19). Symptoms are more frequently reported in males and vary from increased nipple sensitivity to overt gynecomastia.

LEAD. Lead is an extremely common industrial chemical. Occupational exposure has been recognized since ancient times as a reproductive hazard, particularly with regard to the fe-

TABLE 14–2. Hyperestrogenism Recorded in the Thirteen Plants by Company Physicians*

DATE	CASES (MALE AND FEMALE)	NO. OF PLANTS WITH CASES	NO. OF PLANTS PRODUCING ESTROGEN (OF 13)
ca. 1940–1972[†]	58 (DES)	1	—
1955–1978[†]	ca. 20	1	—
1966	1	1	7
1967	2	1	8
1968	0	1	9
1969	1	1	10
1970	18	3	10
1971	2	2	11
1972	5	2	11
1973	13	4	11
1974	14	4	12
1975	16	5	13
1976	15	5	13
1977	8	5	13
1978	8?	4?	13
TOTAL	181		

* From about 1940 to 1978.
[†] The first two lines refer to cases recorded by 2 companies for which a breakdown by year was not available. Reproduced with permission. Zaebst DD, Tanaka S, Haring M. Occupational exposure to estrogens—problems and approaches. In: McLachlan JA, ed. Estrogens in the environment. Amsterdam: Elsevier/North-Holland, 1980:384.)

tus, because transplacental transport readily occurs. Lead exposure is associated with increased rates of spontaneous abortion, perinatal loss, and neurobehavioral problems in the newborn (20). Systemic toxicity is noted with blood levels greater than 50 mcg/100 ml and it is probably unsafe for pregnant women to have levels greater than 30 mcg/100 ml because of the susceptibility of the fetus (21). Elevated lead levels in children have even been noted after ingestion of lead brought home by their parents on articles of clothing (22). With a half-life in bone of 10 years and excretion in breast milk, lead toxicity may persist long after the occupational exposure has ceased.

HALOGENATED POLYCYCLIC HYDROCARBONS. These chemicals, widely used in industry and agriculture, include o,p'DDT, aldrin, Agent Orange, polychlorinated biphenyls (PCBs), heptachlor, and hexachlorophene. They persist for extended periods of time in animals in the food chain, probably because of their high fat solubility. The widely reported thinning of egg shells induced by DDE, a metabolite of DDT (23), attests to its adverse effects on reproduction in predatory birds, including the Bald Eagle. After banning its use, residues of DDE in eggs declined and the reproductive performance of the endangered birds improved (24). An episode of rice oil contamination in Japan demonstrated human fetal toxicity as well as menstrual cycle abnormalities (25). The ubiquitous contamination of the environment with these agents, as well as their persistence in nature, make them of particular long-term concern.

POLYCYCLIC AROMATIC HYDROCARBONS. Fossil fuel combustion, syn-fuel synthesis, and cigarette smoking result in release of a variety of polycyclic aromatic hydrocarbons. These have been demonstrated to induce ovarian tumors in mice, an event preceded by oocyte destruction (26). In the murine paradigm, these compounds require metabolic activation to reactive electrophilic intermediates in the ovary in order to destroy oocytes. Obviously, these studies have not been corroborated in humans, but cigarette smoking provides an opportunity to study intense exposure to polycyclic aromatic hydrocarbons. Increased rates of infertility in smokers have been reported (27), but the number of studies is small and the results less than definitive. The possible mechanism of infertility is obscure, but smoking changes the amplitude of uterine contractions as well as the resting tone (28). As a result, smokers are more likely to have abnormal hysterosalpingograms (29). More relevant to the observations in animals, cigarette smoking has been associated with a decrease in the age of menopause (30). This may be a dose-dependent effect, since those who smoke more than 1 pack per day have an earlier menopause than those who never smoked or quit (Fig. 14–2). Similarly, abnormal sperm morphology and decreased sperm concentration have been observed in male smokers (31). Serum testosterone levels are also reduced in smokers (32), suggesting either a direct effect on Leydig cells

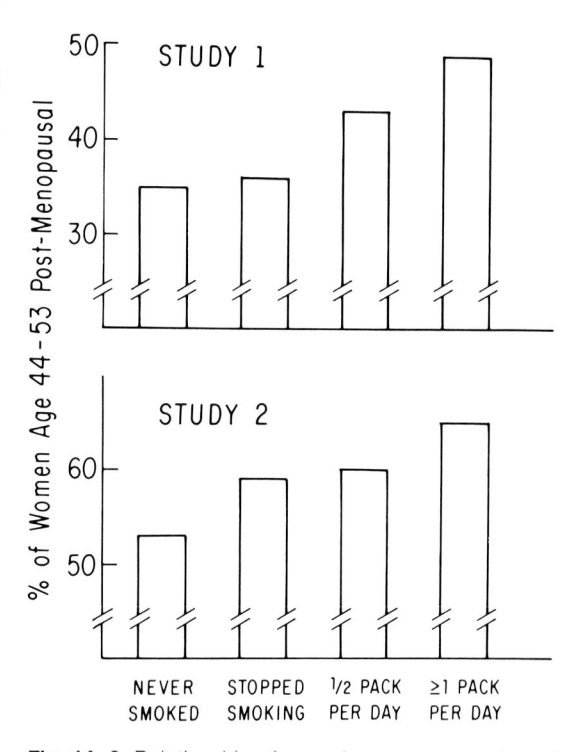

Fig. 14–2. Relationship of age of menopause and smoking. Two studies are presented that correlate the percentage of women between the ages of 45 and 53 years who were postmenopausal with their smoking history. In both studies, the highest percentage of women between 45 and 53 years who were menopausal were those who smoked more than 1 pack per day. The percentage of women who were menopausal was intermediate for the group that smoked half a pack per day. This suggests a dose-dependent relationship. (Modified and reproduced with permission. Jick H et al. Relation between smoking and age of natural menopause. The Lancet 1977;1354–1355.)

or interference with hypothalamic-pituitary-testicular function. With over 3,000 compounds identified in cigarette smoke, it remains difficult to identify the specific active agent(s) responsible, but polycyclic aromatic hydrocarbons, nicotine, and carbon monoxide are the most likely candidates. The effects of automobile exhaust and smokestack emissions on the general population are potentially similar even in nonsmokers in high pollution areas. With an increase in the number of women smoking cigarettes at young ages (33), the reproductive consequences of smoking are of considerable interest.

CARBON MONOXIDE. Carbon monoxide is another byproduct of fossil fuel combustion and smoking. It readily displaces oxygen from hemoglobin by shifting the dissociation curve for oxyhemoglobin to the left and thereby decreasing oxygen tension. Carbon monoxide crosses the placenta and, in experimental animals, causes low-birth-weight infants and fetal death (1). Whether carbon monoxide is the active toxin in cigarette smoke has long been debated, but concentrations as high as 50 to 100 parts per million (ppm) are found in cigarette smoke. Such concentrations can increase the carboxyhemoglobin in smokers to levels of 4% to 10% (34). Smog is another important source of environmental exposure to carbon monoxide and contains as much as 50 ppm. With a relatively short half-life of 4 to 5 hours, sustained inhalation is probably required for significant effects. Even nonsmokers in relatively smog-free environments can be exposed to significant concentrations. Emissions from kerosene space heaters in relatively confined spaces result in levels of carbon monoxide in excess of ambient air quality and safe occupational standards (35).

Environmental Hazards in Men

Males are not immune to environmental effects and may actually be at greater risk because of the high concentrations of chemicals associated with occupational exposures. Spermatogenesis is suppressed by a variety of xenobiotics including many therapeutic agents (Table 14–3). For example, salicylazosulfapyridine, a drug useful in ulcerative

TABLE 14–3. Environmental Agents Known to Inhibit Spermatogenesis in Humans

Kepone (chlordecone)
DBCP (1,2-dibromo-3-chloropropane)
Organic solvents
  Toluene
  Benzene
  Xylene
Lead
Boron
Cadmium
Methylmercury
Cigarettes
Alcohol
Gossypol
Pharmaceutical drugs
  Cimetidine
  Salicylazosulfapyridine
  Alkylating agents
  Vincristine
Prenatal diethylstilbestrol exposure

colitis, may induce infertility as a result of oligospermia, decreased sperm motility, and increased numbers of abnormal spermatozoa (36). Similarly, many industrial and agricultural chemicals are injurious to testicular function. Dibromochloropropane (DBCP), a soil fumigant, has been associated with infertility and lowered sperm counts in farm workers (37). The mechanism of action of this agent is unclear as no change in testosterone production has been demonstrated despite a decrease in gonadotropins. Humans appear to be more sensitive to DBCP than animals and oligospermia occurs at factory levels below 1 ppm. As with many other xenobiotics, this compound was, unfortunately, not recognized as a toxicant until farm workers were noted to become infertile after agricultural exposure to DBCP. Similarly, occupational exposure to lead has been noted to cause decreases in sperm concentrations, abnormal sperm morphology, and loss of libido (38). Occupational exposure to Kepone® has resulted in a syndrome consisting of a variety of neurologic symptoms, joint pains, loss of libido, and oligospermia (39). Alcoholism may lead to significant reproductive problems. Heavy sustained alcohol ingestion results in testicular atrophy (40) with recent data suggesting that this may be a direct effect on the testes (41).

Recently, 2 unrelated therapeutic agents have been associated with gynecomastia. The first is cimetidine, a histamine H-2 receptor antagonist marketed for the treatment of ulcers (42). The presumed mechanism of action is felt to be an antagonism of the androgen receptor (43). In experimental animals, prenatal exposure to cimetidine causes a lower testicular production of testosterone in the adult and a concomitant decline in sexual performance (44). While serum testosterone levels are not decreased in men, lowered sperm concentrations (45) and impotence (46) have been observed. Spironolactone, a potassium-saving diuretic, is thought to cause gynecomastia by inhibiting steroidogenic enzymes necessary for testosterone production (47). The end result of both drugs is a diminution in androgen action allowing the low levels of circulating estrogens in males to induce gynecomastia. Paradoxically, this has been put to therapeutic advantage in decreasing the androgenic manifestations in women with hirsutism and chronic anovulation.

A fascinating account of an environmental agent's effect on male reproduction comes from the Peoples Republic of China and their experience with the yellow pigment gossypol, derived from various cotton species. As reported in a 1957 Chinese journal, a small village in Jaing-su encountered serious reproductive problems:

> At that time, cottonseed oil was far cheaper than bean oil so all of the families used cottonseed oil for cooking. During a period of more than 10 years when everyone ate cottonseed oil, there was not a single child born. . . . About 5 to 6 years before the war, there was a large crop of soybeans in the Northeast provinces. Large amounts of soybean oil were sold to the South. The price of soybean oil became much cheaper than cottonseed oil for cooking and a strange thing happened: every family in the village started to raise children (48).

A change in the oil-processing technology may have contributed to this problem (49). Traditionally, Chinese farmers had first heated cottonseeds and then pressed out the oil with no associated infertility. After the advent of collectivized central processing, the cottonseeds were pressed without heating, which resulted in an increased gossypol content and infertility. In addition to azoospermia in males, women developed amenorrhea, although both effects were reversible after ingestion of cottonseed oil stopped. Subsequent to the discovery of the active agent in cottonseed oil, gossypol has undergone clinical trials as a male contraceptive in the Peoples Republic of China (50). Early results have been promising.

Behavioral Effects of Environmental Agents

The behavioral aspects of reproduction include courtship, sexual, and parental behavior. All are potentially altered by environmental agents. The importance of sexual satisfaction to interpersonal relations is difficult to assess, but intolerance of sexual inadequacy may be a significant contributor to the rising rates of marital discord in our society. The continuing search for newer and safer contraceptive techniques is a testament to the desire to control reproductive output without loss of sexual gratification. Few are willing to abstain from sexual activity as a means of reducing family size. The importance of psychosocial and pathologic factors in sexual dysfunction is difficult to assign, but the significance of these issues to society should not be underestimated.

It is almost impossible to gather epidemiologic data in humans because of the multiple factors known to influence sexual attitudes and behavior. Socioeconomic status, ethnic background, religion, and contraceptive choices are only the most obvious of these factors. Frequency of coitus is a poor index of sexual behavior because other issues such as arousal, initiation, and erotic imagery also influence sexual behavior. The sexual behavior of women fluctuates throughout the menstrual cycle, but the differences did not become apparent until female-initiated coitus rather than coital frequency was examined. Similarly, the frequency of counseling is an unreliable index of sexual dysfunction. Since many aspects of human sexual behavior have no counterpart in animals, the ability to evaluate environmental influences is hampered by the lack of a suitable model system. Agents with potential effects on human sexual behavior include alcohol, cigarette smoking (polycyclic aromatic hydrocarbons), estrogens, and lead. While the endocrinologic changes induced by these agents are well documented, behavioral consequences have not been as thoroughly studied. The possibilities are disturbing.

Permanent alterations in sexual response can be influenced in experimental animals by prenatal or neonatal exposure to compounds that mimic or impede the action of sex steroids that are important in sex differentiation. Women with virilized genitalia secondary to congenital adrenal hyperplasia provide an opportunity to study prenatal androgen exposure. While gender identity in these women is not affected up to the age of early adolescence, subsequent behavior consistent with a male gender role has been reported (51). Similar behavior has been observed in women with genital anomalies who were exposed *in utero* to exogenously administered androgens. These women had no postnatal hormonal exposure and underwent correction of the anomaly prior to gender identification at 18 months of age (52). This suggests that the observed gender role differences were the result of prenatal androgen exposure even though gender identity (i.e., self-perception as a female) was not affected. Psychologic studies of these women have suggested male orientation in adulthood, but the data are not definitive. That treatment of adults with gonadal steroids can alter sexual response is illustrated by a decreased libido noted in men with occupational hyperestrogenism (13). Environmental agents causing subtle behavioral changes mimicking these examples are difficult to detect by traditional epidemiologic methods and, hence, their effect on human sexual behavior is unknown.

Circumstance of Environmental Exposure

The most intense exposure to xenobiotics tends to be occupational, with skin contact and inhalation the most frequent routes. The metabolic fate of these agents is related to the route of exposure; differences in route of exposure may significantly alter the compound and, hence, its action. When 17-beta estradiol is ingested orally, it undergoes conversion to estrone and the ratio of estrone to estradiol that appears in the peripheral circulation is greater than 1 (Fig. 14–3) (53). By contrast, when 17-beta estradiol is administered intravaginally, it predominates in the peripheral blood (Fig. 14–4) (54). Direct absorption into the vascular system, as opposed to transport across the intestinal mucosa and passage through the hepatic portal circulation, probably accounts for

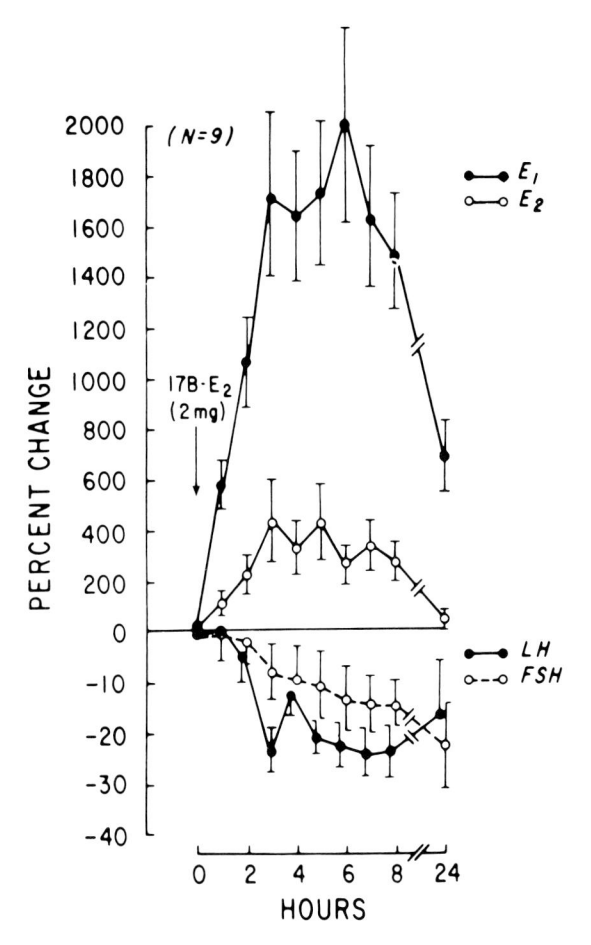

Fig. 14–3. Relationship of serum estradiol (E_2) and estrone (E_1) after oral ingestion of 17-beta estradiol. Graphs of the percent change of serum levels of estradiol, estrone, luteinizing hormone (LH), and follicle-stimulating hormone (FSH) are plotted over 24 hours after ingestion of 2 mg 17-beta estradiol orally. The rise in serum estrone is much more pronounced than that of serum estradiol. This is consistent with the hypothesis that intestinal mucosa possesses the capacity to convert estradiol to estrone. Suppression of gonadotropin concentrations is suggestive of a hypothalamic-pituitary effect. (Reproduced with permission. Yen SSC et al. Circulating estradiol, estrone, and gonadotropin levels following the administration of orally active 17-beta estradiol in postmenopausal women. J Clin Endocrinol Metab 1975;40:518–521.)

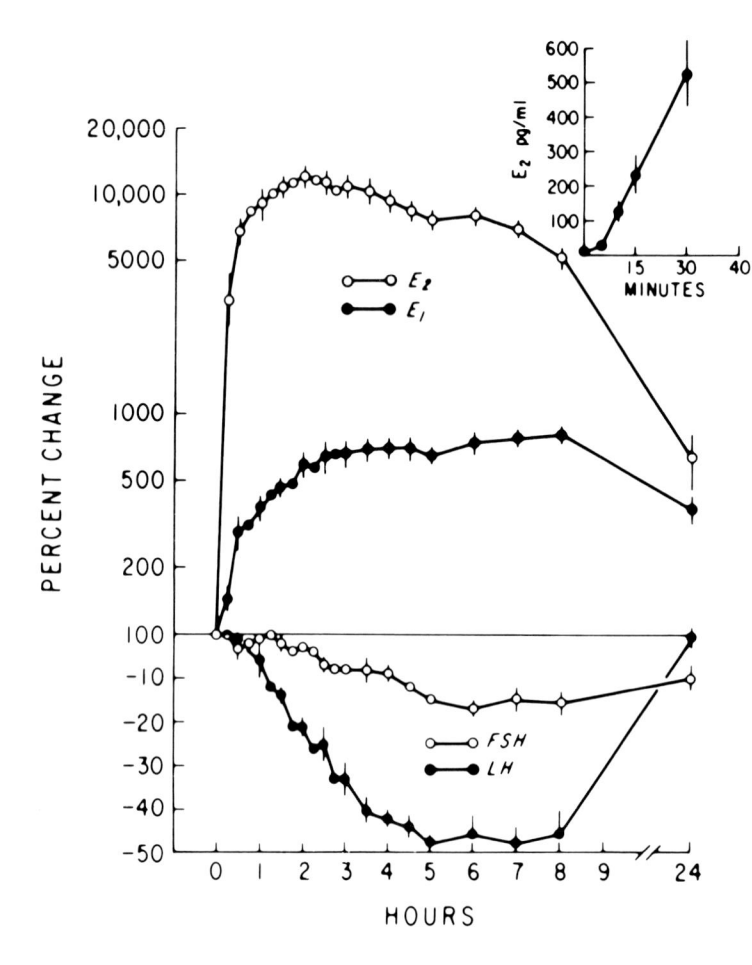

Fig. 14–4. Relationship of serum estradiol (E_2) and estrone (E_1), after intravaginal administration of 17-beta estradiol. This is similar in format to Fig. 14–3. Note the rapid rise of estradiol greater than estrone in serum, which is the reverse of the effect noted with oral administration. Suppression of the gonadotropins occurs and this is suggestive of a hypothalamic-pituitary effect. The greater estradiol-to-estrone ratio suggests direct absorption of the 17-beta estradiol with little conversion at the site of the absorption. (Reproduced with permission. Rigg LA et al. Efficacy of intravaginal and intranasal administration of micronized estradiol 17-beta. J Clin Endocrinol Metab 1977;45:1261–1264.)

the differences. Yet a third pattern of circulating estrogens is observed when 17-beta estradiol is administered intranasally. This is characterized by a rapid, but unsustained, rise in serum estradiol concentrations. The rise in serum estrone was only 60% that of estradiol, but was sustained (Fig. 14–5) (54). These observations suggest that the route of exposure is important when considering the effect of xenobiotic agents.

The temporal aspects of exposure are also critical, as illustrated by the prenatal effects of diethylstilbestrol (DES). Maternal ingestion during the period of genital tract differentiation (approximately 8 to 14 weeks' gestation) induces a myriad of reproductive tract changes, whereas the incidence of such changes is much lower with exposure after termination of organogenesis (55).

Similarly, gender dimorphism can be a significant factor in the response to xenobiotic agents. Women exposed to DES prenatally have a characteristic pattern of vaginal adenosis and cervical and upper genital tract changes, whereas the effect in males (cryptorchid testes, epididymal cysts, and oligospermia) is more variable (2).

The actual compound responsible for an observed effect may be difficult to identify even when the environmental contaminant is known. The herbicide mixture Agent Orange gained notoriety as a defoliant with its use in Vietnam. It has been associated with a syndrome including malaise, psychologic disturbances, liver and immunologic abnormalities, as well as loss of libido and infertility. Agent Orange represents a 1:1 mixture of 2,4-D (dichlorophenoxyacetic acid) and 2,4,5-T (trichlorophenoxyacetic acid), which in the manufacturing process was contaminated by the potent teratogen tetrachlorodibenzo-p-dioxin. Dioxin itself has teratogenic effects in monkeys with levels as low as 50 parts per trillion (10) and as such may be the compound responsible for some of the effects attributed to Agent Orange.

Fig. 14–5. Relationship of serum estradiol (E$_2$) and estrone (E$_1$) after intranasal administration of 17-beta estradiol in saline. The rapid but short-lived rise of E$_2$ and the more sustained rise of E$_1$ suggest either local conversion of E$_2$ to E$_1$ by the nasal membrane or nasal bacterial flora. (Reproduced with permission. Rigg LA et al. Efficacy of intravaginal and intranasal administration of micronized estradiol-17-beta. J Clin Endocrinol Metab 1977;45:1261–1264.)

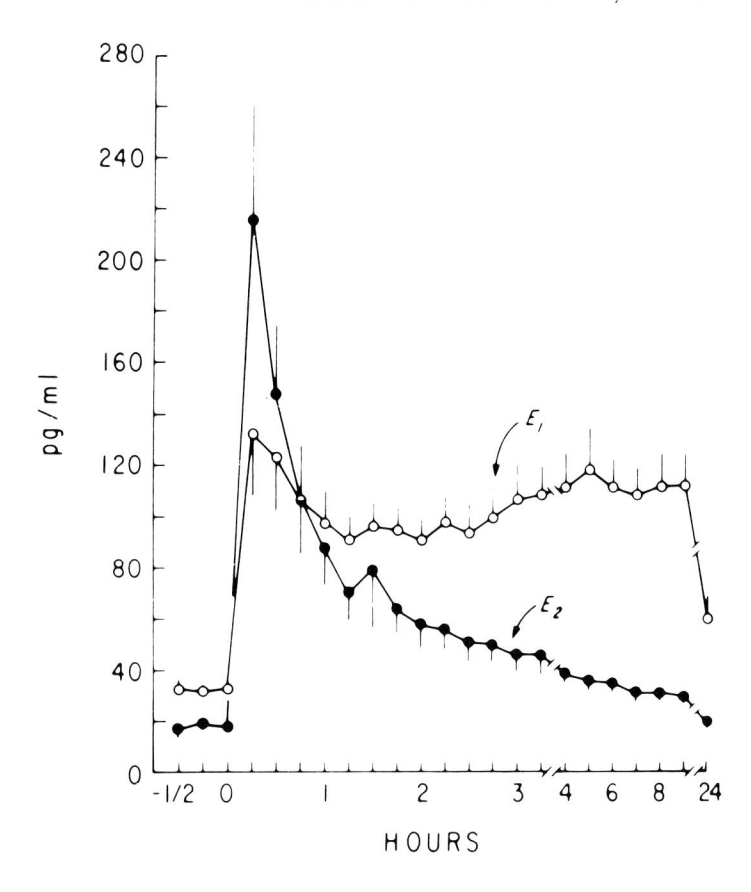

The Fate of Environmental Contaminants

Disturbingly little attention has been paid to the distribution and ultimate fate of industrial chemicals produced on a large scale and ultimately released into the environment. Agents with the widest distribution are pesticides such as organochlorines, organophosphates, carbamates, and herbicides. Many of these compounds are virtually indestructible in nature and persist in the environment for extended periods of time. For example, the breakdown of polychlorinated biphenyls requires incineration in special furnaces at temperatures up to 3,000°C. This is expensive and of limited availability.

As has been noted, an organochlorine, o,p'DDT, bioaccumulates in the food chain because of its lipid solubility. As a result, reproduction in predatory birds is declining. Lipophilic compounds with molecular weights below 700 daltons usually are capable of crossing the placenta and may present hazards to the human fetus. Other examples of this class of compounds include dieldrin, chlordane, and Kepone® (chlordecone).

One of the most instructive environmental contaminations that has been thoroughly evaluated in humans occurred with polychlorinated biphenyls (PCBs). Used for the last 40 years, these compounds have found industrial applications in electric transformers and capacitors as well as lubricants and hydraulic fluids. A related class of compounds, polybrominated biphenyls (PBBs), have been used as fire retardants. Both persist for extremely long periods of time in the environment and are biomagnified in the food chain. Sport fishing in contaminated waters such as Lake Michigan provides direct exposure to humans and secondary exposure through breast milk contamination (56). In monkeys, PCBs have decreased fertility, increased the rate of abortion, caused resorption of embryos, and resulted in low-birth-weight infants (57). No comparable effects have been correlated with PBB exposure to date, but this chemical also crosses the placenta.

Model ecosystems have been developed to evaluate the distribution and metabolic fate of environmental agents in a laboratory setting (58). These have been studied extensively since the early 1970s and provide unique insights into the passage of xenobiotics into the food chain with subsequent bioaccumulation. As depicted in Fig. 14–6, these systems have animal cages for rodents or chickens suspended within a completely enclosed tank containing white quartz sand and sorghum plants simulating a "farm." Standard reference water constitutes a "lake," which is stocked with microorganisms, plankton, snails, and algae. The entire aquarium is covered with Plexiglas® to retard evaporation and maintained at 26°C with a 12-hour daylight cycle.

Radiolabeled xenobiotics such as pesticides, industrial chemicals, energy conversion byproducts, etc. are then introduced into the model ecosystem. The route of exposure can be either in food or water for the animals or by direct application in the "lake" or "farm" consistent with the route of environmental contamination. After equilibration for variable intervals of time, larvae and then fish are added to the "lake." The experiment is then terminated and each component, i.e., water, sand, animals, and plants, is prepared for liquid scintillation counting. The distribution of the radioactivity indicates the spread of the contaminant. Metabolites can be separated by chromatography, giving a clear picture of compartmental metabolism. The ecologic magnification for a variety of compounds in fish in the model ecosystem is illustrated in Fig. 14–7. By these routes, agricultural and industrial chemicals can enter the food chain and ultimately lead to human exposure.

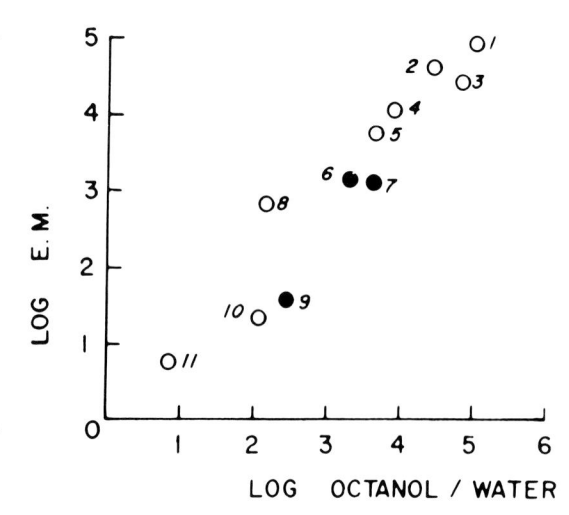

Fig. 14–7. Ecologic magnification of (E.M.) xenobiotics in the model ecosystem. The relationship of the logarithm of ecologic magnification for the fish *Gambusia* to the logarithm of the octanol/water partition coefficient is illustrated. Estrogenic substances (solid circles), methoxychlor (6), chlordecone (7), and DES (9) conform to the general direct relationship as established with DDT (1), hexachlorobiphenyl (2), DDE (3), tetrachlorobiphenyl (4), dieldrin (5), chlorobenzene (8), Anisole (10), and aniline (11). This relationship can be used to predict the propensity for xenobiotic bioaccumulation and food chain transfer. (Reproduced with permission. Metcalf RL. Model ecosystems for environmental studies of estrogens. In: McLachlan JA, ed. Estrogens in the environment. Amsterdam: Elsevier/North-Holland, 1980:209.)

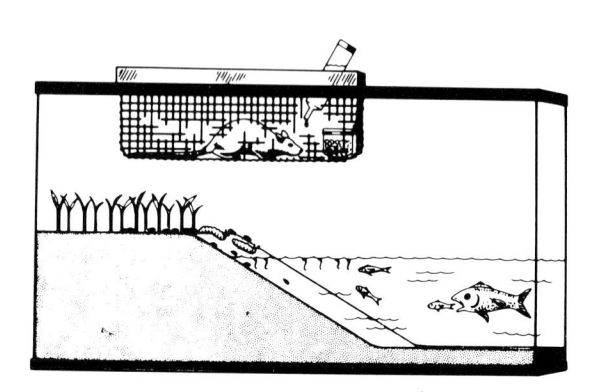

Fig. 14–6. Model ecosystem utilized to evaluate the distribution and metabolism of xenobiotics. Illustrated is a model ecosystem described in the text that allows the evaluation of xenobiotic biodegradeability and ecologic magnification. The contaminant can either be placed in the food and water for the animal or directly on plants or water within the system, depending on the mode of environmental contamination anticipated. (Modified and published with permission. Metcalf RL. Model ecosystems for environmental studies of estrogens. In: McLachlan JA, ed. Estrogens in the environment. Amsterdam: Elsevier/North-Holland, 1980:205.)

Mechanism of Action of Toxicants

Few of the approximately 60,000 currently used industrial chemicals have been screened for genital tract teratogenicity, let alone functional reproductive toxicity. There are many aspects of reproductive toxicology that make evaluation of the mechanism of action of reproductive toxicants difficult. Considerations as to the route of exposure, absorption, transport through the vascular system, interaction with binding proteins, distribution in the body, metabolism, including bioactivation and inactivation, pattern of excretion, gender differences, and the influence of tissue repair must all be considered. Unfortunately, these are difficult to predict for xenobiotics and adequate animal models applicable to humans are not yet available.

Table 14–4 is an outline of mechanisms by which xenobiotics can influence the reproductive process. The effects may be specific for organs in the reproductive tract or more generally on the entire organism, with some selectivity for the reproductive tract. The agent may act at multiple sites, require metabolic activation, or alter physiologic control mechanisms such as enzyme induction at a site distant from the reproductive tract, as, for example, the liver. These combine to make establishment of the exact mechanism of toxicity difficult in many instances.

Reproductive toxicants have been most commonly compounds with structural similarity to endogenous hormones, acting as either agonists or antagonists. This has been most apparent with gonadal steroids, as a wide variety of chemicals are active in bioassays of sex steroids. These include o,p'DDT, polycyclic hydrocarbons, Kepone®, and PCBs, to name a few. Toxins with this action would be classified as direct acting. Larger, more chemically complex hormones, such as the glycoproteins from the pituitary [i.e., follicle-stimulating hormone (FSH) and luteinizing hormone (LH)], are far less likely to be structurally similar to a toxicant and, therefore, have correspondingly lower probability of being mimicked by an environmental agent.

A second pattern of toxicity involves general chemical reactivity with some selectivity for the reproductive tract. Gametes of both males and females seem unusually susceptible. The relatively high lipid content of the gonads may, for example, lead to differential uptake of a lipophilic compound resulting in a greater gonadal injury than would be suggested by systemic toxicity. Examples of chemical reactivity include alkylating agents, cadmium, and boron. These agents demonstrate oocyte toxicity, both in humans and well-studied animal models (59).

A second major category of compounds are those that do not act directly on the reproductive tract either as surrogate hormones or by direct reactivity, but, rather, indirectly impair the reproductive process. The two major mechanisms for indirect-acting toxicants are metabolic conversion of an inactive compound to a toxic metabolite or induction or inhibition of enzymes involved in production or control of reproductive hormones. This may also involve inactivation of detoxification pathways, allowing greater molecular interaction with the toxicant. Polycyclic aromatic hydrocarbons act in this fashion; bioactivation to reactive metabolites is necessary in order to destroy oocytes.

There are several obvious advantages of a thorough understanding of the mechanism of action of a reproductive toxicant. First, it is possible to predict the hazardous nature of compounds that have similar structure-function relationships to known toxins, and thereby aid in the screening of new compounds prior to extensive human exposure. Second, such understanding may suggest chemical modifications of the compound that prevent its metabolism to a toxic intermediate, but do not alter its industrial usefulness. Third, if the mechanism of action is sexually dimorphic, it may yield occupational guidelines for industry, improving the safety of women and their accompanying fetuses in the workplace.

TABLE 14–4. Mechanism of Action of Reproductive Toxicants

MECHANISM	EXAMPLES
Direct acting agents	
Structural analogy	Steroid hormones
	Diethylstilbestrol
	Cimetidine
	Danazol
	o,p'DDT
Chemical reactivity	Alkylating agents
	Cadmium
	Boron
	Lead
	Methylmercury
Indirect acting agents	
Metabolism	Ethanol
	Dibromochloropropane
Disrupted homeostasis	Salicylazosulfapyridine
	Halogenated polycyclic hydrocarbons

Modified from Mattison DR. Mechanisms of action of reproductive toxins. In: Mattison DR, ed. Reproductive toxicology. New York: Alan R. Liss, 1983:65–81.

Screening for Reproductive Toxicity

While carcinogenicity and mutagenicity have been extensively studied, a comparable data base for reproductive toxicology does not exist. No single test system can be expected to detect all reproductive hazards and there is a definite need for development of a coordinated strategy for identification of potential toxicants and defined limits to human exposure. Recently, a screening system has been proposed that integrates a computerized structure-function analysis with predictions of which compounds might act like known toxicants of similar structure. A multigenerational animal study is incorporated as a final screen. More detailed *in vivo* and *in vitro* investigation would be reserved for compounds felt to be possible reproductive toxicants on the basis of the preliminary evaluation (60).

Selecting animal species for testing can be perplexing, as species differences may be dramatic. An illustrative example of species-specific teratology is the phocomelia associated with thalidomide ingestion. Thalidomide does not cause abnormalities in rats or mice, but rabbits and primates are exquisitely sensitive to its effects (3). These species differences led to invalid conclusions as to the safety of thalidomide in humans and it was recognized as a teratogen only after extensive human use with tragic consequences.

Species differences also exist with regard to hormone metabolism as observed with the male sexual response to testosterone. In the rat and hamster, testosterone is aromatized in the central nervous system to estradiol, a potent stimulator of male sexual behavior in the adult castrate. This suggests that estrogens are the virilizing agent in the developing central nervous system in the neonate and fetus. By contrast, estradiol is not effective in producing male sexual activity in castrated adult guinea pigs. It is likely that conversion of testosterone to its 5-alpha-reduced metabolite, dihydrotestosterone, is important in influencing male sexual behavior of the guinea pig (61). A system similar to the guinea pig appears to be operative in the rhesus monkey and, probably, in humans. Hence, attempts to screen environmental agents using a single animal paradigm are complicated by species differences.

The interval of time between environmental exposure and the expression of the reproductive problem can be critical for detection of a toxicant, as illustrated by the prenatal effects of diethylstilbestrol. While extensive human exposure during pregnancy occurred in the late 1940s and early 1950s, no obvious abnormalities were appreciated until a previously rare clear-cell adenocarcinoma of the vagina was associated with prenatal diethylstilbestrol exposure in the early 1970s (62). Subsequently, genital tract anomalies in both males and females have been described, the reproductive consequences of which are not yet fully appreciated. In women, these anomalies have been associated with an increased frequency of ectopic pregnancies as well as premature deliveries, with correspondingly higher rates of perinatal mortality (63).

All these features make detection of environmentally induced reproductive effects on an individual basis problematic. As a physician treating infertile couples, it may be important to consider their living conditions and occupations as well as any systemic symptoms suggestive of toxic exposure (eye irritation, skin rashes, alopecia, etc.). Similar symptoms in coworkers or neighbors, especially infertility, are probably the most suggestive of an environmental impact, but because of the sensitive nature of these complaints it is rarely obvious. A general appreciation of the environmental and occupational agents known to affect reproduction should be useful to the practicing physician, particularly with large numbers of women entering the workplace.

Summary

Despite many examples of environmental agents affecting human reproduction, there is not a general awareness of this possibility by physicians. Unfortunately, most cases of environmentally induced reproductive toxicity occur after extensive human exposure. This dramatizes the need for surveillance and increased efforts to screen new compounds and reduce the human hazard. Our standard of living is increasingly dependent on sophisticated industrial chemicals that ultimately find their way into our environment. A more thorough understanding of the implications of their production is mandatory to protect the most critical issue to our, or any other species, continued safe reproduction.

REFERENCES

1. Messite J, Bond MB. Reproductive toxicology and occupational exposure. In: Zenz C, ed. Development in occupational medicine. Chicago: Year Book Medical Publishers, 1980:59–129.
2. Bibbo M, Gill WB, Azizi F, et al. Follow-up study of male and female offspring of DES-exposed mothers. Obstet Gynecol 1977;49:1–8.
3. Shepard TH. Catalog of teratogenic agents, 2nd ed. Baltimore: The Johns Hopkins University Press, 1976.
4. Hricko A. Social policy considerations of occupational health standards: the example of lead and reproductive effects. Prev Med 1978;7:394–406.
5. Higmite C, Azarnoff DL. Drugs and drug metabolites as environmental contaminants: chlorophenoxyisobretyrate and salicylic acid in sewage and water effluent. Life Sci 1977;20:337–342.
6. Rall DP, McLachlan JA. Potential for exposure to estrogens in the environment. In: McLachlan JA, ed. Estrogens in the environment. Amsterdam: Elsevier/North-Holland, 1980:199–202.
7. Fry DM, Toon CK. DDT-induced feminization of Gull embryos. Science 1981;213:922–924.
8. McLachlan JA, Korach KS, Metzler M. Bioavailability as a determinant in the transplacental toxicity of diethylstilbestrol. In: Neubert D, Merker H-S, Nault H, Langman J, eds. Role of pharmacokinetics in prenatal and perinatal toxicology. Stuttgart: Georg Thieme Publishers, 1978:147–155.
9. Whorton D, Milby TH, Krauss RM, et al. Testicular function in DBCP exposed pesticide workers. J Occup Med 1979;21:161–166.
10. Grant WF. The genotoxic effects of 2,4,5-T. Mutat Res 1979;65:83–119.
11. Dougherty RC. Sperm density and toxic substances: a potential key to identification of environmental health hazards. In: McKinney JD, ed. The chemistry of environmental agents as potential human hazards. Ann Arbor: Ann Arbor Science publication 1980:263–278.
12. Bourne JP. A zodiac study of infertility: is season of birth associated with dysfunctions in ovulation? Baltimore: Department of Maternal and Child Health. The Johns Hopkins University School of Hygiene and Public Health, May 1974.
13. Zaebst DD, Tanaka S. Haring M. Occupational exposure to estrogens—problems and approaches. In: McLachlan JA, ed. Estrogens in the environment. Amsterdam: Elsevier/North-Holland, 1980:377–388.
14. Goldzieher MA, Goldzieher JW. Toxic effects of percutaneously absorbed estrogens. JAMA 1949;140:1156.
15. Harrington JM, Stein GF, Rivera RO, deMorabes AW. The occupational hazards of formulating oral contraceptives—a survey of plant employees. Arch Environ Health 1978;33:12–15.
16. Katzenellenbogen I. A dermato-endocrinological syndrome and problems connected with the production and use of stilbestrol. Harefuah 1956;50:239–242.
17. Hertz R. Personal experiences emphasizing the environmental impact of estrogens. In: McLachlan JA, ed. Estrogens in the environment. Amsterdam: Elsevier/North-Holland, 1980:347–352.
18. Hertz R. Accidental ingestion of estrogens by children. Pediatrics 1958;21:203–206.
19. Stoppleman MRH, van Valkenburg RA. Pigmentation and gynecomastia in children caused by hair lotion containing stilbestrol. Dutch J Med 1955;99:3925–3926.
20. Rom WN. Effects of lead on reproduction. In: Infante PF, Legator MS, eds. Proceedings of a workshop on methodology for assessing reproductive hazards in the workplace. Washington, DC: NIOSH, 1980:33–42.
21. Bridbord K. Occupational lead exposure and women. Prev Med 1978;7:311–321.
22. Chisholm JJ. Fouling one's own nest. Pediatrics 1978;62:614–617.
23. Peakall DB, Linger JL, Risebrough RW, Pritchard JB, Kintner WB. DDT-induced eggshell thinning: structural and physiological effects in these species. Comp Gen Pharmacol 1973;4:305–313.
24. Grier JW. Ban of DDT and subsequent recovery of reproduction in bald eagles. Science 1982;218:1232–1234.
25. Kimbrough RD. The toxicity of polychlorinated polycyclic compounds and related chemicals. CRC Crit Rev Toxicol 1974;2:445–498.
26. Karup T. Oocyte destruction and ovarian tumorigenesis after direct application of a chemical carcinogen (9:10-dimethyl-1:2-benzanthracene) in the mouse ovary. Int J Cancer 1969;4:61–75.
27. Tokuhata GM. Smoking in relation to infertility and fetal loss. Arch Environ Health 1968;17:353–359.
28. Neri A, Eckerling B. Influence of smoking and adrenaline (epinephrine) on the uterotubal insufflation test (Rubin test). Fertil Steril 1969;20:818–828.
29. Drac P, Kopecny J. Sterilitat bei Raucherinnen

und Nichtraucherinnen. Zentralbl Gynakol 1970;27:865–866.
30. Jick H, Porter J, Morrison SA. Relation between smoking and age of natural menopause. Lancet 1971;1:1354–1355.
31. Campbell JM, Harrison KL. Smoking and infertility. Med J Aust 1979;1:342–343.
32. Briggs WJ. Cigarette smoking and infertility in men. Med J Aust 1973;1:616–617.
33. The health consequences of smoking for women: a report to the surgeon general. Washington, D.C.: U.S. Department of Health and Human Services, Public Health Service, 1980.
34. National Academy of Sciences. Carbon monoxide, medical and biological effects of environmental pollutants. Washington, D.C.: National Research Council, 1977.
35. Leaderer BP. Air pollutant emissions from kerosene space heaters. Science 1982;218:1113–1115.
36. Levi AJ, Fisher AM, Hughes L, Hendry WF. Male infertility due to sulphasalazine. Lancet 1979;2:276–278.
37. Whorton D, Drauss RM, Marshall S, Milby TH. Infertility in male pesticide workers. Lancet 1977;2:1259–1261.
38. Lancranjan I, Popescu HI, Gavanescu O, et al. Reproductive ability of workmen occupationally exposed to lead. Arch Environ Health 1975;30:396–401.
39. Cannon SB, Vreazey JM, Jackson RS, et al. Epidemic kepone poisoning in chemical workers. Am J Epidemiol 1978;107:529–537.
40. Lloyd CW, Williams RH. Endocrine changes associated with Laennec's cirrhosis of the liver. Am J Med 1948;4:315–330.
41. Van Thiel DH, Gravaler JS, Cobb CF, Sherins RJ, Lester R. Alcohol-induced testicular atrophy in the adult male rat. Endocrinology 1979;105:888–895.
42. Hall WH. Breast changes in males on cimetidine. N Engl J Med 1976;295:841.
43. Winters SJ, Banks JL, Loriaux DL. Cimetidine is an antiandrogen in the rat. Gasteroenterology 1979;76:504–508.
44. Anand S, Van Thiel DH. Prenatal and neonatal exposure to cimetidine results in gonadal and sexual dysfunction in adult males. Science 1982;218:493–494.
45. Van Thiel DH, Gavaler JS, Smith WI, Paul G. Hypothalamic-pituitary-gonadal dysfunction in men using cimetidine. N Engl J Med 1979;300:1012–1015.
46. Wolf MM. Impotence on cimetidine treatment. N Engl J Med 1979;300:94.
47. Loriaux DL, Menard R, Taylor A, Pita JC, Sauten R. Spironolactone and endocrine dysfunction. Ann Intern Med 1976;85:630–636.
48. Lin BS. Suggestion of feeding on crude cottonseed oil for contraception. Shang-hai I Hsuch Hsueh Pao 1957;6:43.
49. Lobl TJ, Bardin CW, Chang CC. Pharmacologic agents producing infertility by direct action on male reproductive tract. In: Zatuchni GL, Labbok MH, Sciarra JJ, eds. Research frontiers in fertility regulation. Hagerstown, Md.: Harper & Row, 1980:146–168.
50. Liu ZQ, Liu GZ, Hei LS, Zhang RA, Yu LZ. Clinical trial of gossypol as a male infertility agent. In: Feu CC, Griffin D, eds. Recent advances in fertility regulation. Beijung: Geneva Atar SA, 1981:160–163.
51. Ehrhardt AA, Epstein R, Money J. Fetal androgens and female gender identity in the early treated andrenogenital syndrome. Johns Hopkins Med J 1968;123:160–167.
52. Ehrhardt AA, Money J. Progestin-induced hermaphroditism: IQ and psychosexual identity in a study of ten girls. J Sex Res 1967;3:83–100.
53. Yen SSC, Martin PL, Burmier AM, Czekala NM, Greaney MO Jr, Callantine MR. Circulating estradiol, estrone, and gonadotropin levels following the administration of orally active 17-beta-estradiol in postmenopausal women. J Clin Endocrinol Metab 1975;40:518–521.
54. Riggs LA, Milanes B, Villaneuva B, Yen SSC. Efficacy of intravaginal and intranasal administration of micronized estradiol-17-beta. J Clin Endocrinol Metab 1977;45:1261–1264.
55. Kaufman RH, Binder GL, Gray PM, Adam E. Upper genital tract changes associated with exposure in utero to diethylstilbestrol. Am J Obstet Gynecol 1977;128:51–59.
56. Rogan WF, Bagniewska A, Damstra T. Current concepts: pollutants in breast milk. N Engl J Med 1980;302:1450–1453.
57. Allen JR, Barsotti DA. The effects of transplacental and mammary movement of PCB's on infant rhesus monkeys. Toxicology 1976;6:331–340.
58. Metcalf RL, Sangha GK, Kapoor IP. Model ecosystem for the evaluation of pesticide biodegradability and ecological magnification. Environ Sci Technol 1971;5:709–713.
59. Mattison DR. How xenobiotic compounds can destroy oocytes. Contemp Obstet Gynecol 1980;15:157–169.
60. Clark JH, McNulty W, Ross GT, Haney AF, Porter JC, Sakai C. Assessment of risks to human reproduction and to development of the human conceptus from exposure to environmental substances. In: Galbraith W, Voytek P, Ryon M, eds. Advances in modern environmental toxicology, Vol. 3. Oakridge, TN: Oakridge National Laboratories-EPA publication, 1983:3–40.

61. Beach FA. Animal models for human sexuality. In: Sex, hormones, and behavior. London, England: CIBA Foundation Symposium No. 62, 1978. New York: Elsevier/North-Holland, 1979:133–144.
62. Herbst AL, Ulfelder H, Poskanser DC. Adenocarcinoma of the vagina: association of maternal stilbestrol therapy with tumor appearance in young women. N Engl J Med 1971;284:878–881.
63. Herbst AL, Hubby MM, Blough RR, Azizi F. A comparison of pregnancy experience in DES-exposed and DES-unexposed daughters. J Reprod Med 1980;24:62–69.

Habitual Abortion 15

Barry E. Schwarz

The problem of repeated early pregnancy wastage as a cause of infertility has long been recognized, and, in general, is adequately discussed in standard textbooks of gynecology. While sequential abortion is a rare cause of infertility, those couples who do have this problem often present as very anxious and frustrated people who deserve a reasonable assessment based on current knowledge and opinion. Thus, a brief discussion of sequential abortion is an appropriate inclusion in a general consideration of infertility.

The diagnosis of sequential abortion may often be made simply on the basis of history. While 1 spontaneous abortion does not constitute a sequence, the traditional requirement of 3 or more consecutive spontaneous abortions may be waived if the physician discerns an obvious etiology. Occasionally, detection of the beta subunit of human chorionic gonadotropin in a woman's serum will be appropriate if the spontaneous abortions are occurring so early in pregnancy as to make the clinical diagnosis of pregnancy doubtful and/or the obtaining of histologic evidence of pregnancy impractical. It is important to be able to document both repeated pregnancy and consistent ovulation. Women with chronic anovulation may have menstrual histories characterized by sporadic episodes of amenorrhea of short duration; and since urine pregnancy tests are fraught with technical error, many of these women may report a false positive pregnancy test. Therapy for sequential abortion will have a depressingly low success rate when applied to women with chronic anovulation.

The Probability of Sequential Abortion—The Malpas Model

In 1938, Percy Malpas wrote his classic "Study of Abortion Sequences" (1), in which he applied elementary algebra to construct a mathematical model for the problem of sequential abortion. Malpas' model predicted that 73% of women who had 3 consecutive spontaneous abortions would abort in their next pregnancy, or, conversely, that only 27% of women who had 3 consecutive spontaneous abortions would carry their next pregnancy to viability. Eastman also employed a mathematical approach to the problem (2). Using the same basic assumptions as Malpas, he arrived at essentially the same prediction. For the next quarter of a century, few investigators attempted to validate the Malpas-Eastman Model. Instead, many investigators used the Malpas prediction of outcome as a standard to which they compared their results of clinical trials of therapy for sequential abortion. These modes of therapy included thyroid replacement (3,4), local anesthetic injected near the thyroid (5), chorionic gonadotropin injection, progesterone and progestin therapy (6–8), estrogen therapy (9), psychotherapy (10–13), antibiotic therapy, vitamins and other food supplements, and various combinations of these modes (14–17). Compared to the Malpas prediction, all of these modes of therapy produced encouraging results. Interestingly, they all produced approximately the same result; that is, 75% to 80% of women with 3 consecutive spontaneous abortions carried to viability in the next pregnancy regardless of the choice of therapy. This was pointed out in studies in which a placebo produced results equal to hormonal therapy, but nevertheless much better than Malpas' prediction (18–20). Finally, the Malpas model itself was challenged by an analysis of clinical data suggesting that one could expect about 75% of women to carry to viability in the pregnancy following 3 consecutive spontaneous abortions (21).

Malpas and Eastman have been appropriately challenged on the basis of the 3 assumptions they used to construct mathematical models and because their predictions do not correspond to clinical observations. An analysis of Malpas' assumptions is useful, not only to indicate wherein he erred, but also as a background for a reasonable approach to this unusual, but difficult, problem in infertility. Malpas' first assumption was that the spontaneous abortion rate was known and did not vary with age or parity. It is remarkable that almost all studies of the incidence of spontaneous abortion done in the last 25 years have yielded essentially the same number in spite of the fact that a wide variety of clinical groups and analytic methods have been employed (21–23). There is general agreement that relying on patient histories will result in a significant underestimate of the number of early abortions (24). An intriguing approach to this problem has been the use of life table analysis (25,26). This last approach has suggested at least a 20% chance that a fetus living at the time of the first missed menses will die within the next 16 weeks. Malpas used an abortion rate of 18% in his calculations based on a clinical study of a large population of British women, but he cited 2 other British studies in which the abortion rates were 17.6% and 20% (27,28).

Malpas' second assumption was that women abort either for random or recurrent reasons. Malpas realized that recurrent abortion might have many etiologies and that a woman successfully treated for recurrent abortion could still abort for some random reason. In fact, he warned future investigators (to no avail) to be highly suspicious of clinical trials of therapy for recurrent abortion that yielded results that were too good. It seems obvious that therapy aimed at one suspected etiology of recurrent abortion could not be expected to have an impact either on other etiologies of recurrent abortion or on random causes for spontaneous abortion.

Malpas' third and final assumption was that a woman who had aborted once for a recurrent reason would abort in a subsequent pregnancy with a known probability equal to 1. This is the assumption least consistent with current knowledge, in that it implies that all etiologies of recurrent abortion are maternal and that no etiology could be responsible for a high, but less than 100%, risk of abortion.

Malpas also had to estimate the incidence of recurrent reasons for abortion in order to perform his calculations. He estimated that 1% of all pregnancies ended in abortion for recurrent reasons. Using this estimate, his mathematical model produced predicted proportions of women having a given number of consecutive abortions that was modestly consistent with clinical observations cited by him (26). Interestingly, had he estimated the incidence of recurrent abortion as 1 per 1,000 pregnancies, his mathematical predictions would have been moderately consistent with modern clinical numbers (21); all of the attempts at therapy previously cited would have been declared ineffective initially, and we might still be using his seriously flawed model as a standard.

Causes of Repetitive Abortion

INFECTIONS. The accepted and likely causes of repetitive spontaneous abortion may be grouped into 4 major categories: hormonal, anatomic, chromosomal, and immunologic. Because of experience in animal husbandry, it has been tempting to incriminate some infectious agent as a cause of recurrent abortion in women. Viruses such as the rubella virus, cytomegalovirus, and herpes simplex virus are known to be capable of causing human abortion, but these are usually single abortions rather than repetitive events. Other infectious agents such as *Listeria*, *Toxoplasma*, *Brucella*, *Chlamydia*, and *T-Mycoplasma* (29–42) have been suggested as causes of recurrent abortion, but the evidence to support these suggestions is unimpressive. Nevertheless, some reliable authors suggest, perhaps out of desperation, a course of therapy with 1 of the tetracyclines for women who have otherwise unexplained recurrent abortions.

TOXINS. Any factor that increases the risk of spontaneous abortion significantly may, by chance, be responsible for recurrent abortion in a given couple. Exposure to volatile chemicals and other toxins may, rarely, be incriminated (43,44). Careful history and subsequent elimination of the potentially offending chemical from the environment, when possible, should clarify this issue as it may apply to any particular couple.

CHRONIC DISEASE. Although chronic disease states, particularly hepatic or renal disease, are more likely to result in anovulation, it is possible that some diseases such as lupus erythematosus, a disease reportedly associated with a 40% spontaneous abortion rate, may be responsible for occasional instances of recurrent abortion (45).

HYPOTHYROIDISM. As stated earlier, hormonal therapy for unselected patients with habitual abortion has proven to be uniformly successful or unsuccessful depending on the choice of controls or expected rates of response regardless of the choice of hormone. Nevertheless, there is reasonable evidence that hypothyroidism may result in increased rates of spontaneous abortion and, thus, in habitual abortion (46–48). Thyroid replacement is obviously indicated, although there is no convincing evidence that pregnancy performance is improved.

PROGESTERONE DEFICIENCY. Progesterone produced by the corpus luteum is necessary for the maintenance of early human pregnancy. It seems reasonable to expect any early human pregnancy characterized by insufficient progesterone action (whether by virtue of decreased gonadotropic stimulation of the corpus luteum, decreased response of the corpus luteum to gonadotropin, or decreased response of the uterus to progesterone) to end in spontaneous abortion. Measurements of urinary pregnanediol concentrations or serum progesterone concentrations in early pregnancy, and progesterone or progestin therapy for progesterone-deficient pregnancies, have proven to be of no value (6–8,49,50). Inadequate corpus luteum function prior to implantation and extending into early pregnancy has been proposed as a mechanism by which progesterone deficiency might be responsible for habitual abortion (51–53). There is some argument as to whether serial measurement of serum progesterone concentrations, or an endometrial biopsy histologically 3 or more days behind dates as determined from the onset of menses following biopsy (54–56) is the more appropriate method of making the diagnosis. An abnormality should be observed on at least 2 occasions since luteal phase inadequacy may be observed as an isolated, sporadic event in some women (57). Accepted therapy must begin prior to the establishment of pregnancy. Clomiphene citrate in the early follicular phase, human chorionic gonadotropin at midcycle or shortly after ovulation, and preimplantation progesterone therapy have all been used (47,58,59). It is not clear that any of these forms of therapy are of consistent and predictable value in selected cases of habitual abortion. The use of progestins and estrogens postconception is contraindicated in all pregnancies.

INCOMPETENT CERVIX. An incompetent cervical os should be suspected in all women with a history of repeated abortion in the second trimester of pregnancy (60–62). The cervical defect may be associated with trauma or may be congenital (63–65). Typically, painless dilation and effacement of the cervix is followed by prolapse of the intact membranes into the vagina. Expulsion of the intact sac containing a normal fetus may occur, or membranes may rupture and premature labor ensue with or without concomitant chorioamnionitis. Several surgical procedures have been described as appropriate therapy for an incompetent cervix (66). The trachelorrhapy procedure described by Lash (67) has the advantage of being an interval, elective procedure. The Lash procedure is useful in the instance of known traumatic injury to the cervix, particularly if a lesion or defect in the cervix is palpable. Such a lesion is most likely to be detectable at the time of abortion. The cerclage procedures of McDonald (68) or of Shirodkar (69) have more general applicability, but must be performed in the early second trimester of pregnancy (to avoid random first trimester abortions), and preferably prior to the onset of dilation and effacement of the cervix. An incompetent cervical os can be treated with enforced bed rest beginning at the twelfth to fourteenth week of pregnancy, but compliance with this regimen for 26 to 28 weeks is understandably poor.

UTERINE ANOMALIES AND MYOMAS. Uterine anomalies may be associated with an increased abortion rate—34% with a bicornuate uterus, 22% with a septate uterus, and 35% with a unicornuate uterus (70–72). Most women with uterine anomalies will not have recurrent abortion, but some will. Similarly, most women with uterine leiomyomata, even large or multiple submucous leiomyomata, will have normal reproductive performance, but some will have repetitive pregnancy wastage. A hysterogram is the only consistently reliable method currently available for making the diagnosis of a uterine anomaly or of distortion of the endometrial cavity by leiomyomata. Surgical correction of the uterine anomaly is indicated and is often beneficial when the anomaly is associated with repeated early pregnancy wastage (73). The benefits of myomectomy for patients with significant leiomyomata are less clearly established.

GENETIC CAUSES OF ABORTION. Chromosomal anomalies in the conceptus are responsible for 50% to 60% of early spontaneous abortions (74–76), and up to 90% of these chromosomal anomalies represent an abnormal total number of chromosomes (aneuploidy) (75–78). Aneuploidy may occur sporadically as a result of nondisjunction during meiosis in either the father or the mother. Cytogenetic studies of consecutive abortuses have demonstrated a good correlation between the chromosonal status of the second abortus with that of the first (79–81). Thus, if the first abortus was karyotypically normal, 73% of the second abortuses were also karyotypically normal; and if the first abortus was karyotypically abnormal, 72% of the second abortuses were also karyotypically abnormal. In spite of this correlation, aneuploidy of the conceptus must not be a very common cause of recurrent abortion, since there is a greater tendency for couples that have had 2 consecutive chromosomally normal abortuses to have a subsequent abortion than there is for a couple that has had 2 consecutive chromosomally abnormal abortuses.

Three factors could influence the tendency to produce a chromosomally abnormal conceptus repetitively and thus produce habitual abortion: a balanced reciprocal translocation, a genetic tendency favoring nondisjunction, and an environmental influence favoring nondisjunction. Balanced reciprocal translocation carriers are found in about 5% of couples with 2 or more abortions and in about 27% of couples with a history of abortion plus fetal malformation (82). This compares to the estimated 0.2% incidence of balanced reciprocal translocation carriers in couples generally. Since karyotyping is an expensive procedure, and since a couple in which 1 individual is a carrier of a balanced reciprocal translocation would be expected to produce a phenotypically normal child one third of the time (half of these "normal" children would be translocation carriers like the parent), one may wish to reserve karyotyping for couples who have had 3 or more consecutive abortions. Most geneticists, however, currently recommend karyotyping a couple after 2 consecutive abortions.

Genes that causes nondisjunction are known to exist in *Drosophila* (83,84) and in plants (85), but have not been described in man. Nevertheless, in most instances in which 2 consecutive abortions are both genetically abnormal, the actual karyotypes are usually different (76,79,80). The incidence of Down's syndrome among viable siblings of trisomic abortuses is 10 times the expected value (79) and there is an unexpectedly high incidence of X-chromosome mosaicism in women who habitually abort (86,87). Each of these observations suggests that there may, indeed, be some people who have an increased tendency to nondisjunction. Whether this tendency can be inherited or induced environmentally is unknown.

IMMUNOLOGIC CAUSES. The relationship between immunology, spontaneous abortion, and recurrent abortion is controversial but indirectly supported by the observation that the risk of spontaneous abortion in general is proportional to gravidity, but independent of maternal age (88). Some authors have linked certain ABO blood group incompatibilities with an increased incidence of spontaneous abortion and with recurrent fetal wastage (89–94), while others have been unable to show any effect of ABO incompatibility on abortion rates

(95). No other blood-group incompatibilities have consistently been associated with early fetal wastage (96,97). The presence of sperm antibodies in either parent has been linked to an increased incidence of abortion, although this correlation has been disputed (98–100).

Several groups have recently reported an intriguing association between maternal-paternal sharing of major histocompatability antigens and recurrent abortion (101–103). These reports are intriguing, not only because there was no other known etiology for the recurrent abortions (couples with known etiologies for recurrent abortion were excluded), but also because in those instances in which chromosomal studies of the abortuses were available the abortuses were karyotypically normal. Two groups (102,103) have employed innovative and aggressive therapy (immunization with, or repeated infusion of, paternal leukocytes), and both groups have reported great success. The number of patients involved is small and the success rate may be "too good." Nevertheless, this important research may lead to important and significant advances in the diagnosis and management of habitual abortion.

Summary

A careful history and physical examination followed by a hysterogram, karyotyping of the couple, and an evaluation for inadequate luteal phase when appropriate will usually reveal the more probable causes of repeated abortion. Hospital records of previous abortions should be reviewed for the histopathology, the operative description (for clues to cervical incompetence or an anomalous uterus), and for any cytogenetic studies performed. This evaluation should then guide the physician's approach to a distraught couple presenting with the difficult and frustrating problem of habitual abortion.

REFERENCES

1. Malpas P. A study of abortion sequences. J Obstet Gynaecol Br Empire 1938;45:932–949.
2. Eastman NJ. Habitual abortion. In: Meigs JV, Sturgis S, eds. Progress in gynecology. New York: Grune & Stratton, 1946:262–275.
3. Pyle LR. The role of thyroid feedings in pregnancy. J Kans Med Soc 1951;52:589–597.
4. Dowling J, Freinkel N, Ingbar S. Thyroxine-binding by sera of pregnant women, newborn infants, and women with spontaneous abortion. J Clin Invest 1956;35:1263–1276.
5. Mink E. Relief of therapy resistance in habitual abortion by neural therapy of the thyroid gland. Zentalbl Gynakol 1959;81:1311–1318.
6. Bishop P, Richards N. Habitual abortion. Prophylatic value of progesterone pellet implantation. Br Med J 1950;2:130–133.
7. Nilsson L. Treatment of threatened abortion with progesterone. Acta Obstet Gynecol Scand (Suppl 6) 1963;42:128–135.
8. LeVine L. Habitual abortion. A controlled study of progestational therapy. West J Surg 1964;72:30–36.
9. Smith OW. Diethylstilbestrol in the prevention and treatment of complications of pregnancy. Am J Obstet Gynecol 1948;56:821–834.
10. Bevis DCA. Treatment of habitual abortion. Lancet 1951;2:207.
11. Weil RJ, Stewart LC. The problem of spontaneous abortion. Am J Obstet Gynecol 1957;73:322–327.
12. Mann EC. Psychotherapy. Habitual abortion. A report in two parts on 160 patients. Am J Obstet Gynecol 1959;77:706–718.
13. Tupper C, Weil RJ. The problem of spontaneous abortion. IX. The treatment of habitual aborters with psychotherapy. Am J Obstet Gynecol 1962;83:421–424.
14. Collins CG, Weed JC, Collins JH. The treatment of spontaneous, threatened, or habitual abortion. Surg Gynecol Obstet 1940;70:783–786.
15. Vaux NW, Rakoff AE. Estrogen-progesterone therapy: a new approach in the treatment of habitual abortion. Am J Obstet Gynecol 1945;50:353–366.
16. Javert CT. Stress and habitual abortion: their relationship and the effect of therapy. Obstet Gynecol 1954;3:298–306.
17. Wilson RB. Habitual abortion: hormonal physiology and a suggested endocrine treatment for selected patients. Am J Obstet Gynecol 1955;69:614–628.
18. Speert H. Pregnancy prognosis following repeated abortion. Am J Obstet Gynecol 1954;68:665–673.
19. Shearman RP, Garrett WJ. Double-blind study of the effect of 17-hydroxyprogesterone caproate on abortion rate. Br Med J 1963;1:292–295.
20. Goldzieher JW. Double-blind trial of a progestin in habitual abortion. JAMA 1964;188:651–654.

21. Warburton D, Fraser FC. Spontaneous abortion risks in man: data from reproductive histories collected in a medical genetics unit. Am J Hum Genet 1964;16:1–25.
22. Erhardt CL. Pregnancy losses in New York City, 1960. Am J Public Health 1963;53:1337–1352.
23. Tietze C. Introduction to the statistics of abortion. In: Engle ET, ed. Pregnancy wastage. Springfield, Ill.: Charles C Thomas, 1953: 135–145.
24. Braunstein GD, Karrow WG, Gentry WD, et al. Subclinical spontaneous abortion. Obstet Gynecol 1977;50:41s–44s.
25. French FE, Bierman JM. Probabilities of fetal mortality. Public Health Rep 1962;77:835–847.
26. Shapiro S, Jones EW, Densen PM. A life table of pregnancy terminations and correlates of fetal loss. Milbank Mem Fund Q 1962;40:7–45.
27. Whitehouse B. Obstetrics and gynaecology, and comparative medicine. Proc R Soc Med 1929–30;23:241–248.
28. Mall FP. On the frequency of localized anomalies in human embryos and infants at birth. Am J Anat 1917;22:49–72.
29. Nahmias AJ, Josey WE, Naib ZM, et al. Perinatal risk associated with maternal genital herpes simplex virus infection. Am J Obstet Gynecol 1971;110:825–837.
30. Rappaport F, Rubinovitz M, Toabb R, et al. Genital listeriosis as a cause of repeated abortion. Lancet 1960;1:1273–1275.
31. Ruffolo EH, Wilson RB, Weed LA. Listeria monocytogenes as a cause of pregnancy wastage. Obstet Gynecol 1962;19:533–536.
32. Rabau E, David A. Listeria monocytogenes in abortion. J Obstet Gynaecol Br Comm 1963;70:481–482.
33. Kimball AC, Kean BH, Fuchs F. The role of toxoplasmosis in abortion. Am J Obstet Gynecol 1971;111:219–226.
34. Southern PM Jr. Habitual abortion and toxoplasmosis. Obstet Gynecol 1972;39:45–47.
35. Giorgino FL, Mega M. Toxoplasmosis and habitual abortion. Clin Exp Obstet Gynecol 1981;8:132–135.
36. Mardh PA, Ripa T, Svensson L, et al. Chlamydia trachomatis infection in patients with acute salpingitis. N Engl J Med 1977; 296:1377–1379.
37. Driscoll SG, Kundsin RE, Horne JW Jr, et al. Infections and first trimester losses: possible role of mycoplasmas. Fertil Steril 1969; 20:1017–1019.
38. Foy HM, Kenny GE, Wentworth BB, et al. Isolation of Mycoplasma hominis, t-strains and cytomegalovirus from the cervix of pregnant women. Am J Obstet Gynecol 1970;106:635–643.
39. Caspi E, Solomon F, Sompolinsky D. Early abortion and Mycoplasma infection. IGR J Med Sci 1972;8:122–127.
40. Stray-Pedersen B, Eng J, Reikvam TM. Uterine t-Mycoplasma colonization in reproductive failure. Am J Obstet Gynecol 1978;130:307–311.
41. Friberg J. Genital mycoplasma infections. Am J Obstet Gynecol 1978;132:573–578.
42. Gracea E, Botez D, Ioanid L, et al. Genital mycoplasmas and chlamydiae in infertility and abortion. Arch Roum Pathol Exp Microbiol 1981;40:107–112.
43. Cohen EN. Occupational disease among operating room personnel: a national study. Anesthesiology 1974;41:321–340.
44. Moore MR. Prenatal exposure to lead and mental retardation. In: Needleman HL, ed. Low level lead exposure: the clinical implications of current research. New York: Raven Press, 1980:53–65.
45. Fraga A, Mintz G, Orozco J. Systemic lupus erythematosis: fertility, fetal wastage and survival rate with treatment. A comparative study. Arthritis Rheum 1973;16:541.
46. Delfs E, Jones GES. Thyroid, progesterone. Some aspects of habitual abortion. South Med J 1948;41:809–814.
47. Jones GES, Delfs E. Endocrine patterns in term pregnancies following abortion. JAMA 1951;146:1212–1218.
48. Burrow GN. The thyroid gland in pregnancy. Philadelphia: WB Saunders, 1972.
49. Yip SK, Surg ML. Plasma progesterone in women with a history of recurrent early abortions. Fertil Steril 1977;28:151–155.
50. Radwanska E, Frankenberg J, Allen EI. Plasma progesterone levels in normal and abnormal early human pregnancy. Fertil Steril 1978;30:398–402.
51. Grant A, McBride WG, Moyes JM. Luteal phase defects in abortion. Int J Fertil 1959;4:323–329.
52. Horta JLH, Fernandez JG, Soto de Leon B, et al. Direct evidence of luteal insufficiency in women with habitual abortion. Obstet Gynecol 1977;49:705–708.
53. Keller DW, Wiest WG, Askin FB, et al. Pseudocorpus luteum insufficiency: a local defect of progesterone action on endometrial stroma. J Clin Endocrinol Metab 1979; 48:127–132.
54. Botella-Llusia J. The endometrium in repeated abortion. Int J Fertil 1962;7:147–154.
55. Jones GS, Madrigal-Castro V. Hormonal find-

ings in association with abnormal corpus luteum function the human: the luteal phase defect. Fertil Steril 1970;21:1–13.
56. Abraham GE, Maroulis GB, Marshall JR. Evaluation of ovulation and corpus luteum function using measurements of plasma progesterone. Obstet Gynecol 1974;44:522–525.
57. Murthy YS, Arronet GH, Parekh MC. Luteal phase inadequacy. Obstet Gynecol 1970;36:758–761.
58. Garcia J, Jones GS, Wentz AC. The use of clomiphene citrate. Fertil Steril 1977;28:707–717.
59. Jones GS, Aksel S, Wentz A. Serum progesterone values in the luteal phase defects: effect of chorionic gonadotropin. Obstet Gynecol 1974;44:26–34.
60. Neser FN. Cervical incompetence and second trimester abortion. S Afr Med J 1959;2:722–726.
61. McDonald IA. Incompetent cervix as a cause of recurrent abortion. J Obstet Gynaecol Br Comm 1963;70:105–109.
62. Cousins L. Cervical incompetence, 1980: a time for reappraisal. Clin Obstet Gynecol 1980;23:467–479.
63. Singer MS, Hochman M. Incompetent cervix in a hormone exposed offspring. Obstet Gynecol 1978;51:625–626.
64. Goldstein DP. Incompetent cervix in offspring exposed to diethylstilbestrol in utero. Obstet Gynecol 1978;52:73s–75s.
65. Nunley WC, Kitchin JD. Successful management of incompetent cervix in a primigravida exposed to diethylstilbestrol in utero. Fertil Steril 1979;31:217–219.
66. Barter RH, Dusabek JA, Riva HL, et al. Surgical closure of incompetent cervix during pregnancy. Am J Obstet Gynecol 1958;75:511–524.
67. Lash AF, Lash SR. Habitual abortion: the incompetent internal os of the cervix. Am J Obstet Gynecol 1950;59:68–76.
68. McDonald IA. Suture of the cervix for inevitable miscarriage. J Obstet Gynaecol Br Comm 1957;64:346–352.
69. Shirodkar VN. Contributions to obstetrics and gynecology. Baltimore: Williams & Wilkins, 1960:65.
70. Jones HW Jr, Jones GES. Double uterus as an etiological factor in repeated abortion: indications for surgical repair. Am J Obstet Gynecol 1953;65:325–339.
71. Jones WS. Obstetric significance of female genital anomalies. Obstet Gynecol 1957;10:113–127.
72. Andrews MC, Jones HW. Impaired reproductive performance of the unicornuate uterus: intrauterine growth retardation, infertility, and recurrent abortion in five cases. Am J Obstet Gynecol 1982;144:173–176.
73. Strassman EO. Fertility and unification of double uterus. Fertil Steril 1966;17:165–176.
74. Lauritsea JW, Jonasson J, Therkelsen AJ, et al. Studies on spontaneous abortions. Fluorescence analysis of abnormal karyotypes. Hereditas 1972;71:160–163.
75. Kajii T, Ohama K. Niikawa N, et al. Banding analysis of abnormal karyotypes in spontaneous abortion. Am J Hum Genet 1973;25:539–547.
76. Boue J, Boue A, Lazar P. Retrospective and prospective epidemiological studies of 1500 karyotypes in spontaneous human abortions. Teratology 1975;12:11–26.
77. Lauritsen JG. Genetic aspects of spontaneous abortion. Dan Med Bull 1977;24:169–189.
78. Thiede HA, Salm SB. Chromosome studies of human spontaneous abortions. Am J Obstet Gynecol 1964;90:205–215.
79. Boue J, Boue A. Chromosomal analysis of two consecutive abortuses in each of 43 women. Humangenetik 1973;19:275–280.
80. Alberman E, Elliott M, Creasy M, et al. Previous reproductive history in mothers presenting with spontaneous abortions. Br J Obstet Gynaecol 1975;82:366–373.
81. Lauritsen JG. Aetiology of spontaneous abortion. A cytogenetic and epidemiological study of 288 abortuses and their parents. Acta Obstet Gynecol Scand (Suppl) 1976;52:1–29.
82. Byrd JR, Askew DE, McDonough PG. Cytogenetic findings in fifty-five couples with recurrent fetal wastage. Fertil Steril 1977;28:246–250.
83. Gowen JW. Meiosis as a genetic character in drosophila melanogaster. J Exp Zool 1933;65:83–106.
84. White MJD. Animal cytology and evolution, 2nd ed. London and New York: Cambridge University Press, 1954.
85. Khush GS. Cytogenetics of aneuploids. London and New York: Academic Press, 1973.
86. Michels VV, Medrano C, Venne VL, et al. Chromosome translocations in couples with multiple spontaneous abortions. Am J Hum Genet 1982;34:507–513.
87. Hecht F. Unexpected encounters in cytogenetics: repeated abortions and parental sex chromosome mosaicism may indicate risk of nondisjunction. Am J Hum Genet 1982;34:514–516.
88. Naylor AF, Warburton D. Sequential analysis of spontaneous abortion. II. Collaborative study data show that gravidity determines a

very substantial rise in risk. Fertil Steril 1979;31:282–286.
89. Matsunaga E, Itoh S. Blood groups and fertility in a Japanese population with special reference to intrautuerine selection due to maternal-foetal incompatibility. Ann Hum Genet 1958;22:111–131.
90. Reed TE, Kelly L. The completed reproductive performances of 161 couples selected before marriage and classified by ABO-blood group. Ann Hum Genet 1958;22:165–184.
91. Behrman SJ, Buettner JJ, Heglar R, et al. ABO(H) blood incompabilitv as a cause of infertility: a new concept. Am J Obstet Gynecol 1960;79:847–855.
92. Wren BG, Vos GH Blood group incompatibility as a cause of spontaneous abortions. J Obstet Gynaecol Br Comm 1961;68:637–647.
93. Morton NE, Krieger H. Natural selection on polymorphisms in northeastern Brazil. Am J Hum Genet 1966;18:153–171.
94. Cohen BH. ABO and Rh incompatibility. 1. Fetal and neonatal mortality with ABO and Rh incompatibility: some new interpretations. Am J Hum Genet 1970;22:412–440.
95. Hiraizumi Y, Spradlin CT, Ito R, et al. Frequency of prenatal deaths and its relationship to the ABO blood groups in man. Am J Hum Genet 1973;25:362–371.
96. Lauritsen JG, Jorgenson J, Kissmeyer-Nielsen F. Significance of HLA and blood-group incompatibility in spontaneous abortion. Clin Genet 1976;9:575–582.
97. Carapella-deLuca E, Purpura M, Coghi I, et al. Blood groups and histocompatibility antigens in habitual abortion. Haemotologica 1980;13:105–111.
98. Jones WR. Immunological aspects of female infertility. Aust NZ J Obstet 1973;13:219–223.
99. Isojima S, Koyama K, Tsuchiya K. The effect on fertility in women of circulating antibodies against human spermatozoa. J Reprod Fertil (Suppl) 1974;21:125–150.
100. Schwimmer WB, Ustay KA, Behrman SJ. An evaluation of immunologic factors of infertility. Fertil Steril 1967;18:167–180.
101. Komolos L, Zmir R, Joshua H, et al. Common HLA antigens in couples with repeated abortions. Clin Immunol Immunopathol 1977;7:330–335.
102. Taylor C, Faulk P. Prevention of recurrent abortion with leucocyte transfusions. Lancet 1981;2:68–69.
103. Beer AE, Quebbeman JF, Ayers JWT, et al. Major histocompatibility complex antigens, maternal and paternal immune responses and chronic habitual abortions in humans. Am J Obstet Gynecol 1981;141:987–999.

Endometriosis 16

Lewis Russell Malinak and James M. Wheeler

Histogenesis

Endometriosis is defined as aberrant islands of endometrium found in extrauterine locations that exhibit the histology and hormone responsiveness of the functional layer of the native endometrium (1–3). In the 1890s, the pathology of endometriosis was described by von Recklinghausen (4) and Russell (5). However, definitive investigation of this interesting disease began with Sampson's classic papers (3,6–21). Early studies focused on histopathology, natural history, and speculation as to etiology (3–23). Although the etiology of endometriosis remains unknown, the main theories of histogenesis can be summarized:

1. *Transtubal regurgitation and implantation.* This was initially proposed by Sampson (13,15), with experimental and clinical support by TeLinde and Scott (24,25), and others (26–33).
2. *Celomic metaplasia.* Ivanoff (34) and Meyer (35) theorized that repeated inflammation could induce metaplasia of celomic epithelium to endometrial epithelium. Novak suggested that hormonal stimuli might be the activating factor (2,36,37). Endometrium may contain an inducer of celomic metaplasia that does not require implantation for activity (38).
3. *Lymphatic (23,29,40) and/or hematogenous (16,41,42) spread* may be necessary to explain extraperitoneal endometriosis (23, 39–50), although thoracic lesions may be caused by peritoneal seeding through known diaphragmatic fenestrations (48,49).

Sampson concurred that regurgitation/implantation could not explain all tissue involvement (2,16).

Incidence

The reported incidence of endometriosis varies from 1.6% (51) to 50% (52) of women in their childbearing years. The discrepancy in these figures reflects differences in patient population, awareness of the possibility of the disease, and variability in gross and/or histologic diagnosis. Experienced clinicians have estimated that 5% to 15% of premenopausal women can be expected to harbor endometriosis (53–58). Endometriosis is the most common finding in infertile women over 25 years of age (57,59,60), and is found in 40% to 50% of infertile women at surgery (52,61–63).

Demography

The average age at the time of diagnosis is 28 years (57,63), and 75% of the women are between 24 and 50 years (2). However, endometriosis may exist in postpubertal teenagers (30,64–68) and postmenopausal women (69–72); the reported age range is from 10 to 83 years (65,73). Endometriosis has been found in women after hysterectomy, whether or not they had bilateral oophorectomy or received exogenous estrogen therapy (74–80).

There are reports of 3 men with endometriosis who were treated medically for prostatic cancer (81–83). Theoretically, the endometriosis was caused by estrogen-induced hyperplasia of the vestigial prostatic utricle (84).

Initially thought to be predominantly a disease of white women, endometriosis is found in a similar proportion of black (85,86) and Oriental (87) women.

Pregnancy and Endometriosis

Meigs contended that pregnancy is prophylactic therapy of endometriosis (88). The observed proportion of women with endometriosis who are infertile varies, although infertility is recognized as a common complaint (1,51–53,56–63,89–91). In our experience, 90% of women with endometriosis complained of infertility—60% presented with primary infertility, and 30% with secondary infertility (63). Others have found that previously gravid women with endometriosis have spontaneous abortion rates of 20% to 60% (91–97). The unusually high abortion rates had occurred as long as 10 years before the diagnosis (94,97). Following treatment, abortion rates returned to those of the general population (91,94–97).

Pathophysiology

The mechanism(s) by which endometriosis causes symptoms, including infertility, is unknown. Sampson and Meyer both noted the inflammation associated with endometriosis, but differed as to whether this was cause or effect. Formation of adhesions is associated with moderate and severe endometriosis, and their presence explains both pain and infertility (98–102). Anatomic distortion does not occur in mild forms of the disease, yet the symptoms of endometriosis may be severe (98,102, 103). Prostaglandins have been implicated as the cause of both somatic symptoms and infertility (104–106). Peritoneal fluid volume is significantly increased (107) and concentrations of certain prostaglandins are elevated in women (107–113) with endometriosis. These hormones have known effects on tubal motility, ovum release, and ovarian steroidogenesis (114–121), and their presence in increased concentration could explain infertility with even minimal endometriosis (101,103). In addition, abnormalities of prostaglandin metabolism may explain the inordinately high spontaneous abortion rate in women with endometriosis presenting with secondary infertility (94–97).

Endocrine dysfunction has also been observed. Anovulation exists in 17% of women (122) and many have presumed abnormalities of corpus luteum function (123–126). Recently, the absence of ovulation stigmata has been reported in women with mild and moderate endometriosis, biphasic basal body temperature charts, and secretory endometrium (124,127,128). Luteinization of unruptured follicles associated with endometriosis may be the cause of infertility (89,127,128). On the basis of recent prospective data, this thesis has been challenged (129).

Hyperprolactinemia has been reported in infertile women with endometriosis (103,130, 131), although regression of lesions following danazol (Danocrine®) therapy was not associated with a concomitant drop in serum prolactin (130). The relationship of endometriosis to prolactin secretion remains obscure (103).

History and Physical Examination

There is no symptom complex typical of endometriosis. Furthermore, there is no necessary correlation between severity of symptoms and extent of disease. A thorough medical history remains the best screening method for endometriosis.

PAIN. Dysmenorrhea is present in 28% to 63% of women with endometriosis (52,57,132, 133). Classically, women present with progressive secondary dysmenorrhea and are nulligravid or have not conceived for 3 or more years after pregnancy or puberty (133). Six percent of women with endometriosis will have primary dysmenorrhea (132). Deep dyspareunia occurs in 12% to 27% of women (52,57, 133). Sacral backache, accentuated during menses, is present in 25% to 31% of women (132–134). Rectal pain, suggestive of bowel involvement, is present in 4% of women (132,133). Perimenstrual dysuria or hematuria is not common, but endometriosis must be considered (74,135). Inguinal or thigh pain may be a presenting complaint (136,137).

INFERTILITY. Infertility was present in 20% to 50% of women with endometriosis in early studies that described the natural history of the disease (132,133). In later studies, 90% (63) to 100% (57) of women with endometriosis were infertile; two thirds had primary infertility (57,63). There is frequently a history of early spontaneous abortions (91–97).

ABNORMAL BLEEDING. Premenstrual spotting occasionally occurs (136). Hypermenorrhea or intermenstrual bleeding has been reported in 12% to 74% of patients (52,57,132, 133,138,139).

OTHER SYMPTOMS AND SIGNS. Contact bleeding (cervical and vaginal endometriosis) (22,140,141), monthly vulvar swelling (endometriosis extending along the round ligament to the mons pubis) (142), and acute abdomen (due to ruptured endometriomata or bowel involvement) are unusual presenting signs (143–145). Catamenial pneumothorax (pleural endometriosis) (41,46,48,49) and subarachnoid hemorrhage (dura mater endometriosis) (47) have also been reported. Perimenstrual hematuria can signal ureteral, bladder, or kidney involvement (43,78,146,147). In general, any complaint temporally related to menses should raise a suspicion of endometriosis.

PAST HISTORY. A history of any procedure involving manipulation of the genital tract must be sought. Procedures such as a laparotomy, laparoscopy, curettage, episiotomy, cervical cauterization, conization, and amniocentesis have been associated with endometriosis, apparently caused by mechanical transplantation (33,148–154). A previous pelvic operation was performed in 9% (57) to 17% (63,155) of women later diagnosed as having endometriosis. Signs or symptoms in a woman with previous surgery for endometriosis should suggest recurrent disease (155).

FAMILY HISTORY. The familial tendency to develop endometriosis is now without doubt (22,54,156–158). Eight percent to 10% of first-degree relatives of women with endometriosis have the disease (54,157,158). Inheritance is either polygenic or multifactorial (158). Moreover, affected first-degree relatives are twice as likely to have severe endometriosis, develop it at an earlier age, and have a greater risk for recurrence following treatment as are women without a family history of the disease (157,158).

SOCIAL HISTORY. Several authors have described a personality profile of the "typical" woman with endometriosis (57,89). Clinical experience has not been consistent with this stereotype, as the disease occurs across the entire social spectrum of women (85–87).

PHYSICAL EXAMINATION. General examination does not usually suggest the presence of endometriosis, although half of the women with it weigh less than normal and only 13% weigh more than normal (57).

All abdominal and perineal scars should be inspected for endometriotic foci (148,154). A cervical or vaginal exam may reveal the disease (140,141,149–153). Adnexal masses brought on by endometriosis are usually asymmetric, fixed, and cystic or indurated. Masses representing ovarian endometriosis have been found in 3% (132) to 55% (52) of women. Retroversion of the uterus with or without retroflexion exists in 42% (57) to 46% (132) of women. The presence of an immobile uterus suggests severe posterior cul-de-sac disease. The uterus may be displaced anteriorly in 20% of women and be fixed by involvement of the anterior cul-de-sac (132). Cardinal ligament involvement causes lateral uterine and cervical displacement (159).

Rectovaginal examination is essential because the posterior cul-de-sac and uterosacral ligaments are commonly involved. Tenderness and/or nodularity may be detected only by rectal exam. The uterosacral ligaments should be palpated 8 cm from the anus by sweeping the examining finger laterally to medially (89). They are indurated, tender, or nodular in 34% of women with endometriosis (57). Narrowing of the rectal lumen or tenderness are additional findings.

Differential Diagnosis

Several conditions mimic endometriosis. Pain, infertility, and abnormal bleeding occur with leiomyomata uteri. The uterus, however, is enlarged and irregularly shaped. Salpingitis usually causes symmetric adnexal enlargement and distortion with fever and leukocytosis. Unilateral salpingitis associated with intrauterine devices is an exception. The differential diagnosis of an adnexal mass, rectal pain, rectal bleeding, or hematuria all include malignancy. Endometriosis associated with malignancy was known even in Sampson's day (11,160–163). Therefore, definitive diagnosis is imperative before treatment is begun.

Concomitant Disease

Anovulation exists in 17% of women with endometriosis (122). Leiomyomata of the uterus are present in 15% (61,63) and pelvic adhesions are found in 24% to 50% of these women (63,164). Müllerian fusion defects coexist in 5% of women (63,66,67). As these processes also affect treatment and prognosis, knowledge of their presence is an essential part of the woman's management.

Diagnosis

A noninvasive technique such as a pelvic ultrasound may be helpful. The finding of a cul-de-sac or adnexal mass, or excessive peritoneal fluid, is common in women with endometriosis (107,165). An ovarian endometrioma typically appears cystic without septa, has a "shaggy" appearance, and is often associated with adhesions. Extensive endometriosis mimics the "frozen pelvis" of severe chronic pelvic inflammation, adhesive disease, or malignant neoplasms.

A barium enema is useful when colonic involvement is suspected (166,167). Colonoscopy with directed biopsy of mucosal lesions should be performed when a woman complains of premenstrual tenesmus, diarrhea, or hematochezia. A positive histologic diagnosis is helpful in planning surgery since preoperative bowel preparation should be done.

Intravenous pyelography, nucleotide renal scan, or renal ultrasound may reveal hydronephrosis or renal atrophy owing to ureteral obstruction (74,78,135). The presence or absence of renal involvement should be documented prior to surgery.

Laparoscopy is the most valuable diagnostic tool in any woman suspected of having endometriosis (55,57,59–62,65,66,103). It is particularly useful in infertile women who have no other symptoms or findings (59,101). The appearance of endometriosis varies considerably. The earliest macroscopic findings are shaggy, brownish or blue-black raised lesions on peritoneal surfaces. The size of the lesions varies from 2 mm to 5 mm to 10 mm superficial, blood-filled areas. Lesions present for a long time cause fibrosis and adjacent peritoneal "puckering." Advanced disease develops into nodules that invade affected structures. Severe ovarian disease appears as an enlarged cystic mass with a smooth but fibrotic and avascular capsule. The ovary is frequently adherent to other viscera. Dense adhesions are frequently present in advanced endometriosis. "Burned out" or inactive endometriosis appears as a fibrotic area. These may have dark hemosiderin deposits or have no pigmentation. Previous therapy may alter the appearance of any lesion.

Laparoscopic findings should be recorded in a detailed note dictated immediately after the procedure and sketched on a diagram of the pelvis (Fig. 16–1) (168). Such documentation minimizes the errors of future recall, permits classification of disease, and is useful in describing the operative findings to the referring physician and the woman. Intraoperative photography provides even better documentation of findings (169).

The most common sites of involvement of endometriosis are the ovaries (61% to 78% of women) and posterior cul-de-sac (14% to 34%) (51,132). It has been our experience that the posterior cul-de-sac is involved more often than the ovaries. The surface of the uterus is involved in 17% to 55% (51,132). Intramural sigmoid and rectal involvement is found in 3% to 4% of women (51,132,143–145,166,167) and bladder wall involvement occurs in 1% of women (51,132,146,147). Involvement of the bladder serosa is much more common. The cervix, vagina, and vulva are the most frequent sites of extraperitoneal disease, although such involvement is unusual (140–142). Disease in all extraperitoneal sites is uncommon. Distant foci in the thorax, arms, legs, etc. are even less common.

Classification of Endometriosis

Name:

Stage	Score
Stage I (mild)	1-5
Stage II (moderate)	6-15
Stage III (severe)	16-30
Stage IV (extensive)	31-54

Total:

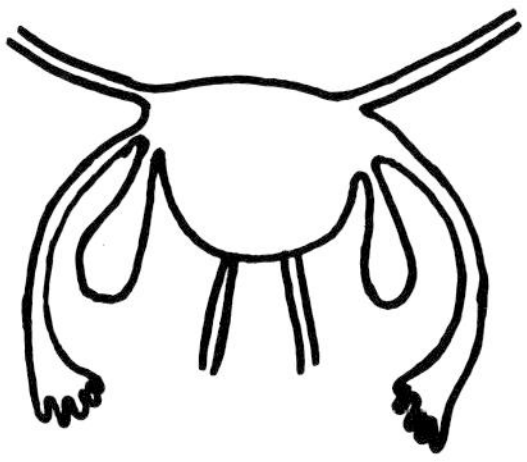

PERITONEUM

Endometriosis	<1 cm	1 cm-3 cm	>3 cm
(Score)	1	2	3
Adhesions	Filmy	Dense with Partial Cul-de-sac Obliteration	Dense with Complete Cul-de-sac Obliteration
(Score)	1	2	3

OVARY

Endometriosis	<1 cm	1 cm-3 cm	>3 cm
(Score) R	2	4	6
L	2	4	6
Adhesions	Filmy	Dense, with Partial Ovarian Enclosure	Dense, with Complete Ovarian Enclosure
(Score) R	2	4	6
L	2	4	6

FALLOPIAN TUBE

Endometriosis	<1 cm	>1 cm	Tubal Occlusion
(Score) R	2	4	6
L	2	4	6
Adhesions	Filmy	Dense with Tubal Distortion	Dense with Tubal Enclosure
(Score) R	2	4	6
L	2	4	6

ASSOCIATED PATHOLOGY:

Fig. 16–1. Classification of endometriosis. (Reproduced with permission. The American Fertility Society. Fertil Steril 1979;32:633–634.)

Cytologic smears of pelvic washings are generally not helpful (170). However, the concentration of prostaglandins in peritoneal fluid is frequently increased (110). The diagnosis of endometriosis is unequivocal only when confirmed histologically (1,2,110). In most instances, excised lesions contain endometrial glands and/or stroma (1,2,57,63,110). Occasionally, a lesion is interpreted as "fibrosis with hemosiderin-laden macrophages" or "mesothelial reaction" and these are compatible with the diagnosis of endometriosis (63,171). Communication between the surgeon and the pathologist increases diagnostic certainty. Understanding the various stages in the natural history of endometriosis will aid pathologists and clinicians in recognizing the disease. Typical peritoneal lesions should be excised with minimal tissue trauma as these are most likely to reveal the expected histology. As the amount of fibrosis increases, the number of endometrial glands decreases and, occasionally, only stroma may be identified. The avascular walls of an ovarian endometrioma ("chocolate cysts") rarely contain glands or stroma, but often contain hemosiderin-laden macrophages that represent a reaction to recurrent hemorrhage. A biopsy of several lesions will improve diagnostic accuracy and the presence of 2 out of the 3 typical elements (endometrial glands, stroma, or hemosiderin-laden macrophages) should be considered diagnostic (171).

Atypical peritoneal lesions should be biopsied as well. Endometriosis is found in 20% of petechial lesions (65). Greenblatt first proposed the existence of microscopic endometriosis and described a method of treatment that is frequently successful (65,103,110,172–174).

Classification

It is difficult to analyze and interpret the results of retrospective clinical studies since the location and extent of lesions are not uniformly described (175). Thus, a practical classification system is necessary to compare treatment results. In 1949, Wicks and Larson proposed a histologic criterion for staging the severity of endometriosis (176). In 1961, Riva et al. described a simple system to stage endometriosis clinically (177). Numerous other classifications have been proposed but a uniform and comprehensive classification does not yet exist (93,98,99,168,176–185). The classification proposed by the American Fertility Society (Fig. 16–1) should probably be used in future studies (61,184,185). A comparative study of 3 contemporary classification systems failed to demonstrate an advantage of any in predicting pregnancy rates (93). In addition, no current classification includes the clinically severe endometriosis of surgical scars, the vulva, cervix, vagina (140–142,148–153,186), or distant organ foci (41–50). None of the classification systems includes microscopic endometriosis (65,110) or malignant transformation of endometriotic foci (11,160–163).

Medical Therapy

EXPECTANT THERAPY. Expectant therapy is a reasonable option in young, infertile women with mild disease diagnosed at laparoscopy (58). This approach dictates a complete infertility evaluation and treatment of all other infertility factors (58,61,89,187–189). Expectant treatment is, thus, *not* synonymous with "no treatment" (89,188). Because of the possibility of progression, a woman treated expectantly should be evaluated regularly (187,189). Expectant therapy in women with mild endometriosis has resulted in pregnancy rates of 31% to 75% (98,190–194) and correction of anovulation coexisting with endometriosis has produced pregnancy rates of 62% to 72% (192, 195). Medical or surgical alternatives are indicated if pregnancy does not occur within 6 to 12 months of expectant therapy or if the woman prefers immediate treatment (192–194).

PREGNANCY AND MENOPAUSE. Hormonal therapy was initially based on observations that the disease regressed during pregnancy and menopause. Sampson (8) and Meigs (88) proposed that early childbearing prevented endometriosis and Goodall suggested that active endometriosis could not coexist with pregnancy (22). Sampson proposed that "retrogression" of the disease occurred during pregnancy (10). Symptomatic improvement and regression of endometriotic foci during pregnancy and the puerperium is a common experience (10,22,140,196,197). Improvement is due, presumably, to decidual change and subsequent atrophy of the ectopic endometrium (198,199). However, endometriosis may progress during pregnancy and an endometrioma may rupture as a result of softening of the capsule caused by the hormones of pregnancy (200–207). The behavior of endometriosis during pregnancy is extremely variable (208–210)—the first trimester is commonly associated with worsening of symptoms, whereas symptoms tend to regress later in pregnancy (209). Postpartum lactation and amenorrhea probably extends the period of "benefit" (89,211). From the results of studies with longitudinal follow-up, only short-term benefits are derived from a pregnancy. Endometriosis usually persists and/or recurs after delivery (155,209,210,212).

Endometriotic lesions usually undergo atrophy after menopause (198). However, active disease is occasionally present in the postmenopausal woman (69–72,74,77–80) and has been attributed to exogenous estrogen replacement or retained ovarian tissue (69,71,72,74). The disease, however, may occur in a postmenopausal woman who has had no exogenous estrogen therapy (70,74,213).

ANDROGENS. Androgens were first used in 1939 for relief of dysmenorrhea that may have been related to endometriosis (214). Despite reports of visible regression of implants (215), most studies failed to demonstrate histologic change after androgen therapy (216,217). Nonetheless, symptomatic improvement often occurs with oral or parenteral testosterone (217–221). Sublingual methyltestosterone, 5 mg to 10 mg daily for 2 to 3 months, may relieve the pelvic pain associated with endometriosis (217). Approximately 15% of women conceive shortly after completion of androgen treatment (220,221). Side effects such as hirsutism and acne coupled with low pregnancy rates and early recurrence of symptoms after treatment have prompted the use of other, more effective agents (217–221).

ESTROGENS. Stilbestrol therapy was first advocated by Karnaky (222,223) in 1948. Doses as high as 400 mg/day were associated with pain relief. However, severe nausea and breakthrough bleeding requiring transfusion were common (224,225). Anaplastic endometrial hyperplasia has occurred in monkeys (216) and women (224). A pregnancy rate of 25% and an 18-month recurrence rate of 27% have been reported (226). Estrogen therapy produces relief of symptoms (221–227) and histologic regression of nodules (226). However, estrogens are rarely recommended because of the frequency and severity of side effects, low pregnancy rates, and the availability of more efficacious medical therapy.

PROGESTINS. Medroxyprogesterone acetate is the most common progestin used (217,225, 228–231). Either oral (10 mg 3 times a day for 3 months) or parenteral (100 mg intramuscularly every 2 weeks for 3 months, followed by 200 mg every month for 3 to 4 months) administration inhibits gonadotropin secretion and induces endometrial gland atrophy (57,217). The major disadvantages of progestin therapy are persistent anovulation for 6 to 12 months following parenteral use and irregular breakthrough bleeding (217). Relief of pain and an increased pregnancy rate occur with oral medication.

ESTROGEN-PROGESTIN ("PSEUDOPREGNANCY") THERAPY. Kistner was the first to report success using high-dose estrogen-progestin combination therapy that simulated the hormonal milieu of pregnancy (232,233). Endometriotic foci develop a decidual reaction, then an inflammatory reaction, and finally undergo necrosis, fibrosis, and eventual scarring (232–236).

Complete or partial resolution of symptoms occur in 53% and in 97% of women, respectively (217). Pregnancy rates are 40% to 50% (61,76,217,232,233). Sixty-two percent of women had some form of recurrence following therapy, and 14 of 31 women with previous surgery for endometriosis required additional surgery after pseudopregnancy (212,217). Side effects include severe nausea, depression, breakthrough bleeding, fluid retention, and breast soreness with enlargement (212,217, 232,233). Thrombophlebitis has not been observed (212,217). Following cessation of estrogen-progestin therapy, ovulation and menses resume in 4 to 6 weeks (57).

Recent studies demonstrate higher pregnancy rates and more prolonged pain relief with surgical therapy than with pseudopregnancy (212,237). In addition, the frequency of side effects and the advent of danazol therapy further diminish the clinical usefulness of high doses of estrogen-progestin. However, lower-dose cyclic combination oral contraceptives commonly relieve pain in young women with suspected or proven mild endometriosis who are not attempting pregnancy (57,58,238).

DANAZOL THERAPY. Danazol is a synthetic derivative of 17-alpha-ethinyl testosterone (239). Greenblatt was the first to describe the clinical applications of danazol, including treatment of women with endometriosis (172). It has been studied and used extensively since 1975 (57,89,198,240).

Initially termed an antigonadotropin (172, 241), danazol has multiple sites of action (242). Inhibition of gonadotropin release (243–246) and synthesis (247,248) occur secondarily to inhibition of hypothalamic and/or pituitary function (246–251). Danazol also affects target organs—specifically, the ovaries (steroidogenesis) (242) and the endometrium (252–253).

Danazol has mild androgenic effects (241–244), probably because it displaces testosterone from sex-hormone-binding globulin, and this results in an increase in the serum concentration of free testosterone (253). An "atypical progestational effect" has been reported (243, 254).

Histologically, danazol-treated endometriosis appears similar to the small atrophic glands and dense inactive stroma of menopausal endometrium (172). Small to medium-sized thin-walled lesions regress in many women (198). Similar lesions in others do not respond. Large, thick-walled endometriomata are refractory to danazol, although a slight decrease in size may occasionally occur (173,198,255,256). The drug reduces vascularity and inflammation and promotes sclerosis (89). Adhesions may replace endometriotic foci after danazol treatment (198,257).

This medication is rapidly absorbed and more slowly metabolized (198). Peak serum levels occur within 2 hours of administration (258) and it has a half-life in serum of 4.5 (258) to 25 (242) hours. Metabolites, thought not to be biologically active (241,258), have tissue half-lives measured in days (242).

Definitive diagnosis is mandatory before danazol is started (242,259). Treatment should begin on the fifth day of spontaneous or induced menses to minimize the risk of treatment early in a pregnancy (198). The optimal dosage of danazol remains controversial and doses from 0.2 mg to 1,000 mg daily have been recommended (260,261). The current package insert recommends 800 mg each day, although there is disagreement as to whether taking the drug 2 or 4 times daily is best (198,242,262). Most early clinical studies reported results with 800 mg daily (255,257,263–265). Danazol may be started at 800 mg daily, but reduced in a stepwise fashion to 400 mg provided the woman remains amenorrheic (193,242). Others begin with 200 mg twice a day and increase to 600 mg, then 800 mg daily if breakthrough bleeding occurs (173,266–268). Since side effects appear to be dose related (242, 262), the authors of recent studies have used daily doses of 100 mg and 200 mg, with variable clinical results (268–270).

The average duration of therapy is 6 months (173,242,262–265,269,270). However, perioperative therapy may be as brief as 12 weeks (173,262,271). If side effects are bearable and liver function tests are monitored, a longer duration of treatment may be considered (272). Treatment for 78 consecutive weeks has been reported (242,262). Women should be urged to wait 1 full menstrual cycle before attempting to conceive because of the risk of pregnancy wastage in conceptions that occur in the first posttreatment cycle (198,242,255,273,274). Contraception is optional when doses greater than 200 mg daily are used since ovulation is inhibited (172,198,242,260). The optimum dosage and duration is, as yet, not determined.

Side effects of danazol are common, but rarely prompt discontinuation of the drug (173,242,266,271,275). The most common side effects are weight gain (2 kg to 10 kg in 3% to 15% of women), edema (6% to 10%), irregular bleeding (8%), gastrointestinal complaints (5% to 8%), vasomotor instability (7% to 8%), dizziness and weakness (7% to 12%), change in libido (6%), decreased breast size (4%), acne (4% to 13%), hirsutism (2% to 6%), and deepening of the voice (1% to 2%) (242,266,275, 276). Women with hepatic dysfunction (242, 272), hypertension (277), heart failure, or renal insufficiency (242) may experience progression of their medical condition during danazol treatment. In our experience, weight gain and edema occur in many women, but these disappear within the first month after cessation of treatment (173).

The experience with danazol is insufficient to define the rate of recurrence of endometriosis (173). Annually, 5% to 15% of all women have a recurrence (242,262).

Danazol therapy alone is most beneficial for women with mild or moderate disease. Relief of pain occurs in 72% to 100% of such women, and laparoscopic improvement of disease has been observed in 85% to 95% of women (242, 255,257,263–265). Reported pregnancy rates following danazol vary from 41% to 51% (180, 255,257,263–265,278). This drug is less effective in relieving symptoms of severe endometriosis, particularly when ovarian involvement is extensive (173,242,255,256,279–281). Danazol has been successful in the treatment of tubal (33), gastrointestinal (242), and ureteral (282) obstruction caused by endometriosis. Also, pulmonary disease has been treated successfully (283).

Danazol may also be used in recurrent disease, either as a second course of medical therapy (198,242) or after initial surgical therapy (173). It has been used successfully in women with unexplained infertility—treatment of microscopic endometriosis has been postulated (172).

ANTIESTROGEN/ANTIPROGESTERONE. Estrogen and progestin receptors have been quantified in endometriotic lesions and are comparable to those in native endometrium (284). Treatment with gestrinone (R-2323), an antiestrogen/antiprogesterone, has resulted in 100% resolution of symptoms and a 67% pregnancy rate (285).

Surgical Therapy

CONSERVATIVE SURGICAL THERAPY. Early advocates of surgery for the treatment of endometriosis recommended removal of the source of the ectopic endometrium (the uterus) as well as the source of its presumed hormonal support (the ovaries) (286,287). A few recommended preservation of some ovarian tissue (132,203,287–290). Many women have been treated with a conservative surgical procedure since the 1950s (53,91,208,291–302), in part because of the side effects of estrogen-progestin therapy (56,57,61,62,89,102, 212,237).

Laparoscopy for fulguration of endometriosis and lysis of adhesions is an acceptable form of treatment for women with mild or moderate endometriosis (273,281,303–305). However, this method is insufficient for women with severe or extensive disease. Because of the well-known risks of bowel, bladder, and ureteral injury (63,190,306–310), selective cautery of lesions is mandatory. Use of the argon laser at laparoscopy may lessen the operative risk because the depth of tissue necrosis is minimal, as is damage to underlying tissue (305). There is, however, insufficient data at this time to conclude that laser fulguration of endometriosis is superior.

A second-look laparoscopy may be useful to evaluate operative success, lyse filmy adhesions, or coagulate small foci of recurrent endometriosis (257,311–314).

INDICATIONS FOR CONSERVATIVE SURGERY (102,299,301,304,306,315). The indications for conservative surgical therapy include:

1. The presence of symptoms, including infertility, that are refractory to expectant or medical therapy.
2. Severe endometriosis.
3. Concomitant impediments to fertility that are best treated surgically (e.g., leiomyomata, müllerian fusion defects, adnexal adhesions).
4. The woman's desires, which are influenced by her age, duration of infertility, obstetric history, and career and life goals.

When laparoscopy provides the diagnosis, definitive surgical therapy may be performed immediately or may be delayed (316). With an immediate laparotomy only 1 hospitalization and anesthetic is necessary. In preoperative counseling, the woman should be given the option of immediate or delayed surgery. Ninety percent of our patients choose immediate surgery (316) and we have not observed a greater risk of complications with immediate laparotomy (63) despite previous reports to the contrary (89,317,318).

Cervical dilatation and endometrial biopsy or curettage should be performed prior to laparoscopy. A No. 8 pediatric Foley catheter should be inserted into the uterine cavity if peritubal surgery or a tuboplasty is likely. This allows intraoperative chromopertubation.

Exposure is usually adequate with a low transverse incision. A vertical incision is preferred in obese women or women with a vertical scar. Gentle handling of tissue throughout the procedure is imperative. The incision edges are draped with laparotomy packs to prevent blood and tissue products from entering the peritoneal cavity. Prior to opening the peritoneum, the surgeons' gloves should be rinsed with sterile irrigation solution to remove all talc powder (319,320). A 4-way self-retaining retractor provides reasonable access without undue pressure on the wound edges. Omental and bowel adhesions are lysed with meticulous attention to hemostasis. The bowel is packed carefully to avoid any contact of abrasive laparotomy packs with the internal genitalia. Grasping instruments and "sponge sticks" should not be used; gentle retraction with the surgeons' fingers or Teflon-coated malleable retractors is preferable. All pelvic organs are kept moist with intermittent irrigation of lactated Ringer's solution containing 5,000 units of heparin and 40 mg dexamethasone per liter that has been warmed to body temperature (306,313,321).

A stay suture placed at the junction of the

uterosacral ligaments and the cervix will afford mobility of the uterus without the use of clamps. We usually perform a presacral neurectomy and have found that this procedure consistently relieves central pelvic pain. However, a presacral neurectomy probably does not improve pregnancy rates (89,102,306,315, 322–325). The peritoneal suture line rarely provides a site for adhesions of any clinical significance. As in any retroperitoneal dissection, ureteral or vascular injury may occur, but these complications are rare in the hands of experienced surgeons (63,322–326).

Endometriotic implants are fulgurated or excised. Superficial implants may be fulgurated, but large or deeply invasive implants must be excised. A traction suture in uninvolved peritoneum adjacent to a nodule aids dissection. Electrocautery near the bladder, bowel, or a ureter may injure these structures and excision is preferable (307–310). Adequate reperitonealization of surgical defects, either with primary closure or with a free peritoneal graft, is important. We prefer the latter over a free omental graft. The round ligaments may be utilized to cover peritoneal defects such as those present following salpingo-oophorectomy or fundal myomectomy.

The extent of ovarian endometriosis varies from pinpoint lesions, which may be safely fulgurated, to invasive nodules or endometriomata, which may compromise ovarian blood supply. The decision to "shell out," resect, or perform a unilateral oophorectomy must be decided on an individual basis and depends upon the integrity of the ovarian blood supply, the amount of normal ovarian cortex remaining, the presence of ipsilateral tubal disease or lack thereof, and the condition of the contralateral tube and ovary. There is evidence that resection of a severely diseased adnexum results in improved pregnancy rates and less chance for recurrence, provided the opposite ovary is not severely involved (57,155). The ovarian cortex should be closed in 2 layers with fine, absorbable suture. Rupture of an ovarian endometrioma is common and the chocolate-like material must be irrigated copiously from the pelvis to minimize subsequent inflammation.

Patency of the fallopian tubes following careful release of periadnexal adhesions must be verified. If the dye (introduced through the No. 8 Foley catheter) does not spill from the fimbria, the possibility of tubal spasm can be eliminated by injecting 1 mg of glucagon intravenously.

The uterosacral ligaments are resected only if they are significantly involved with endometriosis (57,89,306). Plication of the uterosacral ligaments aids in uterine suspension and creates a peritoneal shelf to keep the adnexa from the depths of the cul-de-sac. This, together with presacral neurectomy, aids in relieving deep dyspareunia. Plication of the uterosacral ligaments is a simple but important step in the conservative operation. Complications are rare (63).

An appendectomy should be performed only if the appendix appears diseased (89,306) Appendiceal endometriosis is uncommon (less than 3% of women) (57), and an incidental appendectomy may complicate an otherwise sterile abdominal procedure.

Gastrointestinal endometriosis is usually superficial and rarely penetrates to the mucosa. Therefore, excision of lesions is usually adequate and a bowel resection is infrequently necessary. If a barium enema or colonoscopy with biopsy suggest mucosal disease, a preoperative bowel preparation is necessary.

Invasive lesions of the bladder must be excised entirely even if transmural resection is required. Closure of the bladder with 2 or 3 layers of fine absorbable suture will prevent leakage of urine.

Prior to closure of the abdomen, hemostasis is verified and the peritoneal cavity is irrigated. Irrigation with 100 ml to 200 ml of Hyskon®, a 32% dextran-70 solution, may reduce the frequency and extent of postoperative adhesions (327–330). Finally, the use of antibiotics, antihistamines, and corticosteroids postoperatively may also minimize adhesion formation (331–334). These medications are routinely employed in infertility surgery, and are rarely associated with complications, most of which are minor (63,335).

Conservative surgical treatment of endometriosis is associated with few operative complications (63). Subsequent pregnancy rates are 13% (288) to 94% (336) with an average of 55% to 65% (306). The severity of endometriosis affects the prognosis (180,184,185). Seventy percent to 80% of women with mild endometriosis, 55% to 60% of women with moderate disease, and 40% of women with severe disease conceive after surgery (57,61,89,93, 102,184,190–192,306,315,326,337). Approximately 80% of women conceive within 18 months of operation (63) and these women should be considered to be at high risk for obstetric complications (338). Furthermore, women who required extensive tubal repair have a greater risk for ectopic pregnancy (339–341).

Rates of recurrence are 0.9% for women followed 1 year postoperatively and 13% for those in their eighth postoperative year (155). Recurrence is independent of the severity of disease (155). Pregnancy following surgery appears to delay recurrence, but not prevent it (155,209,210).

COMPLETE OPERATIONS. Endometriosis is a benign disease that commonly exhibits malignant clinical behavior. Hysterectomy is indicated for women with severe disease that is refractory to medical therapy or conservative surgery. It is also the initial operation of choice in women who have completed their families. Ovarian tissue is preserved only if the blood supply is not impaired and the ovaries are not diseased or compromised by adhesions (70,75). Exogenous estrogen replacement should be prescribed for women whose ovaries were removed. The risk of recurrent disease with estrogen replacement (1% to 3%) is the same as that when estrogen therapy is withheld (57, 155).

Hysterectomy should be performed by the abdominal route, since careful inspection of the ovaries is important and surgical injuries are minimized.

COMBINED MEDICAL/SURGICAL THERAPY. Early studies of therapy with androgens or estrogen-progestin combined with surgery failed to demonstrate a significant advantage of this combined approach (212,217,221,237).

Postoperative danazol, however, has demonstrated promise of improved pregnancy rates (257,264,265,279,280,342–344). Many express concern at "wasting" the immediate postoperative period when conception is precluded owing to ovulation suppression with danazol. A preliminary study of infertile women with severe endometriosis, however, demonstrated a pregnancy rate of 79% following 3 to 6 months of postoperative danazol (173). The majority of conceptions occurred within 18 months of surgery postoperatively in both danazol-treated and surgery-only groups. Danazol may be indicated following conservative surgery, particularly in women with severe disease or those with known residual lesions (57,173,198,304). The rationale for postoperative danazol when gross disease is not observed following surgery is the concern that microscopic foci of endometriosis may be present (65,110,172,303,345,346).

Preoperative use of danazol may facilitate surgical removal of endometriosis and diminish postoperative adhesion formation (271). Recurrence and pregnancy rates after preoperative danazol and surgery are unknown.

Summary

Individualization is the hallmark of successful treatment of endometriosis. The young woman with significant pelvic pain should be considered for oral contraceptive therapy, particularly if she has a positive family history. Any finding on pelvic exam that suggests endometriosis should prompt laparoscopic evaluation. Failure to achieve pain relief with oral contraceptives is another indication for laparoscopy.

Infertile women require a laparoscopic diagnosis of endometriosis to stage the disease, document the presence or absence of other factors, and guide the selection of optimal therapy. Young, infertile women with mild disease have the option of expectant therapy. If this fails or is inappropriate because of the woman's age, duration of infertility, frustration, or preference, laparoscopic fulguration, danazol, or laparotomy are indicated.

The best treatment of moderate disease is usually laparotomy, although laparoscopic surgery with or without danazol may be beneficial. Severe endometriosis is a surgical disease and the postoperative use of danazol seems to improve the results.

It is important to emphasize that the management of endometriosis must be integrated into the overall management of the couple's infertility.

REFERENCES

1. Gardner GH. Endometriosis: comments on its pathology. Transaction of the Fifth American Congress of Obstetrics and Gynecology, 1952.
2. Jones HW, Jones GS. Novak's textbook of gynecology, 10th ed. Baltimore: Williams & Wilkins, 1981.
3. Sampson JA. The development of the implantation theory for the origin of peritoneal endometriosis. Am J Obstet Gynecol 1940; 40:549–557.
4. Von Recklinghausen F. Adenomas and cystadenomas of the wall of the uterus and tube; their origin as remnants of the wolffian body. Wier Nisc Wschr 1896;8:530–550.
5. Russell WW. Aberrant portion of the mullerian duct in an ovary. Bull Johns Hopkins Hosp 1899;10:8–18.
6. Sampson JA. Perforating hemorrhagic (chocolate) cysts of the ovary; their importance and especially their relation to pelvic adenomas of endometrial type (adenomyoma of the uterus, rectovaginal septum, sigmoid, etc.). Arch Surg 1921;3:245–323.
7. Sampson JA. Ovarian hematomas of endometrial type (perforating hemorrhagic cysts of the ovary) and implantation adenomas of endometrial type. Boston Med Surg J 1922; 186:445–456.
8. Sampson JA. Life history of ovarian hematomas. Am J Obstet Gynecol 1922;4:451–512.
9. Sampson JA. Intestinal adenomas of endometrial type, their importance, and their relation to ovarian hematomas of endometrial type (perforating hemorrhagic cysts of the ovary). Arch Surg 1922;5:217–280.
10. Sampson JA. Benign and malignant endometrial implants in peritoneal cavity, and their relation to certain ovarian tumors. Surg Gynecol Obstet 1924;38:287–311.
11. Sampson JA. Endometrial carcinoma of the ovary, arising in endometrial tissue in that organ. Arch Surg 1925;10:1–72.
12. Sampson JA. Inguinal endometriosis (often reported as endometrial tissue in groin, adenomyoma in groin, and adenomyoma of round ligament). Am J Obstet Gynecol 1925; 10:462–502.
13. Sampson JA. Heterotopic or misplaced endometrial tissue. Am J Obstet Gynecol 1925; 10:649–664.
14. Sampson JA. Endometriosis of sac of right inguinal hernia associated with pelvic peritoneal endometriosis and endometrial cyst of ovary. Am J Obstet Gynecol 1926;12:459–483.
15. Sampson JA. Peritoneal endometriosis due to menstrual dissemination of endometrial tissue into peritoneal cavity. Am J Obstet Gynecol 1927;14:422–469.
16. Sampson JA. Metastatic or embolic endometriosis, due to menstrual dissemination of endometrial tissue into venous circulation. Am J Pathol 1927;3:93–110.
17. Sampson JA. Endometriosis following salpingectomy. Am J Obstet Gynecol 1928; 16:461–499.
18. Sampson JA. Infected endometrial cysts of ovaries: a report of three cases, two of which were bilateral. Am J Obstet Gynecol 1929; 18:1–16.
19. Sampson JA. Postsalpingectomy endometriosis (endsalpingiosis). Am J Obstet Gynecol 1930;20:443–480.
20. Sampson JA. Pelvic endometriosis and tubal fimbriae. Am J Obstet Gynecol 1932;24:497–542.
21. Sampson JA. Pathogenesis of postsalpingectomy endometriosis in laparotomy scars. Am J Obstet Gynecol 1945;50:597–620.
22. Goodall JR. A study of endometriosis, endosalpingiosis, endocervicosis, and peritoneoovarian sclerosis: a clinical and pathologic study. Philadelphia: JB Lippincott, 1943.
23. Javert CT. Pathogenesis of endometriosis based on endometrial homeoplasia, direct extension, exfoliation and implantation, lymphatic and hematogenous metastasis (including five case reports of endometrial tissue in pelvic lymph nodes). Cancer 1949;2:399–410.
24. TeLinde RW, Scott RB. Experimental endometriosis. Am J Obstet Gynecol 1950; 60:1147–1173.
25. Scott RB, TeLinde RW, Wharton TR Jr. Further studies on experimental endometriosis. Am J Obstet Gynecol 1953;66:1082–1099.
26. Ridley JH, Edwards IK. Experimental endometriosis in the human. Am J Obstet Gynecol 1958;76:783–789.
27. TeLinde RW. The background of studies on experimental endometriosis. Am J Obstet Gynecol 1978;130:570–571.
28. Ridley JH. The histogenesis of endometriosis. A review of facts and fancies. Obstet Gynecol Surv 1968;23:1–35.
29. Hanton EM, Malkasian GD Jr, Dockerty MB, Pratt JH. Endometriosis in young women. Am J Obstet Gynecol 1967;98:116–120.
30. Moore JG, Schiffrin BS, Erez S. Ovarian tumors in childhood and adolescence. Am J Obstet Gynecol 1967;99:913–922.
31. Schenken RS, Asch RH. Surgical induction of endometriosis in the rabbit: effects on fertility and concentrations of peritoneal fluid prostaglandins. Fertil Steril 1980; 34:581–587.

32. Ridley JH. Correspondence. Am J Obstet Gynecol 1981;140:233.
33. Stock RJ. Postsalpingectomy endometriosis: a reassessment. Obstet Gynecol 1982;60:560–570.
34. Ivanoff NSK. Voprosu ob adenomimakh matki. St. Petersburg K 1907;897–920.
35. Meyer R. Metaplasia theory with inflammation as a primary inducing factor: adenomyosis, adenofibrosis, and adenomyoma. In: Veit-Stoekel, ed. Handbuch der Gynakologic. Munich: Bergmann, 1930.
36. Novak EA, Hoge AF. Endometriosis of the lower genital tract. Obstet Gynecol 1958;12:687–693.
37. Novak EA. Pathology of endometriosis. Clin Obstet Gynecol 1960;3:413–428.
38. Merrill JA. Endometrial induction of endometriosis across Milipore filter. Am J Obstet Gynecol 1970;106:516–523.
39. Halban J. The lymphatic origin of endometriosis. Arch Gynaekol 1925;124:457–482.
40. Koss LG. Miniature adenoacanthoma arising in an endometriotic cyst in an obturator lymph node. Cancer 1963;16:1369–1372.
41. Lattes R, Shepard F, Tovell H, Wylie R. A clinical and pathological study of endometriosis of the lung. Surg Gynecol Obstet 1956;103:552–558.
42. Hartz PH. Occurrence of decidual-like tissue in the lung. J Clin Pathol 1956;9:48–49.
43. Hajdu SI, Koss LG. Endometriosis of the kidney. Am J Obstet Gynecol 1970;106:314–315.
44. Labay GR, Femen F. Malignant pleural endometriosis. Am J Obstet Gynecol 1971;109:478–480.
45. Sensenig DM, Serlin O. Hawthorne HR. Pericardial endometriosis: an experimental study in dogs. JAMA 1966;198:645–647.
46. Shearin RPN, Hepper NG, Payne WS. Recurrent spontaneous pneumothorax concurrent with menses. Mayo Clin Proc 1963;46:415–416.
47. Lombardo L, Mateos JH, Barroeta FF. Subarachnoid hemorrage due to endometriosis of the spinal canal. Neurology 1968;18:423–426.
48. Foster DC, Stern JL, Buscema J, Rock JA, Woodruff JD. Pleural and parenchymal pulmonary endometriosis. Obstet Gynecol 1981;58:552–556.
49. Slasky BS, Siewers RD, Lecky JW, Zajko A, Burkholder JA. Catamenial pneumothorax: the roles of diaphragmatic defects and endometriosis. Am J Reprod Med 1982;138:639–643.
50. Felson H, McGuire J, Wasserman P. Stromal endometriosis involving the heart. Am J Med 1960;29:1072–1076.
51. Fallus R, Rosenblum G. Endometriosis: a study of 260 private hospital cases. Am J Obstet Gynecol 1940;39:964–975.
52. Williams TJ, Pratt JH. Endometriosis in 1000 consecutive celiotomies: incidence and management. Am J Obstet Gynecol 1977;129:245–250.
53. Gray LA. Surgical treatment of endometriosis. Clin Obstet Gynecol 1960;3:472–491.
54. Ranney B. Endometriosis: IV, hereditary tendency. Obstet Gynecol 1971;37:734–737.
55. Hasson HM. Incidence of endometriosis in diagnostic laparoscopy. J Reprod Med 1976;16:135–138.
56. Williams TJ. The role of surgery in the management of endometriosis. Mayo Clin Proc 1975;50:198–203.
57. Buttram VC Jr, Betts JW. Endometriosis. Curr Probl Obstet Gynecol 1979;2:1–58.
58. Ranney B. Etiology, prevention and inhibition of endometriosis. Am J Obstet Gynecol 1975;123:778–785.
59. Peterson EP, Behrman SJ. Laparoscopy of the infertile patient. Obstet Gynecol 1970;36:363–367.
60. Katayama KP, Ju KS, Manuel M, Jones GS, Jones HW Jr. Computer analysis of etiology and pregnancy rates in 636 cases of primary infertility. Am J Obstet Gynecol 1979;135:207–214.
61. Kistner RW. Endometriosis and infertility. In: Behrman SJ, Kistner RW, eds. Progress in infertility, 2nd ed. Boston: Little, Brown & Co., 1975.
62. Wharton LR. Endometriosis. In: TeLinde RW, Mattingly, RF, eds. Operative Gynecology, 4th ed. Philadelphia: JB Lippincott, 1970.
63. Wheeler JM, Meacham RB, Malinak LR. Complications of infertility surgery. Submitted 1983.
64. Schrifin BS, Erez S, Moore JG. Teenage endometriosis. Am J Obstet Gynecol 1973;116:973–980.
65. Goldstein DP, DeCholnoky C, Emons SJ. Adolescent endometriosis. J Adolesc Health Care 1980;1:37–41.
66. Huffman JW. Endometriosis in young teenage girls. Pediatr Ann 1981;10:44–49.
67. Baker ER, Horger EO III, Williamson HO. Congenital atresia of the uterine cervix: two cases. J Reprod Med 1982;27:39–43.
68. Chatman DL, Ward AB. Endometriosis in adolescents. J Reprod Med 1982;27:156–160.
69. Kempers RD, Dockerty MB, Hunt AB, Symmonds RE. Significant postmenopausal endometriosis. Surg Gynecol Obstet 1960;111:348–356.
70. Ranney B. Endometriosis III: complete opera-

tions. Am J Obstet Gynecol 1978;109:1137–1144.
71. Punnonen R, Klemi P, Nikkanen V. Postmenopausal endometriosis. Eur J Obstet Gynaecol Reprod Biol 1980;11:195–200.
72. Djursing H, Peterson K, Weberg E. Symptomatic postmenopausal endometriosis. Acta Obstet Gynecol Scand 1981;60:529–530.
73. Henrikson E. Endometriosis. Am J Surg 1955;90:331–337.
74. Sen SK, Treherne CA, Perry FA, Ashhurst JC. Endometriosis of the ureter in a post-hysterectomy patient. J Natl Med Assoc 1967;59:327–329.
75. Hofmeister FJ. Discussion. In: Ranney B, ed. Endometriosis IV: complete operations. J Obstet Gynecol 1971;109:1137–1144.
76. Kistner RW. Management of endometriosis in the infertility patient. Fertil Steril 1975;26:1151–1165.
77. Venter PF, Anderson JD, Van Weldon DJJ. Postmenopausal endometriosis: a case report. S Afr Med J 1977;56:1136–1138.
78. Stewart WW, Ireland GW. Vesical endometriosis in a postmenopausal woman: a case report. J Urol 1977;188:480–481.
79. Schram JD. Endometriosis after "pelvic cleanout." South Med J 1978;71:1419–1420.
80. Kistner RW. Written communication to Schram JD, February 1979. In: Schram JD. Endometriosis after "pelvic cleanout." South Med J 1978;71:1419–1420.
81. Oliker AJ, Harns AE. Endometriosis of the bladder in a male patient. J Urol 1971;106:858–861.
82. Pinkert TC, Catlon EE, Stransh S. Endometriosis of the urinary bladder in a man with prostatic carcinoma. Cancer 1979;43:1562–1567.
83. Schrodt GR, Alcorn MD, Ibanez J. Endometriosis of the male urinary system: a case report. J Urol 1980;124:722–723.
84. Melicow MM, Pachter MR. Endometrial carcinoma of prostatic utricle (uterus masculinus). Cancer 1967;20:1715–1722.
85. Lloyd FP. Endometriosis in the Negro woman. Am J Obstet Gynecol 1964;89:468–469.
86. Chatman DL. Endometriosis in the black woman. J Reprod Med 1976;16:303–306.
87. Miyazawa K. Incidence of endometriosis among Japanese women. Obstet Gynecol 1976;48:407–409.
88. Meigs JV. The medical treatment of endometriosis and the significance of endometriosis. Surg Gynecol Obstet 1949;89:317–321.
89. Batt RE, Naples JD. Conservative surgery for endometriosis in the infertile couple. Curr Probl Obstet Gynecol 1982;6:1–98.
90. Strathy JH, Molgaard CA, Coulam CB, Melton LJ III. Endometriosis and infertility: a laparoscopic study of endometriosis among fertile and infertile women. Fertil Steril 1982;38:667–672.
91. Petersohn L. Fertility in patients with ovarian endometriosis before and after treatment. Acta Obstet Gynecol Scand 1970;49:331–333.
92. Jones GS, Jones HW Jr. Editorial. Obstet Gynecol Surv 1971;26:539.
93. Rock JA, Guzick DS, Sengos C, Schweditsch M, Sapp KC, Jones HW Jr. The conservative surgical treatment of endometriosis: evaluation of pregnancy success with respect to the extent of disease as categorized using contemporary classification systems. Fertil Steril 1981;35:131–137.
94. Naples JD, Batt RE, Sadigh H. Spontaneous abortion rate in patients with endometriosis. Obstet Gynecol 1981;57:509–512.
95. Stohs GF, Roberts DK, Franklin RR. Relationship between endometriosis and spontaneous abortion. Presented to District VII ACOG Annual Meeting Oct. 3–4, 1981.
96. Olive DL, Franklin RR, Gratkins LV. The association between endometriosis and spontaneous abortion: a retrospective clinical study. J Reprod Med 1982;27:333–338.
97. Wheeler JM, Johnston B, Malinak LR. The relationship of endometriosis to spontaneous abortion. Fertil Steril 1983;39:656–660.
98. Acosta AA, Buttram VC Jr, Besch PK, Malinak LR, Franklin RR, Vanderheyden JD. A proposed classification of pelvic endometriosis. Obstet Gynecol 1973;42:19–25.
99. Buttram VC Jr. An expanded classification of endometriosis. Fertil Steril 1978;30:240–242.
100. Ohtsuka N. Study on pathogenesis of adhesions in endometriosis. Acta Obstet Gynecol Japan 1980;32:1758–1763.
101. Moghissi KS, Wallach EE. Unexplained infertility. Fertil Steril 1983;39:5–21.
102. Buttram VC Jr. Conservative surgery for endometriosis in the infertile female: a study of 206 patients with implications for both medical and surgical therapy. Fertil Steril 1979;31:117–123.
103. Muse KN, Wilson EA. How does mild endometriosis cause infertility? Fertil Steril 1982;38:145–152.
104. Weed JC, Arquembourg PC. Endometriosis: can it produce an autoimmune response resulting in infertility? Clin Obstet Gynecol 1980;23:885–893.
105. Weed JC, Arquembourg PC, Schneider GT. Infertility in endometriosis may be due to autoimmune reaction. Presented at the Annual Meeting of the Central Association of Obstetricians and Gynecologist, 1981.

106. Willman EA, Collins WP, Clayton SG. Studies in the involvement of prostaglandins in uterine symptomatology and pathology. Br J Obstet Gynaecol 1976;83:337–341.
107. Drake TS, Metz SA, Grunert GM, O'Brien WF. Peritoneal fluid volume in endometriosis. Fertil Steril 1980;34:280–281.
108. Meldrum DR, Shamonki IM, Clark KE, Rubinstein LM, Lebherz TB. Prostaglandin content of ascitic fluid in endometriosis: a preliminary report. Presented to the 25th Annual Meeting of the Pacific Coast Fertility Society, Palm Springs, California, October 1977.
109. Drake TS, O'Brien WF, Ramwell PW, Metz SA. Peritoneal fluid thromboxane B_2 and 6-keto-prostaglandin $F_{1\text{-alpha}}$ in endometriosis. Am J Obstet Gynecol 1981;140:401–404.
110. Drake TS, O'Brien WF, Ramwell PR. Elevated peritoneal fluid prostanoids in unexplained infertility—a possible biochemical marker for microscopic endometriosis. Fertil Steril 1982;37:302 (Abs).
111. Moon YS, Leung PCS, Yuen BH, Gomel V. Prostaglandin F in human endometriotic tissue. Fertil Steril 1982;37:303 (Abs).
112. Badawy SZ, Marshall L, Gabal AA, Nusbaum ML. The concentration of 13,14-dihydro-15-keto prostaglandin $F_{2\text{-alpha}}$ and prostaglandin E_2 in peritoneal fluid of infertile patients with and without endometriosis. Fertil Steril 1982;38:166–170.
113. Haney AF, Muscata JJ, Weinberg JB. Peritoneal fluid cell populations in infertility patients. Fertil Steril 1981;35:696–698.
114. Coutinho EM, Maia HS. The contractile response of the human uterus, fallopian tube and ovary to prostaglandins in vivo. Fertil Steril 1971;12:539–543.
115. Wentz AC, Jones GS. Transient luteolytic effect of prostaglandin $F_{2\text{-alpha}}$ in the human. Obstet Gynecol 1973;42:172–181.
116. Sun F, Chapman J, McQuire J. Metabolism of prostaglandin endoperoxide in animal tissues. Prostaglandins 1977;14:1055–1074.
117. Toppozada M, Khowessah M, Shaala S, Osman M, Rahman HA. Aberrant uterine response to prostaglandin E_2 as a possible etiologic factor in functional infertility. Fertil Steril 1977;28:434–437.
118. Lindblom B, Hamberger L, Wiquist N. Differential contractile effects of prostaglandins E and F on the isolated circular and longitudinal smooth muscle of the human oviduct. Fertil Steril 1978;30:553–559.
119. Omini C, Pasargiklian R, Rolco GC, Fano M, Barti F. Pharmacological activity of PGI_2 and its metabolite 6-oxo-$PGF_{1\text{-alpha}}$ on human uterus and fallopian tubes. Prostaglandins 1978;15:1045–1054.
120. Wallach E, Wright K, Hamada Y. Investigation of mammalian ovulation with an in vitro perfused rabbit ovary preparation. Am J Obstet Gynecol 1978;132:728–738.
121. Herman A, Claeys M, Moncada S, Vane JA. Biosynthesis of prostacyclin, PGI_2 and 12-HETE by pericardium, pleura, peritoneum and aorta of the rabbit. Prostaglandins 1979;18:439–452.
122. Soules MR, Malinka LR, Bury R, Poindexter A. Endometriosis and anovulation: a coexisting problem in the infertile female. Am J Obstet Gynecol 1976;125:412–417.
123. Grant A. Additional sterility factors in endometriosis. Fertil Steril 1966;17:514–519.
124. Brosens IA, Koninckx PR, Corveleyn PA. A study of plasma progesterone, estradiol-17 beta, prolactin, and LH levels, and of the luteal phase appearance of the ovaries in patients with endometriosis and infertility. Br J Obstet Gynaecol 1978;85:246–250.
125. Hargrove JT, Abraham GG. Abnormal luteal function in endometriosis. Fertil Steril 1980;34:302.
126. Cheesman KL, Ben-Nun I, Chatterton RT Jr, Cohen MR. Relationship of luteinizing hormone, pregnanediol-3-glucuronide, and estriol-16-glucuronide in urine of infertile women with endometriosis. Fertil Steril 1982;38:542–548.
127. Marik J, Hulka J. Luteinized unruptured follicle syndrome: a subtle cause of infertility. Fertil Steril 1978;29:270–274.
128. Dmowski WP, Ruo R, Scommegna A. The luteinized unruptured follicle syndrome and endometriosis. Fertil Steril 1980;33:30–34.
129. Radwanska E, Dmowski WP. Luteal function in infertile women with endometriosis. Presented to the 28th Annual Meeting of the American Fertility Society, Las Vegas, Nevada, March 20–24, 1982.
130. Hirschowitz JS, Soler NC, Wortsman J. The galactorrhea-endometriosis syndrome. Lancet 1978;1:896–898.
131. Muse K, Wilson EA, Jawad MJ. Prolactin hyperstimulation in response to thyrotropin-releasing hormone in patients with endometriosis. Fertil Steril 1982;38:419–422.
132. Haydon GB. A study of 569 cases of endometriosis. Am J Obstet Gynecol 1942;43:704–709.
133. Smith GVS. Endometrioma. Am J Obstet Gynecol 1929;17:806–814.
134. Chamberlain GV. Backache-II. Br Med J 1971;2:159–160.
135. Bates JS, Beecham CT. Retroperitoneal endo-

135. [continued] metriosis with ureteral obstruction. Obstet Gynecol 1969;34:242–248.
136. Duncan C, Pitney WR. Endometrial tumors in the extremities. Med J Aust 1949;2:715–717.
137. Guiot G, Levy J, Auqmer L. Sciatica caused by endometriosis (catamenial sciatica). Press Med 1965;73:1397–1398.
138. Wentz AC. Premenstrual spotting: its association with endometriosis but not luteal phase inadequacy. Fertil Steril 1980;33:605–607.
139. Cope E. Dysfunctional bleeding. Br Med J 1971;2:631–632.
140. Dilts PV Jr, Greene RR. Multiple areas of endometriosis of the ectocervix and vagina. Am J Obstet Gynecol 1965;91:292–295.
141. Wolfe SA, Mackles A, Greene HJ. Endometriosis of the cervix: classification and analysis of 17 cases. Am J Obstet Gynecol 1961;81:111–123.
142. Malinak LR. Unreported case.
143. Howard RJ, Ellis CMC, Delaney JP. Intussusception of the appendix simulating carcinoma of the cecum. Arch Surg 1970;102:520–522.
144. Meyers WC, Kelvin FM, Jones RS. Diagnosis and surgical treatment of colonic endometriosis. Arch Surg 1979;114:169–175.
145. Malinak LR. Unreported case.
146. Way S, Young JR. Ureteric invasion by endometriosis. Br J Urol 1976;48:38.
147. Abeshouse BS, Abeshouse G. Endometriosis of the urinary tract: a review of literature. J Int Coll Surg 1960;34:43–63.
148. Chatterjee SK. Scar endometriosis: a clinicopathologic study of 17 cases. Obstet Gynecol 1980;56:81–84.
149. Williams GA. Endometriosis of the cervix uteri—a common disease. Am J Obstet Gynecol 1960;80:734–741.
150. Gardner HL. Cervical endometriosis, a lesion of increasing importance. Am J Obstet Gynecol 1962;84:170–173.
151. Allan N, Cowan LE. Primary endometriosis of the cervical remnant following a Manchester repair operation. Obstet Gynecol 1963;22:253–255.
152. Gardner HL. Cervical and vaginal endometriosis. Clin Obstet Gynecol 1966;9:358–372.
153. Bentivoglio G. Histological changes in the uterine cervix after cryotherapy. Minerva Med 1974;65:3674–3675.
154. Gordon PH, Schottler JL, Balcos EG, Goldberg SM. Perianal endometrioma. Dis Colon Rectum 1976;19:260–265.
155. Wheeler JM, Malinak LR. Recurrent endometriosis: incidence, management and prognosis. Am J Obstet Gynecol 1983;146:247–253.
156. Frey GH. The familial occurrence of endometriosis. Am J Obstet Gynecol 1957;73:418–421.
157. Simpson JL, Elias S, Malinak LR, Buttram VC Jr. Heritable aspects of endometriosis: I. Genetic studies. Am J Obstet Gynecol 1980;137:327–331.
158. Malinak LR, Buttram VC Jr, Elias S, Simpson JL. Heritable aspects of endometriosis: II. Clinical characteristics of familial endometriosis. Am J Obstet Gynecol 1980;137:332–337.
159. Manna A, Gorulli R. Infiltration of the parametrium and uterosacral ligaments: a clinical sign of fundamental importance for the diagnosis of endometriosis. Quad Clin Obstet Ginec 1966;21:769–770.
160. Greene JW, Enterline HT. Carcinoma arising in endometriosis. Obstet Gynecol 1957:9:417–421.
161. Scully FR, Richardson GS, Barlow JF. Development of malignancy in endometriosis. Clin Obstet Gynecol 1966;9:384–411.
162. Fathalla MF. Malignant transformation in ovarian endometriosis. J Obstet Gynaecol Br Comm 1967;74:85–92.
163. Mostoufizadeh M, Scully RE. Malignant tumors arising in endometriosis. Clin Obstet Gynecol 1980;23:951–963.
164. Kelly JV, Rock J. Culdoscopy for diagnosis in infertility. Am J Obstet Gynecol 1956;72:523–527.
165. Konincks PA, Renner M, Brosens FA. Origin of peritoneal fluid in women: an ovarian exudation product. Br J Obstet Gynaecol 1980;87:177–183.
166. Culver GJ, Pereira RM, Seibel R. Radiographic features of rectosigmoid endometriosis. Am J Obstet Gynecol 1978;76:1176–1184.
167. Gordon RL, Evers K, Kressel HY, Laufer I, Herlinger H, Thompson JJ. Double-contrast enema in pelvic endometriosis. Am J Radiol 1982;138:549–551.
168. American Fertility Society. Classification of endometriosis. Fertil Steril 1979;32:633–634.
169. Kent PR, Malinak LR. Intraoperative photography: a sterile system. Obstet Gynecol 1978;52:365–368.
170. Portuondo JA, Herran C, Echanojauregui AD, Riego AG. Peritoneal flushing and biopsy in laparoscopically diagnosed endometriosis. Fertil Steril 1982;38:538–541.
171. Robbins SL. Cotran RS. Pathologic basis of disease. Philadelphia: WB Saunders, 1979.
172. Greenblatt RB, Dmowski WP, Mahesh VB, Scholer HFL. Clinical studies with an antigonadotropin: danazol. Fertil Steril 1971;32:102–112.

173. Wheeler JM, Malinak LR. Postoperative danazol therapy in infertility patients with severe endometriosis. Fertil Steril 1981;36:460–463.
174. DeBrux JA, Bret JA, Demay L, Bardiaux M. Recurring pelvic peritonitis: a comment on the Allen-Masters syndrome. Am J Obstet Gynecol 1968;102:501–505.
175. Hammond ED, Rock JA. Endometriosis (letter). Obstet Gynecol 1977;49:383.
176. Wicks MJ, Larson CP. Histologic criteria for evaluating endometriosis. Am J Obstet Gynecol 1949;48:611–614.
177. Riva HG, Kawasaki DM, Messinger AJ. Further experience with norethynodrel in treatment of endometriosis. Obstet Gynecol 1962;19:111–117.
178. Beecham CT. Classification of endometriosis. Obstet Gynecol 1966;28:437 (letter).
179. Beecham CT. Endometriosis: when is surgical treatment indicated? Postgrad Med 1978;63:221–225.
180. Kistner RW, Siegler AM, Behrman SJ. Suggested classification for endometriosis: relationship to infertility. Fertil Steril 1977;28:1008–1010.
181. Andrews WC. Classification of endometriosis. Fertil Steril 1981;35:124–137.
182. Beecham CT. Endometriosis (letter). Obstet Gynecol 1974;44:915.
183. Acosta AA. Endometriosis (author's reply). Obstet Gynecol 1974;44:915.
184. Guzick DS, Bross DS, Rock JA. Assessing the efficacy of the American Fertility Society's classification of endometriosis: application of a dose-response methodology. Fertil Steril 1982;38:171–176.
185. Adamson GD, Frison L, Lamb EJ. Endometriosis: studies of a method for the design of a surgical staging system. Fertil Steril 1982;38:659–666.
186. Wheeler JM, Malinak LR. Unpublished data.
187. Kistner RW. Endometriosis and infertility. Clin Obstet Gynecol 1959;2:877–889.
188. Dmowski WP. Endometriosis and spontaneous abortion (letter). Obstet Gynecol 1981;58:763–764.
189. Ingersoll FM. Selection of medical or surgical treatment of endometriosis. Clin Obstet Gynecol 1977;20:849–864.
190. Garcia CR, David SS. Pelvic endometriosis: infertility and pelvic pain. Am J Obstet Gynecol 1977;129:740–747.
191. Decker HW, Lopez H. Conservative surgical therapy of endometriosis and infertility. Infertility 1979;2:155–164.
192. Schenken RS, Malinak LR. Conservative surgery vs. expectant management for the infertile patient with mild endometriosis. Fertil Steril 1982;37:183–187.
193. Seibel MM, Berger MJ, Weinstein FG, Taymor MC. The effectiveness of danazol on subsequent fertility in minimal endometriosis. Fertil Steril 1982;38:534–537.
194. Portuondo JA, Echanojauregui AD, Herran C, Alijarte I. Early conception in patients with untreated mild endometriosis. Fertil Steril 1983;39:22–25.
195. Dmowski WP, Cohen MR, Wihlen JC. Endometriosis and ovulatory failure: does it occur? In: Greenblatt RB, ed. Recent advances in endometriosis. Amsterdam: Excerpta Medica 1976:129–136.
196. Beischer NO. Endometriosis of an episiotomy scar cured by pregnancy. Obstet Gynecol 1966;28:15–21.
197. Gainey HL, Keele JE, Nicolay KS. Endometriosis in pregnancy: clinical observation. Am J Obstet Gynecol 1965;91:292–295.
198. Dmowski WP. Current concepts in the management of endometriosis. Obstet Gynecol Annu 1981;10:279–311.
199. Mocquot P, Musset R. Remarques sur la physiologie pathologique des endometriosis à propos de trois observations d'endometriose du cul-de-sac postérieur du vagin. Gynecologie et Obstetrique 1949;48:135–154.
200. Fredrickson H. Association of pregnancy and endometriosis. Acta Obstet Gynecol Scand 1957;36:481–491.
201. Anderson M, Edmond RM. Rupture of an endometriotic cyst in late pregnancy. J Obstet Gynaecol Br Comm 1974;81:907–909.
202. Clement PB. Perforation of the sigmoid colon during pregnancy: a rare complication of endometriosis. Br J Obstet Gynaecol 1977;84:548–550.
203. Scott RB. Endometriosis and pregnancy—with a report of two cases. Am J Obstet Gynecol 1944;47:608–632.
204. Pratt JH, Riggins RS, Fourst GT Jr. Ruptured endometrial cysts as a cause of acute abdominal symptoms (endometrial pelvic peritonitis). Am J Obstet Gynecol 1952;63:90–98.
205. Brill HM, Rapaport L, Kaplan S. Intrapartum rupture of bilateral ovarian endometrial cysts—case report. Am J Obstet Gynecol 1957;73:200–201.
206. Noel LFE. Rupture of bilateral endometriotic cysts in later pregnancy simulating accidental haemorrhage. J Obstet Gynaecol Br Comm 1971;68:1051–1053.
207. Tawa K. Ovarian tumors in pregnancy. Am J Obstet Gynecol 1964;90:511–516.
208. Devereux WP. Endometriosis: long-term ob-

servation with particular reference to incidence of pregnancy. Obstet Gynecol 1963; 22:444–450.
209. McArthur JW, Ulfelder H. The effect of pregnancy upon endometriosis. Obstet Gynecol Surv 1965;20:209–233.
210. Walton LA. A reexamination of endometriosis after pregnancy. J Reprod Med 1977;19:341–344.
211. Meigs JV. Endometrial hematomas of the ovary. Boston Med Surg J 1922;187:1–13.
212. Andrews WC, Larsen GD. Endometriosis: treatment with hormonal pseudopregnancy and/or operation. Am J Obstet Gynecol 1979; 118:643–649.
213. Wheeler JM, Malinak LR. Unpublished data.
214. Salmon UJ, Geist SH, Walter RI. Treatment of dysmenorrhea with testosterone propionate. Am J Obstet Gynecol 1939;38:264–273.
215. Creadick RN. The non-surgical treatment of endometriosis. NC Med J 1950;11:576–577.
216. Scott RB, Wharton LR Jr. The effects of testosterone on experimental endometriosis in rhesus monkeys. Am J Obstet Gynecol 1959; 78:1020–1027.
217. Andrews WC. Medical vs. surgical therapy of endometriosis. Clin Obstet Gynecol 1980; 23:917–930.
218. Hamblen EC. Androgenic treatment of women. South Med J 1957;50:743–752.
219. Preston SN, Campbell HB. Pelvic endometriosis treatment with methyltestosterone. Obstet Gynecol 1953;2:152–157.
220. Katayama KP, Manuel M, Jones HW Jr, Jones GS. Methyltestosterone treatment of infertility associated with pelvic endometriosis. Fertil Steril 1976;27:83–86.
221. Hammond MG, Hammond CB, Parker RT. Conservative treatment of endometriosis externa: the effects of methyltestosterone therapy. Fertil Steril 1978;29:651–654.
222. Karnaky KJ. The use of stilbestrol for endometriosis. South Med J 1948;41:1109–1111.
223. Karnaky KJ. Endometriosis (letter). JAMA 1955; 157:267.
224. Douglass CF, Weed JC. Endometriosis treated with prolonged administration of diethylstilbestrol. Obstet Gynecol 1957;13:744–748.
225. Kistner RW. Endometriosis. In: Sciarro JJ, ed. Gynecology and Obstetrics. Hagerstown, Md.: Harper & Row, 1977.
226. Haskins AL, Woolf B. Stilbestrol-induced hyper-hormonal amenorrhea for the treatment of pelvic endometriosis. Obstet Gynecol 1955;5:113–122.
227. Bickers W. Stilbestrol in endometriosis. South Med J 1949;42:229–232.
228. Moghissi KS, Boyce CR. Management of endometriosis with oral medroxyprogesterone acetate. Obstet Gynecol 1976;47:265–267.
229. Gunning JE, Moyer D. The effect of medroxyprogesterone acetate on endometriosis in the human female. Fertil Steril 1967;18:759–774.
230. Timonen S, Johansson CJ. Endometriosis treated with lynestrenol. Ann Chir Gynaecol 1968;57:144–147.
231. Johnston WIH. Dydrogesterone and endometriosis. Br J Obstet Gynaecol 1976;83:77–80.
232. Kistner RW. The use of newer progestins in the treatment of endometriosis. Am J Obstet Gynecol 1958;75:264–278.
233. Kistner RW. The treatment of endometriosis by inducing pseudopregnancy with ovarian hormones: a report of 58 cases. Fertil Steril 1959;10:539–556.
234. Lebherz TB, Fobes CD. Management of endometriosis with norprogesterone. Am J Obstet Gynecol 1961;81:102–110.
235. Andrews MC, Andrews WC, Strauss AF. Effects of progestin-induced pseudopregnancy on endometriosis: clinical and microscopic studies. Am J Obstet Gynecol 1959;78:776–785.
236. Kourides IA, Kistner RW. Three new synthetic progestins in the treatment of endometriosis. Obstet Gynecol 1968;31:821–828.
237. Hammond CB, Rock JA, Parker RT. Conservative treatment of endometriosis: the effect of limited surgery and hormonal pseudopregnancy. Fertil Steril 1976;27:756–766.
238. Buttram VC Jr. Cyclic use of combination oral contraceptives and the severity of endometriosis. Fertil Steril 1979;31:347–348.
239. Manson AJ, Stonner FW, Neumann HC, et al. Steroidal heterocycles: VII. Androstano [2,3-d] isoxozoles and related compounds. J Med Chem 1963;6:1–9.
240. Plano VF. Danazol: review of recent studies. JAOA 1980;79:530–534.
241. Potts O. Pharmacology of danazol. In: Greenblatt RB, ed. Recent advances in endometriosis. Amsterdam: Excerpta Medica 1976:1–13.
242. Barbieri RL, Ryan KJ. Danazol: endocrine pharmacology and therapeutic application. Am J Obstet Gynecol 1982;141:453–463.
243. Dmowski WP, Scholar HFL, Mahesh VB, Greenblatt RB. Danazol: a synthetic steroid derivative with interesting physiologic properties. Fertil Steril 1971;22:9–18.
244. Dmowski WP. Endocrine properties and clinical application of danazol. Fertil Steril 1978;31:237–251.
245. Elridge JC, Dmowski WP, Mahesh VB. Effects of castration of immature rats on serum FSH

and LH, and of various steroid treatments after castration. Biol Reprod 1974;10:438–446.
246. Pedroza E, Vilchez-Martinez JA, Arimura A, Schally AV. Danazol effects on gonadotropin basal levels and pituitary responsiveness to LH-RH in immature male rats. Contraception 1978;17:61–69.
247. Franchimont P, Cramilion C. The effect of danazol on anterior pituitary function. Fertil Steril 1977;28:814–817.
248. Shane JM, Kates R, Barbieri RL, Todd RB, Davis IJ. Pituitary gonadotropin responsiveness with danazol. Fertil Steril 1978;29:637–639.
249. Vilchez-Martinez JA, Pedroza E, Arimura A, Schally AV. Effects of danazol on gonadotropin secretion after ovariectomy in rats. Contraception 1978;17:283–290.
250. Jones GS. Discussion. Am J Obstet Gynecol 1975;121:817.
251. Riedl H-H, Semm K. Mechanism and influence of antigonadotropin—treatment with danazol (Winobanin): clinical experiences with a 3-step-therapy for extragenital endometriosis. In: Semm K, Greenblatt RB, Mettler L, eds. Genital endometriosis in infertility. New York: Thieme-Stratton Inc., 1982:43–54.
252. Woods GP, Wu CH, Flickinger GL, Mikhail G. Hormonal changes associated with danazol therapy. Obstet Gynecol 1975;45:302–304.
253. Stevens SR, Smith RG. Interaction of danazol with steroid receptors and serum binding proteins in the human. Clin Chem 1979;25(6):1108 (Abs).
254. Wentz AC, Jones GS, Sapp KC, King TM. Progestational activity of danazol in the human female subject. Am J Obstet Gynecol 1976;126:378–384.
255. Dmowski WP, Cohen MR. Antigonadotropin (danazol) in the treatment of endometriosis. Am J Obstet Gynecol 1978;130:41–48.
256. Chalmers JA. Danazol in the treatment of endometriosis. Drugs 1980;19:331–341.
257. Dmowski WP, Cohen MR. Treatment of endometriosis with an antigonadotropin, danazol: a laparoscopic and histologic evaluation. Obstet Gynecol 1975;46:147–154.
258. Davison C, Banks W, Fritz A. The absorption, distribution, and metabolic fate of danazol in rats, monkeys, and human volunteers. Arch Int Pharmacodyn Ther 1976;221:294–310.
259. Wallach EE, Buttram VC Jr, Dmowski WP, Hammond CB. Finding the best treatment for endometriosis—a symposium. Contemp Obstet Gynecol 1980;15:70–120.
260. Gambrell AD Jr, Greenblatt RB. Treatment of infertility due to endometriosis with low dosages of danazol. Fertil Steril 1982;37:304 (Abs).
261. Lind T, Cook DB. How does danazol work? Lancet 1976;2:1401 (letter).
262. Barbieri RL, Canick JA, Makris A, Todd RB, Davies IJ, Ryan KJ. Danazol inhibits steroidogenesis. Fertil Steril 1977;28:809–813.
263. Friedlander RL. The treatment of endometriosis with danazol. J Reprod Med 1973;10:197–199.
264. Greenblatt RB, Tzingounis V. Danazol treatment of endometriosis: long term follow-up. Fertil Steril 1979;32:518–520.
265. Lauerson NH, Wilson KH, Birnbaum S. Danazol: an antigonadotropic agent in the treatment of pelvic endometriosis. Am J Obstet Gynecol 1973;123:742–747.
266. Ward GD. Dosage aspects of danazol therapy in the treatment of endometriosis. Postgrad Med J 1977;55:7–9.
267. Biberoglu KO, Behrman SJ. Dosage aspects of danazol therapy in endometriosis: short term and long term effectiveness. Am J Obstet Gynecol 1981;139:645–654.
268. Moore EE, Harger JH, Rock JA, Archer DF. Management of pelvic endometriosis with low dose danazol. Fertil Steril 1981;36:15–19.
269. Dmowski WP, Kapetanakis E, Scommegna A. Variable effects of danazol on endometriosis at 4 low-dose levels. Obstet Gynecol 1982;59:408–415.
270. Chalmers JA. Treatment of endometriosis with reduced dosage schedules of danazol. Scot Med J 1982;27:143–146.
271. Buttram VC Jr, Belue JB, Reiter R. Interim report of a study of danazol for the treatment of endometriosis. Fertil Steril 1982;39:478–483.
272. Pearson K, Zimmerman HJ. Danazol and liver damage. Lancet 1980;1:645–646.
273. Daniell F, Christianson D. Combined laparoscopic surgery and danazol therapy of endometriosis externa. Fertil Steril 1981;35:521–525.
274. Peress MR, Krentner AK, Mathur NS, et al. Female pseudohermaphroditism with somatic chromosomal anomaly in association with in utero exposure to danazol. Am J Obstet Gynecol 1982;142:708–709.
275. Rakoff AE. Side effects of danazol therapy. In: Greenblatt RB, ed. Advances in endometriosis. Amsterdam: Excerpta Medica 1976:108–115.
276. Spooner JB. Classification of side effects to danazol therapy. J Int Med Res 1977;5:15–17.
277. Bretza JA, Novey HS, Vaziri ND, Warner AS. Hypertension, a complication of danazol therapy. Arch Int Med 1980;140:1379–1380.

278. Van Zyl JA, Muller MS, Van Niekerk WA. Danazol in the treatment of endometriosis externa. S Afr Med J 1980;58:591–598.
279. Noble AD, Letchworth AT. Preliminary observation of the use of danazol in endometriosis compared to estrogen/progestin combination therapy. J Int Med Res 1977;5:79–81.
280. Chalmers JA, Shervington PC. Danazol: follow-up of patients with endometriosis treated with danazol. Postgrad Med J 1979;55:44–47.
281. Mettler L, Semm K. Clinical and biochemical experience with danazol in the treatment of endometriosis in cases with female infertility. Postgrad Med J 1979;55:27–30.
282. Gardner B, Whitaker RH. The use of danazol for ureteral obstruction caused by endometriosis. J Urol 1981;125:117–118.
283. Ronnberg Z, Ylostulo P. Treatment of pulmonary endometriosis with danazol. Acta Obstet Gynecol Scand 1981;60:77–78.
284. Janne O, Kauppila A, Kokko E, Lantto T, Ronnberg L, Vihko R. Estrogen and progestin receptors in endometriosis lesions: comparison with endometrial tissue. Am J Obstet Gynecol 1982;141:562–566.
285. Coutinho EM. Treatment of endometriosis with gestrinone (R-2323) a synthetic antiestrogen, antiprogesterone. Am J Obstet Gynecol 1982;144:895–898.
286. Dannreuther WT. The treatment of pelvic endometriosis. Am J Obstet Gynecol 1941;41:461–474.
287. Cashman BZ. Hysterectomy with preservation of ovarian tissue in the treatment of endometriosis. Am J Obstet Gynecol 1942;47:484–493.
288. Holmes WR. Endometriosis. Am J Obstet Gynecol 1942;43:255–266.
289. Payne FL. The clinical aspects of pelvic endometriosis. Am J Obstet Gynecol 1940;39:373–382.
290. Counsellor VS. The clinical significance of endometriosis. Am J Obstet Gynecol 1939;37:788–792.
291. Whitehouse DB, Bates A. Endometriosis: the results of conservative surgery. J Obstet Gynaecol Br Emp 1955;62:378–384.
292. Fallon J. The clinical aspects of endometriosis. Ann West Med Surg 1950;4:321–326.
293. Counsellor V, Crenshaw JL Jr. A clinical and surgical review of endometriosis. Am J Obstet Gynecol 151;62:930–942.
294. TeLinde RW, Scott RB. Diagnosis and treatment of endometriosis. G.P. Am Academy of General Practice 1952;5:61–65.
295. Fearl CL. Endometriosis—will conservative surgery increase fertility? West J Surg Obstet Gynecol 1962;18:96–99.
296. McCoy JB, Bradford WZ. Surgical treatment of endometriosis with conservation of reproductive potential. Am J Obstet Gynecol 1963;87:394–398.
297. Sheets JL, Symmonds RE, Banner EA. Conservative surgical management of endometriosis. Obstet Gynecol 1964;23:625–628.
298. Green TH. Conservative surgical treatment of endometriosis. Clin Obstet Gynecol 1966;9:293–308.
299. Rogers SF, Jacobs WM. Infertility and endometriosis: conservative surgical approach. Fertil Steril 1968;19:529–536.
300. Parsons L. Conservative surgical management of external endometriosis. Obstet Gynecol 1968;32:576–579.
301. Ranney B. Endometriosis I: Conservative operations. Am J Obstet Gynecol 1970;107:743–753.
302. Spangler DB, Jones GS, Jones HW Jr. Infertility due to endometriosis: conservative surgical therapy. Am J Obstet Gynecol 1971;109:850–857.
303. Audebert AJ, Larrne-Charlus S, Emperaire TC. Danazol—endometriosis and infertility, a review of 62 patients treated with danazol. Postgrad Med J 1979;55:10–13.
304. Cohen MR. Laparoscopic diagnosis and pseudomenopause treatment of endometriosis with danazol. Clin Obstet Gynecol 1980;23:901–915.
305. Keye WR Jr, Matson GA, Dixon J. The use of the argon laser in the treatment of experimental endometriosis. Fertil Steril 1983;39:26–29.
306. Malinak LR. Infertility and endometriosis: operative technique, clinical staging and prognosis. Clin Obstet Gynecol 1980;23:925–935.
307. Hasson HM. Electrocoagulation of pelvic endometriotic lesions with laparoscopic control. Am J Obstet Gynecol 1972;135:115–121.
308. Cheng YS. Ureteral injury resulting from laparoscopic fulguration of endometriosis implants. Am J Obstet Gynecol 1976;126:1045–1046.
309. Rioux JE, Yuzpe AA. Electrosurgery untangled. Contemp Obstet Gynecol 1974;4:118–124.
310. Rioux JE, Yuzpe AA. Know thy generator! Contemp Obstet Gynecol 1975;6:52–64.
311. Diamond E. Lysis of postoperative adhesions and infertility. Fertil Steril 1979;31:287–295.
312. Swolin K. Electromicrosurgery and salpingostomy: long term results. Am J Obstet Gynecol 1975;121:418–419.
313. Surrey MW, Friedman S. Second look laparoscopy after reconstructive pelvic surgery for infertility. J Reprod Med 1982;27:658–660.

314. Raj SG, Hulka JF. Second look laparoscopy in infertility. Fertil Steril 1982;37:294 (Abs).
315. Buttram VC Jr. Surgical therapy of endometriosis in the infertile female: a modified approach. Fertil Steril 1979;32:635–640.
316. Malinak LR. Laparoscopy—immediate laparotomy in the infertile female. Presented at the American Fertility Society, New Orleans, Louisiana, March 1978.
317. Garcia CR, Mastrioanni LJ. Microsurgery for treatment of adnexal disease. Fertil Steril 1980;34:413–424.
318. Corson SL. Microsurgery for treatment of adnexal disease. Fertil Steril 1981;35:367 (letter).
319. Yaffe H, Reinhartz T, Laufer N, Beyth Y. Potentially deleterious effect of cornstarch glove powder in tubal reconstructive surgery. Fertil Steril 1978;29:699–701.
320. Tolbert TW, Brown JL. Surface powder on surgical gloves. Arch Surg 1980;115:729–730.
321. Glucksman DL. The effect of topically applied corticosteroid in the prevention of peritoneal adhesions: an experimental approach with a review of the literature. Surgery 1966; 60:352–360.
322. Schmitze HE, Towne JE. The treatment of pelvic endometriosis. Am J Obstet Gynecol 1948;55:583–590.
323. Black WT. Use of presacral sympathectomy in treatment of dysmenorrhea. Am J Obstet Gynecol 1964;89:16–22.
324. Polan ML, DeCherney A. Presacral neurectomy for pelvic pain in infertility. Fertil Steril 1980;34:557–560.
325. Puolakka J, Kauppola A, Ronnberg L. Results in the operative treatment of pelvic endometriosis. Acta Obstet Gynecol Scand 1980; 59:429–431.
326. Hammond CB, Haney AF. Conservative surgical treatment of endometriosis: 1978. Fertil Steril 1978;30:497–509.
327. Dizerega GS, Hodgen GD. Prevention of postoperative tubal adhesions: comparative study of commonly used agents. Am J Obstet Gynecol 1980;136:173–178.
328. Holtz G, Baker ER. Inhibition of peritoneal adhesion reformation after lysis with 32% dextran-70. Fertil Steril 1980;34:394–395.
329. Malinak LR, Buttram VC Jr. Adhesion suppression in infertility surgery: systemic and intraperitoneal therapy following conservative operation for endometriosis. Fertil Steril 1972;28:326–329.
330. Dizerega G, Utian W. Efficacy of 32% dextran-70 in the prevention of peritoneal adhesions and the utility of second look laparoscopy in infertility. Fertil Steril 1982;37:291 (Abs).
331. Horne HW Jr, Jacintho V. A new medical adjuvant to infertility surgery: a preliminary report. Fertil Steril 1966;17:792–796.
332. Horne HW Jr, Clayman M, Debrovner G, et al. The prevention of postoperative pelvic adhesions following conservative operative treatment for human infertility. Int J Fertil 1973; 18:109–115.
333. Replogle RL, Johnson R, Gross RE. Prevention of postoperative intestinal adhesions with combined promethazine and dexamethasone therapy: experimental and clinical studies. Ann Surg 1966:163:580–588.
334. O'Brien WF, Drake TS, Bilro MC. The use of ibuprofen and dexamethasone in the prevention of postoperative adhesion formation. Obstet Gynecol 1982;60:373–378.
335. Magyar DM, Hayes MF, Moghissi KS, Subrammamun MG. Pituitary-adrenal function following administration of the dexamethasone-promethazine antiadhesions regimen. Fertil Steril 1982;37:292 (Abs).
336. Norwood GE. Sterility and fertility in women with pelvic endometriosis. Clin Obstet Gynecol 1960;3:456–471.
337. Sadigh H, Naples JD, Batt RE. Conservative surgery for endometriosis in the infertile couple. Obstet Gynecol 1977;49:562–566.
338. Poulson AM, Bryner WA. The obstetric complications of the infertility patient. Obstet Gynecol 1977;49:174–179.
339. Jansen RPS. Abortion incidence following fallopian tube repair. Obstet Gynecol 1980; 56:499–502.
340. Ranney B, Chastain D. Ovarian function, reproduction and later operations following adnexal surgery. Obstet Gynecol 1978;51:521–527.
341. Wist A. Endometriosis and tubal pregnancy. Ann Chir Gynaecol 1968;57:161–162.
342. Ingerslev M. Experience with danazol in severe and extensive endometriosis. J Int Med Res 1977;5:81–84.
343. Hirschowitz JS, Soler NC, Wortsman J. Sex steroid levels during treatment of endometriosis. Obstet Gynecol 1979;54:448–450.
344. Ronnberg L, Ylostalo P, Jorvineu PA. Effects of danazol in the treatment of severe endometriosis. Postgrad Med J 1979;55:21–23.
345. van Dijk JG, Frolich M, Brand EC, van Hall EV. Treatment of unexplained infertility with danazol. Postgrad Med J 1979;55:79–80.
346. Greenblatt RB. Danazol in the treatment of infertility. Drugs 1980;19:362–369.

Artificial Insemination 17

James Aiman

Artificial insemination is not a treatment for infertility but is usually a means of circumventing an insurmountable barrier to fertility, and, ultimately, a tacit admission that specific therapy has failed or does not exist. Physicians who perform and couples who receive artificial insemination must understand this because of the enormous potential for psychologic trauma and marital stress (Chapter 2).

Counseling

The indications and contraindications, the timing and technique, the probability of success, the risks and complications, the chances of having a child with a birth defect, mechanisms for assuring anonymity, selection of a donor (if the husband's semen is not used), and the cost of artificial insemination should be understood by the couple before they make a decision to begin. The couple should be given sufficient opportunity to ask questions, to voice any concern, and to stipulate any requirements (e.g., physical characteristics of a donor). Most couples are not prepared to accept artificial insemination, especially with donor semen, until they can accept that there is no other means of having a child or of reducing a high risk of transmitting a genetic disorder. Each couple should be told all the options available to them: adoption, medical or surgical therapy of oligospermia or azoospermia, going without (further) children, foster parenthood, or others. In summary, this initial discussion of artificial insemination is an opportunity for the couple to gather information and not a forum to be persuaded to proceed. One-third to one-half of couples choose not to proceed further with artificial donor insemination after receiving this information. Of those couples who sign a consent to proceed, approximately 25% choose not to begin or to stop artificial insemination before pregnancy occurs (Table 17–1) (1). The reasons given by these couples are listed in Table 17–2. Many of these reasons reflect psychologic concerns about the procedure. Donor selection, anonymity, the technique of insemination, fear of the consequences (e.g., malformations and problems during pregnancy), and moral concerns are the topics most frequently raised by these couples (2–5).

Indications

ARTIFICIAL INSEMINATION—HUSBAND'S SEMEN (AIH). Indications for artificial insemination using the husband's semen (AIH) are listed in Table 17–3 (6–9). These can be grouped into 3 categories: subnormal semen, failure to deliver a sufficient number of sperm to the cervical os, and failure of sperm migration in the female genital tract.

Oligospermia is the most frequent indication for AIH and success rates are related to the degree of oligospermia. If the ejaculate volume is greater than 3 ml, the more concentrated portion of a split ejaculate should be inseminated. Since 80% or more of the sperm in an ejaculate appear in the first portion, sperm can be concentrated by requesting the

TABLE 17–1. Outcome of Couples Consenting to Artificial Insemination with Donor Semen (AID)

	NO.	PERCENT
Couples consenting	135	
Couples choosing not to start	14	10.4
Women stopping AID	22	16.3

Reproduced with permission. Aiman J. Fertil Steril 1982;37:94–99.

TABLE 17–2. Reasons for Not Starting or Stopping AID

	NO. NOT STARTING	NO. STOPPING
Moved	5	2
Chose to adopt	0	5
Psychologic problem	0	5
Ethical concern	1	1
Marital problems	1	2
Financial problems	1	1
Pregnancy	1	1
No basal temperatures	1	0
Other infertility factor	0	1
Unknown	4	4

AID = artificial insemination with donor semen.
Reproduced with permission. Aiman J. Fertil Steril 1982;37:94–99.

husband to collect (by masturbation) the first few drops of his ejaculate in 1 jar, squeeze his penis to stop the flow of semen, then allow the bulk of his ejaculate to fall into a second jar. Success with this technique is based on 2 assumptions: It is the concentration of sperm more than the total number that is significant, and placing the sperm directly into the cervix increases the number of sperm that reaches the upper female genital tract.

Small (less than 1 ml) or excessive (over 6 ml) ejaculate volumes result in a diminished number of sperm being trapped by the cervical mu-

TABLE 17–3. Indications for Artificial Insemination, Husband's Semen (AIH)

Oligospermia
Small ejaculate volume
Large ejaculate volume*
Hypomotility
Poor postcoital test
Coital disorder
Induced ovulation
Unexplained infertility

* Using the first portion of the semen, collected as a split ejaculate.

cus. The rationale for AIH in men with an abnormal semen volume is that more sperm reach the uterus and fallopian tubes when the semen is placed against or into the cervix.

Diminished sperm motility (less than 50% of the sperm exhibit active forward progression) is also a stated indication for AIH. Presumably, placing the semen directly into the cervix results in a greater number of motile sperm ascending into the uterus and fallopian tubes. Separation of motile from nonmotile sperm has been attempted with physiologic diluents, albumin columns, and other solutions (10–15). Usually there is a great loss in motile sperm concentration while the percent of motile sperm increases. Use of the first portion of a split ejaculate (9), or the addition of caffeine (8) or kallikrein (16) has been advocated when the husband's sperm are less than normally motile.

When a specific abnormality in a postcoital exam is present, it should be treated and AIH performed only if therapy is unsuccessful. An abnormal postcoital test may be the result of improper timing, a physical or immunologic abnormality of the mucus, a cervical infection, an abnormality of the semen, or a coital factor (see Chapter 7). Antibiotics should be prescribed for a cervical infection, estrogen for a persistently viscous mucus, and glucocorticoids for a sperm antibody. These failing, AIH is a logical procedure although fewer than 20% of these women conceive. Success rates with AIH for an undiagnosed abnormality of the postcoital test are comparable.

Impotence, hypospadias, intractable vaginismus and, possibly, extreme degrees of uterine flexion are coital factors that may be circumvented by AIH. Since the husband's ejaculate is normal, conception rates should be normal unless other impediments to fertility exist.

AIH has also been used when the husband ejaculates in a retrograde direction into his urinary bladder. Retrograde ejaculation is a common sequela of surgery, medication, or diseases that damage the sympathetic nerves (T12 to L3). These nerves stimulate smooth muscle contraction of the epididymis, vas deferens, seminal vesicle and prostate, and closure of the bladder neck (17). Causes of retrograde ejaculation are summarized in Table 17–4. The technique of AIH for retrograde ejaculation involves the application of certain principles—

TABLE 17-4. Causes of Retrograde Ejaculation

Surgery
  Bladder neck
  Prostate
  Rectal
  Lumbar sympathectomy
  Retroperitoneal
    lymphadenectomy
  Aortoiliac
Disease
  Diabetes mellitus
  Demyelinating disease
  Multiple sclerosis
  Amyotrophic lateral sclerosis
  Spinal cord trauma
Medication
  Major tranquilizers
  Antihypertensive drugs

grade ejaculation has been summarized by Collins (18).

AIH is occasionally used when anovulatory women receive clomiphene or gonadotropins. AIH ensures that sperm are present in her genital tract at the expected time of ovulation, but means that the physician is intervening to a much greater extent. While pregnancy may occur in fewer months, the ultimate pregnancy rate is probably no greater than with coitus.

AIH for unexplained infertility must be considered empiric therapy. Occult infections, subtle disorders of ovulation, endometriosis, antibodies to sperm or the zona pellucida, and even emotional factors may cause "unexplained" infertility (19). For many of these, AIH should result in pregnancy no more frequently than by chance, estimated to be 8% to 10% in infertile couples.

fluid restriction to minimize urine output, rendering the urine alkaline, retrieval of sperm, washing of sperm, and, finally, insemination.

Urine can be made alkaline with 300 mg sodium bicarbonate orally, 3 to 4 times a day beginning 1 to 2 days before the first insemination is planned. Alternately, the bladder can be irrigated with a sterile alkaline solution. Two milliliters of the solution are left in the bladder and the husband masturbates immediately after this.

Semen is then collected by voiding or catheterization, washed with an alkaline nutrient solution such as Baker's solution (Table 17-5), then centrifuged for 10 minutes at 1,500 rpm. The supernatant is discarded and the sperm pellet, resuspended in 1 ml to 2 ml of solution, is inseminated.

Antegrade ejaculation can occasionally be achieved with alpha-adrenergic agonists such as ephedrine or phenylpropanolamine. Medication is more successful in men with minimal sympathetic dysfunction. Treatment of retro-

ARTIFICIAL INSEMINATION—DONOR SEMEN (AID). Indications for AID are summarized in Table 17-6 (1,20-23). The variation in reported frequency results partly from differences in the evaluation of male reproductive disorders. Karyotypes and vasograms are less frequently done, so the frequency of chromosomal and obstructive abnormalities may

TABLE 17-6. Indications for AID

INDICATION	FREQUENCY (%)
Oligospermia	29-45
Idiopathic	13-22
Cryptorchidism	1-4
Varicocele	3-18
Orchitis	1
Drugs, alcohol	3
Azoospermia	30-66
Idiopathic	19-28
Cryptorchidism	3-13
Obstructive	3-10
Chromosomal (e.g., Klinefelter's syndrome)	2-12
Orchitis, trauma, drugs	6-12
Endocrine	1-6
Vasectomy	8-30
Genetic	1-4
Sexual	2
Systemic disease	1

AID = artificial insemination with donor semen.
From Aiman J. Fertil Steril 1982;37:94-99; Friedman S and Mattei A et al. In: David G, Price WS, eds. Human artificial insemination and semen preservation. New York: Plenum Press, 1979:223-230 and 313-324; Albrecht BH et al. Fertil Steril 1982;37:792-797; and Edvinsson A et al. Fertil Steril 1983;39:327-332.

TABLE 17-5. Baker's Solution

INGREDIENT	AMOUNT (GM)
Glucose	3.0
Na_2HPO_4	0.6
KH_2PO_4	0.01
NaCl	0.2
H_2O	100.0

actually be higher and the frequency of idiopathic oligospermia or azoospermia correspondingly lower. Other indications for AID include sperm autoimmunization (23), Rh isoimmunization, and cervical factors in infertility. Sex selection has also been proposed as an indication for AID. However, separation of X- and Y-bearing sperm is not sufficiently reliable that the couple can be assured of their preference. Moreover, sex selection without a medical indication seems to be a trivial reason for AID in the face of the large demand when a medical indication does exist and in the face of the social and psychologic implications of the procedure.

Cryptorchidism is found in about 10% of newborn males, but only in 1.7% to 3.0% of males older than 1 year (24). Damage to spermatogenic epithelium is progressive, but the critical age after which fertility will be significantly impaired is uncertain (24,25). Certainly, fertility is reduced if the testes are not brought into the scrotum by the age of puberty, even when the cryptorchidism is unilateral (25).

Steroids and steroid analogues, gonadotropic hormones, chemotherapeutic drugs, heavy metals, prostaglandin antagonists, pesticides, insecticides, and certain antihypertensive drugs are compounds that can adversely affect male reproduction (26) (see also Chapter 14). AID is indicated if the medication cannot be discontinued or damage to the germ cells is permanent.

Chronic systemic disease may impair spermatogenesis, sexual potency, or ejaculation. Diabetes mellitus, cystic fibrosis (27), and chronic alcoholism (28) are only 3 examples of systemic diseases that may permanently impair male fertility.

Evaluation of the Couple

One semen analysis is insufficient to conclude that oligospermia or azoospermia is the cause of the couple's infertility. At least 3 semen analyses should be performed at intervals of at least 1 month to be certain that a reduction in sperm concentration, motility, or other parameter is not a transient effect of an acute illness, medication use, trauma, etc. Because some causes of oligospermia or azoospermia are potentially correctable, the husband should provide a complete medical history and receive a thorough physical examination (29).

Diagnostic procedures should be selected that confirm (or refute) the presence of an abnormality. If there is no apparent cause for oligospermia or azoospermia, then tests of thyroid and adrenal function should be obtained. Diabetes mellitus should be considered and blood glucose concentrations measured. Measurement of serum concentrations of testosterone, estradiol, or gonadotropins are not usually helpful except in men with suspected hypothalamic-pituitary or testicular failure. The diagnosis and management of male reproductive failure is discussed in Chapters 11 and 12.

As many as 20% of infertile couples may have more than 1 cause of infertility. The presence of an additional cause will reduce the probability of pregnancy with AID. For this reason, it is important to document the presence of ovulation and exclude the presence of a cervical, uterine, or tubal abnormality. A basal temperature record (BBT) is a reliable indicator of ovulation (1,30–32), although others have found a BBT unreliable (33) or monophasic in approximately 20% of ovulatory cycles (34). While a BBT may be uninformative, it still is the most convenient means of detecting the approximate day of ovulation in order to time the insemination. Ultrasonography has been shown to be useful in detecting ovulation in women being inseminated and the fecundability rate was improved by its use (35).

Less settled and more controversial is the value of testing for tubal patency before AID is begun. A hysterosalpingogram may suggest proximal tubal obstruction when none exists or miss distal tubal or peritubal disease. Corson achieved a high pregnancy rate after 3 cycles of AID (72% of women who ultimately conceived) without screening for tubal (or uterine) pathology (36). Febrile morbidity due to pelvic infection occurs in 3% of women after a hysterosalpingogram (37). Such infections may create tubal obstruction or necessitate a hysterectomy. Conversely, tubal pathology may be present in as many as 20% to 33% of women failing to conceive with AID and 22% to 75% may conceive after reconstructive surgery (36,38). Women with no history to suggest pelvic disease may not require a hysterosalpingogram before AID. However, women with a history or findings that suggest tubal or uterine pathology should have a hysterosalpingogram and/or laparoscopy to exclude disease that would preclude conception with AID.

No additional diagnostic tests or procedures are necessary for women with a normal history and physical findings. The finding of a specific abnormality that may reduce the chance of success with AID may necessitate additional evaluation, the nature of which is dictated by the abnormal finding.

Donor Selection

The person choosing the donor has an obligation to select one that meets the requirements of the recipient couple (e.g., physical characteristics) and one that has been screened for medical and genetic disease. Obviously, the donor should have a normal fertility potential. Few who perform AID have the luxury of requiring "proven" fertility in their group of donors since most semen donors are medical students who have no children. The donor should have a consistently normal semen analysis.

Few physicians keep accurate records of the number of pregnancies per donor and obtain "very little genetic screening" data (39). On the basis of a single instance of a child conceived by donor insemination with G_{M2}-gangliosidosis, more detailed screening of donors, including carrier testing (Tay-Sachs disease, sickle cell anemia, thalassemia) for donors in a high-risk population, has been advocated (40). Familial histiocytosis (41) and Turner's syndrome (42) have been found in children conceived by donor insemination. These reports refer to instances of Down's syndrome and an abnormality of chromosome 8 in children conceived by AID. The recommendation of a more thorough survey of the family pedigree is a valid one that requires little additional time or expense and may exclude a small number of donors who could transmit a genetic disease. A detailed medical history of all first-degree relatives (parents, siblings, children) is the minimum that should be obtained.

The incidence of genetic abnormalities and birth defects is not higher in the children of women conceiving by donor insemination. The genetic abnormalities reported may not be transmitted from the donor and the insemination itself is unlikely to cause chromosomal damage. For these reasons, a karyotype of potential donors is not routinely necessary. It is more efficient, cost effective, and probably sufficient to exclude a potential donor if he has a mendelian trait, a multifactorial disease (e.g., diabetes mellitus), or a family history of either.

Since most donors are medical students or resident physicians, their participation is usually limited to the duration of their training, and is frequently less. Seventy-seven percent of physicians use a donor for 6 or fewer pregnancies (39). The risk of consanguinity as a result of AID is small and the remoteness of its possibility has been confirmed mathematically (43).

Technique

INSEMINATION. Fresh semen should be allowed to liquefy and frozen semen should be thawed before insemination. The insemination should then be done within 2 hours since sperm motility will decline thereafter. Intravaginal insemination is less successful than cervical placement of semen and should not be done. A glass pipette, cervical cap, or small animal feeding tube are the instruments most commonly used to perform the insemination (Fig. 17–1). After injecting the semen into the cervical canal with the pipette or metal feeding tube, the woman is often kept in a recumbent position for 5 to 25 minutes, although this does not seem to enhance the conception rate (38). The cervical cap is usually removed after several hours, cleaned, and reused.

Intrauterine insemination may be indicated in the presence of antisperm cervical antibodies or other cervical factors such as viscous mucus, cervical infection, or absent mucous production (see Chapter 7). Experience with intrauterine insemination for sperm isoantibodies is limited (44).

TIMING. Correct timing of artificial insemination is complicated by the difficulty in predicting when ovulation is imminent. The mean day of the menstrual cycle on which the basal temperature nadir occurs (determined from previous cycles) is the easiest, yet least precise, method (1,22,36,45,46). Ultrasonic measurement of follicular growth (35) and rapid, semiquantitative assays of luteinizing-hormone (LH) concentrations are more precise methods

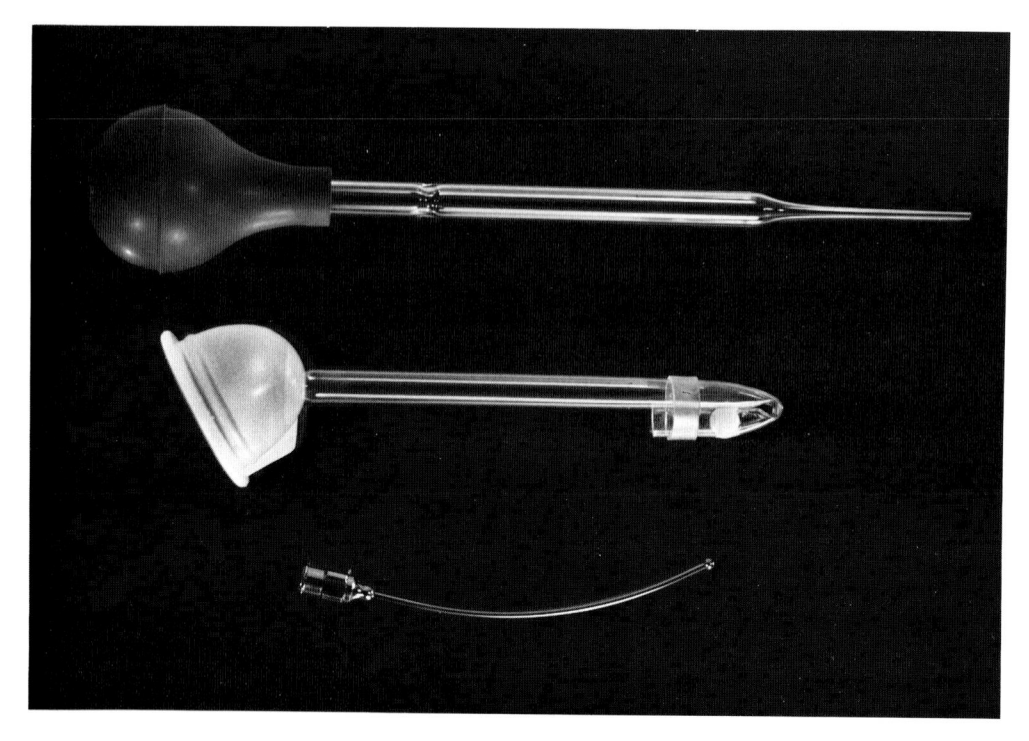

Fig. 17–1. Instruments to perform artificial insemination. A pasteur pipette and bulb (top) is inexpensive, convenient, and does not damage the endocervix. The cervical cap (middle) is placed on the cervix and the semen introduced through a pliable cannula (not shown) through the stem of the cap. An 18-guage small animal feeding tube is shown at the bottom (Popper & Sons, Inc., New Hyde Park, N.Y.).

to detect ovulation. However, they are also more cumbersome and expensive.

Since no method to detect ovulation is absolutely precise and because the moment of ovulation varies from cycle to cycle, the first insemination should be scheduled 1 to 2 days before the expected time of ovulation. The insemination may be performed then if the semen sample has been collected. If it is possible to arrange to have a semen sample on very short notice, then the insemination can be deferred 1 to 2 days, or until the clinical evidence is suggestive that ovulation is imminent. Often, however, arrangements for a semen sample must be made well in advance. If so, the insemination should be performed at the time of the first scheduled visit and the woman asked to return in 2 days if ovulation has not occurred. Since sperm will survive in the female genital tract for several days when the cervical mucus reflects a high estrogen environment, insemination performed 1 to 3 days before ovulation may still result in conception. However, repeating the insemination if ovulation has not occurred improves the probability of conception. Many physicians perform only 2 inseminations per cycle, while others continue to perform inseminations at 2-day intervals until ovulation has occurred. From a review of the literature, Corson concluded that 2 inseminations per cycle were optimal for women who ovulated predictably (47). More than 2 inseminations improve conception rates only in women who ovulate erratically.

The optimal day for insemination seems to be the nadir of the basal temperature (i.e., the last day before the sustained rise in temperature associated with ovulation). Garcia et al. correlated the results of ultrasound, estradiol, progesterone, and LH concentrations in women who were undergoing laparoscopic oocyte retrieval (48). The basal temperature nadir coincided with the day on which the LH peak occurred in the majority of women. Ovulation occurred an average of 10 hours after the LH peak. Estradiol concentrations were not helpful because there was often a double peak. Progesterone concentrations do not increase until after ovulation so this assay is not a useful predictor of ovulation.

Results

Approximately 20% of women conceive each month when artificial insemination is performed (1,36). This is the same as the rate in women conceiving after sexual intercourse (49). While the rate is less with 1 insemination per cycle, it is not increased when more than 2 to 3 inseminations are performed. Most authors perform artificial insemination for 6 months based on observations that the cumulative pregnancy rate approaches 90% to 95% and is increased little by continuing the procedure for significantly longer periods (38,50). In assessing overall results, many authors include the total number of conceptions, including second pregnancies in women. This inflates the cumulative success rate since women of proven fertility are included more than once while women who did not conceive are counted only once. Approximately 25% of women stop artificial insemination before they conceive or before they have reached the 6-month time limit (47). Inclusion of these in calculating the pregnancy rate results in a misleadingly low success rate. Fifty percent to 75% of women destined to conceive do so within 3 months.

In addition to statistical artifacts, other factors also influence the reported success rates with artificial insemination. Other impediments to fertility will reduce the chances of success with artificial insemination and the thoroughness of the medical investigation differs in most reports. Semen quality (51,52), age of the woman (38,50,53), regularity of ovulation (54), and the characteristics of the cervix and its mucus (45) are other factors that influence the outcome of artificial insemination.

Experience with intrauterine insemination is insufficient to give accurate pregnancy rates. Because of the risk of serious complications, intrauterine insemination should be done with caution and only when an indication exists. The small animal feeding tube shown in Fig. 17–1 is useful for this; it can be introduced into the uterine cavity with minimal discomfort and without first sounding the uterus. A cervical tenaculum is not necessary for countertraction since the rounded end of the feeding tube is small enough that it can be inserted with little resistance.

FRESH SEMEN (DONOR). When women discontinuing artificial insemination before the time limit are excluded, approximately 75% of women will conceive. The mean time for conception is approximately 3 months and 85% to 95% of women destined to conceive have done so by the end of 6 cycles. The risk of spontaneous abortion or of bearing a child with a congenital malformation is no greater than that of women conceiving after sexual intercourse (47).

FROZEN SEMEN (DONOR). Pregnancy rates with donor semen that had been frozen and thawed on the day of insemination are only one half to two thirds those of AID with fresh semen (20,55). Sperm motility is reduced by the process of freezing and thawing (56,57). There is also electron microscopic evidence of fragmentation of the acrosomal membrane during the freeze-thaw cycle (58). These observations are the likely explanation for the lower success rates. There is, however, no evidence that these structural and functional changes in sperm increase the risk of bearing a child with a congenital malformation.

INSEMINATION WITH HUSBAND'S SEMEN. Pregnancy rates after artificial insemination with the husband's semen (AIH) are lower than when donor semen is used (6–9). Pregnancy rates of 10% to 20% are rarely exceeded whether the husband's semen is used shortly after ejaculation or has been frozen for later use (59). However, this range is for all indications including oligospermia, ejaculatory disturbances, and the others indicated in Table 17–3. This rate is greatly influenced by the presence of an abnormality in semen, the most frequent indication. Insemination done in conjunction with ovulation induction or because of the presence of hypospadias results in a higher rate of conception (6,7).

Complications of Artificial Insemination

Failure is the most frequent complication of artificial insemination. Others occur infrequently and most are minor.

The most feared complication is the use of the wrong semen sample. However, any program should have a defined protocol for identification of a donor semen sample and a system for double-checking the accuracy of the identification. If there is any doubt, the procedure should not be performed and the sample discarded.

The problem of transmitting a venereal disease is a real one (60) but an unlikely possibility when the donors are chosen from a selected population such as medical or graduate students. Periodic screening for syphilis or gonorrhea assures those involved only that the donor has neither at the time of the screening. It is not possible nor practical to screen each donor each time that he contributes a sample.

The transmission of a genetic disease is infrequent with donor insemination (43,61). Based on the assumptions of Moser (61), the observations of Curie-Cohen (39), and population figures for the United States, the calculated number of consanguinous marriages each year as a result of AID is 0.015 (Table 17–7). It is not feasible to obtain a karyotype from all prospective donors. Moreover, such a practice would not ascertain those with a single gene mutation.

Three complications may occur with intrauterine insemination. Uterine contractions are common; the resulting cramps may be intense and associated with a vagal response (hypotension, bradycardia, diaphoresis, syncope). These are the result of seminal plasma prostaglandins. Aspirin, either before or after the procedure may minimize the severity of uterine cramping. Atropine (0.4 mg to 0.6 mg) should be administered for a severe vasovagal response, while placing the woman in the Trendelenburg position is usually sufficient for mild reactions.

Intrauterine infection is the second potential complication of intrauterine insemination, presumably occurring (infrequently) because vaginal bacteria are carried into the uterine cavity when the internal cervical os is penetrated. Cleansing of the ectocervix may minimize this risk. Transmission of gonorrhea is possible and gonococci survive in ejaculated semen for at least 2 hours (60).

Anaphylaxis caused by the formation of antibodies against sperm or seminal plasma proteins is the third serious complication of intrauterine insemination. The use of no more than 0.3 cc to 0.4 cc of ejaculate or washing the sperm with a physiologic solution (Table 17–5) minimizes this risk, and the frequency and severity of uterine contractions.

TABLE 17–7. Estimated Risk of Consanguinity Due to AID in the United States

N = total annual births (3.4 million)
I = estimated annual number of live births from AID (20,000)
P = % of annual births due to AID (20,000/3.4 million) = 0.59%
O = estimated number of offspring per donor per year = 5
D = annual number of donors required per year (I/O) = 4,000
M = number of marriages per year (= 1/2 or less of N) = 1.7 million, maximum
A = annual number of marriages between AID individuals (= MP^2) = 59
H = estimated number of half-sibling marriages per year due to AID (= A/D)

$H = 0.015$.

AID = artificial insemination with donor semen.
Mathematical construct from Moser H. In: David G, Price WD, eds. Human artificial insemination and semen preservation. New York: Plenum Press, 1979:379–383.

Ethical, Legal, and Psychologic Issues

Understanding the psychology of infertility (Chapter 2) is essential for those who perform artificial insemination because of the potential feelings of guilt and loss of self-esteem of each member of the couple. Each of us is imbued with a set of values, which we use unconsciously as a basis for making judgments and decisions. Recognizing our own ethical and religious precepts is as important as understanding the conflict that artificial insemination may create for couples, many of whom must reconcile their own moral and religious principles with their desire to have children (Chapter 21).

Not only must physicians understand the medical, ethical, and psychologic aspects of artificial insemination, but they must conform to laws that define who may receive artificial insemination, the status of children so conceived, the requirements for obtaining a proper consent, and others (Chapter 22).

REFERENCES

1. Aiman J. Factors affecting the success of donor insemination. Fertil Steril 1982;37:94–99.
2. d'Elicio G, Campana A, Mornaghini L. Psychodynamic discussions with couples requesting AID. In: David G, Price WS, eds. Human artificial insemination and semen preservation. New York: Plenum Press, 1979:407–411.
3. Czyba JC, Chevret M. Psychological reactions of couples to artificial insemination with donor sperm. Int J Fertil 1979;240–245.
4. Harvey B, Harvey A. How couples feel about donor insemination. Contemp Obstet Gynecol 1977;9:93–97.
5. Menning BE. Donor insemination: the psychosocial issues. Contemp Obstet Gynecol 1981; 18:155–172.
6. Sato H, Kobayashi T, Mochimaru F, Iizuka R. Results of AIH in 1475 patients. In: David G, Price WS, eds. Human artificial insemination and semen preservation. New York: Plenum Press, 1979:521–528.
7. Steiman RP, Taymor ML. Artificial insemination homologous and its role in the management of infertility. Fertil Steril 1977;28:146–150.
8. Harrison RF. Insemination of husband's semen with and without the addition of caffeine. Fertil Steril 1978;29:532–534.
9. Nunley WC, Kitchin JD, Thiagarajah S. Homologous insemination. Fertil Steril 1978; 30:510–515.
10. Glass RH, Ericsson RJ. Intrauterine insemination of isolated motile sperm. Fertil Steril 1978;29:535–538.
11. Harris SJ, Milligan MP, Masson GM, Dennis KJ. Improved separation of motile sperm in asthenospermia and its application to artificial insemination homologous (AIH). Fertil Steril 1981;36:219–221.
12. Koper A, Evans PR, Witherow RON, Flynn JT, Bayliss M, Blandy JP. A technique for selecting and concentrating the motile sperm from semen in oligozoospermia. Br J Urol 1979; 51:587–590.
13. Lopata A, Patullo MJ, Chang A, James B. A method for collecting motile spermatozoa from human semen. Fertil Steril 1976;27:677–684.
14. Comhaire F, Vermeulen L, Zegers-Hochschild F. Enhancement of sperm motility: selecting progessively motile spermatozoa. In: Bain J, Schill W-B, Schwarzstein L, eds. Treatment of male infertility. Berlin: Springer-Verlag, 1982: 283–284.
15. Dmowski WP, Gaynor L, Lawrence M, Rao R, Scommegna A. Artificial insemination homologous with oligospermic semen separated on albumin columns. Fertil Steril 1979;31:58–62.
16. Schill WB. Kinin-releasing pancreatic proteinase kallikrein. In: Bain J, Schill W-B, Schwarzstein L, eds. Treatment of male infertility. Berlin: Springer-Verlag, 1982:125–142.
17. Kedia KR, Markland C. The ejaculatory process. In: Hafez ESE, ed. Human semen and fertility regulation in men. St. Louis: CV Mosby Co., 1976:497–503.
18. Collins JP. Retrograde ejaculation. In: Bain J, Schill W-B, Schwarzstein L, eds. Treatment of male infertility. Berlin: Springer-Verlag, 1982: 179–189.
19. Moghissi K, Wallach E. Unexplained infertility. Fertil Steril 1983;39:5–21.
20. Friedman S. Artificial insemination with frozen human semen: 227 cases. In: David G, Price WS, eds. Human artificial insemination and semen preservation. New York: Plenum Press, 1979:223–230.
21. Mattei A, Mattei MG, Laugier P, Mattei JF, Conte-Devoix B, Roulier R. The male factor in AID requests: 558 cases. In: David G, Price WS, eds. Human artificial insemination and semen preservation. New York: Plenum Press, 1979:313–324.
22. Albrecht BH, Cramer D, Schiff I. Factors influencing the success of artificial insemination. Fertil Steril 1982;37:792–797.
23. Edvinsson A, Bergman P, Steen Y, Nilsson S. Characteristics of donor semen and cervical mucus at the time of conception. Fertil Steril 1983;39:327–332.
24. Bardin CW, Paulsen CA. The testes. In: Williams RH, ed. Textbook of endocrinology, 6th ed. Philadelphia: WB Saunders, 1981:336–337.
25. Lipshultz LI, Caminos-Torres R, Greenspan CS, Snyder PJ. Testicular function after orchiopexy for unilaterally undescended testis. N Engl J Med 1976;295:15–18.
26. Aiman J. Infertility. In: Duenhoelter J, ed. Greenhill's office gynecology. Chicago: Year Book Medical Publishers, 1983:188–223.
27. Taussig LM, Lobeck CC, di Sant'Agnese PA, Ackerman ER, Kattwinkel J. Fertility in males with cystic fibrosis. N Engl J Med 1972; 287:586–589.
28. Gordon GG, Altman K, Southren AL, Rubin E, Lieber CS. Effect of alcohol (ethanol) administration of sex-hormone metabolism in normal men. N Engl J Med 1976;295:793–797.
29. How to organize a basic study of the infertile

couple. The American Fertility Society, Birmingham, Ala., 1971.
30. Magyar DM, Boyers SP, Marshall JR, Abraham GE. Regular menstrual cycles and premenstrual molimina as indicators of ovulation. Obstet Gynecol 1979;53:411–414.
31. Hilgers TW, Bailey AJ. Natural family planning II: basal body temperature and estimated time of ovulation. Obstet Gynecol 1980;55:333–339.
32. Newill RGD, Katz M. The basal body temperature chart in artificial insemination by donor pregnancy cycles. Fertil Steril 1982;38:431–438.
33. Bauman JE. Basal body temperature: unreliable method of ovulation detection. Fertil Steril 1981;36:729–733.
34. Moghissi K. Accuracy of basal body temperature for ovulation detection. Fertil Steril 1976;27;1415–1421.
35. Marinho AO, Sallam HN, Goessens LKV, Collins WP, Rodeck CH, Campbell S. Real time pelvic ultrasonography during the periovulatory period of patients attending an artificial insemination clinic. Fertil Steril 1982;37:633–638.
36. Corson SL. Factors affecting donor artificial insemination success rates. Fertil Steril 1980;33:415–422.
37. Stumpf PG, March CM. Febrile morbidity following hysterosalpingography: identification of risk factors and recommendations for prophylaxis. Fertil Steril 1980;33:487–492.
38. Sulewski JM, Eisenberg F, Stenger VG. A longitudinal analysis of artificial insemination with donor semen. Fertil Steril 1978;29:527–531.
39. Curie-Cohen M, Luttrell MS, Shapiro S. Current practice of artificial insemination by donor in the United States. N Engl J Med 1979;300:585–590.
40. Johnson WG, Schwartz RC, Chutorian AM. Artificial insemination by donors: the need for genetic screening. Late-infantile GM_2-gangliosidosis resulting from this technique. N Engl J Med 1981;304:755–757.
41. Shapiro DN, Hutchinson RJ. Familial histiocytosis in offspring of two pregnancies after artificial insemination. N Engl J Med 1981;304:757–759.
42. King CR, Magenis E. Turner syndrome in the offspring of artificially inseminated pregnancies. Fertil Steril 1978;30:604–605.
43. Jacquard A, Schoevaert D. Artificial insemination and consanguinity. In: David G, Price WS, eds. Human artificial insemination and semen preservation. New York: Plenum Press, 1979:385–387.
44. Ingerslev HJ. Antibodies against spermatozoal surface-membrane antigens in female infertility. Acta Obstet Gynecol Scand (Suppl 100) 1981;8–52.
45. Schwartz D, Mayaux M-J, Martin-Boyce A, Czyglik F, David G. Donor insemination: conception rate according to cycle day in a series of 821 cycles with a single insemination. Fertil Steril 1979;31:226–229.
46. Strickler RC, Keller DW, Warren JC. Artificial insemination with fresh donor semen. N Engl J Med 1975;293:848–853.
47. Corson SL, Batzer FR, Baylson MM. Donor insemination. In: Wynne RM, ed. Obstet Gynecol Annu, Vol. 12. Norwalk, Conn.: Appleton-Century-Crofts, 1983:283–309.
48. Garcia JE, Jones GS, Wright GL. Prediction of the time of ovulation. Fertil Steril 1981;36:308–315.
49. Leridon H. The efficacy of natural insemination: a comparative standard for AID. In: David G, Price WS, eds. Human artificial insemination. New York: Plenum Press, 1979:191–196.
50. Glezerman M. Two hundred and seventy cases of artificial donor insemination: management and results. Fertil Steril 1981;35:180–187.
51. Friedman S. Artificial insemination with donor semen mixed with semen of the infertile husband. Fertil Steril 1980;33:125–128.
52. Pfeffer WH, Wallach EE, Beck WW, Barrett ATM. Artificial insemination with husband's semen: prognostic factors. Fertil Steril 1980;34:356–361.
53. Schwartz D, Mayaux MJ. Female fecundity as a function of age. Results of artificial insemination in 2193 nulliparous women with azoospermic husbands. N Engl J Med 1982;306:404–406.
54. Smith KD, Rodriguez-Rigau L, Steinberger E. The influence of ovulatory dysfunction and timing of insemination on the success of artificial insemination donor (AID) with fresh or cryopreserved semen. Fertil Steril 1981;36:496–502.
55. Steinberger E, Smith KD. Artificial insemination with fresh or frozen semen: a comparative study. JAMA 1973;223:778–783.
56. Smith KD, Steinberger E. Survival of spermatozoa in a human sperm bank: effects of long term storage in liquid nitrogen. JAMA 1973;223:774–777.
57. Sherman JK. Synopsis of the use of frozen semen since 1964: state of the art of human semen banking. Fertil Steril 1973;24:397–412.
58. Escalier D, Bisson JP. Quantitative ultrastructural modifications in human spermatozoa after

freezing. In: David G, Price WS, eds. Human artificial insemination and semen preservation. New York: Plenum Press, 1979:107–122.
59. Decker WH. Pooled and frozen homologous (husband) semen for artificial insemination. Infertility 1978;1:25–32.
60. Jennings RT, Dixon RE, Nettles JB. The risks and prevention of *Neisseria gonorrheae* transfer in fresh ejaculate donor insemination. Fertil Steril 1977;28:554–556.
61. Moser H. Population genetics and AID. In: David G, Price WD, eds. Human artificial insemination and semen preservation. New York: Plenum Press, 1979:379–383.

Reproductive Performance of Previously Infertile Couples

Richard J. Worley and William R. Keye, Jr.

Our purpose is to analyze the outcome of conceptions occurring in previously infertile couples. Spontaneous abortion, ectopic pregnancy, premature labor, congenital anomalies, miscellaneous obstetric complications, and normal term pregnancy are some of the possible fates of a conceptus in such couples. Some of these outcomes are applicable only to women with certain disorders, such as the relationship of premature labor to müllerian anomalies. Miscellaneous obstetric complications developing late in pregnancy often bear no obvious relationship to the previous cause of infertility, yet the occurrence of any of these is potentially serious and therefore important to consider.

The Abortion Rate in a Normal Population

Spontaneous abortion is a highly discernible abnormal pregnancy outcome. Before deciding whether the spontaneous abortion rate is increased in previously infertile women, it is essential to define this rate in a normally fertile population. The incidence of abortion is often higher in women who conceive after a variety of treatments for infertility. Hence, an analysis of the abortion incidence in such couples may be a sensitive and objective means of assessing distortions in reproductive physiology that result from treatment or persistence of disease (1).

It is both crucial and difficult to select the appropriate spontaneous abortion rate in a normally fertile population when comparing this to the rate in previously infertile women. Subclinical abortion is as common as clinically apparent abortion in a group of women treated for infertility (2). The subclinical abortions were detected by the presence of human chorionic gonadotropin (hCG) in serum before the gestation was suspected and the total abortion incidence in these women was 37% (2). Total pregnancy loss may be as high as 50% when this figure is added to the incidence of pregnancy loss before implantation. However, if the incidence of spontaneous abortion in women 20 to 29 years old conceiving for the first time is assessed by life table analysis, the incidence of clinical plus subclinical abortion is only about 10% (1). This figure is most appropriate for comparison to that of infertile women conceiving after therapy and we will assume a 10% spontaneous abortion rate for normally fertile women.

Anovulation

CLOMIPHENE THERAPY. When pregnancy follows clomiphene therapy, it is relevant to analyze the ensuing spontaneous abortion rate, the incidence of congenital anomalies, and perhaps also the occurrence of miscellaneous obstetric complications.

Some authors believe the spontaneous abortion rate is increased in pregnancies that follow clomiphene therapy, but others say not. Understandably, investigators who report abortion rates of 8.9% in 45 pregnancies after clomiphene treatment (3), or of *zero* in 96 such pregnancies (4) conclude that the abortion rate is not increased. To the contrary, records of the initial manufacturer of clomiphene citrate indicate that of 2,364 pregnancies occurring after clomiphene treatment, 451, or 19.3% aborted spontaneously (5). This rate, nearly twice that expected, was also borne out both in a subsequent review (6) and in a large independent series (7). By comparison, 28, or 1.2% of the 2,364 pregnancies were ectopic, a figure similar to that of a reference population, suggesting that an increase in early pregnancy wastage following clomiphene therapy is virtually limited to uterine pregnancies.

Faulty ovum formation, multiple pregnancy, and corpus luteum inadequacy are possible consequences of clomiphene use that could increase the abortion rate. Boue and Boue found that the frequency of karyotypic abnormalities in abortuses resulting from either gonadotropin or clomiphene induction, 84%, was higher than the 60% incidence in an unselected population (8). While it is plausible that this observation is relevant to the apparent increase in the spontaneous abortion rate following clomiphene use, there is no good evidence of which we are aware that the incidence of congenital anomalies is increased among children born in the latter half of pregnancies resulting from clomiphene therapy. To the contrary, the widely reported experience is that the incidence and pattern of birth defects in such offspring does not differ from the population at large (3, 4, 9, 10).

Multiple gestation after clomiphene stimulation (5) may also contribute to the spontaneous abortion rate that attends its use. Although widely quoted as 8% to 10%, the incidence of multiple births in recent experience has typically been as low as 2% to 5%, and the pregnancies have consisted almost exclusively of twins (3, 9). These figures may underestimate the magnitude of the problem, however. Perhaps only half of women known sonographically to have multiple gestational sacs in the first trimester of pregnancy have successful live births, and on the contrary, some women who deliver 1 infant were known to have additional gestational sacs earlier in pregnancy (11). Thus, the increased incidence of multiple gestation contributes to the increased abortion rate.

The importance of inadequate luteal function to spontaneous abortion associated with clomiphene therapy is difficult to ascertain. Uniform diagnostic criteria do not exist, nor is there agreement that luteal phase inadequacy results in pregnancy loss. Clomiphene has been suggested as a *cause* of inadequate luteal phase, but clomiphene has also been used to *treat* it. Our own view is that the importance of an inadequate luteal phase to poor reproductive performance may be overestimated since successful pregnancies may ensue without treatment (12), and ". . . there are no controlled studies which conclusively establish either its role as a cause for infertility, or the value of therapy" (13). Although it is commonly asserted that clomiphene is a cause of inadequate luteal phase (4), we and others believe that luteal dysfunction is the consequence of aberrant folliculogenesis, which in turn is most often the result of inadequate gonadotropin stimulation early in the follicular phase of the ovarian cycle (14). Rather than incriminate clomiphene as a cause of an inadequate luteal phase, it is instead rational to employ the agent in an effort to augment FSH release early in the cycle to correct the faulty follicular maturation that results in inadequate luteal function. Several groups have used clomiphene successfully for this purpose (13,15,16). Clomiphene may be more effective in women with marked defects in luteal function than in those with mild defects (17). Conception rates after treatment in 46 women with severe or mild defects were 79% and 8.9%, respectively. In 86 women with disorders of ovulation, clomiphene reduced the rate of pregnancy wastage from 70% to 6.7% (4).

An inadequate luteal phase occurring with clomiphene use may be the result of insufficient medication. Chronic estrus anovulation, luteal dysfunction, fertile ovarian cycles, and superovulation may represent differential thresholds of gonadotropin-dependent ovarian function. Stimulation of the ovaries of women in either of the first 2 categories with sufficient amounts of clomiphene often enhances gonadotropin-dependent ovarian function to the next threshold, or beyond, in a dose-related fashion (14). Inadequate luteal function and ensuing early pregnancy loss after clomiphene is likely the result of suboptimal stimulation of ovarian function and not the consequence of some intrinsic property of clomiphene, such as its antiestrogenic action. The antiestrogenic properties of clomiphene may not be as important in preventing conception or predisposing to pregnancy loss as they are commonly believed to be (9).

At least 3 groups have analyzed the obstetric experiences of a large number of women conceiving with clomiphene (4,10,18). The incidence of prematurity is increased, but this is due solely to an increased incidence of multiple gestation (4). This association is consistent with recognized risk factors for premature delivery: uterine anomaly, history of diethylstilbestrol (DES) exposure, repeated second-trimester abortion, and multiple gestation (19).

Hack and her colleagues (4) also noted that 16.7% of the 96 pregnancies they studied after clomiphene treatment were complicated by pregnancy-induced hypertension, a much higher incidence than the 1.4% reported for the population of Israel, the site of her study. None of the women who developed pregnancy-induced hypertension had a multiple gestation and the authors were unable to account for the relatively frequent occurrence of hypertension. In contrast, neither Adashi et al. (10) nor Poulson and Bryner (18) found an increased incidence of pregnancy-induced hypertension among their patients.

Poulson and Bryner found that 17.5% of women conceiving with clomiphene received oxytocin to augment labor, a 3-fold increase, compared to women not receiving clomiphene (18). Cesarean section rates are also higher (16% and 19%) in women who received clomiphene (4,18). The indications for Cesarean section in these women bear no apparent relationship to clomiphene use and only 2 of 13 Cesarean sections were for twins (4). Other obstetric indications existed in these 2 women. No increase in "gestational maternal disorders" or "perinatal obstetric complications" were found in clomiphene-treated women (10). The reproductive outcome of women after clomiphene therapy is summarized in Table 18–1.

GONADOTROPIN THERAPY. Most of the adverse effects of clomiphene on pregnancy outcome exist with gonadotropin therapy, but often to a greater extent. Whereas clomiphene alters pituitary-gonadal relationships for only a few days and stimulates only early follicular maturation, gonadotropins induce more profound changes in ovarian physiology, follicular maturation, and end organ responses. Estrogen assays, ultrasonic measurement of follicular diameter, and other adjuncts are the only techniques available to monitor gonadotropin induction of ovulation. These are crude means of surveying a complex process that involves many crucial events in the microenvironment of the developing follicle to which we have no access (20).

Thus, it is not surprising that there are a variety of related obstetric consequences. Jansen reviewed the outcome of 884 gonadotropin-induced pregnancies collected from the literature and reported a spontaneous abortion incidence of 22.7% (1). Ben-Rafael and associates noted an abortion rate of 29% in women who conceived after gonadotropin therapy, but a rate of only 8.8% in women who conceived after spontaneous ovulation (21).

Karyotypic abnormalities are one of the causes of an increased incidence of abortion after gonadotropin-induced cycles. The karyotypic incidence is increased in abortuses after gonadotropin therapy just after clomiphene therapy (8). Gratefully, the incidence of congenital malformations in infants born after midpregnancy following gonadotropin therapy is not different from the population at large (22). Inaccurate timing of the ovulating dose of hCG (administered as an LH surrogate) also increases the likelihood of abortion (23).

Estradiol secretion often increases as the result of maturation of multiple follicles. Recognizing that estrogen (and other sex steroids) affect oviductal motility, McBain and associates

TABLE 18–1. Reproductive Outcome after Clomiphene Therapy

Increased spontaneous abortion rate
  Faulty ovum formation
  Multiple gestation
  Inadequate corpus luteum?
Increased incidence of prematurity
  Multiple gestation
No increased incidence of congenital anomalies
---

attributed "an unexpectedly high rate of ectopic pregnancy" after conceptions that follow gonadotropin-induced ovulation to this high rate of estrogen production (24). Six of their 193 pregnancies (3.1%) were tubal gestations. They computed that a urinary estrogen excretion of greater than 200 mcg/24 hours on the day hCG was given was associated with a 10% chance of ectopic pregnancy. A related but rather unusual problem is the occurrence of simultaneous intrauterine and extrauterine pregnancies, a circumstance that may complicate as many as 1% of pregnancies that follow gonadotropin treatment (23). This possibility creates an important obligation for the clinician to differentiate between concurrent intrauterine and extrauterine pregnancy rather than ovarian hyperstimulation syndrome (see below) when investigating adnexal enlargement after gonadotropin-induced ovulation (25).

An inadequate luteal phase could also contribute to early pregnancy wastage after gonadotropin-induced ovulation. This could occur because none of the stimulated follicles may be mature and because hCG may not be given at the right time in the proper dose (26). While it is common practice to give a single 10,000 IU injection of hCG to stimulate ovulation, Gemzell administers 9,000 IU at the time of ovulation, then an additional 6,000 IU 6 or 7 days later "in order to guarantee a luteal phase of normal length" (27). Jansen states that abortion rates are lowest when supplemental hCG is routinely given in the luteal phase (1).

Multiple pregnancy is another cause of increased early pregnancy wastage after gonadotropin therapy. The incidence of multiple pregnancy following gonadotropin treatment is at least 18%, but rates as high as 53% have been reported (23). In general, the highest rates of multiple pregnancy occurred 15 to 20 years ago when gonadotropins were first used to induce ovulation. Refinement of the regimen and the use of estrogen assays to monitor the effects of treatment have led to a reduction in the frequency of multiple pregnancy, but the rate is still more than 10 times the incidence after spontaneous ovulation. Although multiple pregnancy is clearly a cause of early pregnancy wastage (11), Holcberg and associates found that the late outcome of 10 triplet pregnancies that resulted from ovulation induction was better than that of 21 triplet gestations that arose spontaneously (28), and they believed that early recognition was a key factor leading to the difference in outcome. Earlier recognition of multiple gestation led to earlier reduction in physical activity, earlier and longer hospitalization before delivery, longer mean duration of pregnancy, higher mean infant birth weight, a lower perinatal mortality rate, and a lower incidence of pregnancy-induced hypertension.

Maternal consequences of multiple pregnancy may also be dire; one that is nearly unique to pregnancies following ovulation induction is ovarian hyperstimulation. The problem is much more prominent after gonadotropin therapy than after the use of clomiphene (23). The probability of hyperstimulation increases with the number of fetuses. The hyperstimulation syndrome occurred in only 2 of 47 women with singleton gestations, but in 5 of 23 women with twin pregnancies, 2 of 5 with triplet pregnancies, and 1 of 2 with quadruplet gestations (29). Ovarian hyperstimulation resolves with time and conservative management (30) (see also Chapter 6).

The remaining maternal complications of multiple pregnancy following gonadotropin treatment are not unique to ovulation induction. Anemia, pregnancy-induced hypertension, hydramnios, puerperal hemorrhage, and Cesarean section are all more common with multiple gestations (23). The adverse effects of gonadotropins on pregnancy performance are summarized in Table 18–2.

TABLE 18–2. Reproductive Outcome after Gonadotropin-Induced Ovulation

High spontaneous abortion rate
    Faulty ovum formation
    Increased incidence of ectopic pregnancy?
    Multiple pregnancy
    Inadequate luteal phase
Ovarian hyperstimulation syndrome
Increased incidence of prematurity
    Multiple gestation
Other consequences of multiple gestation
    Anemia
    Pregnancy-induced hypertension
    Hydramnios
    Puerperal hemorrhage
    Cesarean section
Incidence of congenital anomalies not increased

BROMOCRIPTINE THERAPY. Two major questions must be addressed in analyzing the outcome of pregnancies that follow bromocriptine therapy. What is the effect of bromocriptine on the pregnancy? What is the effect of pregnancy on unresected, incompletely resected, or recurrent prolactinomas?

Bromocriptine exerts little discernible effect on pregnancies that result from its use. The spontaneous abortion rate in women conceiving with bromocriptine does not differ from the rate in an unselected population (1). While some have questioned whether a luteal phase defect may follow rapid reduction of prolactin concentrations (31), the high pregnancy rate (32) and low abortion rate argue against such a defect. Even when bromocriptine is taken only in the follicular phase, the subsequent luteal phase is normal. Ovulation and conception rates are high despite luteal phase elevations in prolactin concentration (33). Griffith and associates, in a study of 448 pregnancies in women who conceived while taking bromocriptine, also found a low rate of spontaneous abortion and an unaltered incidence of twin pregnancy (1.6%) and congenital anomalies (2.9%) (34). Turkalj and colleagues found similar rates in an analysis of 1,410 pregnancies in 1,335 women who took bromocriptine either during the cycle of conception or later in the pregnancy (35). Large doses of bromocriptine are occasionally given during pregnancy to treat the uncommon complication of a symptomatic, expanding prolactinoma (36). Adverse effects on the fetus have not been described despite the observation that the drug enters the fetus and causes a marked reduction in fetal plasma prolactin concentrations (35). The lack of fetal consequences of maternal bromocriptine ingestion during pregnancy led Canales and associates to adopt bromocriptine as primary therapy in women with pituitary prolactinomas, regardless of size. They also recommended that the drug be continued prophylactically during pregnancy in women with macroadenomas (37).

The other major concern is the effect of pregnancy in women with unresected, incompletely resected, or recurrent prolactinomas. Boyar and others expressed the concern that such lesions might enlarge during pregnancy, even after bromocriptine therapy (36,38–40). Gemzell and Wang collated the data from the responses of 25 groups responding to a questionnaire and summarized the outcome of 217 pregnancies in women with a pituitary adenoma (Table 18–3) (41). Of 91 pregnancies that occurred in women with untreated microadenomas, 95% had no signs or symptoms of tumor enlargement. However, 36% of the 56 pregnancies in women with untreated macroadenomas were complicated by headaches, visual disturbances, diabetes insipidus, or a combination of symptoms. Sixty percent of the women who developed symptoms required surgery, radiation, or bromocriptine during or shortly after pregnancy. The experience of women with previously treated adenomas was similar to that of women with untreated microadenomas—5 of 70 pregnancies (7.1%) were complicated by headache and/or visual disturbances, although only 1 of these women required treatment (irradiation) during pregnancy. The benign course of pregnancy in

TABLE 18–3. Reproductive Outcome after Bromocriptine Therapy: The Effect of Pregnancy on Pituitary Adenomas

	NO. OF PREGNANCIES	SYMPTOMS* No.	SYMPTOMS* %	CONSERVATIVE THERAPY	DEFINITIVE THERAPY†
Untreated microadenomas	91	5	5.5	5	0
Untreated macroadenomas	56	20	36	13	9
Treated adenomas	70	5	7.1	4	1

* Headache, visual disturbance, or diabetes insipidus.
† Bromocriptine, hypophyseal surgery, or irradiation.
Adapted from Gemzell C, Wang CF. Outcome of pregnancy in women with pituitary adenoma. Fertil Steril 1979; 31:363–372.

about 95% of women with pituitary microadenomas and the far greater rate of tumor complications among women with macroadenomas is confirmed by others (32,39,42,43). From these data, we suggest that women with microadenomas receive bromocriptine but those with macroadenomas have their tumors resected. Should surgery become necessary, there is evidence that prolactinomas treated with bromocriptine may be more difficult to resect transsphenoidally than untreated tumors (44).

Tubal Disease

It is nearly impossible to produce an accurate, meaningful analysis of reproductive outcome after treatment of tubal disease because there are so many different types of tubal pathology with varying degrees of severity. The problem of deriving accurate information is compounded by the multitude of procedures used to restore tubal anatomy. Recognizing these difficulties, we have chosen to summarize most of the available information about pregnancy outcome after salpingostomy, uterotubal implantation, tubal anastomosis, and salpingolysis. When possible, we have assessed the impact of microsurgical techniques in improving reproductive performance. Data regarding live births, spontaneous abortions, and ectopic pregnancies after tubal surgery are summarized in Table 18-4.

The abortion rate of intrauterine pregnancies is higher (16.6% to 26.7%) than the reference rate (10%) following most tubal surgical procedures (45–47). Gamete aging may be partly reponsible for this increase. While loculations within the tubal lumina resulting from tubal disease or corrective surgery may cause ectopic implantation, it is also possible that ovum transport may be delayed and the ovum aged when it is fertilized. Postovulatory aging of the secondary oocyte leads to embryonic wastage in lower animals (48), and perhaps in women (49). The tubal isthmus may contribute to the selection of sperm that will fertilize an ovum; hence, sperm selection may be impaired in women with abnormal tubal function (1). Abnormal tubal function may also contribute to the increased abortion rate, perhaps by allowing larger numbers of karyotypically abnormal spermatozoa to fertilize an ovum (1).

The ectopic pregnancy rate following tubal plastic or lytic procedures (9% to 15.5%) is approximately 10 times higher than the rate in an unselected population. The cause of ectopic implantation after tubal plastic surgery is almost certainly altered transport of the conceptus in tubes damaged by disease but only partially restored by surgery.

Diamond has compared the pregnancy rates in 2 groups of women (360 total) operated upon for infertility attributed to postoperative pelvic adhesions (50). Two hundred and twenty of the women underwent surgery by conventional techniques (1968 to 1974) and 140 by microsurgical techniques (1974 to 1977). In addition to an improved pregnancy rate, there was a reduction in the incidence of fetal wastage (spontaneous abortion, ectopic pregnancy, molar gestation) from 26.7% to 7% after adopting microsurgical techniques. In studies of this kind, however, it is difficult to know whether the improved outcome resulted from use of the microscope or to the impact of numerous other improvements in surgical instruments, suture, and technique that were introduced along with the operating microscope. Siegler and Kontopoulos achieved a 28% pregnancy rate in 80 women who underwent microsurgical tuboplasty, a figure more than twice that in 80 women after conventional surgery (51). However, the ectopic pregnancy rate after microsurgery (11%) was not strikingly

TABLE 18-4. Pregnancy Outcome after Tubal Operations Collated from Published Reports

TREATMENT	PREGNANCY OUTCOME		
	SUCCESSFUL	ABORTION	ECTOPIC
Salpingostomy	352	121 (26.7%)	87 (15.5%)
Uterotubal implantation	265	77 (22.4%)	49 (12.5%)
Tubal anastomosis	97	19 (17.9%)	20 (14.7%)
Salpingolysis	531	98 (16.6%)	62 (9.0%)

Modified from Jansen RPS. Spontaneous abortion incidence in the treatment of infertility. Am J Obstet Gynecol 1982;143:451–473. Reproduced with permission.

lower than after conventional surgery (17%). Gomel reported a pregnancy rate after microsurgical reanastomosis of previously ligated tubes that was more than twice the rate reported after conventional surgery (52). Only 1 of the 118 women in his series had a tubal pregnancy, and the incidence of spontaneous abortion (9.4%) was not increased. For comparison, he cited tubal pregnancy rates as high as 21% after conventional reanastomosis (52). These data suggest that microsurgery for infertility not only results in an increased pregnancy rate, but also improves pregnancy outcome. However, Garcia and Mastroianni cite evidence that the rate of tubal pregnancy after microsurgical salpingostomy (reported as high as 12%) is considerably higher than the lowest rate reported after either conventional surgery (3%) or use of the Rock-Mulligan hood (6% to 10%) (53). The reasons for these differences are not presently apparent, but the observation underscores the need for a continuing appraisal of the relative benefits of modified conventional techniques versus the more expensive microsurgical procedures.

Pregnancy rates in women undergoing conservative surgery for tubal pregnancy are surprisingly high. One third of 352 women whose tube was conserved while removing a tubal pregnancy subsequently achieved an intrauterine pregnancy, while 15% of those who conceived had a repeat ectopic pregnancy (54). Jones and Rock, however, collected data from 129 women with conservatively managed tubal pregnancies and reported a lower repeat ectopic pregnancy rate (7%) (55). Valle and Lifchez performed conservative surgery in 13 women with tubal pregnancies; all 11 of the 13 who were available for follow-up and had tried to conceive have had at least 1 term pregnancy (56). Thus, conservative surgery using microsurgical techniques when possible is justified in the management of ectopic pregnancy in women who wish to conceive again.

Uterine Abnormalities

Leiomyomata, congenital malformations, and uterine synechiae interfere with reproductive performance by causing abortion or premature labor. Other complications ascribed to uterine malformations include limb reduction anomalies from early limb compression *in utero* (57), implantation of the pregnancy in the uterine angle medial to the uterotubal junction (58), abnormal fetal presentation in labor, a resultant increased Cesarean section rate, and a 3-fold increase in the incidence of low-birth-weight infants with an increased perinatal loss (59). Complications more closely related to uterine synechiae are placenta previa and placenta accreta (60).

UTERINE LEIOMYOMATA. A term pregnancy rate of 40% to 50% follows myomectomy in women with primary infertility (61–63). The pregnancy rate in women with myomata not undergoing myomectomy is unknown. The incidence of spontaneous abortion after myomectomy is approximately 17% (1). Despite the lack of extensive supporting data, most authorities recommend myomectomy in women with otherwise unexplained primary infertility when the uterus is 2 or more times the normal size, and whenever leiomyomata are discovered in women with recurrent midpregnancy loss. It is commonly recommended that Cesarean section be performed instead of allowing labor in women who have undergone myomectomy (64). Jones and Rock, however, delivered 16 of 28 such women vaginally. They recommend that vaginal delivery be anticipated unless the uterine scars may have been weakened by postoperative infection or multiple incisions were made in the uterus during an extensive myomectomy (63).

CONGENITAL UTERINE ANOMALIES. Among the numerous variations and degrees of müllerian anomalies, only 2 have important influences on reproductive performance: septate uterus and bicornuate uterus (65–67). The mechanism of early pregnancy wastage in women with one of these conditions is presumed to be defective implantation. Later in pregnancy physical constraint and distortion of the enlarging gestational sac may lead to prostaglandin generation and premature labor. Regardless of the mechanism, the rate of pregnancy wastage in untreated women is as high as 70% to 80%. Musich and Behrman reported a successful pregnancy outcome in 28% of women with a uterine anomaly (66). Most, however, had a didelphic uterus. The rate of pregnancy loss was 90% in women with septate or bicornuate anomalies. Approximately 75%

of women will deliver a viable infant after metroplasty for a septate or bicornuate uterus (66,68).

In contrast to the septate and bicornuate anomalies, didelphic anomalies infrequently impair reproductive performance and rarely require surgical correction (65–67). Other obstetric complications appear to occur no more frequently than normal in women with uterine anomalies.

UTERINE SYNECHIAE. Spontaneous abortion, premature delivery, ectopic pregnancy, placenta accreta, and placenta previa are the principal adverse effects of intrauterine adhesions on pregnancy outcome (60). Unfortunately, many of these outcomes are cited only anecdotally, so it is difficult to analyze the impact of therapy on their occurrence rates. In addition, so many treatments have been implemented in the management of uterine synechiae that it is often difficult to collate data in a useful fashion.

Despite these difficulties, estrogen therapy after lysis or removal of adhesions appears to reduce significantly the rate of spontaneous abortion. The composite spontaneous abortion rate after lysis of intrauterine adhesions in women who did not receive estrogen supplementation was 35.4% (1). In contrast, the abortion rate in women treated with estrogen after lysis of synechiae was 7.5%. The overall success of pregnancy after treatment of uterine synechiae does not seem to depend on the extent of disease (69).

March and colleagues were able to accomplish complete lysis of adhesions in 61 of 66 women with uterine synechiae (70). After completing surgical and hormonal therapy, 98% of these women had normal menses and the uterine cavity was normal at the time of repeat hysteroscopy in 32 of 34 women. Seven of 10 women who desired to become pregnant had done so. While these results are encouraging, the role of hysteroscopy in improving pregnancy outcome must be assessed with additional studies.

Cervical Factor

Two types of cervical abnormalities impair reproductive performance. The first is cervical hostility, a term that encompasses a variety of disorders that result in lack of sperm penetration into mucus or immobilization of spermatozoa in mucus. An inadequate quantity or quality of cervical mucus, endocervical infection, and the presence of antisperm antibodies are examples of cervical hostility. (Treatment of these is discussed in Chapter 7.) The incidence of spontaneous abortion may be high in some women who produce antisperm antibodies when conception does occur. Over 50% of women who were infertile more than 3 years because of the presence of sperm-immobilizing or sperm-agglutinating antibodies aborted their next conception (71). Only 10% to 12% of those with infertility caused by other factors did so (71). Otherwise, these disorders do not appear to alter reproductive performance once conception occurs.

An incompetent cervix is the other major cervical cause of poor reproductive performance. This problem does not constitute a barrier to conception, and hence, it is not traditionally considered a principal cause of infertility, per se. An incompetent cervix instead leads to midpregnancy loss or premature delivery as a result of passive cervical dilatation. Cerclage of the incompetent cervix results in a successful outcome in 85% to 90% of women who subsequently conceive (72). In addition to other abnormalities, women exposed as fetuses to diethylstilbestrol may also have an incompetent cervix (73). Women at risk for cervical incompetence should be examined carefully and often during the first half of their pregnancies so that cerclage can be performed when cervical dilatation is first observed (74). The procedure should be performed prophylactically in women who had cervical incompetence in a previous pregnancy.

Endometriosis

It is commonly assumed that pregnancy ameliorates persistent or recurrent endometriosis and that the pregnancy is not at increased risk. Both assumptions are incorrect.

The composite spontaneous abortion rate in 98 pregnancies following pseudopregnancy therapy was 18%, nearly twice the normal rate in a reference population and twice the rate in 769 pregnancies after surgical treatment of endometriosis (9.3%) (1). The abortion rate in

97 pregnancies following danazol therapy, 10.6%, was no different than normal (1). Petersohn apparently was the first author to document an increased incidence of abortion in women with endometriosis (75). Naples and associates also found a high abortion rate in a retrospective analysis of 214 pregnancies that occurred before endometriosis was recognized; the rate increased rapidly as the disease became clinically recognizable (76). After treatment, the abortion rate fell and the term pregnancy rate rose, but the outcome of pregnancy was better after surgical than nonsurgical therapy. Of the 50 pregnancies that followed surgical resection of endometriosis, 46 resulted in live births (44 delivered at term) and 4 ended in spontaneous abortion. In contrast, only 36 of the 51 pregnancies that followed nonsurgical treatment delivered at term. Four percent of the pregnancies ended prematurely and 25.5% aborted spontaneously. Wheeler and associates reported a similarly salutary effect of conservative surgery; the spontaneous abortion rate fell from 34% to 9% after surgery (77). They speculated that the abortion rate may be increased as the result of tubouterine effects produced by prostaglandins from the endometriosis.

These reports provide evidence that conservative surgical procedures, and perhaps also danazol, may lead to a better pregnancy outcome than pseudopregnancy regimens. This view is consistent with the observation that pregnancy may not exert the therapeutic impact on endometriosis that has been traditionally taught (78). In fact, endometriomas occasionally enlarge and rupture during pregnancy, causing a hemorrhagic crisis (79).

Male Factor

There is no evidence that seminal or spermatozoal abnormalities influence the reproductive outcome after the first half of pregnancy.

Seminal factors may influence the abortion rate. The composite abortion incidence in pregnancies resulting from artificial insemination of fresh donor semen, 11% to 14%, is not significantly different from the reference population (1). In contrast, the incidence of abortion is probably increased in pregnancies that occur after insemination of the husband's semen (AIH). Jansen computed a composite abortion incidence of 24.3% in 264 such pregnancies (1). Since AIH is most commonly performed for such reasons as oligospermia or poor sperm motility, the chance that an ovum may be fertilized by an intrinsically abnormal sperm could thereby be increased. Whatever the mechanism, the increased abortion incidence after AIH is the only evidence that defective spermatozoa increase the likelihood of early pregnancy wastage.

In Vitro Fertilization

Two of the first 4 pregnancies Steptoe and Edwards achieved by *in vitro* fertilization (IVF) were chromosomally defective (80). There are still too few reported pregnancies to assess reproductive performance. Nevertheless, the apparent abortion incidence may be somewhat increased after IVF and embryo transfer; this may be the result of the detection bias guaranteed by the intensely close surveillance of each treatment cycle. In contrast to the early experience in England, the late outcome of pregnancies reported thus far seems similar to an unselected population of women (81–83).

Recurrent Abortion

Schwarz has discussed the flawed assumptions in defining the risk of yet another abortion in women who have habitually miscarried in the past (Chapter 15). Warburton and Fraser computed a 32% risk of a fourth abortion in women with 3 previous consecutive abortions (84). Despite relative agreement about the validity of this computed risk, it is crucial to recognize that the causes of abortion are varied and that the chances of a subsequent abortion depend greatly on the cause(s) of the previous ones. Tho et al. reported that recurrent pregnancy wastage was associated with genetic disorders in 25% of couples, with müllerian anomalies in 15%, and with luteal phase dysfunction or other endocrine abnormalities in 23% (85,86). In 37% of couples, the reason for recurrent abortion is unknown. Thirty-two percent of those with a genetic basis for abortion subsequently had a living child; 60% of women with a müllerian anomaly, 91% of those with an endocrine abnormality, and 62% with unexplained recurrent abortion did likewise (86).

Reproductive Performance After Age Thirty-five

Tulandi and colleagues analyzed the reproductive performance of 93 infertile couples in whom the female partner was older than 36 years (87). A tubal factor was the most commonly identified cause of infertility in women between 36 and 40 years. After age 40, the infertility was most often unexplained. These observations contradict the widespread belief that ovulatory dysfunction is the most common cause of infertility in women older than 35 years. Only 33% of women older than 36 years conceived (87). Thirty-one percent of the conceptions ended as a spontaneous abortion.

Declining reproductive performance in the fifth decade of life is not exclusively the fault of women. Friedman computed that the frequency of autosomal dominant disease among the offspring of fathers who are 40 years of age or older is at least 0.3% to 0.5%, a figure similar to the risk of Down's syndrome in the offspring of 35- to 40-year-old mothers (88).

Despite the poor outlook for correcting infertility in couples after the age of 35, pregnancy is not clearly contraindicated solely on the basis of age in healthy women. The principal problems of such pregnancies are prematurity and an increased perinatal mortality rate, but many admonitions about the risks of circulatory disorders, hypertension, diabetes mellitus, and others have not proved to be sufficiently problematic to advise against pregnancy (89). The reproductive outcome of women older than 35 years is summarized in Table 18–5.

TABLE 18–5. Reproductive Performance after Age Thirty-five

1. The spontaneous abortion rate is increased 200%.
2. There is an increased incidence of autosomal dominant disease in offspring of fathers over age 40.
3. Prematurity and perinatal mortality rates are increased.

Conclusion

Our care of infertile couples does not end at the moment of conception. The risk of spontaneous abortion is increased with many disorders that cause infertility. Problems late in pregnancy may also occur more frequently in these women, but their occurrence is related to 2 factors—the cause of infertility and the age of the couple at the time of conception.

REFERENCES

1. Jansen RPS. Spontaneous abortion incidence in the treatment of infertility. Am J Obstet Gynecol 1982;143:451–473.
2. Chartier M, Roger M, Barrat J, Michelon B. Measurement of plasma human chorionic gonadotropin (hCG) and beta-hCG activities in the late luteal phase: evidence of the occurrence of spontaneous menstrual abortions in infertile women. Fertil Steril 1979;31:134–137.
3. Gorlitsky GA, Kase NG, Speroff L. Ovulation and pregnancy rates with clomiphene citrate. Obstet Gynecol 1978;51:265–269.
4. Hack M, Brish M, Serr DM, Insler V, Salomy M, Lunenfeld B. Outcome of pregnancy after induced ovulation. Follow-up of pregnancies and children born after clomiphene therapy. JAMA 1972;220:1329–1333.
5. Clomid. Product information with illustrations and commentary. Cincinnati: Merrell-National Laboratories, 1972.
6. Asch RH, Greenblatt RB. Update on the safety and efficacy of clomiphene citrate as a therapeutic agent. J Reprod Med 1976;17:175–180.
7. Garcia J, Jones GS, Wentz AC. The use of clomiphene citrate. Fertil Steril 1977;28:707–717.
8. Boue JG, Boue A. Increased frequency of chromosomal anomalies in abortions after induced ovulation. Lancet 1973;1:679–680.
9. Gysler M, March CM, Mishell DR, Bailey EJ. A decade's experience with an individualized clomiphene treatment regimen including its effect on the postcoital test. Fertil Steril 1982;37:161–167.
10. Adashi EY, Rock JA, Sapp KC, Martin EJ, Wentz AC, Jones GS. Gestational outcome of clomiphene-related conceptions. Fertil Steril 1979;31:620–626.
11. Varma TR. Ultrasound evidence of early pregnancy failure in patients with multiple conceptions. Br J Obstet Gynaecol 1979;86:290–292.
12. Driessen F, Holwerda PJ, Putte SCJ, Kremer J. The significance of dating an endometrial bi-

opsy for the prognosis of the infertile couple. Int J Fertil 1980;25:112–116.
13. Speroff L, Glass RH, Kase NG. Clinical gynecologic endocrinology and infertility, 3rd ed. Baltimore: Williams & Wilkins, 1983:480.
14. DiZerega GS, Hodgen GD. Luteal phase dysfunction infertility: a sequel to aberrant folliculogenesis. In: Wallach EE, Kempers RD, eds. Modern trends in infertility and conception control. Philadelphia: Harper & Row, 1982:12–22.
15. Echt CR, Romberger FT, Goodman JA. Clomiphene citrate in the treatment of luteal phase defects. Fertil Steril 1969;20:564–571.
16. Quagliarello J, Weiss G. Clomiphene citrate in the management of infertility associated with shortened luteal phases. Fertil Steril 1979;31:373–377.
17. Downs KA, Gibson M. Clomiphene citrate therapy for luteal phase defect. Fertil Steril 1983;39:34–38.
18. Poulson AM, Bryner WA. The obstetric complications of the infertility patient. Obstet Gynecol 1977;49:174–179.
19. Creasy RK, Gummer BA, Liggins GC. System for predicting spontaneous preterm birth. Obstet Gynecol 1980;55:692–695.
20. Speroff L, Glass RH, Kase NG. Clinical gynecologic endocrinology and infertility, 3rd ed. Baltimore: Williams & Wilkins, 1983:75–100.
21. Ben-Rafael Z, Mashiach S, Oelsener G, Farine D, Lunenfeld B, Serr DM. Spontaneous pregnancy and its outcome after human menopausal gonadotropin/human chorionic gonadotropin-induced pregnancy. Fertil Steril 1981;36:560–564.
22. Brown JB, Evans JH, Adey FD, Taft MP, Townsend L. Factors involved in the induction of fertile ovulation with gonadotropins. J Obstet Gynaecol Br Comm 1969;76:289–307.
23. Schenker JG, Yarkoni S, Granat M. Multiple pregnancies following induction of ovulation. In: Wallach EE, Kempers RD, eds. Modern trends in infertility and conception control. Philadelphia: Harper & Row, 1982:134–152.
24. McBain JC, Evans JH, Pepperell RJ, Robinson HP, Smith M, Brown JB. An unexpectedly high rate of ectopic pregnancy following the induction of ovulation with human pituitary and chorionic gonadotropin. Br J Obstet Gynaecol 1980;87:5–9.
25. Granat M, Evron S, Navot D. Pregnancy in heterotopic fallopian tube and unilateral ovarian hyperstimulation. Acta Obstet Gynecol Scand 1981;60:215–217.
26. Olson JL, Rebar RW, Schreiber JR, Vaitukaitis JL. Shortened luteal phase after ovulation induction with human menopausal gonadotropin and human chorionic gonadotropin. Fertil Steril 1983;39:284–291.
27. Gemzell CA, Roos P, Loeffler FE. Follicle-stimulating hormone extracted from human pituitary. In: Behrman SJ, Kistner RW, eds. Progress in infertility, 2nd ed. Boston: Little, Brown & Co., 1975:486.
28. Holcberg G, Biale Y, Lewenthal H, Insler V. Outcome of pregnancy in 31 triplet gestations. Obstet Gynecol 1982;59:472–476.
29. Hack M, Brish M, Serr DM, Insler V, Lunenfeld B. Outcome of pregnancy after induced ovulation. Follow-up of pregnancies and children born after gondotropin therapy. JAMA 1970;211:791–797.
30. Speroff L, Glass RH, Kase NG. Clinical gynecologic endocrinology and infertility, 3rd ed. Baltimore: Williams & Wilkins, 1983:539–541.
31. Schulz KD, Geiger W, del Pozo E, Kunzig HJ. Pattern of sexual steroids, prolactin, and gonadotropic hormones during prolactin inhibition in normally cycling women. Am J Obstet Gynecol 1978;132:561–566.
32. Crosignani PG, Ferrari C, Scarduelli C, Picciotti MC, Caldara R, Malinverni A. Spontaneous and induced pregnancies in hyperprolactinemic women. Obstet Gynecol 1981;58:708–713.
33. Coelingh Bennink HJT. Intermittent bromocriptine treatment for the induction of ovulation in hyperprolactinemic patients. Fertil Steril 1979;31:267–272.
34. Griffith RW, Turkalj I, Braun P. Outcome of pregnancy in mothers given bromocriptine. Br J Clin Pharmacol 1978;5:227–231.
35. Turkalj I, Braun P, Krupp P. Surveillance of bromocriptine in pregnancy. JAMA 1982;247:1589–1591.
36. van Roon E, van der Vijver JCM, Gerretsen G, Hekster REM, Wattendorff RA. Rapid regression of a suprasellar extending prolactinoma after bromocriptine treatment during pregnancy. Fertil Steril 1981;36:173–177.
37. Canales ES, Garcia IC, Ruiz JE, Zarate A. Bromocriptine as prophylactic therapy in prolactinoma during pregnancy. Fertil Steril 1981;36:524–526.
38. Boyar RM, Kapen S, Weitzman ED, Hellman L. Pituitary microadenoma and hyperprolactinemia. N Engl J Med 1976;294:263–265.
39. Bergh T, Nillius SJ, Wide L. Clinical course and outcome of pregnancies in amenorrhoeic women with hyperprolactinaemia and pituitary tumours. Br Med J 1978;1:875–880.
40. Van Dalen JTW, Greve EL. Rapid deterioration of visual fields during bromocryptine-induced pregnancy in a patient with a pituitary adenoma. Br J Ophthalmol 1977;61:729–733.

41. Gemzell C, Wang CF. Outcome of pregnancy in women with pituitary adenoma. Fertil Steril 1979;31:363–372.
42. Jewelewicz R, Vande Wiele RL. Clinical course and outcome of pregnancy in twenty-five patients with pituitary microadenomas. Am J Obstet Gynecol 1980;136:339–343.
43. Shewchuk AB, Adamson GD, Lessard P, Ezrin C. The effect of pregnancy on suspected pituitary adenomas after conservative management of ovulation defects associated with galactorrhea. Am J Obstet Gynecol 1980;136:659–666.
44. Landolt AM, Keller PJ, Froesch ER, Mueller J. Bromocriptine: does it jeopardise the result of later surgery for prolactinomas? Lancet 1982;2:657–658.
45. Crane M, Woodruff JD. Factors influencing the success of tuboplastic procedures. Fertil Steril 1978;19:810–825.
46. David A, Nagar H, Sheer DM. Tubal plastic surgery at the Tel Hashomer Hospital: a critical study. Fertil Steril 1976;27:511–516.
47. Jansen RPS. Abortion incidence following fallopian tube repair. Obstet Gynecol 1980;56:499–502.
48. Lanman JT. Delays during reproduction and their effects on the embryo and fetus. 2. Aging of eggs. N Engl J Med 1968;278:1047–1054.
49. Guerrero R, Rojas OI. Spontaneous abortion and aging of human ova and spermatozoa. N Engl J Med 1975;293:573–575.
50. Diamond E. Lysis of postoperative pelvic adhesions in infertility. Fertil Steril 1979;31:287–295.
51. Siegler AM, Kontopoulos V. An analysis of macrosurgical and microsurgical techniques in the management of the tuboperitoneal factor in infertility. Fertil Steril 1979;32:377–383.
52. Gomel V. Microsurgical reversal of female sterilization: a reappraisal. Fertil Steril 1980;33:587–597.
53. Garcia C-R, Mastroianni L. Microsurgery for treatment of adnexal disease. In: Wallach EE, Kempers RD, eds. Modern trends in infertility and conception control. Philadelphia: Harper & Row, 1982:258.
54. Hallatt JG. Repeat ectopic pregnancy: a study of 123 consecutive cases. Am J Obstet Gynecol 1975;122:520–523.
55. Jones HW, Rock JA. Surgery of the oviduct. In: Reparative and constructive surgery of the female generative tract. Baltimore: Williams & Wilkins, 1983:109.
56. Valle JA, Lifchez AS. Reproductive outcome following conservative surgery for tubal pregnancy in women with a single fallopian tube. Fertil Steril 1983;39:316–320.
57. Graham JM, Miller ME, Stephan MJ, Smith DW. Limb reduction anomalies and early in utero limb compression. J Pediatr 1980;96:1052–1056.
58. Jansen RPS, Elliott PM. Angular intrauterine pregnancy. Obstet Gynecol 1981;58:167–175.
59. Pritchard JA, MacDonald PC. Williams obstetrics, 16th ed. New York: Appleton-Century-Crofts, 1980:629.
60. Forssman L. Posttraumatic intrauterine synechiae and pregnancy. Obstet Gynecol 1965;26:710–713.
61. Rubin IC. Uterine fibromyomas and sterility. Clin Obstet Gynecol 1958;1:501–518.
62. Barter RH, Parks J. Myoma uteri associated with pregnancy. Clin Obstet Gynecol 1958;1:519–533.
63. Jones HW, Rock JA. Surgery of the body of the uterus. In: Reparative and constructive surgery of the female generative tract. Baltimore: Williams & Wilkins, 1983:61–71.
64. Pritchard JA, MacDonald PC. Williams obstetrics, 16th ed. New York: Appleton-Century-Crofts, 1980:850–851.
65. Rock JA, Jones HW. The clinical management of the double uterus. Fertil Steril 1977;28:798–806.
66. Musich JR, Behrman SJ. Obstetric outcome before and after metroplasty in women with uterine anomalies. Obstet Gynecol 1978;52:63–66.
67. Buttram VC, Gibbons WE. Mullerian anomalies: a proposed classification (an analysis of 144 cases). Fertil Steril 1979;32:40–46.
68. Jones HW, Rock JA. Anomalies of the mullerian ducts. In: Reparative and constructive surgery of the female generative tract. Baltimore: Williams & Wilkins, 1983:185.
69. Bergquist CA, Rock JA, Jones HW. Pregnancy outcome following treatment of intrauterine adhesions. Int J Fertil 1981;26:107–111.
70. March CM, Israel R, March AD. Hysteroscopic management of intrauterine adhesions. Am J Obstet Gynecol 1978;130:653–657.
71. Jones WR. Immunological aspects of infertility. In: Scott JS, Jones WR, eds. Immunology of human reproduction. New York: Grune & Stratton, 1977:375.
72. Kuhn RPJ, Pepperell RJ. Cervical ligation: a review of 242 pregnancies. Aust NZ Obstet Gynaecol 1977;17:79–83.
73. Rosenfeld DL, Bronson RA. Reproductive problems in the DES-exposed female. Obstet Gynecol 1980;55:453–456.
74. Nunley WC, Kitchin JD. Successful management of incompetent cervix in a primigravida exposed to diethylstilbestrol in utero. Fertil Steril 1979;31:217–219.

75. Petersohn L. Fertility in patients with ovarian endometriosis before and after treatment. Acta Obstet Gynecol Scand 1970;49:331–333.
76. Naples JD, Batt RE, Sadigh H. Spontaneous abortion rate in patients with endometriosis. Obstet Gynecol 1981;57:509–512.
77. Wheeler JM, Johnston BM, Malinak LR. The relationship of endometriosis to spontaneous abortion. Fertil Steril 1983;39:656–660.
78. Walton LA. A reexamination of endometriosis after pregnancy. J Reprod Med 1977;19:341–344.
79. Pritchard JA, MacDonald PC. Williams obstetrics, 16th ed. New York: Appleton-Century-Crofts, 1980:635–636.
80. Steptoe PC, Edwards RG, Purdy JM. Clinical aspects of pregnancies established with cleaving embryos grown in vitro. Br J Obstet Gynaecol 1980;87:757–768.
81. Wood C, Trounson A, Leeton J, et al. A clinical assessment of nine pregnancies obtained by in vitro fertilization and embryo transfer. Fertil Steril 1981;35:502–508.
82. Wood C, Trounson A, Leeton JF, et al. Clinical features of eight pregnancies resulting from in vitro fertilization and embryo transfer. Fertil Steril 1982;38:22–29.
83. Jones HW, Jones GS, Andrews MC, et al. The program for in vitro fertilization at Norfolk. Fertil Steril 1982;38:14–21.
84. Warburton D, Fraser FC. Spontaneous abortion risks in man: data from reproductive histories collected in a medical genetics units. Am J Hum Genet 1964;16:1–25.
85. Glass RH, Golbus MS. Habitual abortion. Fertil Steril 1978;29:257–265.
86. Tho PT, Byrd JR, McDonough PG. Etiologies and subsequent reproductive performance of 100 couples with recurrent abortion. Fertil Steril 1979;32:389–395.
87. Tulandi T, Arronet GH, McInnes RA. Infertility in women over the age of 36. Fertil Steril 1981;35:611–614.
88. Friedman JM. Genetic disease in the offspring of older fathers. Obstet Gynecol 1981;57:745–749.
89. Kessler I, Lancet M, Borenstein R, Steinmetz A. The problem of the older primipara. Obstet Gynecol 1980;56:165–169.

Primary Amenorrhea 19

James Aiman

Menarche occurs at a mean age of 12.8 to 13.5 years (1,2) and 95% of normal women have begun to menstruate by the age of 15.5 to 16 years. After 16 years of age, women who have never menstruated may be normal but are more likely to have a genetic, developmental, or endocrinologic abnormality that warrants a careful evaluation. A comprehensive evaluation is not necessary for most women under the age of 16 years, but is for women over 16 years, especially if there is a family history of primary amenorrhea, ambiguous genitalia, or evidence of an endocrinopathy that may affect menstrual function. An abbreviated evaluation without extensive hormonal studies or karyotype is often sufficient to relieve the adolescent's or her parents' concern that something other than delayed puberty is the cause of primary amenorrhea. Thus, there are 3 indications to evaluate a woman who has never menstruated—age over 16 years, a positive family history of amenorrhea or genital abnormality, and patient or parental concern.

In the first part of this chapter, a practical, efficient, and economical approach to the diagnosis of primary amenorrhea is described. This approach relies on a careful history, a thorough physical examination, and a minimum of laboratory tests. The last part of this chapter contains a description of the conditions that cause primary amenorrhea, their unique diagnostic features, and their therapy. Each cause is described within its appropriate diagnostic category.

General Observations

There are a series of observations that relate certain clinical features to the embryology, genetics, or endocrinology of normal sexual differentiation and maturation (Table 19–1).

A. *Sexual infantilism means no exposure to androgen or estrogen.* Sexual infantilism refers to the prepubertal appearance of a girl. Breast growth or other signs of sexual maturation are absent. The presence or absence of pubic hair is not included in the list of features used to define sexual infantilism since this will frequently be present as a manifestation of adrenal function even though ovarian function may be absent.

B. *Breast development in a woman with primary amenorrhea means estrogen exposure.* The estrogen exposure may be the result of current ovarian secretion or prior secretion from ovaries that no longer produce estrogen. A drug history that excludes prior estrogen therapy is essential before concluding that the breast development resulted from endogenous estrogen production.

C. *Genital ambiguity means abnormal testosterone and dihydrotestosterone representation* in utero. The presence of ambiguous genitalia in a newborn that was genetically destined to be a female means that the fetus was exposed to excessive testosterone from the ovaries or adrenal glands of the fetus or her mother. Additionally, maternal ingestion of drugs with androgenic effects during

TABLE 19–1. General Observations

A. Sexual infantilism means no androgen or estrogen exposure.
B. Breast development means estrogen exposure.
C. Genital ambiguity means abnormal testosterone and dihydrotestosterone representation *in utero*.
D. Hirsutism and clitoral enlargement mean excessive testosterone and dihydrotestosterone exposure.
E. No uterus means müllerian duct regression factor *in utero*.
F. Müllerian agenesis is the only condition where the uterus is absent and the karyotype is 46,XX.
G. Hypertension in a woman with primary amenorrhea suggests 17-alpha-hydroxylase deficiency.
H. Internal genital anomalies are often associated with urinary tract anomalies.
I. The presence of a Y chromosome in a woman with primary amenorrhea is associated with an increased risk of a gonadal tumor.
J. Any sex steroid activity in a woman with primary amenorrhea due to gonadal dysgenesis is also associated with a risk of a gonadal tumor.
K. Gonadal dysgenesis is the cause of primary amenorrhea in chromatin negative (45,X or 46,XY) women with a uterus.

pregnancy may cause virilization of the genitalia of a fetus destined to be a female.

Genital ambiguity in a fetus genetically destined to be a male is the result of deficient testosterone (or dihydrotestosterone) synthesis or deficient testosterone action *in utero*. Deficient synthesis of testosterone may be due to congenital absence of the testes (3), absence of Leydig cells (4), or an enzymatic defect that precludes normal testosterone synthesis (5–11). Each of these enzyme defects is inherited as an autosomal recessive trait.

Variable degrees of genital ambiguity are found in genetic males with one of the androgen-resistant syndromes caused by a deficiency of the cytosolic receptor in androgen target tissues (12). These are inherited as X-linked recessive traits, although affected subjects with no family history have also been described.

D. *Hirsutism and clitoral enlargement mean excessive testosterone and dihydrotestosterone exposure.* Although the production of several other androgens is often increased in hirsute women, the biologic potency of these is less than 10% to 20% that of testosterone or dihydrotestosterone. Testosterone excess in a hirsute woman may be due to a functional or neoplastic disorder of the ovary or adrenal gland.

E. *No uterus means müllerian duct regression factor was present* in utero. Müllerian duct regression factor is a peptide hormone produced by Sertoli cells that locally suppresses the development of the müllerian duct. Given the testicular source of this substance, the absence of a uterus in a woman with primary amenorrhea suggests the presence of testes and implies a 46,XY karyotype. There is 1 exception to this association of no uterus and the presence of testes.

F. *Müllerian agenesis is the only condition where the uterus is absent and the karyotype is a normal 46,XX.* Since ovarian function in these women is normal, documentation of ovulation proves this cause of primary amenorrhea and excludes any cause of male pseudohermaphroditism. Most true hermaphrodites have a 46,XX karyotype and may not have a uterus (though more than one half do) (13). However, most true hermaphrodites will be Y-antigen positive, which suggests that genetic information on the Y chromosome has been translocated to another chromosome (14).

G. *Hypertension in a woman with primary amenorrhea suggests 17-alpha-hydroxylase deficiency.* Subjects with 17-alpha-hydroxylase deficiency are sexually infantile because androgen and estrogen secretion is decreased or absent. Cortisol secretion is also decreased and ACTH concentrations are increased. Hypertension occurs in these subjects as a consequence of an ACTH-stimulated increase in the secretion of 11-desoxycorticosterone, a potent mineralcorticoid.

H. *Internal genital tract anomalies are often associated with urinary tract anomalies.* The presence of an anomaly in one system is an indication to evaluate the other. For example, an intravenous pyelogram will reveal an abnormality of the kidneys in approximately 30% of women with a transverse vaginal septum, no uterus, or an abnormally developed uterus (e.g., a bicornuate uterus) (15).

I. *The presence of a Y chromosome in a woman with primary amenorrhea is associated with the development of a dysontogenetic gonadal tumor.* The gonads of such women ought to be removed since 25% to 40% will develop a tumor (16–18), although usually not until the third decade of life (19). The streak gonads of a woman with 46,XY gonadal dysgenesis should be removed at the time of diagnosis since the streaks will never produce sex steroids. Removal of the testes from a subject with complete testicular feminization may be deferred until the end of puberty since these women will feminize (i.e., develop breasts), but not virilize. To prevent virilization at the time of puberty, the testes of a subject with an incomplete form of androgen resistance should be removed when the diagnosis is certain.

J. *Any endocrine activity in a woman with primary amenorrhea is also associated with an increased risk of a dysontogenetic gonadal tumor.* Nine women with gonadal dysgenesis and a gonadal tumor but no Y chromosome had evidence of feminization (e.g., breast growth or uterine bleeding) or masculinization (17,20). Since these signs have also been reported in women with dysgenetic gonads containing hyperplastic hilus cells (21–23), the association of endocrine activity and a gonadal tumor is less frequent or certain than the association of such tumors with a Y chromosome.

K. *Any woman with primary amenorrhea who is chromatin negative and has a uterus has gonadal dysgenesis.* Women with a 45,X or a 46,XY karyotype will have streak gonads and a uterus. Presumably, the gonads of a woman with 46,XY gonadal dysgenesis are so dysgenetic (or "malformed") that they fail to produce müllerian duct regression factor as well as steroids. The only exception to this general observation is true hermaphroditism, in which it is possible to have a 46,XY karyotype and a uterus (13).

Evaluation of Primary Amenorrhea

The cause of primary amenorrhea can be learned by answering 4 questions:

a. Which sex steroid is expressed?
b. Does she have a uterus?
c. What is her karyotype?
d. What are the serum concentrations of LH and FSH?

The approach to a woman with primary amenorrhea described here depends upon answering these questions in this sequence (Fig. 19–1).

A. *Which sex steroid is represented?* The answer to this question is "none" for the woman who is sexually infantile and *sexual infantilism* is the first of 4 categories based on hormonal expression (Fig. 19–1, top left). For the woman with primary amenorrhea who has breast growth, the answer to this question is "estrogen" and she is categorized as having *incomplete puberty* (Figure 19-1, top right). Testosterone is the hormone represented in women with *congenital genital ambiguity*, which is defined by the presence of posterior labial fusion and/or phallic enlargement noted at birth or before the onset of puberty (Fig. 19–1, bottom right). Testosterone is also the hormone represented in a woman who develops signs of masculinization at or after the onset of puberty and these women are categorized as having *acquired androgen excess* (Fig. 19–1, bottom left). These definitions are based on the general observations described in the previous section.

B. *Does she have a uterus?* A pelvic examination will provide the answer to this question. The implications of no uterus in a woman with primary amenorrhea are summarized by general observations E and F (Table 19–1).

C. *What is her karyotype?* The presence or absence of a Barr body is used as a visual substitute for a karyotype in Fig. 19–1. While a buccal smear is rapid and inexpensive, it may be inaccurate and misleading owing to technical problems. Moreover, a chromatin-negative buccal smear does not distinguish between a 45,X and a 46,XY karyotype. For these reasons, a karyotype of peripheral lymphocytes should be performed to answer this third question. The presence of a Y chromosome implies the presence of testes and increases the risk of a dysontogenetic gonadal tumor—a risk that is absent in women with a 45,X karyotype.

D. *What are the serum concentrations of luteinizing hormone (LH) and follicle-stimulating hormone (FSH)?* The answer to this question is nec-

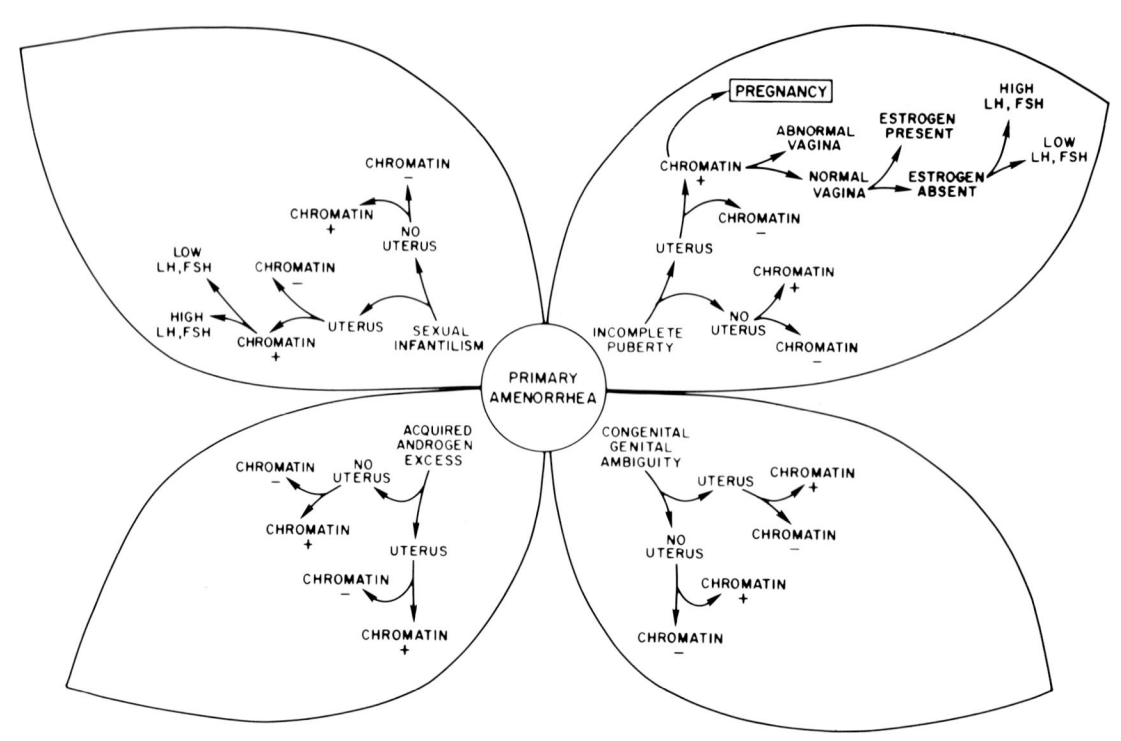

Fig. 19–1. Diagnostic approach to primary amenorrhea. After categorizing the woman according to her hormonal status, she is sequentially subcategorized by the presence or absence of a uterus, her karyotype, and her LH and FSH concentrations.

essary only for women with primary amenorrhea who have a uterus and a 46,XX karyotype. Low concentrations of LH and FSH are found in women with hypothalamic or pituitary failure. High concentrations of LH and FSH occur in women with ovarian failure who lack estradiol secretion to inhibit pituitary gonadotropin secretion.

Causes of Primary Amenorrhea

The reported causes of primary amenorrhea are summarized in Table 19–2. The statistics of Ross (24) are a review of the literature through 1972 whereas the reports of Kallio (25) and Maschak (26) represent individual studies. Because of the difference in the nature of these reports and in how the women were evaluated, the percentages in Table 19–2 are only approximate estimates of the causes of primary amenorrhea.

SEXUAL INFANTILISM.

Gonadal Dysgenesis (Turner's Syndrome). Women with gonadal dysgenesis are sexually infantile and have a uterus. Serum LH and FSH concentrations are increased, usually to levels greater than 50 mIU/ml because ovarian secretion of estradiol is absent (23). Gonadal dysgenesis is the most frequent cause of ovarian failure and primary amenorrhea (Table 19–2). In addition to the presence of streak gonads (Fig. 19–2), these women have a characteristic appearance, the features of which are summarized in Table 19–3 (27). Monosomy for the short arm of the X chromosome is present in all of these women. However, the presence of these clinical features is sufficient to make the diagnosis of gonadal dysgenesis and a karyotype is useful only for confirmation.

Germ cells are present in the gonads at the time of birth and approximately 40 women with Turner's syndrome have conceived (28–30). Most of these women had a mosaic karyotype, occasionally demonstrated only after cytogenetic analysis of gonadal tissue (31). However, fertility is rare in these women, who should receive estrogen to stimulate breast growth and enhance pubic hair development. Estrogen will also stimulate a growth spurt, although adult height is rarely greater than 5 feet. Because endometrial cancer may develop

TABLE 19–2. Causes of Primary Amenorrhea

	FREQUENCY (%)		
	Ross (24)	Kallio (25)	Maschak (26)
Gonadal dysgenesis	29	36	27
Testicular feminization	11*	2	6
Steroid enzyme deficiency	—	1	2
Polycystic ovarian disease	8	3	3
Ovarian failure	—	—	6
Congenital anorchia	—	—	2
Delayed puberty	6	—	—
Hypogonadotropic hypogonadism	8	9	19
Hypothalamic/pituitary tumor	—	2	8
Hypothalamic dysfunction	—	—	8
Hypothalamic/pituitary failure	0.2	—	10
Müllerian/urogenital abnormality	18	27	10
Miscellaneous	16	2	—
Unknown	4	18	—
Number of patients	538	100	62

* Frequency of genetic males: includes testicular feminization, gonadal dysgenesis (46,XY), congenital anorchia, and steroid enzyme defects in unknown proportion.

with estrogen therapy, a combination of estrogen and progestin should be prescribed once maximal stimulation of puberty has occurred. Endometrial cancer has also been reported with estrogen-progestin therapy (32).

The streak gonads do not need to be removed because the occurrence of a gonadal tumor is extremely rare in women with gonadal dysgenesis who do not have a Y chromosome. Evidence of sex steroid activity is usually present in women with Turner's syndrome who have a gonadal tumor not associated with the presence of a Y chromosome (17,20).

Pure Gonadal Dysgenesis. Sexual infantilism, the presence of a uterus and streak gonads, and increased serum concentrations of LH and FSH are also features of women with pure go-

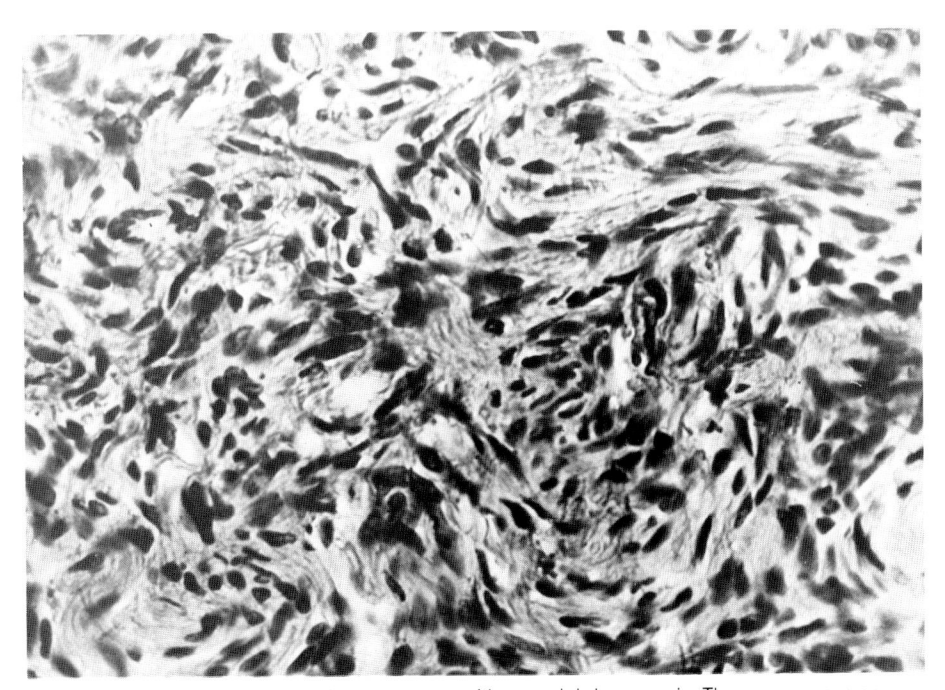

Fig. 19–2. A streak gonad from a woman with gonadal dysgenesis. There are no ova or follicles.

TABLE 19-3. Frequency of Turner Features in Gonadal Dysgenesis*

	45,X	45,X/46,XX	46,XX (p−)	46,XisoX (q+)
Short stature	96%	76%	83%	50%
Webbed neck	46	26	4	5
Low hairline	72	48	17	18
Shield chest	53	55	22	19
Pigmented nevi	63	49	17	14
Cubitus valgus	54	54	34	14
Short fourth metacarpal	47	40	17	24
Lymphedema	38	26	—	—
Cardiac abnormality	16	7	4	0
Renal abnormality	39	16	0	0
Hearing abnormality	54	30	0	5

* All values are percentages. 45,X/46,XX is a mosaic karyotype; 46,XX (p−) is deletion of the short arm of 1 X chromosome; 46,XisoX (q+) is an isochromosome of the long arm of 1 X chromosome. (From Simpson JL. Gonadal dysgenesis and sex chromosome abnormalities: phenotypic-karyotypic correlations. In: Vallet HL, Porter IH, eds. Genetic mechanism of sexual development. New York: Academic Press, 1979:365–405.)

nadal dysgenesis. However, these women have few or none of the somatic abnormalities of Turner's syndrome (33–35). There is often a family history of primary amenorrhea in women with pure gonadal dysgenesis. A 46,XY karyotype is present in approximately 30% of these subjects and there is a high risk for the development of a gonadal tumor (16,17,36). Gonadal tumors are rare in these women when they are sexually infantile and have no Y chromosome. Breast development, phallic enlargement, or other signs of sex steroid secretion may be caused by a tumor-induced secretion of estrogen or testosterone, but these signs have also been observed in affected women without a tumor (23). Fertility is not possible and these women should receive estrogen plus a progestin.

Mixed Gonadal Dysgenesis. The syndrome of mixed gonadal dysgenesis is characterized by the presence of a testis or gonadal tumor (usually intraabdominal) on one side, a streak gonad on the other side, and persistent müllerian structures (37,38). Masculinization of the external genitalia occurs at puberty when a testis is present. Feminizing signs such as breast growth suggest that the testis has been replaced by a gonadal tumor. Less than 50% of affected individuals have any of the phenotypic features of gonadal dysgenesis described in Table 19-3. The karyotype in most of these women is 45,X/46,XY. Despite the presence of a testis on one side, müllerian duct structures are usually present bilaterally. Presumably, the testis did not produce müllerian duct regression factor. An epididymis and vas deferens are usually found on the side of the testis. As with other forms of gonadal dysgenesis, serum concentrations of LH and FSH are usually increased. Because of the presence of a testis or a tumor, these women may not present as sexually infantile, but rather as having congenital genital ambiguity or precocious sexual development.

Sexually infantile women with mixed gonadal dysgenesis require estrogen to induce breast growth. Since fertility is not possible and masculinization of the external genitalia is likely to occur at puberty, the testis should be removed. One fourth of patients will develop a gonadal tumor, which appears before puberty in most subjects. This would also favor removal of the testis once the diagnosis of mixed gonadal dysgenesis is made. Women who develop a gonadal tumor are less virilized at birth and have fewer masculinizing signs at puberty, while feminizing signs such as breast growth are common.

17-Alpha-Hydroxylase Deficiency. This enzyme is required for conversion of pregnenolone and progesterone to 17-alpha-hydroxypregnenolone and 17-alpha-hydroxyprogesterone (Fig. 19–3). Congenital deficiency of this enzyme is inherited as an autosomal recessive trait and genetic males and females are affected with equal frequency. Synthesis of androgens, estrogens, and cortisol is deficient (6,7,39,40). Regardless of the karyotype, af-

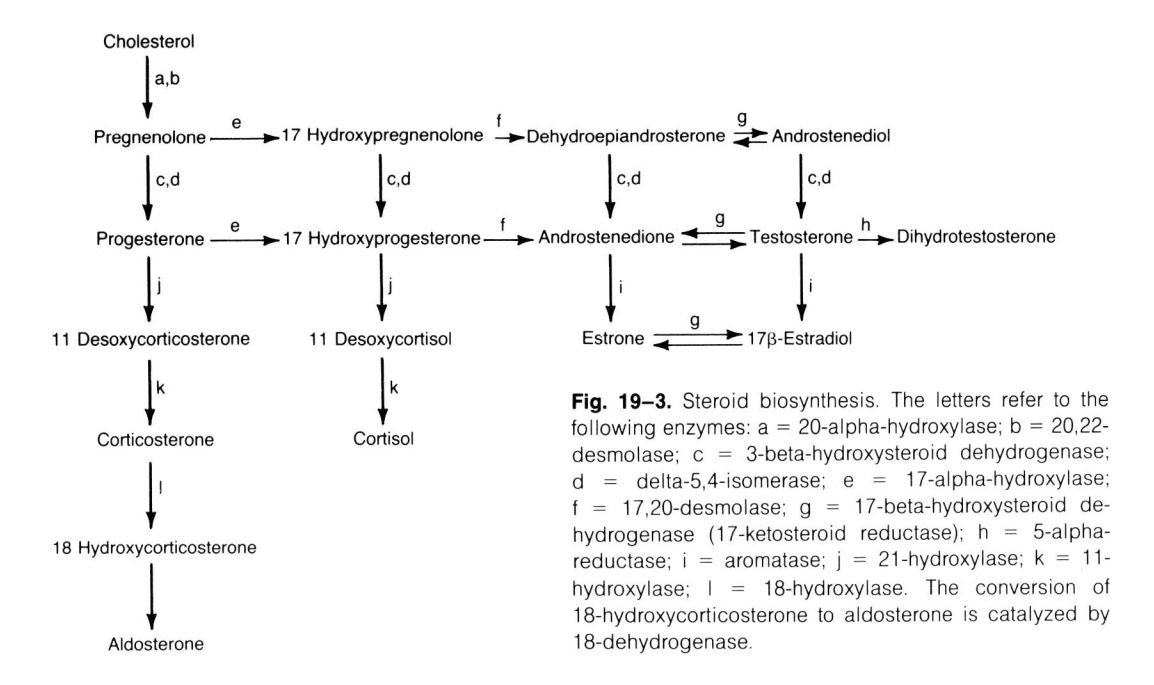

```
Cholesterol
   │ a,b
   ▼
Pregnenolone ──e──▶ 17 Hydroxypregnenolone ──f──▶ Dehydroepiandrosterone ⇌g⇌ Androstenediol
   │ c,d                │ c,d                        │ c,d                      │ c,d
   ▼                    ▼                            ▼                          ▼
Progesterone ──e──▶ 17 Hydroxyprogesterone ──f──▶ Androstenedione ⇌g⇌ Testosterone ──h──▶ Dihydrotestosterone
   │ j                  │ j                          │ i                        │ i
   ▼                    ▼                            ▼                          ▼
11 Desoxycorticosterone  11 Desoxycortisol         Estrone ⇌g⇌ 17β-Estradiol
   │ k                  │ k
   ▼                    ▼
Corticosterone         Cortisol
   │ l
   ▼
18 Hydroxycorticosterone
   │
   ▼
Aldosterone
```

Fig. 19–3. Steroid biosynthesis. The letters refer to the following enzymes: a = 20-alpha-hydroxylase; b = 20,22-desmolase; c = 3-beta-hydroxysteroid dehydrogenase; d = delta-5,4-isomerase; e = 17-alpha-hydroxylase; f = 17,20-desmolase; g = 17-beta-hydroxysteroid dehydrogenase (17-ketosteroid reductase); h = 5-alpha-reductase; i = aromatase; j = 21-hydroxylase; k = 11-hydroxylase; l = 18-hydroxylase. The conversion of 18-hydroxycorticosterone to aldosterone is catalyzed by 18-dehydrogenase.

fected subjects are phenotypic females with primary amenorrhea, delayed puberty, and sexual infantilism. Because cortisol secretion is low, ACTH concentrations are increased, resulting in increased adrenal secretion of pregnenolone, progesterone, and 11-desoxycorticosterone. Affected individuals are hypertensive because of the excessive mineralcorticoid secretion. Serum concentrations of LH and FSH are increased because of the diminished secretion of testosterone or estradiol. Subjects with a 46,XX karyotype will have a cervix, uterus, and fallopian tubes, whereas those with 46,XY karyotype will have a blind-ending vagina without müllerian duct structures.

The testes of 46,XY subjects should be removed for 2 reasons. First, the enzyme deficiency is rarely complete and some signs of virilization may occur at puberty. Second, there is an increased risk for the development of a testicular tumor.

These women, regardless of karyotype, require glucocorticoid therapy (hydrocortisone, 20 mg to 40 mg/day or cortisone acetate, 25 mg to 37.5 mg/day) to suppress ACTH and mineralcorticoid secretion. Lowering of blood pressure and reduction of the serum progesterone concentration to preovulatory values should occur with adequate therapy.

These women also require estrogen (e.g., conjugated estrogens, 1.25 mg to 5 mg/day) to stimulate breast growth. Once puberty is complete, these women, especially those with a uterus, should receive cyclic estrogen-progestin therapy.

Hypothalamic Amenorrhea. In addition to secreting gonadotropin-releasing hormone (GnRH), the hypothalamus also regulates hunger and satiety, body temperature, and serum osmolality. A disorder in any of these functions suggests that hypothalamic dysfunction is the cause of primary amenorrhea in a woman with low serum concentrations of LH and FSH (41). Hypothalamic dysfunction beginning before puberty will result in sexual infantilism. Onset of the abnormality may occur after the onset of puberty and cause primary amenorrhea in a woman who has developed breasts. These women will have a cervix and uterus and their karyotype is 46,XX. Clinic findings in women with lesions of the hypothalamus are summarized in Table 19–4 (42).

Weight reduction below 90% of ideal body weight can cause amenorrhea and extreme weight loss results in the more complex metabolic changes characteristic of *anorexia nervosa* (43–48). With simple weight loss or anorexia nervosa, thermoregulation is abnormal and partial diabetes insipidus occurs. Clinical signs and symptoms and biochemical abnormalities of anorexia nervosa are summarized in Tables 19-5 and 19-6.

Other causes of hypothalamic amenorrhea are categorized in Table 19-7. Disorders of the hypothalamus and their treatment are described in Chapter 3. If the abnormality cannot be corrected and the woman desires fertility, then stimulation of ovulation with gonadotropins or gonadotropin-releasing hormone is necessary (see Chapter 6).

Pituitary Disorders. A disorder of the pituitary gland is the cause of primary amenorrhea in approximately 10% to 15% of women (Table 19-2). Conversely, 3% to 4% of women with a pituitary tumor will never have menstruated (49). Most women with primary hypopituitarism have a craniopharyngioma (50). Von Recklinghausen's disease, astrocytomas, germinomas, and other infiltrating lesions of the pituitary account for many of the remaining women with primary hypopituitarism and amenorrhea. In many of these instances, the abnormality may not be unique or specific to the pituitary and there may be concomitant involvement of the hypothalamus. Categorical causes of amenorrhea due to pituitary dysfunction are listed in Table 19-8.

Women with pituitary causes of amenorrhea will have a uterus, no evidence of current es-

TABLE 19-4. Clinical Features of Women with a Hypothalamic Lesion*

	AGE	
	½–15 years (n = 9)	23–67 years (n = 11)
Precocious puberty	4	—
Hypogonadism	2	5
Obesity	3	4
Emaciation	0	2
Dysthermia	1	6
Somnolence	2	6
Diabetes insipidus	2	5
Oliguria	1	0
Psychiatric disturbances	1	5
Other	1	1

* Values are number of women.
From Bauer HG. Endocrine and other clinical manifestations of hypothalamic disease: a survey of 60 cases with autopsies. J Clin Endocrinol Metab 1954;14:13–31.

TABLE 19-5. Signs and Symptoms of Anorexia Nervosa

	FREQUENCY (%)
Symptoms	
Amenorrhea	100
Constipation	62
Preoccupation with food	45
Abdominal pain	19
Cold intolerance	19
Vomiting	5
Signs	
Hypotension	86
Hypothermia	64
Dry skin	62
Lanugo hair	52
Bradycardia	26
Edema	26
Systolic murmur	14
Petechiae	10

From Warren MP, Vande Wiele RL. Clinical and metabolic features of anorexia nervosa. Am J Obstet Gynecol 1973;117:435–449.

TABLE 19-6. Biochemical Abnormalities in Anorexia Nervosa

Hypothalamus
  Partial diabetes insipidus
  Prepubertal or pubertal pattern of LH secretion
  Abnormal thermoregulation
  Cachexia
Pituitary
  Low LH and FSH concentrations
  Reduced response of LH and FSH to gonadotropin-releasing hormone
  High basal growth hormone concentrations
  Reduced growth hormone response to hypoglycemia
  Delayed TSH response to thyroid-releasing hormone (TRH)
Ovary
  Low estradiol secretion
  Increased 2-hydroxylase activity (increased catechol estrogen formation)
  Decreased 16-hydroxylase activity
Adrenal
  Increased plasma cortisol concentrations
  Decreased metabolic clearance rate of cortisol (production rates of cortisol are normal)
  Decreased 11-oxidation
Thyroid
  Low to normal thyroxine (T_4) concentrations
  Low conversion of T_4 to triiodothyronine (T_3)
  Low T_3 concentrations
Other
  Decreased 5-alpha-reductase activity
  Increased insulin binding to receptors

trogen production, a 46,XX karyotype, and low serum concentrations of LH and FSH. Failure of LH and FSH concentrations to increase following the administration of GnRH distinguishes these women from those with hypothalamic dysfunction. However, administration of GnRH for 3 to 7 days may be necessary before an increase in LH and FSH concentrations occurs. Failure to recognize the need to "prime" the pituitary leads to the diagnosis of primary pituitary failure more frequently than it actually exists. Because these women may have a pituitary tumor, measurement of the serum prolactin concentration and computerized tomography are useful adjuncts. Disorders of the pituitary and their management are discussed in Chapter 4.

Delayed Puberty. Women older than 16 years with sexual infantilism and absent menses are 2.5 standard deviations beyond the mean age of the onset of puberty. Constitutional (idiopathic) delay of puberty occurs in 0.5% to 1% of girls older than 13 years old, who are usually shorter than 95% of their peers of the same chronologic age. Bone age lags significantly behind chronologic age and is a more precise indicator of sexual maturation. Growth velocity (i.e., increase in height per unit of time) is normal for the patient's bone age. As a result of physiologic immaturity, hypothalamic secretion of gonadotropin-releasing hormone (GnRH) is low. Consequently, serum LH and FSH concentrations are low. The presence of normal olfaction, absence of hypertension, a normal phenotype, the presence of a uterus, and, finally, a normal 46,XX karyotype distinguish girls with constitutionally delayed puberty from those with other causes of sexual infantilism and primary amenorrhea. Moreover, there is often a family history of delayed puberty.

Sexual maturation will begin when the young woman achieves a bone age of 11 to 13 years. The girl and her parents should be reassured that puberty and subsequent development will be normal, although she may ultimately be 1 inch to 2 inches shorter than her peers. Also, secondary sexual characteristics usually appear within 1 year if LH concentrations increase following the administration of 100 mcg GnRH or if estradiol concentrations begin to increase spontaneously. However, reassurance alone may be insufficient therapy when the stigma of appearing less mature than her peers causes psychologic stress. For these women, a 3- to 6-month course of ethinyl estradiol (10 mcg to 50 mcg/day) or conjugated estrogens (0.3 mg to 1.25 mg/day) should induce the development of secondary sexual characteristics. If puberty does not ensue or serum estradiol concentrations do not increase spon-

TABLE 19–7. Hypothalamic Causes of Amenorrhea

CATEGORY	EXAMPLES
Obesity syndromes	Fröhlich's syndrome
	Prader-Willi syndrome
	Laurence-Moon-Biedl syndrome
Weight loss	Simple weight loss
	Anorexia nervosa
Olfactory-genital dysplasia	Kallman's syndrome
Inflammation	Meningitis, encephalitis
Granulomatous disease	Sarcoidosis, syphilis, tuberculosis
Tumor	Meningioma, craniopharyngioma, optic glioma
Vascular abnormality	Aneurysm, arteriovenous malformation, pituitary stalk section
Systemic disease (51)	Inflammatory bowel disease, chronic renal disease, Bartter's syndrome

TABLE 19–8. Pituitary Causes of Amenorrhea

CATEGORY	EXAMPLES
Tumor	Meningioma, optic nerve glioma, craniopharyngioma, prolactinoma
Infiltrating lesion	Von Recklinghausen's disease, sarcoidosis, tuberculosis, hemochromatosis
Vascular abnormality	Aneurysm, A-V malformation, pituitary stalk section
Necrosis	Diabetes mellitus, post-infectious hydrocephalus
Hypopituitarism	Isolated gonadotropin deficiency, panhypopituitarism, intrasellar cysts, empty sella syndrome
Autoimmunity	

taneously after cessation of therapy, a second 3- to 6-month course of estrogen therapy should be prescribed. Only 1 or 2 courses of estrogen therapy are usually necessary (2).

Congenital Anorchia. This rare entity has been reviewed by Coulam and Edman and co-workers (3,52). These women are genetic males (46,XY) with no uterus and increased serum concentrations of LH and FSH. Affected subjects will be sexually infantile phenotypic females if the gonads regress before testosterone secretion begins at 8 to 9 weeks of embryonic life. Testicular regression later in embryonic life will result in variable degrees of genital ambiguity. The concentration of testosterone and its precursors is low, whereas in subjects with an enyzme deficiency the concentration of the enzyme precursor is increased. Unfortunately, it is usually necessary to perform a laparotomy to confirm the absence of testes since abdominal testes are at risk for malignancy. Estrogen replacement and surgical correction of ambiguous genitalia complete the therapy of these subjects.

Leydig Cell Agenesis. Subjects with testes that contain seminiferous tubules but no interstitial cells have a rare form of male pseudohermaphroditism (4). Affected subjects will be sexually infantile with primary amenorrhea because steroid-producing cells in the testes are absent. The karyotype is 46,XY. A cervix, uterus, and fallopian tubes are absent because müllerian duct regression factor was secreted *in utero*. The testes in the subject reported (4) were palpable along the inguinal canals. Because of the presence of a Y chromosome, women with this disorder should be explored and the testes removed. Sexual maturation will occur with estrogen replacement therapy, but fertility is not possible.

The differential diagnosis of primary amenorrhea in sexually infantile women is summarized in Table 19–9.

INCOMPLETE PUBERTY.

Pregnancy. Approximately 10% of girls 13 years of age or less are sexually active and 30,000 infants will be born annually to these women. While most of these young women have begun to menstruate before they conceive, a small percentage will become pregnant before their first menses. Pregnancy should be included in the differential diagnosis of young women with breast growth who have a uterus and a 46,XX karyotype who have not yet menstruated. This is an important first consideration since diagnostic tests that are potentially harmful to a fetus can be avoided.

Vaginal Abnormalities. Abnormalities of the vagina may result in an apparent lack of menstruation. However, these women may have cryptomenorrhea, or "hidden menses." Labial agglutination, an imperforate hymen, or a transverse vaginal septum will obstruct the outflow of menses and cause retrograde menstruation. The presence of cyclic lower abdominal

TABLE 19–9. Causes of Primary Amenorrhea and Sexual Infantilism

UTERUS	KARYOTYPE	LH AND FSH CONCENTRATIONS	CAUSE
Present	45,X;46,XY	(High)*	Gonadal dysgenesis
	46,XX	High	Pure gonadal dysgenesis
			17-hydroxylase deficiency
			Prepubertal ovarian failure
		Low	Hypopituitarism
			Pituitary tumor
			Delayed puberty
			Hypothalamic dysfunction
Absent	46,XY	(High)	17-hydroxylase deficiency
			Congenital anorchia
			Leydig cell agenesis
	46,XX		(No diagnosis)

* When the concentrations of LH and FSH are in parentheses, they are not essential to make the diagnosis.

pain suggests this diagnosis, especially when a speculum cannot be inserted.

Women with labial agglutination often have a history of poor perineal hygiene and/or perineal trauma. Topical estrogen cream is usually sufficient to separate the labia and surgery should be reserved for those women in whom estrogen was not successful.

An imperforate hymen will bulge outward between the labia minora and will often have a bluish discoloration caused by an accumulation of menstrual blood in the vagina. Needle aspiration will confirm this diagnosis. Stellate incisions of the hymen correct the problem.

A transverse vaginal septum represents failure of vaginal canalization between the urogenital and müllerian portions of the vagina. The septum is usually present one half to two thirds the distance from the vaginal introitus to where the cervix should be visualized. Thus, a vaginal speculum can be inserted, but only partially, and a cervix cannot be visualized. However, the uterus can be palpated on rectal examination.

Associated abnormalities of the urinary tract and skeleton are common in women with congenital absence of the vagina (Mayer-Rokitansky-Kuster-Hauser syndrome) (53). Surgical correction is necessary to provide any chance of future fertility, although the uterus is frequently hypoplastic and nonfunctioning (54).

Chronic Estrous Anovulation. This is often a variant of constitutional delayed puberty. These women are normal in that they have breast growth and pubic hair, a uterus, and a 46,XX karyotype, although they have not yet begun to menstruate. Their ovaries are secreting estrogen, but normal ovulatory menses have not developed. A 1- to 2-year interval between the onset of puberty and the initiation of menstruation is typical and these women should begin to menstruate within 6 to 12 months of the initial examination. Hormonal therapy should be delayed until a diagnosis other than chronic estrous anovulation is certain.

Polycystic ovarian disease is the cause of primary amenorrhea in 3% to 8% of women (Table 19-2). Many pubertal girls with polycystic ovarian disease are obese and often give a history of premature adrenarche (e.g., growth of pubic and axillary hair). Hirsutism may be present, although this is not a universal feature of polycystic ovarian disease. The ovaries may be slightly enlarged. If fertility is not desired, menses should be induced with a progestin or oral contraceptive at least every 3 to 4 months because these women appear to have an increased risk for endometrial cancer (55,56). Induction of ovulation for those women desiring fertility is discussed in Chapter 6.

Systemic illnesses such as diabetes mellitus, hepatic disease, or thyroid dysfunction may cause primary amenorrhea in a woman with incomplete puberty (51). Symptoms, physical findings, and laboratory results consistent with any of these disorders should be sought in evaluating these causes of primary amenorrhea. Specific therapy of any of these should induce ovulation and menstruation.

Acyclic gonadotropin secretion is one of several terms applied to a poorly understood disorder that expresses itself as primary or (more commonly) secondary amenorrhea and is associated with normal concentrations of LH and FSH. However, midcycle surges of LH and FSH do not occur. Yen has classified this disorder as hypothalamic chronic anovulation or psychogenic amenorrhea (57). Evidence of estrogen effect may be absent and there is no other physical explanation for the amenorrhea. The role of the hypothalamus in this disorder is discussed in Chapter 3. These women may ovulate upon removal of any stress factors, but they may require clomiphene or gonadotropins (see Chapter 6).

Ovarian Failure. Premature ovarian failure is a rare cause of primary amenorrhea in sexually infantile women or women with incomplete puberty. Concentrations of LH and FSH are increased. Premature menopause and the gonadotropin-resistant ovary syndrome are distinct causes of premature ovarian failure in women with incomplete puberty and primary amenorrhea. If ovarian failure occurs before the onset of puberty, affected women may be sexually infantile. Coulam has recently surveyed the literature and proposed a classification of gonadal failure (58). Estrogen replacement is necessary and pregnancy is unlikely. However, a few women with gonadotropin-resistant ovaries have conceived during estrogen therapy (58).

CNS-Hypothalamic-Pituitary Failure. These disorders have been discussed under the category of sexual infantilism. The onset of hypothalmic or pituitary failure probably occurred later in women with incomplete puberty to explain the breast growth.

Müllerian Agenesis. This is the only condition in which the karyotype is 46,XX and the uterus is absent. The cause of this disorder is unknown. It occurs sporadically and the family history of affected women is normal. Normal pubic hair development distinguishes this from testicular feminization. Since women with müllerian agenesis have normal ovarian function, a biphasic basal temperature chart or a serum progesterone concentration greater than 5 ng/ml will document the presence of ovulation. Fertility is not possible and no therapy, other than counseling, is required.

Testicular Feminization. Women with the complete form of testicular feminization have well-developed breasts and a normal female phenotype despite the presence of a 46,XY karyotype. Sexual hair is absent or sparse. The vagina is short and ends blindly because there is no cervix or uterus. Testes are present intraabdominally or within hernial sacs along the inguinal canals. The testes produce normal (male) quantities of testosterone but excessive quantities of estradiol (59).

Most women with complete testicular feminization have a reduced quantity of the cytoplasmic receptor for testosterone and dihydrotestosterone in androgen target tissues (12). This is apparently the result of a single gene defect, which is inherited as an X-linked recessive trait. Thus, genetic males are affected and genetic females are carriers of the gene but are unaffected and normally fertile. Qualitative abnormalities of the androgen receptor have also been described (60–62). The mechanism of testosterone action is illustrated in Figure 19–4.

Treatment consists of removal of the gonads and subsequent estrogen replacement. Surgery may be delayed until completion of puberty since feminization but no masculinization will occur. The testes should be removed before the age of 25 to 30 years because of the risk of malignancy (19). Despite the presence of a male karyotype, these subjects should be considered women because their psychosexual

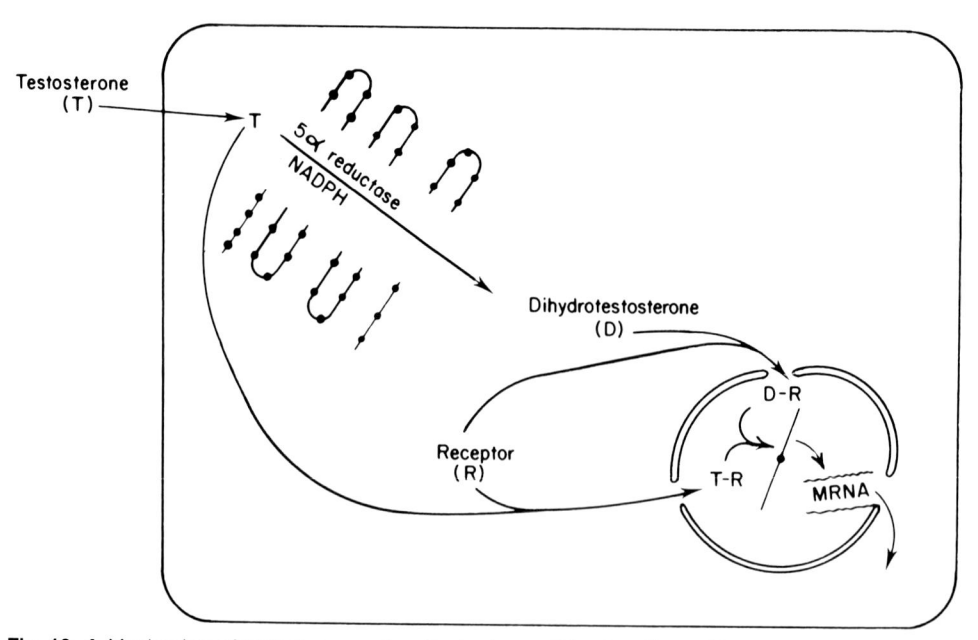

Fig. 19–4. Mechanism of testosterone action. Testosterone (T) enters the cell by diffusion. Testosterone may be converted to dihydrotestosterone (D) and either steroid can combine with the cytoplasmic androgen receptor (R). After a conformational change in the receptor, the androgen-receptor complex is translocated to the nucleus where it occupies acceptor sites on chromatin or nuclear proteins. Messenger RNA (mRNA) synthesis is followed by ribosomal protein synthesis (not shown) and other androgen responses.

orientation is feminine. They should be told that fertility is not possible, but that they will otherwise function as normal women. They should not be told that they "should have been a man" or that they have testes. Rather, the need to remove their "ovaries" or "gonads" is explained. Nonspecific descriptions of the gonads help to preserve the self-esteem of these women while conveying the necessity for surgery.

The causes of primary amenorrhea in women with incomplete puberty are summarized in Table 19–10.

CONGENITAL GENITAL AMBIGUITY. Congenital genital ambiguity means abnormal testosterone representation *in utero*. Posterior fusion of the labia and marked phallic enlargement are the most common presenting manifestations. Clitoral enlargement alone is insufficient to conclude that testosterone representation was abnormal *in utero* since this may occur with an acquired form of androgen excess. The assessment of a woman with ambiguous genitalia is outlined in Fig. 19–5.

It is first necessary to decide if the woman was destined *in utero* to be a male or a female. The presence of a Y chromosome, the absence of a cervix and uterus, and the presence of testes suggest that the woman was destined to be a male and her genital ambiguity was the consequence of insufficient testosterone synthesis or action. Partially or completely descended gonadal masses imply that they are testes since normal ovaries are always located intraabdominally. Conversely, the absence of a Y chromosome (e.g., 46,XX or 45,X), the presence of a cervix and uterus, and the absence of testes suggest that the woman was destined to be a female but was exposed to excessive testosterone *in utero*.

There are 3 categorical diagnoses for subjects with genital ambiguity. Male pseudohermaphroditism exists when genital ambiguity has developed in a male. The gonads are testes and the karyotype is 46,XY. Female pseudohermaphroditism is the categorical diagnosis when genital ambiguity has occurred in a woman. The karyotype may be 46,XX but any karyotype except one that contains a Y chromosome may be present. The gonads are ovaries or streaks. True hermaphroditism is defined by the presence of both ovarian and testicular tissue in the same individual (13).

A diagnostic approach to a woman with female pseudohermaphroditism is illustrated in Fig. 19–6. The source of the excessive testosterone may be the fetus or her mother. Neither functional nor neoplastic disorders of a fetal ovary that cause genital ambiguity have been described. The most common cause of genital ambiguity in a newborn is congenital adrenal hyperplasia, which, if untreated, also causes postnatal and prepubertal virilization, heterosexual precocious puberty, and primary amenorrhea.

TABLE 19–10. Causes of Primary Amenorrhea and Incomplete Puberty (Breast Growth)

UTERUS	KARYOTYPE	VAGINA	ESTROGEN*	LH AND FSH	CAUSE
Present	45,X or 46,XY	(Normal)	0	(High)	Gonadal dysgenesis
	46,XX	Normal	+		Polycystic ovarian disease
					Acyclic gonadotropin secretion
					Delayed menarche
			0	High	Ovarian failure
					Gonadal dysgenesis
			0	Low	Pituitary tumor
					Hypopituitarism
					Hypothalamic dysfunction
			+	Low	Pregnancy
Present	46,XX	Abnormal			Imperforate hymen
					Transverse vaginal septum
					Congenital absence of the vagina
Absent	46,XX	Normal	+	Normal	Müllerian agenesis
Absent	46,XY	Short	+	(High)	Testicular Feminization

* Estrogen effect is present or serum estradiol concentrations exceed 50 pg/ml. Observations in parentheses are not essential to establish the diagnosis.

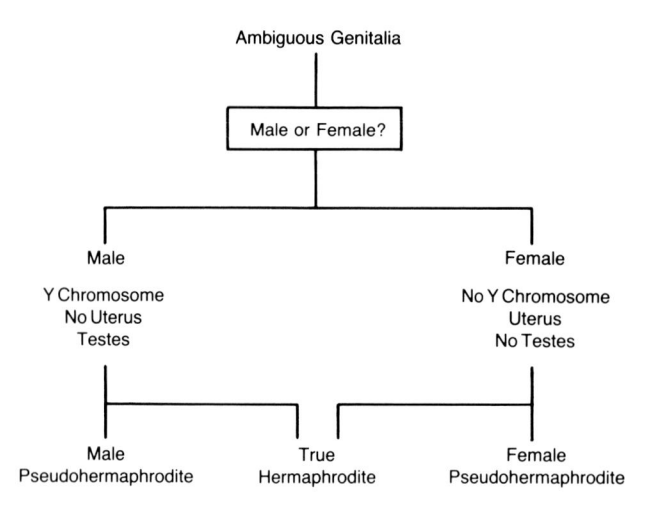

Fig. 19–5. Evaluation of ambiguous genitalia. Essential to the final diagnosis is the decision whether the affected person was destined to be a male or female. The presence or absence of a Y chromosome, a uterus, and testes make this decision.

Congenital Adrenal Hyperplasia (63). Deficiency of 21-hydroxylase or 11-hydroxylase is the most common cause of female pseudohermaphroditism. These disorders are inherited as autosomal recessive traits and the gene for 21-hydroxylase is closely linked to the HLA complex on chromosome 6 (64). The gene for 11-hydroxylase has, however, not been linked to the HLA complex or to any specific chromosome (65).

Subjects with congenital virilizing adrenal hyperplasia will be born with genital ambiguity. Untreated, they will progessively virilize in infancy, have precocious heterosexual puberty, and have a shorter adult height because of early epiphyseal closure induced by excessive adrenal androgen secretion. The diagnosis of a deficiency of either enzyme is suggested by the presence of these signs in an amenorrheic woman who has a cervix and uterus and who relates a history of affected family members. Precursors of these enzymes are secreted in excess of normal. Serum concentrations of progesterone, 17-hydroxyprogesterone, dehydroepiandrosterone sulfate, and androstenedione are markedly elevated as a consequence (see Fig. 19–3). The serum concentration of testosterone is also increased, but this may be less helpful since women with an ovarian cause of androgen excess may also have high testosterone concentrations.

Salt wasting (i.e., hyponatremia and increased sodium excretion) may occur in subjects with 21-hydroxylase deficiency since 11-desoxycorticosterone and aldosterone synthesis is impaired. With complete loss of 21-hydroxylase deficiency, salt wasting may be so pronounced that this becomes life threatening in the neonatal period.

In subjects with 11-hydroxylase deficiency, the synthesis and secretion rate of 11-desoxycorticosterone (DOC) is increased. Because DOC is a potent mineralcorticoid, there is no salt wasting, but hypertension may be severe.

Treatment with cortisol or other glucocorticoids is necessary to suppress the elevated

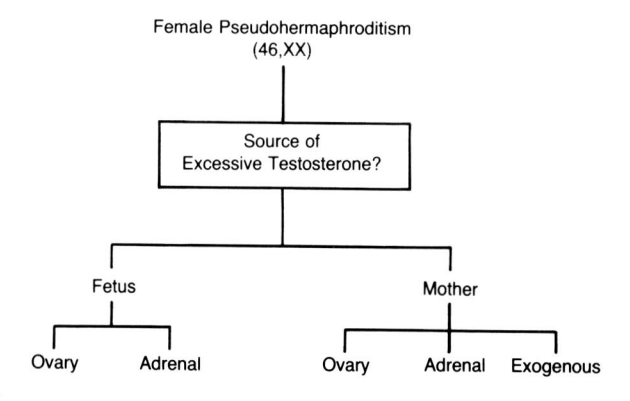

Fig. 19–6. Female pseudohermaphroditism. These are genetic females exposed to excessive testosterone *in utero*. The testosterone can originate from the fetus or the mother.

ACTH concentrations. Effective therapy arrests the progression of virilization by suppressing the ACTH-induced increases in adrenal androgen secretion. Approximately 25 mg cortisol/m^2 of body surface, or equivalent doses of related glucocorticoids, are usually sufficient. Stabilization of the signs of androgen excess, resumption of ovulatory menses, and normalization of other clinical manifestations are evidence of effective therapy. Serum concentrations of 17-hydroxyprogesterone, dehydroepiandrosterone sulfate, or testosterone should decrease to normal and are useful adjuncts in monitoring therapy (63,66).

Adrenal Tumor (67,68). Tumors of the adrenal cortex occur with a frequency of 1 in 500,000 and the ratio of females to males is approximately 2:1. While virilization or signs of Cushing's syndrome are frequently present, genital ambiguity is rare because *in utero* exposure to excessive adrenal steroids will not occur unless the fetus or her mother develops the tumor during pregnancy. In addition to very high concentrations of adrenal androgens, lack of adrenal cortical suppression with high doses of dexamethasone helps to differentiate a neoplasm from a functional adrenal disorder. Selective venous catheterization of each adrenal vein and computerized tomography are also useful diagnostic tools. Treatment is surgical resection of the tumor. Survival following removal of an adrenal carcinoma is poor. Small tumor size and benign histologic features are poor criteria to predict the clinical outcome following removal.

Maternal Adrenal Disorders. Uncontrolled 21-hydroxylase or 11-hydroxylase deficiency in a pregnant woman may cause virilization of a female fetus. However, such women are usually anovulatory and will not conceive unless their disease is controlled with glucocorticoid therapy. This also pertains to women with an adrenal tumor.

Maternal Ovarian Disorders. Hyperreactio luteinalis (69,70) is an infrequent cause of maternal virilization during pregnancy and a rare cause of virilization of a female fetus. Benign hyperplasia and luteinization of ovarian theca cells are the histologic correlates in affected women. Most of these women have a clinical condition of pregnancy associated with an enlarged placenta and high hCG concentrations (e.g., multiple pregnancy and Rh isoimmunization). Fetal virilization is uncommon because testosterone secretion from affected maternal ovaries is only moderately increased and the placenta can convert large amounts of testosterone to estradiol before the testosterone enters the fetus. For this reason, few women should have primary amenorrhea since they are unlikely to be virilized *in utero* by their mother's hyperreactio luteinalis.

Luteomas in pregnancy also tend to occur in women with excessive placental hCG secretion. These tumors are frequently solid and unilateral, in contrast to hyperreactio luteinalis, which is usually cystic and bilateral. Regression after pregnancy occurs. Virilization of a female fetus or the mother occurs in 10% to 30% of pregnancies complicated by a luteoma (70–72). Polycystic ovarian disease may be a predisposing factor to the development of a luteoma (73). While virilization of a female fetus is a recognized effect, the occurrence of amenorrhea when that newborn reaches the age of puberty has not been described because no one has followed these infants through the age of puberty. However, amenorrhea remains a possibility because antenatal androgen exposure can permanently alter hypothalamic-pituitary function. Unfortunately, virilized women with an adnexal mass must be explored because other benign or malignant ovarian tumors may stimulate excessive ovarian androgen secretion. Fortunately, ovarian tumors in pregnancy are rare and infrequently cause signs of androgen excess (73,74).

Maternal Drug Ingestion. Drugs with androgenic side effects are listed in Table 19–11. While these drugs may virilize a female fetus, it is unknown if their antenatal effect will produce amenorrhea in adolescence or adulthood.

Male pseudohermaphroditism results when a fetus destined to be a male produces insufficient quantities of testosterone and dihydrotestosterone to virilize the genitalia or when testosterone action is impaired. The diagnostic approach to such a patient is illustrated in Fig. 19–7. The extent of genital ambiguity depends upon the severity of the abnormality and variation in the degree of ambiguity is the norm even within the same category.

TABLE 19-11. Drugs with Androgenic Side Effects

Testosterone
Synthetic progestins
Danocrine
Glucocorticoids
Diazoxide
Minoxidil
Phentoin sodium
Hexachlorobenzene
Streptomycin
Penicillamine

Deficient Testosterone Synthesis. The pathway of testosterone synthesis from cholesterol is illustrated in Fig. 19-3. Deficiency of 20,22-desmolase (cholesterol to pregnenolone), 3-beta-hydroxysteroid dehydrogenase (pregnenolone to progesterone), 17-hydroxylase (progesterone to 17-hydroxyprogesterone), 17,20-desmolase (17-hydroxyprogesterone to androstenedione), 17-hydroxysteroid dehydrogenase (androstenedione to testosterone), and 5-alpha-reductase (testosterone to dihydrotestosterone) may each cause male pseudohermaphroditism and genital ambiguity (5-11,63,75-78). Each of these disorders is transmitted as an autosomal recessive trait.

Subjects with a deficiency of 20,22-desmolase or 3-beta-hydroxysteroid dehydrogenase usually die in infancy, but adolescent and adult subjects with a deficiency of any of the other enzymes have been described. The diagnosis should be suspected in a woman with primary amenorrhea who has genital ambiguity, no uterus, and a family history of similarly affected relatives. The specific enzyme that is deficient can be determined by measuring the concentration of the steroid precursor and product of that enzyme. The concentration of the precursor will be elevated, while that of the product hormone will be low to normal.

If the concentration of testosterone and all its precursors is low, the testes may be absent (3,52), or lack interstitial cells (4). Such conditions are uncommon and the degree of genital ambiguity depends upon the duration of interstitial cell function during embryonic life. Disappearance of the testes or interstitial cells before 8 to 9 weeks of pregnancy may result in sexual infantilism and not genital ambiguity.

The testes of subjects with male pseudohermaphroditism must be removed for 2 reasons. Because an enzyme deficiency is rarely complete, virilization may occur at the time of puberty. Secondly, the testes are at risk for malignancy when they are incompletely descended

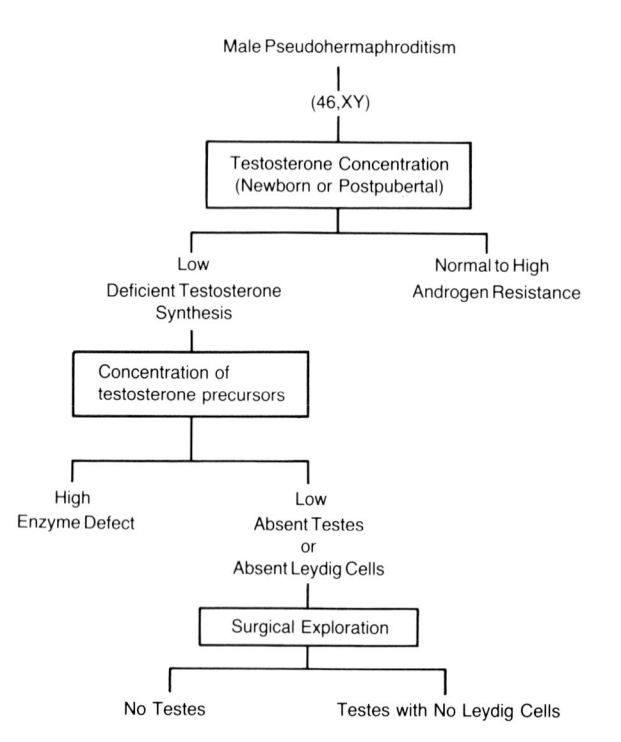

Fig. 19-7. Male pseudohermaphroditism. These are genetic males whose genitalia failed to virilize normally. This will result when testosterone synthesis is impaired or testosterone action is deficient. Testosterone synthesis is impaired with certain enzyme defects (see Fig. 19-3) or when testosterone-producing cells are absent.

into the scrotum. Correction of genital ambiguity and estrogen replacement complete the therapy. Fertility is not possible.

Partial Androgen Resistance. Syndromes described by Lubs, Gilbert-Dreyfus, Madden, and Reifenstein (12,79–81) include genetic males with a reduced quantity of the cytoplasmic androgen receptor. Since levels of androgen receptor binding are comparable to those of women with complete androgen resistance, receptor binding capacity is not the sole factor that controls the phenotypic expression of external genital virilization.

These women have a 46,XY karyotype, testes that secrete normal male quantities of testosterone, and no cervix or uterus. Because the testes secrete an increased quantity of estradiol, breast growth is also found in all affected subjects (80,81). As with the complete form of androgen resistance, the testes are located within the abdomen or hernial sacs along the inguinal ligaments. Androgen resistance occurs once every 2,000 to 64,000 male births. Incomplete forms of androgen resistance comprise about 10% of these.

Treatment of women with incomplete androgen resistance is slightly different from that of women with the complete form. The testes must be removed at the time of diagnosis and before puberty if possible. Partial virilization of the external genitalia will occur at the time of puberty and can be prevented by early removal. These testes are at risk for malignancy. Correction of the genital ambiguity to create a labia and vagina should be done for all subjects except these who have only penile hypospadias as evidence of defective virilization. After removal of the testes, estrogen replacement is necessary. Fertility is not possible.

True Hermaphroditism (13). The presence of both ovarian and testicular tissue in the same individual defines true hermaphroditism (Fig. 19–8). The gonadal composition may be any combination of ovarian and testicular tissue—an ovary with a testis or ovotestis on the opposite side, a testis with an ovary or ovotestis, or bilateral ovotestes. Most true hermaphrodites are raised as females, although only 10% will have normal-appearing female genitalia. Most will have a uterus despite the presence of testicular tissue. Breasts are usually present. The karyotype is most often 46,XX, although the presence of Y-chromosomal material on an autosomal or X chromosome is suggested by the

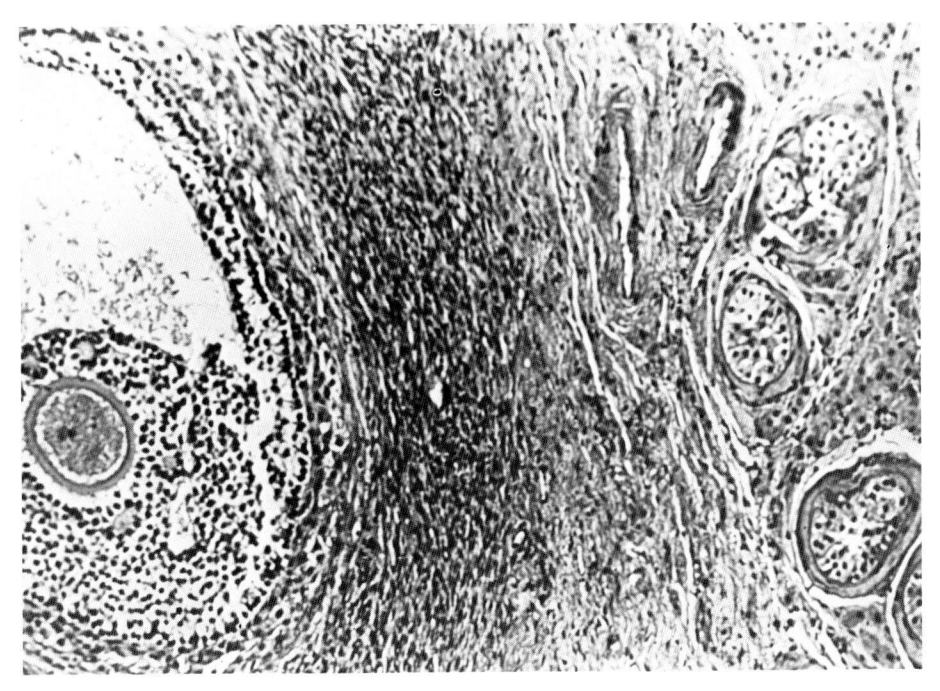

Fig. 19–8. Ovotestis. A graafian follicle is on the left and seminiferous tubules are on the right. The presence of ovarian tissue (containing follicles) and testicular tissue in the same person defines true hermaphroditism.

finding of the Y antigen on somatic cell membranes (14). The extent of virilization and breast growth at puberty appears to be related to the gonadal secretion rates of testosterone and estradiol (82). True hermaphrodites have occasionally ovulated and conceived. The offspring have been normal. One true hermaphrodite has fathered a child (83).

Because the presence of a Y chromosome or genetic information from a portion of the Y chromosome confers an increased risk of a gonadal malignancy, the testicular component of the gonads must be removed. Approximately 60% of subjects with a testicular neoplasm will have detectable quantities of hCG, although an assay more sensitive than a slide pregnancy test is required to detect most of these (84). It is unknown if ovulation would occur if only the testicular tissue were removed and the ovarian tissue was not.

The genital ambiguity must be corrected surgically to create a functional vagina and reduce phallic enlargement. In all subjects with pseudo- or true hermaphroditism, I have emphasized that surgery for genital ambiguity that creates a female anatomy is the procedure of choice. This pertains regardless of the karyotype, the presence or absence of a uterus, or the type of gonads that are present. The reason for this emphasis is that creation of a functional vagina and a clitoral-like phallus is much easier than creation of an anatomically acceptable and functional penis. There are 2 exceptions to this dictum—the presence of penile hypospadias as the only manifestation of genital ambiguity, and a subject whose psychosexual orientation is so masculine that gender reversal is impossible. The causes of primary amenorrhea and congenital genital ambiguity are summarized in Table 19–12.

ACQUIRED ANDROGEN EXCESS. Women who become hirsute, develop clitoral enlargement, lose scalp hair and develop male-pattern balding, and acquire other signs of androgen excess represent the final category in considering the etiology of primary amenorrhea (Fig. 19–1, bottom left). These women are not sexually infantile nor do they have genital ambiguity or prepubertal virilization. Signs of androgen excess in these women usually begin during puberty or shortly thereafter. The extent of hirsutism provides few clues to the eti-

TABLE 19–12. Causes of Primary Amenorrhea and Genital Ambiguity

UTERUS	KARYOTYPE	CAUSE
Present	45,X/46,XY	Mixed gonadal dysgenesis
	46,XY;46,XX	Gonadal dysgenesis with a tumor or hilus-cell hyperplasia
	46,XX	Congenital adrenal hyperplasia
		Adrenal tumor
		Ovarian tumor
		Luteoma
		Hyperreactio luteinalis
		Medication (Table 19–11)
		True hermaphroditism
Absent	46,XY	Steroid enzyme deficiency
		Partial androgen resistance
		Congenital anorchia
		Leydig cell agenesis
		True hermaphroditism
	46,XX	(No diagnosis)

ology since the degree of androgen excess correlates with the production rate of testosterone, but does not relate to the source of that testosterone or the disorder causing the increased production (85). Serum testosterone concentrations are often less than expected for the degree of androgen excess and do not always reflect the production rate of testosterone since the rate of removal of testosterone from the serum (the metabolic clearance rate) increases when the production rate increases. To illustrate this, a hirsute or virilized woman may produce twice as much testosterone as does a normal woman. While her testosterone concentration may increase, it will be less than twice normal because the metabolic clearance rate increases and this causes the testosterone concentration to return toward normal.

Gonadal Dysgenesis. This has already been described in the categories of sexual infantilism and incomplete puberty. These women have streak gonads, a cervix and uterus, and high concentrations of FSH and LH. Any karyotype may be found in these women, although 46,XY and 46,XX are probably the most common. The appearance of signs of androgen excess in a woman with gonadal dysgenesis is ominous and a dysontogenetic tumor such as a gonadoblastoma may be the cause of the virilizing signs (Fig. 19–9). Although benign hyperplasia of hilus cells may be the cause

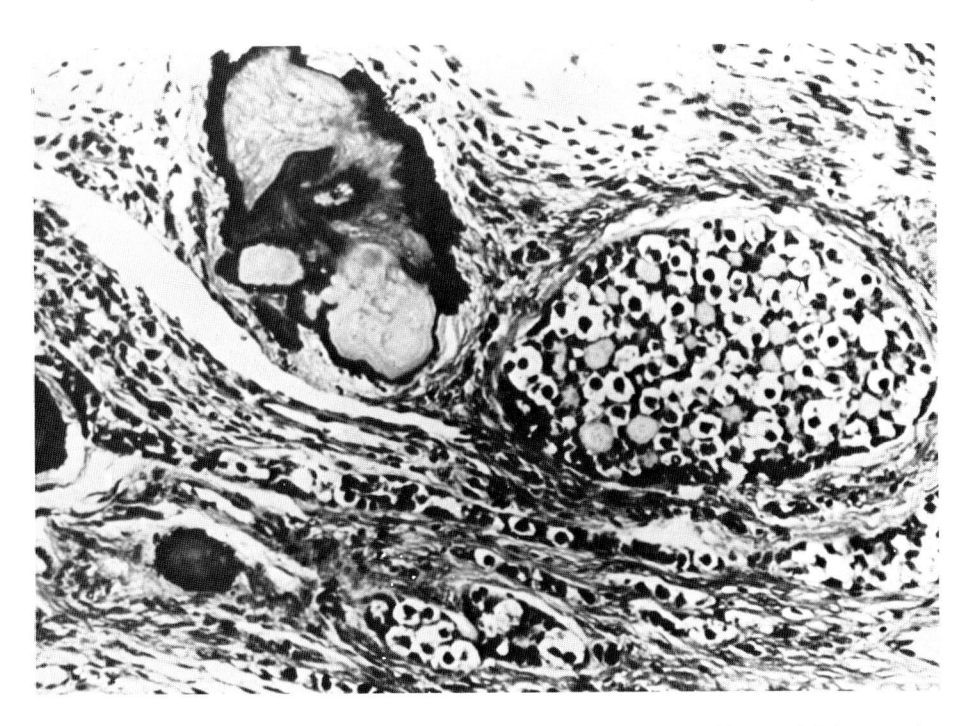

Fig. 19–9. Gonadoblastoma. This is the most common tumor of women with gonadal dysgenesis. Solid nests of cells contain both germ cells and sex cord derivatives (Sertoli-granulosa cells). These solid nests are surrounded by a fibrous stroma that often contains foci of calcification. A dysgerminoma will be found in approximately 50% of women with a gonadoblastoma.

of the androgen excess, it is impossible to distinguish this from a tumor. For this reason, women with gonadal dysgenesis who develop signs of androgen excess should be explored and the streak gonads removed. A gonadal tumor can occur in women with gonadal dysgenesis who do not have a Y chromosome, but it is rare (17,20). Each of the 9 women described had signs of feminization or masculinization.

Polycystic Ovarian Disease. This and the next 5 causes of acquired androgen excess (hyperthecosis, ovarian tumor, attenuated adrenal hyperplasia, Cushing's syndrome, and adrenal tumors) occur in women who have a uterus and a 46,XX karyotype (see Fig. 19–1). Polycystic ovarian disease is probably the most frequent cause of oligomenorrhea or secondary amenorrhea, but is the apparent cause of primary amenorrhea in 3% to 8% of women (Table 19–2). The degree of androgen excess is variable and many women with polycystic ovarian disease have no hirsutism. Obesity is a common feature of these women. Whether these women become obese because of the anabolic effect of testosterone or produce excessive quantities of testosterone because they are obese is a dilemma that cannot be resolved at present. Bates has shown that weight loss alone is sufficient to cause a reduction in serum testosterone concentrations and restore ovulation and fertility in obese women with polycystic ovarian disease (86). These women also produce increased quantities of androstenedione, a weak androgen but an important prehormone for estrone formation in extraglandular tissues (87). For this reason, estrogen effects such as vaginal rugosity and cervical mucous production are present despite signs of androgen excess. Thus, a woman with primary amenorrhea, breast growth and other signs of estrogen effect, hirsutism developing at the time of puberty, a cervix and uterus, and symmetric ovaries probably has polycystic ovarian disease. The condition most similar to this is attenuated adrenal hyperplasia, which can be distinguished from polycystic ovarian disease by the presence of higher dehydroepiandrosterone sulfate concentrations, and increased basal or ACTH-stimulated concentrations of 17-hydroxyprogesterone.

If fertility is desired, induction of ovulation

with clomiphene is often successful (see Chapter 6). Periodic induction of uterine bleeding (every 2 to 4 months) is necessary for these women who do not wish to conceive because their risk of endometrial cancer is increased (55,56). Goldzieher has reviewed polycystic ovarian disease recently (88).

Hyperthecosis. Hyperthecosis is probably a variant of polycystic ovarian disease that differs from it only by the severity of the clinical signs and symptoms. Women with hyperthecosis are more hirsute and often virilized (e.g., clitoromegaly). While hyperthecosis may result in primary amenorrhea, oligomenorrhea or secondary amenorrhea are more common. Compared to women with polycystic ovarian disease, those with hyperthecosis have longer menstrual intervals and may only bleed 1 to 2 times per year. Production rates of testosterone are higher, as are extraglandular production rates of estrone (89). Whereas the ovaries of women with polycystic ovarian disease have multiple dilated subcortical follicles with hyperplasia of the theca cells, diffuse stromal hyperplasia with few follicles is the histologic pattern in hyperthecosis. Because of the high rates of extraglandular estrogen production, women with hyperthecosis also have a greater risk for endometrial cancer, which occurs at a younger age (89).

For women not desiring fertility, uterine bleeding should be induced with a synthetic progestin (e.g., medroxyprogesterone acetate, 10 mg to 20 mg daily for 5 to 10 days) or an oral contraceptive at least every 2 to 4 months. This may protect these women against the increased risk of endometrial cancer. Ovulation induction with clomiphene or gonadotropins is usually unsuccessful and a wedge resection of the ovaries may be necessary. Reports of pregnancy in women with hyperthecosis are scarce so the probability of successful induction of ovulation is unknown.

Virilizing Ovarian Tumors. Sudden onset and rapid progression of masculinizing signs, concentrations of testosterone greater than 2 ng/ml, and asymmetric enlargement of 1 ovary are suggestive that acquired androgen excess is caused by an ovarian tumor that is secreting testosterone. Functioning ovarian tumors occur infrequently in children and adolescents, so these are uncommon causes of primary amenorrhea. Only 28% of masculinizing ovarian tumors reported by Ireland and Woodruff occurred in women under 20 years old (90). Gonadal stromal tumors and Sertoli-Leydig cell tumors accounted for 55% of the tumors in this age group. In most instances, the tumor cells themselves appear to be the source of excessive testosterone secretion. However, any ovarian tumor may cause masculinization by stimulating surrounding ovarian stroma to secrete testosterone in greater quantities. The mechanism of this stromal stimulation is unknown.

Resection of the tumor usually results in the resumption of ovulation and menstruation within 4 to 8 weeks. The hirsutism is unlikely to disappear, especially if it is pronounced or has been present for more than 6 months. Conservative surgery that preserves the woman's potential for fertility is sufficient unless the tumor is malignant and has extended beyond its capsule.

Attenuated Adrenal Hyperplasia. Within the last several years a form of 21-hydroxylase or 11-hydroxylase deficiency has been described in which affected subjects present with a clinical syndrome closely resembling polycystic ovarian disease (64,91–93). These women have no genital ambiguity but develop signs of androgen excess at the time of expected puberty. Serum concentrations of dehydroepiandrosterone, androstenedione, and testosterone are elevated but often not sufficiently to distinguish these women from those with polycystic ovarian disease. However, serum concentrations of 17-hydroxyprogesterone are often 50 to 100 times greater than normal and are useful in establishing the diagnosis of attenuated adrenal hyperplasia (Fig. 19–10). Moreover, there is usually a family history of affected relatives since deficiency of either enzyme is inherited as an autosomal recessive trait.

Treatment is the same as that for the congenital virilizing forms of adrenal hyperplasia (see the earlier section on congenital adrenal hyperplasia under "Congenital Genital Ambiguity"). Since cortisol synthesis is deficient, replacement therapy with physiologic doses of cortisol or equivalent doses of any other glucocorticoid should restore ovulation. Serum concentrations of 17-hydroxyprogesterone should

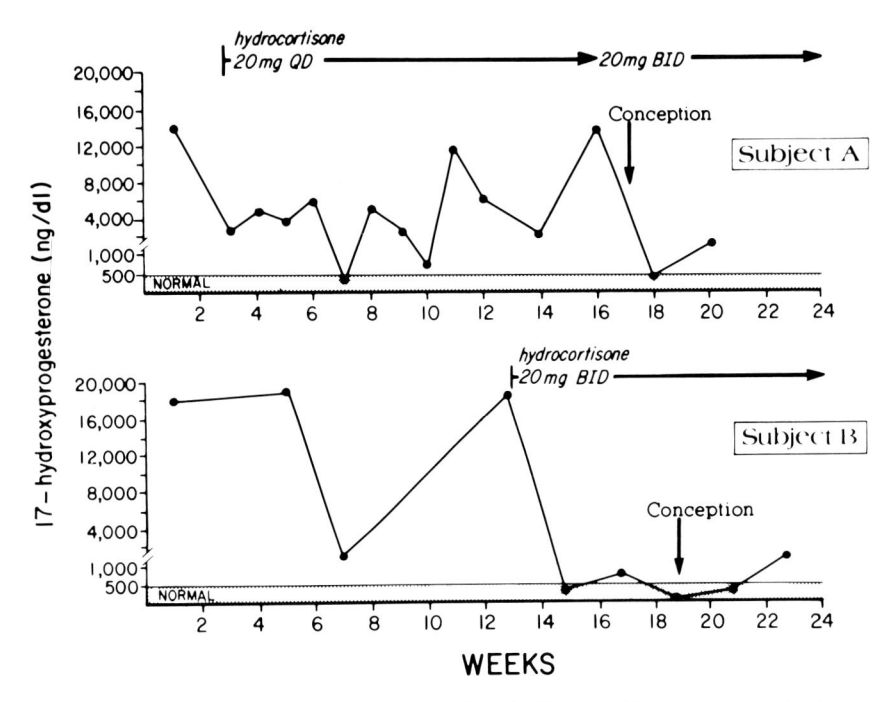

Fig. 19-10. 17-hydroxyprogesterone concentrations in 23-year-old monozygous twin sisters with attenuated (cryptic) 21-hydroxylase deficiency. Both presented with a syndrome very similar to polycystic ovarian disease—mild hirsutism, oligomenorrhea, anovulation, and infertility. Treatment with only hydrocortisone rapidly restored ovulation.

decrease to the normal range and are useful to monitor therapy (Fig. 19-10).

Adrenal Tumors. These are extremely rare causes of androgen excess. Occurring in a pregnant woman, virilization of a female fetus is likely. When one occurs in a prepubertal woman, acquired androgen excess and primary amenorrhea will be present. Diagnosis and management of these tumors have already been discussed in the section on adrenal tumor under "Congenital Genital Ambiguity." The use of a dexamethasone suppression test to distinguish an adrenal tumor from a pituitary tumor or functional adrenal disorder is described in the appendix of Chapter 4.

Cushing's Syndrome. Cushing's syndrome occurs when cortisol secretion by the adrenal cortex is chronically increased. This may occur with an autonomous adrenal tumor or excessive stimulation of the adrenal cortex by ACTH. Increased concentrations of ACTH occur with a hypersecretory state of the pituitary gland, an ACTH-secreting pituitary adenoma (Cushing's disease), or secretion of ACTH from an ectopic source. The most common source of ectopic ACTH is a carcinoma of the lung and a neoplasm here or in the thymus, pancreas, thyroid, or derivatives of neural crest tissue (e.g., a pheochromocytoma or neuroblastoma) should be suspected when high concentrations of cortisol are not suppressed by dexamethasone and there is no evidence of a pituitary or adrenal tumor (94). Primary amenorrhea will be a presenting complaint only when Cushing's syndrome develops before puberty or during its early stages. Pituitary causes of amenorrhea and the manifestation of Cushing's syndrome are described more completely in Chapter 4.

Treatment is dictated by the cause of the Cushing's syndrome but, if successful, ovulation, menstruation, and fertility should become normal.

Androgenic Drugs. Medications that may cause hirsutism or other manifestations of acquired androgen excess are summarized in Table 19-11. A careful history of drug use and elimination of any of these should allow menstruation to begin. As with all causes of androgen excess, the hirsutism may not disappear if it has been present for more than 6 months or it became extensive.

5-Alpha-Reductase Deficiency. This disorder, like deficiencies of other enzymes necessary for normal steroidogenesis, is inherited as an autosomal recessive trait. Affected males will usually have evidence of congenital genital ambiguity, although this may not be pronounced. However, virilization of the genitalia occurs at the time of puberty and has been so pronounced in some that the affected subject switched from a female to a male gender role (76). Genetic males have no cervix or uterus and testes are present that secrete normal male quantities of testosterone. Breast growth does not occur. Conversion of testosterone to dihydrotestosterone normally occurs in the genitalia and other androgen target tissues. Lacking normal enzyme activity, these subjects cannot virilize their genitalia in a normal fashion during intrauterine life. Presumably, testosterone itself is sufficient to virilize the genitalia at the time of puberty.

The testes should be removed at the time of diagnosis to prevent further genital virilization. Reduction of an enlarged phallus and creation of a functional vagina should be done at the same time. Fertility is not possible.

Causes of primary amenorrhea and acquired androgen excess are summarized in Table 19–13.

TABLE 19–13. Causes of Primary Amenorrhea and Acquired Androgen Excess

UTERUS	KARYOTYPE	CAUSE
Present	46,XY	Gonadal dysgenesis with a tumor or hilus-cell hyperplasia
	46,XX	Polycystic ovarian disease
		Hyperthecosis
		Ovarian tumor
		Attenuated adrenal hyperplasia
		Cushing's syndrome
		Adrenal tumor
		Medication (Table 19–11)
Absent	46,XY	5-alpha-reductase deficiency
	46,XX	(No diagnosis)

Summary

The diagnostic approach to a woman with primary amenorrhea is based on the application of embryologic and endocrinologic principles to clinical medicine. The assessment of such a woman requires a disciplined approach that results in the sequential segregation of the causes of primary amenorrhea according to the sex steroid manifested, the presence or absence of müllerian derivatives, the karyotype, and the serum concentrations of LH and FSH.

REFERENCES

1. Wyshak G, Frisch RE. Evidence for a secular trend in age of menarche. N Engl J Med 1982;306:1033–1035.
2. Styne DM, Grumbach MM. Puberty in the male and female: its physiology and disorders. In: Yen SSC, Jaffe RB, eds. Reproductive endocrinology: physiology, pathophysiology and clinical management. Philadelphia: WB Saunders, 1978:189–240.
3. Coulam CB. Testicular regression syndrome. Obstet Gynecol 1979;53:44–49.
4. Berthezene F, Forest MG, Grimaud JA, Claustrat B, Mornex R. Leydig-cell agenesis: a cause of male pseudohermaphroditism. N Engl J Med 1976;295:969–972.
5. Schneider G, Genel M, Bongiovanni AM, Goldman AS, Rosenfield RL. Persistent testicular delta 5-isomerase, 3 beta-hydroxysteroid dehydrogenase (delta 5,3 beta-HSD) deficiency in the delta 5,3 beta-HSD form of congenital adrenal hyperplasia. J Clin Invest 1975;55:681–690.
6. Bricaire H, Luton JP, Laudat P, et al. A new male pseudohermaphroditism associated with hypertension due to a block of 17 alpha-hydroxylation. J Clin Endocrinol Metab 1972;35:67–72.
7. New MI. Male pseudohermaphroditism due to 17-alpha-hydroxylase deficiency. J Clin Invest 1970;49:1930–1941.
8. Zachmann M, Vollmin JA, Hamilton W, Prader A. Steroid 17,20-desmolase deficiency: a new cause of male pseudohermaphroditism. Clin Endocrinol 1972;1:369–385.
9. Goebelsmann U, Horton R, Mestman JH, et al. Male pseudohermaphroditism due to testicular 17-beta-hydroxysteroid dehydrogenase deficiency. J Clin Endocrinol Metab 1973;36:867–879.

10. Saez JM, de Peretti E, Morera AM, David M, Bertrand J. Familial male pseudohermaphroditism with gynecomastia due to a testicular 17-ketosteroid reductase defect: I. Studies in vivo. J Clin Endocrinol Metab 1971;32:604–610.
11. Imperato-McGinley J, Guerrero L, Gautier T, Peterson RE. Steroid 5 alpha-reductase deficiency in man: an inherited form of male pseudohermaphroditism. Science 1974;186:1213–1215.
12. Griffin JE, Wilson JD. The syndromes of androgen resistance. N Engl J Med 1980;302:198–209.
13. van Niekerk WA. True hermaphroditism, an analytic review with a report of 3 new cases. Am J Obstet Gynecol 1976;126:890–907.
14. Saenger P, Levine LS, Wachtel SS, et al. Presence of H-Y antigen and testis in 46,XX true hermaphroditism, evidence for Y-chromosomal function. J Clin Endocrinol Metab 1976;43:1234–1239.
15. Simpson JL. Anomalies of internal ducts. In: Simpson JL, ed. Disorders of sexual differentiation, etiology and clinical delineation. New York: Academic Press, 1976:341–359.
16. Scully RE. Gonadoblastoma, a review of 74 cases. Cancer 1970;25:1340–1356.
17. Schellhas HF. Malignant potential of the dysgenetic gonad. Obstet Gynecol 1974;44:298–309,455–462.
18. Simpson JL. Gonadal dysgenesis. In: Simpson JL, ed. Disorders of sexual differentiation, etiology and clinical delineation. New York: Academic Press, 1976:259–302.
19. Manuel M, Katayama KP, Jones HW. The age of occurrence of gonadal tumors in intersex patients with a Y chromosome. Am J Obstet Gynecol 1976;124:293–300.
20. Warren JC, Erkman B, Cheatum S, Holman G. Hilus-cell adenoma in a dysgenetic gonad with XX/XO mosaicism. Lancet 1964;1:141–143.
21. Bardin CW, Rosen S, LeMaire WJ, et al. In vivo and in vitro studies of androgen metabolism in a patient with pure gonadal dysgenesis and Leydig cell hyperplasia. J Clin Endocrinol Metab 1969;29:1429–1437.
22. Judd HL, Scully RE, Atkins L, Neer RM, Kliman B. Pure gonadal dysgenesis with progressive hirsutism: demonstration of testosterone production by gonadal streaks. N Engl J Med 1970;282:881–885.
23. Carr BR, Aiman J. Steroid production in a woman with gonadal dysgenesis, breast development, and clitoral hypertrophy. Obstet Gynecol 1980;56:492–498.
24. Ross GT, Vande Wiele RL. The ovaries. In: Williams RH, ed. Textbook of endocrinology, 5th ed. Philadelphia: WB Saunders, 1974:368–422.
25. Kallio H. Cytogenetic and clinical study on 100 cases of primary amenorrhoea. Acta Obstet Gynecol Scand (Suppl) 1973;24:7–78.
26. Mashchak CA, Kletzky OA, Davajan V, Mishell DR Jr. Clinical and laboratory evaluation of patients with primary amenorrhea. Obstet Gynecol 1981;57:715–721.
27. Simpson JL. Gonadal dysgenesis and sex chromosome abnormalities: phenotypic-karyotypic correlations. In: Vallet HL, Porter IH, eds. Genetic mechanism of sexual development. New York: Academic Press, 1979:365–405.
28. Nakashima I, Robinson A. Fertility in a 45,X female. Pediatrics 1971;47:770–773.
29. Reyes FI, Koh KS, Faiman C. Fertility in women with gonadal dysgenesis. Am J Obstet Gynecol 1976;126:668–670.
30. Philip J, Sele V. 45,XO Turner's syndrome without evidence of mosaicism in a patient with 2 pregnancies. Acta Obstet Gynecol Scand 1976;55:283–286.
31. Goldstein DE, Kelly TE, Johanson AJ, Blizzard RM. Gonadal dysgenesis with 45,XO/46,XX mosaicism demonstrated only in a streak gonad. J Pediatr 1977;90:604–605.
32. van Campenhout J, Choquette P, Vauclair R. Endometrial pattern in patients with primary hypoestrogenic amenorrhea receiving estrogen replacement therapy. Obstet Gynecol 1980;56:349–355.
33. Sohval AR. The syndrome of pure gonadal dysgenesis. Am J Med 1965;38:615–625.
34. Boczkowski K, Teter J. Clinical, histological and cytogenic observations in pure gonadal dysgenesis. Acta Endocrinol 1966;51:497–510.
35. McDonough PG. Amenorrhea—etiologic approach to diagnosis. Fertil Steril 1978;30:1–15.
36. Schellhas HF, Trujillo JM, Rutledge FN, Cork A. Germ cell tumors associated with XY gonadal dysgenesis. Am J Obstet Gynecol 1971;109:1197–1204.
37. Davidoff F, Federman DD. Mixed gonadal dysgenesis. Pediatrics 1973;52:725–742.
38. Zah W, Kalderon AE, Tucci JR. Mixed gonadal dysgenesis. Acta Endocrinol (Suppl 197): 1975;1–39.
39. Biglieri EG, Herron MA, Brust N. 17-Hydroxylation deficiency in man. J Clin Invest 1966;45:1946–1954.
40. Goldsmith O, Solomon DH, Horton R. Hypogonadism and mineralcorticoid excess: the 17-hydroxylase deficiency syndrome. N Engl J Med 1967;277:673–677.
41. Homburg R, Potashnik G, Lunenfeld B, Insler V. The hypothalamus as a regulator of repro-

ductive function. Obstet Gynecol Surv 1976; 31:455–471.
42. Bauer HG. Endocrine and other clinical manifestations of hypothalamic disease: a survey of 60 cases with autopsies. J Clin Endocrinol Metab 1954;14:13–31.
43. Bates GW, Bates SR, Whitworth NS. Reproductive failure in women who practice weight control. Fertil Steril 1982;37:373–378.
44. Frisch RE, Wyshak G, Vincent L. Delayed menarche and amenorrhea in ballet dancers. N Engl J Med 1980;303:17–19.
45. Vigersky RA, Andersen AE, Thompson RH, Loriaux DL. Hypothalamic dysfunction in secondary amenorrhea associated with simple weight loss. N Engl J Med 1977;297:1141–1145.
46. Frisch RE, McArthur JW. Menstrual cycles: fatness as a determinant of minimum weight for height necessary for their maintenance or onset. Science 1974;185:949–951.
47. Warren MP, Vande Wiele RL. Clinical and metabolic features of anorexia nervosa. Am J Obstet Gynecol 1973;117:435–449.
48. Wentz AC. Body weight and amenorrhea. Obstet Gynecol 1980;56:482–487.
49. Coulam CB, Laws ER Jr, Abboud CF, Randall RV. Primary amenorrhea and pituitary adenomas. Fertil Steril 1981;35:615–619.
50. Brasel JA, Wright JC, Wilkins L, Blizzard RM. An evulation of seventy-five patients with hypopituitarism beginning in childhood. Am J Med 1965;38:484–498.
51. Morley JE, Melmed S. Gonadal dysfunction in systemic disorders. Metabolism 1979;28:1051–1073.
52. Edman CD, Winters AJ, Porter JC, Wilson J, MacDonald PC. Embryonic testicular regression: a clinical spectrum of XY agonadal individuals. Obstet Gynecol 1977;49:208–217.
53. Griffin JE, Edwards C, Madden JD, Harrod MJ, Wilson JD. Congenital absence of the vagina: the Mayer-Rokitansky-Kuster-Hauser syndrome. Ann Intern Med 1976;85:224–236.
54. Jones HW, Rock JA. Reparative and constructive surgery of the female generative tract. Baltimore: Williams & Wilkins, 1983.
55. McDonald TW, Malkasian GD, Gaffey TA. Endometrial cancer associated with feminizing ovarian tumor and polycystic ovarian disease. Obstet Gynecol 1977;49:654–658.
56. Fechner RE, Kaufman RH. Endometrial adenocarcinoma in Stein-Leventhal syndrome. Cancer 1974;34:444–452.
57. Yen SSC. Chronic anovulation due to CNS-hypothalmic-pituitary dysfunction. In: Yen SSC, Jaffe RB, eds. Reproductive endocrinology: physiology, pathophysiology and clinical management. Philadelphia: WB Saunders, 1978: 349–352.
58. Coulam CB. Premature gonadal failure. Fertil Steril 1982;38:645–655.
59. MacDonald PC, Madden JD, Brenner PF, Wilson JD, Siiteri PK. Origin of estrogen in normal men and women and in women with testicular feminization. J Clin Endocrinol Metab 1979;49:905–916.
60. Brown TR, Marc M, Rothwell SW, Migeon CJ. Human complete androgen insensitivity with normal dihydrotestosterone receptor binding capacity in cultured genital skin fibroblasts: evidence for a qualitative abnormality of the receptor. J Clin Endocrinol Metab 1982;55:61–69.
61. Amrhein JA, Klingensmith GJ, Walsh PC, McKusick VA, Migeon CJ. Partial androgen insensitivity: the Reifenstein syndrome revisited. N Engl J Med 1977;297:350–356.
62. Griffin JE. Testicular feminization associated with a thermolabile androgen receptor in cultured human fibroblasts. J Clin Invest 1979;64:1624–1631.
63. Bongiovanni AM. Congenital adrenal hyperplasia and related conditions. In: Stanbury JB, Wyngaarden JB, Frederickson DS, eds. The metabolic basis of inherited disease, 4th ed. New York: McGraw-Hill, 1978:868–893.
64. Migeon CJ, Rosenwaks Z, Lee PA, Urban MD, Bias WB. The attenuated form of congenital adrenal hyperplasia as an allelic form of 21-hydroxylase deficiency. J Clin Endocrinol Metab 1980;51:647–649.
65. Brautbar C, Rosler A, Landau H, et al. No linkage between HLA and congenital adrenal hyperplasia due to 11-beta-hydroxylase deficiency. N Engl J Med 1979;300:205–206.
66. Lee PA, Plotnick LP, Kowarski AA, Migeon CJ, eds. Congenital adrenal hyperplasia. Baltimore: University Park Press, 1977.
67. Hutter AM, Kayhoe DE. Adrenal cortical carcinoma: clinical features of 138 patients. Am J Med 1966;41:572–580.
68. Bertagna C, Orth DN. Clinical and laboratory findings and results of therapy in 58 patients with adrenocortical tumors admitted to a single medical center (1951 to 1978). Am J Med 1981;71:855–875.
69. Girouard DP, Barclay DL, Collins CG. Hyperreactio luteinalis: review of the literature and report of 2 cases. Obstet Gynecol 1964;23:513–525.
70. Hensleigh PA, Woodruff JD. Differential maternal-fetal response to androgenizing luteoma or hyperreactio luteinalis. Obstet Gynecol Surv 1978; 33:262–271.
71. Garcia-Bunuel R, Berek JS, Woodruff JD. Lu-

teomas of pregnancy. Obstet Gynecol 1975;45:407–414.
72. Verkauf BS, Reiter EO, Hernandez L, Burns SA. Virilization of mother and fetus associated with luteoma of pregnancy: a case report with endocrinologic studies. Am J Obstet Gynecol 1977;129:274–280.
73. Verhoeven ATM, Mastboom JL, Van Leusden HAIM, Van Der Velden WHM. Virilization in pregnancy coexisting with an (ovarian) mucinous cystadenoma: a case report and review of virilizing ovarian tumors in pregnancy. Obstet Gynecol Surv 1973;28:597–622.
74. Chung A, Birnbaum SJ. Ovarian cancer associated with pregnancy. Obstet Gynecol 1973;41:211–214.
75. Griffin JE, Wilson JD. Hereditary male pseudohermaphroditism. Clin Obstet Gynecol 1978;5:457–479.
76. Peterson RE, Imperato-McGinley J, Gautier T, Sturla E. Male pseudohermaphroditism due to steroid 5-alpha-reductase deficiency. Am J Med 1977;62:170–191.
77. Imperato-McGinley J, Peterson RE. Male pseudohermaphroditism: the complexities of male phenotypic development. Am J Med 1976;61:251–272.
78. Imperato-McGinley J, Peterson RE, Stoller R, Goodwin WE. Male pseudohermaphroditism secondary to 17-beta-hydroxysteroid dehydrogenase deficiency: gender role change in puberty. J Clin Endocrinol Metab 1979;49:391–395.
79. Wilson JD, MacDonald PC. Male pseudohermaphroditism due to androgen resistance: testicular feminization and related syndromes. In: Stanbury JB, Wyngaarden JB, Frederickson DS, eds. The metabolic basis of inherited disease, 4th ed. New York: McGraw-Hill, 1978:894–913.
80. Wilson JD, Harrod MJ, Goldstein JL, Hemsell DL, MacDonald PC. Familial incomplete male pseudohermaphroditism, type 1: evidence for androgen resistance and variable clinical manifestations in a family with the Reifenstein syndrome. N Engl J Med 1974;290:1097–1103.
81. Madden JD, Walsh PC, MacDonald PC, Wilson JD. Clinical and endocrinologic characterization of a patient with the syndrome of incomplete testicular feminization. J Clin Endocrinol Metab 1975;41:751–760.
82. Aiman J, Hemsell DL, MacDonald PC. Production and origin of estrogen in two true hermaphrodites. Am J Obstet Gynecol 1978;132:401–409.
83. Shannon R, Nicolaides NJ. True hermaphroditism with oogenesis and spermatogenesis. Aust NZ J Obstet Gynaecol 1973;13:184–187.
84. Braunstein GD, Vaitukaitis JL, Carbone PP, Ross GT. Ectopic production of human chorionic gonadotrophin by neoplasms. Ann Intern Med 1973;78:39–45.
85. Aiman EJ, Edman CD, Sitteri PK, MacDonald PC. Androgen production and origin of estrogen in three groups of hirsute or virilized women. Gynecol Invest 1975;6:21.
86. Bates GW, Whitworth NS. Effect of body weight reduction on plasma androgens in obese, infertile women. Fertil Steril 1982;38:406–409.
87. Aiman J. Age, estrogen, and the endometrium. Clin Obstet Gynecol 1981;24:193–202.
88. Goldzieher JW. Polycystic ovarian disease. Fertil Steril 1981;35:371–394.
89. Aiman J, Edman CD, Worley RJ, Vellios F, MacDonald PC. Androgen and estrogen formation in women with ovarian hyperthecosis. Obstet Gynecol 1978;51:1–9.
90. Ireland K, Woodruff JD. Masculinizing ovarian tumors. Obstet Gynecol Surv 1976;31:83–111.
91. Levine LS, Dupont B, Lorenzen F, et al. Genetic and hormonal characterization of cryptic 21-hydroxylase deficiency. J Clin Endocrinol Metab 1981;53:1192–1198.
92. Kohn B, Levine LS, Pollack MS, et al. Late-onset steroid 21-hydroxylase deficiency: a variant of classical congenital adrenal hyperplasia. J Clin Endocrinol Metab 1982;55:817–827.
93. Zachmann M, Tassinari D, Prader A. Clinical and biochemical variability of congenital adrenal hyperplasia due to 11 beta-hydroxylase deficiency. A study of 25 patients. J Clin Endocrinol Metab 1983;56:222–229.
94. Odell WD. Humoral manifestations of cancer. In: Williams RH, ed. Textbook of endocrinology, 6th ed. Philadelphia: WB Saunders, 1981:1228–1241.

Adoption 20

Mary Reistroffer

Adoption is a familiar word to most adults in contemporary America but we should not assume any genuine depth or breadth of knowledge, because our perception depends upon our perspective. Adoption may be an alternative and a solution for childless couples and parentless children. For many, this is the limit of perception about adoption. Yet, adoption is an institution that is responsive to the mores and cultural pressures of society as a whole and to the dictates of other institutions in our society.

We cannot assume any genuine knowledge about adoption for another reason. Adoption today is different from adoption as it has existed in the past. Adoption in the future will be different from adoption today because of important and ever-changing norms dictated by the will of society. In the past, adoption may have meant the healthy white couple choosing the healthy white newborn. The common perception was that this was a solution for childless couples and parentless children that merely required the approval of a judge who followed the dictates of laws that demanded little in the process.

The purpose of this chapter is to trace the history of adoption and show how adoption today is a result of a cultural evolution. The basic structure of adoption today will be described and reference to adoption resource contacts made.

Adoption in History

Although Sargon, King of Babylonia in 2800 B.C., described his own adoption by Akki, the water carrier (1), the oldest written laws of adoption are those by Hammurabi in the Babylonian empire of 2000 B.C. In the 286 codes of Hammurabi, those that concerned adoption dealt with issues that are germaine today: Will the child be treated differently from a natural child? Will the child suffer from a change in caretaker? Will the adopted child and family be suited to each other? Courtiers in Babylonian society were prevented by law (and occasionally by castration) from fathering children. Adoption was the only means of passing on their high social status. Adoption by a courtier in Babylonia was a distinct honor and a great leap in the social status of the child. Boys were also adopted by free craftsmen to learn and inherit the adoptive father's trade. The main object of adoption was to acquire a son to perpetuate the family and to perform the religious rites due to the adoptive father after his death. Most ancient civilizations sanctioned adoption and its practice is mentioned in the Bible—Pharoah's daughter adopted Moses and Mordecai adopted Esther.

However, adoption was only one of several ways of obtaining heirs. Polygamy, legitimation, and the levirate were additional means and only the last has died out. The levirate law allowed a man to inherit his brother's widow and raise children in his name. The legitimation of children by concubines or maids was apparently common and was represented in the book of Genesis by the history of Jacob and Rachel. However, adoption does not seem to exist in Jewish law.

Roman law developed over many centuries and came to include laws of adoption. Patricians adopted successors to eliminate claimants of whom they disapproved, and Marcus Aurelius even adopted a son to inherit the crown of the empire. Roman adoption law was complicated by the concept of *paterfamilias*. This was a social manifestation of a cult of ancestor worship in which a family's ancestors conferred social rank and a member of 1 family was inextricably bound to that family. By the reign of Justinian, Roman law had reconciled this dilemma by creating 2 types of adoption: *adrogatio* and *adoptio*. Adrogatio was possible only for a person who was *sui iuris*, that is, a member of no family but his own. A child whose father died was considered *sui iuris*. If such a full adoption took place, the adoptee and all his descendants belonged to his new family. His previous cult was destroyed and he worshipped his new ancestors. *Adoptio*, or simple adoption, was permissible even to one who had heirs and the adoptee was considered *alieni iuris*, a subordinate member of the family. The problem of *adoptio* was the residual power of the *paterfamilias* over the person to be adopted. This power, or *potestas*, had to be renounced 3 times before the child was free for adoption.

China is most widely known for its ancestor cult and adoption also flourished there. One manifestation of this ancestor worship is the desire to have one's tablet placed in the hall of ancestors. This required a descendant to place it there and to carry out the prescribed worship since "Heaven awaits no one who has no male issue" (1). Adoption provided such a successor for those who had no children. Adopted children in China were almost always boys because of religious requirements and because girls were only temporary residents in the natal family. Once a girl married, her descendants became a part of her husband's lineage.

Islam is either indifferent or opposed to adoption because polygamy and easy divorce are traditional. The patriarchal nature of Islam militates against adoption and a man can legitimate his own child merely by acknowledgement; marriage to the child's mother is not required.

Hindu law describes at least 12 types of adoption. The degree of closeness between adoptee and adopter is prescribed. The adopted should be of the same family but not within prohibited degrees of kinship. Adoption was a form of exchange and as such required a transaction to occur between the adopter and the adoptee's parents. Hence the provision, curious to Westerners, that an orphan cannot be adopted—there is no one to give him in adoption. Hindu laws of inheritance are immensely complex and more so for the person dying without an heir. Adoption solved many inheritance problems when no natural sons existed.

The feudal system was introduced to England at the time of the Norman conquest. One consequence of this system was that everyone had a place in society and orphans were easily absorbed into large aristocratic households. With the disintegration of the feudal system, parentless children were no one's responsibility. England's first Poor Law was passed in 1597 and contained provisions for orphaned children. This and the subsequent Poor Laws were administered locally by parishes. This meant that every parish was inclined to keep its poor rate down by hounding the poor out of the district. Mothers of illegitimate children were held responsible and assigned to work houses. Their children were often placed in other institutions until they were old enough for the work houses. Adoption was accepted *de facto* but not *de jure* in England at this time. England first passed an Adoption Act in 1926.

In the United States, Massachusetts was the first state to pass an adoption law in 1851. This law required a joint petition by the adopting mother and father, written consent of the child's natural parents, and a written decree by a judge if he was satisfied that the adoption was "fit and proper." Other states followed by passing individual adoption laws modeled on that of Massachusetts, and by 1923 all states had passed an adoption law. Many of the early adoption laws were intended merely to provide evidence of the legal transfer of a child from the biologic to adoptive parents. Michigan was one of the first states that mandated an investigation when it passed its law in 1891. By 1938, 24 states required that all adoption petitions be referred to a local agency or the state department of public welfare (2). Each law reflects the heritage of past customs and concerns for heirs, class structure, racial restrictions, age requirements, and kinship limitations.

In this brief history of adoption (1,2), the traditions of family, religion, race, social class, relinquishment of parental rights, and legal assumption of parental responsibilities that confer rights of inheritance on the adopted child are powerful ones that influence adoption as it exists today. But the evolution of legislation in the United States clearly reflects a shifting of emphasis from the good of the state to the welfare and protection of those affected by adoption.

Adoption Today

The basis of adoption today is state law and each is unique in defining who may and may not adopt, the mechanism for terminating parental rights, and the assessment process that must occur. In short, each law mandates how the adoption of a minor child occurs and defines the minimum protection required by the courts before allowing the adoption to occur.

Most states require some investigative procedures before an adoption decree is granted. For governmental and voluntary child placement agencies, this usually means that the adoptive parents complete an application that describes their personal, social, and medical situation. Each agency usually defines guidelines for accepting an adoption application. State residency, marital status, church affiliation if the agency is a denominational one, age, health, and psychologic stability are but a few of the possible guidelines. These guidelines are often a result of legal requirements and adoptive agencies, either governmental or voluntary, must adhere to defined minimum standards, rules, regulations, and other administrative policies.

Despite its primary legal base, adoption is also a social process, emotionally charged and heavily laden with folklore, hearsay, and myths of gigantic proportions. Important societal and institutional trends have converged to prompt a rapid and dynamic, even radical, change in adoption, especially nonrelative ones. Illegitimacy, the right to legal abortion, medical advances that enable previously infertile couples to have children, the growing number of adolescent pregnancies, the astounding accumulation of nearly one-half million children and youth in "temporary placement" service systems, and required time-limited intervention in reported instances of child abuse and neglect are but some of the factors that are shaping and changing adoption today (3,4).

Deinstitutionalization is a contrived word to describe a policy that has emerged in response to the "warehousing" of children and adults in need that occurred around 1900. Institutions for the care of the mentally ill, developmentally disabled, ill, aged, incarcerated nonfelons, or orphaned children were often large, impersonal, and located in places remote from the home community. Deinstitutionalization was a growing cause in the 1960s, but became public policy by 1970. This policy included 2 aims: dispersal and discharge of current cases to community-based care, and diversion of all new candidates to home community care. The resulting endeavor in this area nearly overwhelmed local community services that were charged with investigating and intervening in instances of child abuse and neglect.

The impact of these societal forces caused a protracted crisis in communities that had limited placement resources. These forces were important in shaping adoption as it now is. By 1975, as many as 525,000 children in the United States were in family foster care or institutional placement. Many of these were captive of a system that perceived such placement as a protective solution and not a temporary mechanism for providing care. Many of these children became victims of a series of temporary court orders which resulted in "temporary placement" for years. Thus, "temporary" meant placement of a child without termination of parental rights and had little relation to the duration of the placement.

Because of the large and growing number of children in so-called temporary placement, a concept of permanency planning was formulated and developed into a working model in Oregon from 1971 to 1972. Permanency planning required the coordinated efforts of the legal system and social agencies to provide a review, a plan for permanent placement, and implementation and conclusion of the plan within 2 years. In 1978, the Oregon model became national policy; with the passage of Public Law 96–272 in 1980, implementation was assured. In essence and intent, permanency planning incorporates a plan and a timetable for implementation of the plan so that children are not kept in a limbo of "temporary placement" for more than 2 years. An important provision of permanency planning is the federal mandate to *prevent* children from coming to placement by providing services to the child within his or her own family. Placement occurs only when the problems are so severe that removing the child from the birth or extended family is best for the child.

As a result of all these forces, there is now a growing emphasis on screening-in, rather than screening-out adoptive candidates (5). This has fostered one of the myths of adoption—the "waiting list." While every agency has an approved group of homes, any responsible agency takes care not to expand its pool of available homes beyond the number in which they expect to place a child within 2 years. No agency manipulates the group waiting for placement of a child by asking them to "take a number and wait your turn." Most agencies have a timetable for *each* approved family and try to meet that timetable in their planning. The duration until placement of a child is, and should be, modified by other factors such as a family illness, job changes, unemployment, or other crisis situations. Other than crisis situations, factors such as parental termination, sudden intervention by the extended family, divorce of applicants or marriage of single applicants, and a medically complicated birth of a child that is to be placed for adoption also modify the timetable until placement. Any one or all of these keep the approved applications in a state of flux. Many couples may not recognize these factors and interpret the time until placement as an inflexible "waiting list." Adoptive parents should understand that such adjustments are more responsible than irresponsible.

While the placement of a healthy white infant will continue, such placements have become a miniscule part of the adoption effort. The focus of governmental and voluntary agencies doing child placement is and will continue to be directed toward the achievement of permanent placement of children and youth now in temporary situations. This may be done by early reunification with birth families. In instances of a child born to an unwed mother, the putative father is acknowledged as having rights, and services to both parents are offered. Long-term contractual care, including guardianship with foster parents and placing children for adoption, are alternatives when reunification with the birth family is not best for the child.

Much of the confusion that currently exists stems from the fact that both the courts and the service agencies are *simultaneously* establishing procedures to manage existing caseloads and stem the influx of children needing care and placement. While their policies and procedures are occasionally contradictory, the aim of the legal system and the social agencies is clearly the same—the welfare of the child.

Because social service agencies are now beginning to screen in the persons seeking to adopt, how adoptive parent candidates approach a placement resource and how they are received is changing. A common misconception is that an agency uses the "home study" to select only those with ideal personal qualifications and that the selection process is based on a subjective assessment of parenting potential. In fact, agencies today, as in the past, are seeking applicants who can nurture a child by making a life long commitment and who can respond and grow as they manage the demands that being a parent imposes.

While the initial process of application remains much the same as in the past, the emphasis on screening in of the applicants means the home study is less a unilateral process in which a decision is made after an investigation and more a mutual decision and a preparation for the parenting experience. This change in emphasis is having a strong impact on the reception that adoptive candidates receive in their overture to placement services (6,7).

Applicants for adoption today will find nearly insurmountable barriers and agencies that are unable to take their application if they are willing to consider *only* an infant or young child. Because of the paucity of such children for adoption, the emphasis now is on placement of older children and those with special needs. Applicants can expect to be invited to an initial interview or a group meeting session unless their stipulation for an infant is nonnegotiable. An invitation to attend an interview or group meeting should be seized upon by adoptive applicants, even though they retain a strong preference for an infant or young child. This initial contact can be a learning experience for the person or couple wishing to adopt. Often, candidates for adoption are reacting to the fact that they cannot have their own child and have proceeded too hastily to adoption. This is a viable alternative, but only after the infertile couple has resolved their grief over the loss of the children they will never have (see Chapter 2). Agencies have focused on the couples that are ready, but are now beginning to assist these couples to work through their grief and choose alternatives.

The Adoption Process

Many agencies will continue to use the traditional format of office and home interviews rather than group meetings. These agencies place a high value on the privacy of the applicants and the relationship that they develop with the professional assigned to work with them. The intent of the initial contacts is to arrive at a decision to proceed or not, to define the circumstances of an adoption, and to support the applicants with information. The number of interviews is dictated by the individual situation. This format, however, is expensive because of the professional's time, and accounts for the fees commonly charged for adoption services. The initial contact is often by telephone and followed by a joint interview. One or more interviews with each applicant usually precedes a visit to the applicants' home. This initial screening process includes a consideration of the applicants' agreement to pursue adoption and of not responding to a current family crisis. Physical health necessary to meet the demands of parenting is also an important consideration in this initial screening, as is the absence of obvious psychologic problems that should delay or preclude the application.

Separate interviews with each member of an applicant couple are important because 1 spouse is often the spokesperson for both. The application is considered in the context of the whole family and the home interview takes into account the presence of other children. No matter how well prepared for these initial interviews, the applicants will be anxious because they feel they are being evaluated and they recognize the importance of the step they are taking.

There is a confusion in the variety of procedures, practices, and contacts in the home study process. One agency may have a very sophisticated system of practice that is implemented by an experienced and well-trained professional staff, while another may use a different procedure that is carried out by a staff that is inexperienced and undertrained. It is in the applicants' best interest to gather information from those close to adoption (e.g., an organization such as Resolve, those who have adopted, a physician who works closely with infertile couples, or a social worker with an interest in adoption). Many communities have social organizations of couples who have adopted. These and organizations such as Resolve provide information and support to their own members but welcome couples who are pursuing or considering adoption.

The responsibility of the professional assigned to the applicant is to represent the agency to the applicants and to represent the applicants in regard to their desires, their potential as adoptive parents, and their choice of an appropriate child. The intent of this process is for the agency and the applicants to know each other well. The interval from the acceptance to approval of the application is approximately 9 months in most situations. The thrust of the interview process is an acceleration of the time usually required to know someone and not a mechanism for entrapment. For example, an adoptive applicant may be confounded by an inquiry into how he or she expresses anger. The agency worker does not value one behavior or expression as healthier than another (except when a behavior pattern suggests the possibility of abuse); rather, the worker uses this as an avenue to discuss the degree to which a parent is a model for a child and to point out that the prospective parent should not expect a better level of expression or behavior than he or she tolerates in himself or herself. As another example, the worker may note that the adoptive parent completed only 2 years of high school. The fact is unimportant in itself but may have implications in a parenting role. The circumstances may have been an economic necessity or a personal preference. If economic, does the applicant feel cheated, overvalue education, or tend to exert undue pressure on a child to achieve academically? It is the attitude and residual feelings behind many simple facts that are important and not the facts themselves. The worker does not expect to find adults who have had a trouble-free life experience, but looks for their basic satisfactions and dissatisfactions and how they have grown in response to these. Applicants who cling to perceptions they had as children and who fail to mature in response to life experiences may have difficulty functioning as parents.

In any agency with a quality adoption program, the decision to approve or terminate the application is not a unilateral privilege of the assigned worker. The study is carefully monitored by consultant and supervisory staff, who direct the proceedings and share the ultimate decision. This is intended to ensure fairness because no agency wishes to subject the applicants or a child to an experience of failure.

Once approved, childless couples will be projected into the parenting role by simulation and will be encouraged to seek out experiences with children. These experiences should be more than casual encounters with the children of friends. This prepares applicants for the remarkable upheaval wrought by the placement of a child and begins to establish rituals of living with a child.

The study process should be a rewarding and meaningful experience for applicants if they have been prepared for what it is intended to accomplish by a skilled professional.

In all but a few rare instances, an adoption is not finalized by court action until 6 months after placement of the child. This 6-month period is intended to be a time for relationships to develop before the final step and not a trial period. An agency has contact during this period but is geared more to support of the placement than removal of the child for cause. No agency would remove a child from the adoptive home unless there were clear indications of child abuse, gross failure of adjustment, or a request for removal by the adoptive parents. Indications of trouble in the placement would prompt any agency to resolve the problems rather than remove the child hastily.

Adoption today includes the controversy of the "open record," fears that the natural parents will attempt to recover the child, and opposition to adoption by influential members of the candidates' extended families. All pose a threat that warrants discussion in an applicant group or during the study interviews.

The "open record" controversy developed in the last 10 years as a byproduct of objections that military, investigative, and credit records were not shared or available to the subjects of those records. Proponents of open records argued that all records should be available. In 1975 Great Britain passed a statute that enabled adult adoptees to examine records that had previously been sealed by the court and held confidential. Subsequently, some states and courts have softened their statutory provisions to allow access to medical information concerning an adopted child. Presently, the trend is to permit the opening of records for the necessary medical information, for determination of inheritance, or for other equally compelling reasons, but to allow access to the record only through the court. It is difficult to speculate if this is a first step in eventually allowing complete open records in matters of adoption (8,9). Increasingly, birth parents who surrendered children for adoption and adult adoptees are joining groups that are nominally mutual support groups, but are becoming involved in the open record controversy.

Appeals to set aside a final adoptive decree and return the child to the birth parents do occur. Some states are changing their laws to reduce the period of time that such an action is allowed. In most states, the time limit for appeal is as short as 6 months, but in some states it remains 5 years. The shortening of the time until the adoption is granted and the time for a recovery action is closed is taking place while efforts are being made to make termination of parental rights a court action rather than a process of affidavit. The latter is a response, in part, to the growth of a black market in adoption over the past several years. All of these efforts indicate a concern for protecting the rights of *all* the parties to adoption.

Independent Adoptions

Another facet of adoption is the independent adoption, one that has been arranged by "facilitators" to avoid agency services and involvement. Subsidized adoptions are also being promoted in certain circumstances and these are funded by the federal government (in part). Many states prohibit nonagency or unprotected adoptions and impose stiff penalties on "facilitators." Other states impose only modest misdemeanor level penalties and expect adverse publicity and professional embarrassment to act as a deterrent (10).

While independent placements escalate risk, it is dismaying to discover that these are often prompted by the challenge of the pursuit provoked by the shortage of infants for adoptive placement rather than a deep-seated yearning for a child. This translates into securing a child as quickly as possible and by any means possible. Agencies are wary of applicants who engage in strategies such as simultaneous applications to several placement services, working toward an independent placement by arrangements with a physician and attorney, or unilaterally approaching a pregnant woman. While overtures to several agencies may be necessary to initiate an application, it is likely that this avid shopping and arranging will be discovered and will prompt closure of all avenues.

Subsidized adoption began in the last decade to offer ongoing payments to parents who adopt children expected to have substantial medical expenses over several years. It has now been expanded to include payments when the financial resources of the adopting family are limited and would otherwise preclude the adoption. Subsidy arrangements are important in achieving permanent placement for the impaired or special needs child.

Adoption Resources

1. Candidates and counselors can purchase the current issue of the Child Welfare League of America *CWLA Directory of Member and Associate Agencies*, which is published in January of each year. CWLA is a national standard-setting organization with public and voluntary child welfare service member agencies throughout the United States and Canada. The Directory is arranged by states and provinces and is coded to identify services that are offered (e.g., adoption). This is available from CWLA, 67 Irving Place, New York, New York 10003 (about $10.00).
2. Candidates can write the state department of social services or public welfare in the capital of the state in which they reside. If that department is not involved directly in adoption services, it should be able to provide information about adoption services within the state. Correspondence should be addressed to "Adoption Service" and should include the candidates' telephone number to enable an early reply. It is helpful if the inquiry letter includes religious affiliation, and indicates any preferences as to age and sex of a child.
3. Candidates living in larger cities should look in the yellow page telephone book under "Social Service Agencies." Any agency noting "child or family services" in their name can be helpful in providing local information. Agencies that have a religion as part of their name do not necessarily restrict applications to members of that religion. Many agency names include this because of their founding and support constituency, but offer services on a nonsectarian basis.
4. Candidates in all of the more than 4,200 counties in the United States have a county department of social services with offices located in the county seat. These agencies can identify local and nearby adoptive placement services, and may offer such services themselves. Applicants should call the "Child Placement" or "Foster Care Services" division of the county.

REFERENCES

1. Kadushin A. Substitute care: adoption. In: Child welfare services. New York: Macmillan and Co., 1967.
2. Abbott G. The child and the state. Chicago: University of Chicago Press, 1938:164–171.
3. Cole ES. Adoption services today and tomorrow. In: DPHEW publication #78–30158. Child welfare strategy in the coming years. Washington, DC, 1978:132–168.
4. Bedger JE. Teenage pregnancy: Research related to clients and services. Springfield, Ill.: Charles C Thomas, 1980.
5. Stein TJ, Gambril ED, Wiltse KT. Children in foster homes: achieving continuity of care. New York: Praeger, 1978.
6. Tremitiere BT. Adoption of children with special needs—the client-centered approach. Child Welfare 1979;10:681–688.

7. Jewett CL. Adopting the older child. Cambridge: Harvard Common Press, 1978.
8. Libman ET, Lubimiv GP, Schlesinger B. Know and tell: Adoption disclosure in Canada. Toronto: University of Toronto School of Social Work, 1978.
9. Sorosky AD, Baran A, Pannor R. The adoption triangle. New York: Doubleday, 1976.
10. Meezan W, Katz S, Russo EM. Adoption without agencies: a study of independent adoptions. New York: Child Welfare League of America, 1978.

The Ethics of Reproductive Intervention

21

Dennis J. Doherty

The ethical dimension of any issue is the one about which people tend to argue the most. While people understandably find medical and scientific advances fascinating and any legal ramifications interesting, it is the ethical or moral (the terms may be used interchangeably) aspects of these advances that are often the most controversial. This is so because people have ideas and beliefs about what is right and wrong, even though they may not completely understand the technology or the laws that are constructed in the wake of these technologic developments.

Something is not moral simply because it is possible. Because something *can* be done does not mean that it *may* or *should* be done. It is possible to prolong human life almost indefinitely, but at times it would be wrong to do so. Most people accept this since most understand the meaning of, and wish for themselves, "death with dignity." That it is possible to conceive a child without intervention by a physician does not mean that it is moral or even desirable to do so unless certain other conditions exist, notably the ability to care for a child. Because of medical intervention, procreation is possible for many couples who would otherwise have to accept a life without children. This gives birth to a number of questions relating to the ethical dimensions of reproduction.

The Task of Ethics

Before considering those questions, a brief overview of the task of ethics is in order. The purpose of ethical inquiry is to make value judgments, to determine whether an actual or proposed activity is truly commensurate with being human. Since this is the purpose of the discipline of ethics, by obvious inference ethics is concerned also with prohibitions (of activities which would be dehumanizing). Ethical analysis is therefore positive; its focus is on that which will enhance life. Attempts to determine if an activity is commensurate with being human will generate much disagreement, but it is through such disagreement that value (ethical) judgments become more refined. Ethical dilemmas exist when values come into conflict; admittedly, it would be easier (and more satisfying to many) if the answers were clearly defined and available for ready reference (1). But this is not so. In reality, solutions to ethical dilemmas are not as easily achieved as are the results of a blood test or an X-ray (and even these are subject to interpretation).

The work of ethics might be compared to making and reading maps. A direct map is ordinarily more readable than one which features every aspect of the terrain. In comparison, both physicians and patients know that an on-the-spot diagnosis with a simple prescription for a medication is certainly preferable to (and less costly than) a lengthy evaluation and course of therapy. Precision in diagnosis is essential to good patient care, but it happens at times that a battery of tests must be run in order to arrive at a precise diagnosis. The same is true of ethical analysis. Traditional maps in life must be carefully reviewed and new maps drawn to include recent technologic advances. Even the Ten Commandments, the basis of Judaeo-Christian moral teaching, are, at best, signposts that imply more than they literally express. As such, they are not only to be read, but also read into (which is the root meaning of the verb, "to understand"). For example, one of the Commandments prohibits adultery, and people argue whether artificial insemination by a donor (AID) is prohibited by this Commandment (i.e., Is AID adultery?). The Hippocratic oath tells us to "do no harm," but this dictum is often too broad to be immediately applicable. Whether a proposed medical or surgical procedure is harmful can be determined only when the circumstances are given.

When ethicians (ethicists, moralists), with either a philosophic or theologic persuasion, ply their craft, they argue theories of interest to other ethicians. Their arguments are often in a jargon only other ethicians can understand. But these theories and the language in which they are expressed (e.g., deontology, act-utilitarianism, etc.) are probably of little interest to practicing physicians whose own ethical sensitivities have been molded by the realities of clinical practice. The physician, however, can be as helpful to the ethicist as the ethicist can be to the physician. The conclusions (value judgments) derived by ethicians are only as good as the evidence that supports them. This evidence comes from 2 sources—argument and authority (expert opinion). Both sources are usually incomplete because the data are incomplete and are perceived and interpreted differently by each individual. To the extent that the evidence is persuasive, it provides a degree of certainty sufficient to act on—ethical or moral certainty. From the nature of moral certainty, it is possible for individuals with opposing viewpoints to act ethically, in good conscience. Thus, those who, in conscience, object to military conscription and those who, in conscience, accept it are both acting ethically. For some, the weight of authority (e.g., religion or traditional teaching) will be decisive without further question; for others, a certain amount of rational analysis, supported by their professional experience, will be conclusive.

In any event, ethical certainty is, at best, relative since there are always many contingencies. Ethical certainty is equivalent to the medical certainty of a consulting physician who states, "In my best judgment . . . ," even though other physicians might reach a different conclusion from the same data. It is also comparable to the legal doctrine of "beyond a reasonable doubt," even though one jury will acquit and another convict someone on the basis of the same evidence (not a hypothetical situation). That ethical judgments vary should surprise no one. Ethical theory cannot require absolute certainty since, as noted, there are too many uncertainties and contingencies. At times we just cannot be absolutely certain which course of action is right. Relative certainty is adequate if we are to make value judgments in the face of conflicting evidence and values, and essential if we are to act conscientiously (ethically).

We may now consider the ethics of artificial insemination by a donor (AID), surrogate motherhood, and *in vitro* fertilization (IVF). What may now appear to be science fiction will surely become scientific fact. Human genetic manipulation and cloning are 2 examples of technology on the horizon. AID, surrogate motherhood, and IVF are actualities. They are not, by their existence, moral (or immoral), but because they are techniques that are now used, they are worthy of consideration. I believe that all 3 techniques share 1 pivotal question: Granted that reproductive technologies make parenthood possible, does such scientific intervention enhance or debase the meaning of parenthood, as we understand it? There are other related questions, of course, but they are reducible to this one. If the nature of parenthood is enhanced, the use of scientific knowhow is ethical; if, on the contrary, becoming a parent in this way somehow degrades those involved, scientific procreation is unethical. Hence, each person's understanding of the meaning of parenthood will be the basis of the value judgment concerning AID, surrogate motherhood, and IVF.

Does parenthood mean the physical capacity to procreate or does it mean the emotional capacity to nurture—to love and provide for the well-being of nascent human life? Does it mean both? If so, is each capacity a coequal consideration or does 1 enjoy a decisive priority in the making of a moral judgment about scientific intervention? From an ethical standpoint, must the begetting of new life be in the actual psychophysical context of an act of lovemaking with all the affective overtones which that humanly connotes? Stated otherwise, is becoming a parent ethical only within the framework of a stable union between a husband and wife whose child is their love personified?

Each of these technologies is separate and multidimensional, although all devolve on the concept of parenthood. We may proceed concisely in our ethicizing as follows: Consider the principal arguments for and against each, then reach an ethical judgment or practical resolution of the moral problems posed by the issue.

Artificial Insemination with Semen from a Donor (AID)

ANALYSIS. Some argue that procreation is moral only between a husband and wife who are able to impregnate and conceive in the natural way and to assume the responsibility entailed. Should either be sterile or otherwise incapacitated medically, that is unfortunate. But marriage is "for better or for worse" and their desire to have children can be satisfied only through adoption, if that is possible. If it is not, they must channel their creative desire in other legitimate directions. In other words, if the couple is unable to have children naturally, for whatever reason, they have no moral right to request outside intervention. In this way, their integrity as a married couple is maintained, their marital union is undefiled (preserved from adulterous intrusion), and the difficulties created by insemination of donor sperm (questionable genealogy, legitimacy, the possibility of incest) are avoided and the situation is better all around. This is the official teaching of both Roman Catholicism (2) and Orthodox Judaism (3). Respected Protestant authors are divided on the subject.

Roman Catholic teaching regards AID as immoral because it is depersonalizing. Even artificial insemination with the husband's semen is considered immoral. Sexual impotence and sterility following cancer therapy do not modify the Catholic proscription against artificial insemination with either a donor's or the husband's sperm because the integrity of the marriage is undermined. From this view, artificial insemination makes marriage "nothing more than a biological laboratory" whereas the marriage union by its very nature requires the personal activity of the spouses (4). By contrast, Jewish teaching permits the use of the husband's sperm for artificial insemination provided certain conditions are met (5). Rabbinic teaching, however, is not uniform regarding the method used to obtain the sperm (6).

What is the persuasive force of this prohibition of AID? Surely there is merit in portraying marriage as such an intensely personal union (and in religious terms, an exclusive covenant) that only within its confines is it moral to use one's lifegiving potential. But is this ideal situation a moral imperative? Just as ideally one might observe that marriage should be "till death," but divorce is a fact of life tolerated by both church and temple. Does this ideal situation place undue emphasis on the physical or material aspects of fertility?

Recalling our questions about parenthood, the husband is not the genetic or biologic father when AID is successful. Other than his genetic contribution, the donor is not involved and is hardly entitled to be called a parent in any meaningful sense. The ordinary understanding of parenthood looks to the ability to nurture and, for this reason, members of an adoptive couple are more truly parents than the biologic father and mother who do not assume the lifelong obligation of nurturing the child. On occasion, the court will place a child with foster parents (see Chapter 20). Further, in blended or reconstituted family situations (that is, remarriage by persons, each of whom has children by a prior marriage), the love provided by the stepparent fulfills the obligation of parenthood, even though the stepparent is not the genetic progenitor. There is a considerable difference between being able to sire a child and to care for a child—the difference is the nature of parenthood.

What then is the morality of AID from the standpoint of marital exclusiveness? Is the donor, whose fathering function is limited only to a seminal presence, to be regarded as an adulterous intruder? Is the wife an adulteress? Indeed, are all who cooperate somehow guilty?

Traditionally, adultery (meaning actual physical intercourse) has been prohibited for at least 2 reasons. First, paternity is uncertain; if a wife were to become pregnant by another man without her husband's knowledge (and clearly without his consent), it would be an injustice to her husband to expect him to assume the responsibility for a child not his own. Indeed, she herself could not be sure who impregnated her. Moreover, any other children fathered by the husband would thereby be deprived of a portion of their legitimate inheritance. Distasteful though it may seem to us today, this understanding of sexual exclusivity was linked with the idea of ownership; wives were considered property. From this concept of wife as property, there was a legal double standard regarding punishment of an adulterer and an adulteress. So sexual fidelity was intended to ensure legal justice. Secondly, adultery was regarded as a clear manifestation of a disordered desire for sexual pleasure that would jeopardize the marital bond.

Neither of these reasons applies in AID. Although the donor's identity is protected, the husband knows that he is not the biologic father and he and his wife are willing to accept this arrangement. He is willing to become a parent in the manner of an adoptive father. Nor does AID have anything to do with an inordinate desire for sexual pleasure. It has everything to do with enhancing the situation of a childless couple who can, thanks to modern reproductive intervention, become parents; one of them (the wife) bears a child that is biologically related. At times, AID is offered because of a high risk of passing on a detrimental genetic trait.

Because of other considerations, AID can be unethical in individual instances. In cultures where the ability to father children is a proof of masculinity, the psychologic damage done to a sterile husband and the subsequent adverse impact on the marriage would be a sufficient reason to prohibit AID. Serious instability in any marriage would be sufficient reason to dissuade a couple from having a child naturally. AID could be unethical on the basis of the process of donor selection and the use of 1 donor too frequently (thereby increasing the risk of incest). The process of donor selection invites the charge of selective breeding, but this can also be said of preconceptive genetic counseling or of choosing a mate on the basis of that person's "good breeding." The risk of incest in the next generation because 1 donor was used too frequently is of special concern in Jewish teaching (3). In a highly mobile society this risk is mathematically remote, and probably less than the risk of children in a blended family becoming sexually active with each other, a situation that does not seem to cause undue concern. But the anonymity involved in the use of donors can pose a formidable problem regarding the best interests of the child who, at present, is not entitled to learn of his genetic makeup, his paternal biologic roots. Adopted children, except in certain jurisdictions, are unable to find out anything about either birth parent and this need for identity is, reportedly, causing problems. But no one is arguing against adoption for that reason. In AID, then, much depends on the discretion of the physician in screening the possible donors (7).

EVALUATION. In the preceding discussion, the arguments favor the view that AID, properly circumscribed, is ethical when it is lifegiving, not only in the sense of being procreative, but also when it enhances the lives of those couples who cannot otherwise conceive their own child. The cogency of the arguments for and against AID, whether taken singly or collectively, will be perceived differently and some degree of ethical certainty (for or against AID) follows. However, an evaluation of the argumentation is subject not only to theoretical objections regarding the nature of parenthood (the unbreakable linkage between the biologic capacity to procreate and the psychologic ability and responsibility to nurture), but more, I think, to each physician's own experiential awareness of dealing with childless couples who can have a child only in this way. If an individual physician cannot, in conscience, cooperate in the AID procedure, he or she might at least refer such a couple to a physician who, in conscience, can assist the couple.

We have considered AID in the usual circumstances of a marriage, and the presumption has been that the couple is willing and able to care for a child. But other factors exist that have ethical ramifications. If some persons are understandably concerned about donor selection, it is also an understandable concern how recipients are selected for insemination. Should a single woman be inseminated? Or one just living with a man? What if she is single and on welfare? Or a lesbian? Perhaps a moral principle could be formulated to the effect that the less convinced the doctor is that the best interests of the (potential) child will be served, the greater is his or her obligation not to cooperate. This is the same view that is surely operative in dealing with a married couple. It is, of course, a subjective judgment and leaves the doctor open to the charge that he is practicing discrimination, that he is imposing his own values on someone else. Nonetheless, he is acting ethically; when such doubts persist he can hardly abdicate his own conviction simply to satisfy someone's desire to get pregnant—someone, it may be noted, who has the physical (if not moral or psychologic) option of arranging for natural insemination.

Surrogate Motherhood

ANALYSIS. Surrogate motherhood is an ethical issue related to AID. There are, however, several important differences. Although some consider it to be the female counterpart of AID since the surrogate is artificially inseminated with sperm from a donor (the husband of an infertile woman), the woman who is impregnated is obviously more involved than the anonymous sperm donor used for artificial insemination. In the situation of surrogate motherhood the sperm donor is not anonymous. The surrogate mother surrenders the child to the infertile couple, whereas the biologic mother conceiving by AID keeps her child. The payment involved reflects the degree of involvement—perhaps $75.00 for a sperm donor versus $10,000.00 for a surrogate mother. A woman with blocked oviducts or who is otherwise sterile and who receives a mature ovum from an anonymous donor is the true counterpart to AID. The comparison is complete when the woman conceives after coitus with her husband. Our concern at the moment, however, is surrogate motherhood as this is ordinarily understood.

The use of the terms *surrogate* or *host* or *stand-in* mother is revealing; she is the biological mother, but the *real* mother in human terms is the woman who accepts (adopts) the child as her own. To my understanding, again, parenthood is primarily psychologic, a matter of disposition or orientation to nurture; it is a matter of bonding, not blood. But what kind of a person would endure (or enjoy) a pregnancy and then, as a matter of contractual agreement, hand her baby over to someone else? That someone else, of course, is the child's biologic father who, along with his wife, is receiving the child into a loving environment. The idea of pregnancy for profit (or "womb rent") raises interesting legal questions but, from an ethical standpoint, the motivation of the surrogate mother does not make a given childless couple's desire to have a baby unethical. The motivation of a physician or lawyer who engages the services of a surrogate mother is also irrelevant in considering the morality of an infertile couple who are considering this procedure. In fact, some women volunteer their bodies as a service to others with no real thought that the baby will be theirs. It is easy to envision a situation in which a woman (perhaps even a twin) would want to do this for her sterile sister.

Motivation apart, the objection to surrogate motherhood is still a fundamental one—that procreation is separated from the physical expression of love (coitus) and from the nurturing during the pregnancy. Even leading theologians cannot agree on what God intends in this regard. Hence, one's understanding of the nature of parenthood is again pivotal in moralizing about scientific intervention. Perhaps it is the emotional aura that surrounds conception, pregnancy, and childbirth that genuinely specifies what becoming parents means. Coitus as a reproductive endeavor is not specifically human. People respond to the idea of "having a baby" from the perspective of starting or adding to a family and not with the view that the baby is a visible product of the union of ovum and sperm. Indeed, unplanned pregnancies usually do not evoke primordial feelings of parental fulfillment, even though parenthood is beginning because of a biologic (genetic) fusion.

Technically, the physician who artificially inseminates a surrogate mother is performing the same procedure as insemination of a woman with donor sperm when her husband is infertile. Many of the objections are the same—the psychologic state of a sterile spouse or one who is at genetic or medical risk, the subsequent impact of this procedure on the marriage, the selection of the surrogate parent, and others. These objections will be evaluated in different ways, as will the allegation of the intrinsic unity between lovemaking and procreation, and procreation and nurturing.

EVALUATION. Ethical issues that have differing moral evaluations should not prevent the creation of a uniform legal regulation. Until the existing legal ambiguity is eliminated, surrogate motherhood, I believe, is unethical. Ideally, the function of law is to enshrine societal values. Because of the rapidity of technologic advances, law will always lag. This is not to criticize lawyers or lawmakers, but, rather, to point out that technology influences our values and we have not yet had time to legislate this recent phenomenon. As a result, the child's status and that of the others involved are at risk until the rights and responsibilities of all parties are legislatively defined and enforced.

What if the surrogate mother wants to keep the baby? Could she be enjoined from doing so by reason of an overriding legal right of the biologic father who has contracted with her? Can she be successfully sued by the biologic father if she absconds with the baby? If she miscarries, is the payment to be prorated? If the father/husband and his wife divorce or separate, who will be awarded custody of the child? Are they both free to change their minds in that event? What if either becomes widowed? What if the child is less than perfect? Can a biologic father (and his wife if she is a coequal party to the contract) require or prevent an amniocentesis? What if abortion is morally repugnant to the surrogate? If the expectant mother contracts a serious disease or gets a job offer, can she invoke her constitutional right to privacy (to abort)? May she do so, despite an existing agreement? Who is responsible if the baby survives an abortion attempt? These are some of the questions that await legislative answers that define the will of society.

Because of these questions, the issue of surrogate motherhood must still be regarded as socially experimental and, in the absence of legal safeguards, unethical. The conscientious physician, if he or she is not to be regarded as a mere technician, must be satisfied that these safeguards are in effect before cooperating in the conception of a child in a surrogate mother situation.

In Vitro Fertilization (IVF)

ANALYSIS. When science fiction becomes fact, people understandably become excited. Since July 1978, when Louise Brown was born in England, *in vitro* fertilization has become another way to overcome infertility. Now that it can be done and has been done, the ethical question persists with all the more urgency: Should it (continue to) be done?

The procedure raises 2 highly debatable questions. First, since IVF is still considered by many to be experimental and since, as is obvious, informed consent cannot be obtained directly, is the proxy consent of the would-be parents acceptable? In my opinion, such a consent is acceptable because IVF parallels the natural situation regarding the beginning of life. That is, conception through natural sexual intercourse is accompanied by a certain amount of risk which science should help to reduce. The procedure itself is becoming less experimental. At the time that Louise Brown was making headlines, one physiologist at Michigan State University is reported to have observed that British scientists had not tried *in vitro* fertilization in nonhuman primates and stated that "the work by Steptoe and Edwards should do a lot to help those of us who experiment with monkeys" (8).

Second, what, if any, moral issues exist when a fertilized ovum is discarded? The answer to this question will devolve on one's view of the morality of abortion. Namely, is the discarding of an ovum fertilized *in vitro* the destruction of a human being? (If this life is not yet regarded as personal, the question of informed consent does not arise.) What I am suggesting, therefore, is that the controversy surrounding IVF is fully understandable since the question of when human life begins is insoluble. It can be argued, for example, that natural pregnancies often end in spontaneous abortions, but that is no reason to destroy life deliberately that is created (procreated) in a test tube. But it can also be argued that human life is not present until the activity of the heart or brain begins since human life ends when this activity ceases. The uncertainty of when humanhood begins versus the certainty of a couple producing a child by *in vitro* fertilization is the dilemma that is central to the ethical concern of discarding a fertilized ovum. In the United States, and probably elsewhere, ova fertilized *in vitro* are reportedly not discarded (see Chapter 13).

For many of the other concerns, the arguments are the same as in AID and surrogate motherhood. However, IVF does occasion more possibilities for, and hence more objections to, the prepackaging or prefabrication of babies. Some would draw the moral line at IVF only when it is the wife's ovum and the sperm is her husband's, and subsequent implantation is within the wife's uterus; others would accept donor sperm or donor ova. Other scenarios are not unimaginable: *in vitro* fertilization of donor ova by donor sperm and subsequent implantation in a different woman for ultimate delivery to another couple. The legal quagmire that this could create, akin to that encountered in surrogate motherhood, should certainly be addressed before going much beyond the usual husband-wife arrangement.

EVALUATION. It seems to me that *in vitro* fertilization is moral, granted that the couple is otherwise suited to become parents. To be imaginative for a moment, space colonization is on the horizon and it is reasonable to assume that ova fertilized *in vitro* could be frozen and stored aboard spacecraft for future population of space colonies. We may object, of course, but this is what will surely happen and, in time, it will be seen as morally acceptable. We or our children will live to see it! Back on earth, a more pressing concern is the priority that *in vitro* fertilization should be given in the face of competing advances in medicine that will benefit more people. The answer to this will help to place the morality of *in vitro* fertilization in perspective.

Conclusion

Speaking very humanly, who of us would tell Louise Brown or any other child of *in vitro* fertilization, any child born of a surrogate mother, or one whose father is an anonymous sperm donor that they should never have been brought into existence? This is, to be sure, an *ad hominem* argument and it may be, in the final analysis, that only an argument such as this will tip the scale in favor of a sufficient degree of moral certainty. I referred earlier (in the context of surrogate motherhood) to the "primordial feelings of parental fulfillment." Arguments *ad hominem* appeal to feelings that are deep within us. These feelings constitute what Peter Medawar refers to as "a certain natural sense of the fitness of things, a feeling that is shared by most kind and reasonable people even if we cannot define it in philosophically defensible or legally accountable terms" (9). The discipline of ethics both respects and probes these feelings in an ongoing effort to refine our appreciation of basic human values, the most basic of which is veneration for life, *the* value which confronts us dramatically in the area of scientific reproduction.

REFERENCES AND FOOTNOTES

1. Page IH. Ethical troubles; who's making the rules? Modern Medicine 1974;April 15:32–33.
2. Pope Pius XII. An address to the Fourth International Convention of Catholic Doctors, September 29, 1949. Catholic Mind 1950;48:252.
3. Rosner F. Test tube babies, host mothers and genetic engineering in Judaism. Tradition 1981;Summer:142.
4. Pope Pius XII. An address to the Italian Catholic Union of Midwives, October 29, 1951. Catholic Mind 1952;50:61.
5. Rosner F. Test tube babies, host mothers and genetic engineering in Judaism. Tradition 1981;Summer:142. "For example, there must be a reasonable period of waiting after the marriage vows or proof of infertility and, according to many authorities, the insemination may not be performed during a wife's period of ritual impurity." See also Jakobovits I. Judaism. In: Reich WT, ed. Encyclopedia of bioethics, Vol. 2. New York: The Free Press, 797 & 800.
6. Rosner F. ibid. "According to the rabbis, masturbation should be avoided, if possible. *Coitus interruptus*, retrieval of sperm from the vagina, or the use of a condom, are the preferred methods."
7. Nelson JB. Human medicine: ethical perspectives on new medical issues. Minneapolis: Augsburg Publishing House, 1973:62. Nelson cites an instance of medical-legal-ethical analysis that appeared in the Minneapolis Tribune on September 20, 1971. A man used a sperm bank as insurance against the possibility of his young son being sterile; in which case the father's semen

would be used to impregnate his future daughter-in-law "in order that the family blood line might be preserved." (This would make the son, in some jurisdictions, the "natural" father of his own half-brother! See, for example, Wisconsin Statutes, section 891.40.)

8. All about that baby. Newsweek 1978; August 7:70.
9. Medawar PB. The hope of progress: a scientist looks at problems in philosophy, literature, and science. Garden City, New York: Doubleday & Co., 1973:84.

ously unrecognized legal theories such as wrongful life and wrongful birth. ("Wrongful life" usually refers to an action brought by a child born with birth defects as a result of a physician's negligence. "Wrongful birth" usually refers to an action brought by the parents of an unwanted child or a child born with birth defects.) Additionally, courts
Legal Issues in Reproduction

Peggy A. Hardwick

In many respects, the law has failed to keep pace with the rapid advances being made in reproductive technology. New procedures for infertility treatment create legal issues that courts and legislatures have not addressed, and that existing law cannot address adequately. As a result, there is a great deal of uncertainty as to the physician's legal duties in treating an infertile couple and his or her potential liability for such treatment (1).

An increasing number of courts are allowing plaintiffs to recover damages for malpractice under previously unrecognized legal theories such as wrongful life and wrongful birth. ("Wrongful life" usually refers to an action brought by a child born with birth defects as a result of a physician's negligence. "Wrongful birth" usually refers to an action brought by the parents of an unwanted child or a child born with birth defects.) Additionally, courts have expanded existing theories, such as mental and emotional distress and outrage, to encompass actions arising from new reproductive technology (2). Finally, in some cases, the physician could be subject to criminal prosecution for performing a procedure or failing to comply with statutory provisions.

Because many types of infertility treatment are new or have only recently become widespread, there is little legal authority, either statutory or decisional, to guide the physician as to the legal standards required in the diagnosis and treatment of infertility. It is possible, however, to anticipate the issues likely to arise and the precautions the physician should take in order to avoid liability. Generally, the physician should be aware of the standard of care required in the performance of a particular procedure and the requirement of informed consent. The physician should also be aware of the potential problems associated with each treatment. Finally, the physician should be aware of any statutes in his or her state that will affect his or her civil or criminal liability.

In this chapter we will discuss the standard of care required of physicians, informed consent, and then relate these and other legal issues to artificial insemination, *in vitro* fertilization, and surrogate mother contracts.

Standard of Care

In order to prove that a physician performed a procedure negligently, a plaintiff must show that the physician failed to meet the legally required standard of care. There are 2 theories as to the standard of care required of the physician. The first is the "locality rule" or "community standard." The second is the "national standard."

The community standard holds that a physician must exercise the degree of care and skill ordinarily exercised by other reasonably prudent physicians in the community or in a similar locality. The policy behind this rule is to prevent small-town practitioners from being held to the same standards as practitioners in urban areas, with access to more modern information and facilities. Implicit in this rule is the assumption that some characteristics of a certain locality or type of community justify a lower standard of care than is required in a different type of locality. Recently, however, courts have challenged the validity of this assumption in view of modern communication networks, the increasing standardization of medical training, and increasing specialization in the medical profession. Consequently, many courts have adopted the national standard.

The national standard requires a physician to exercise that degree of care and skill ordinarily exercised by a reasonably competent practitioner in the same speciality who is acting under the same or similar circumstances. This rule requires a higher standard of care than the community standard. Even jurisdictions that have not adopted the national standard in all cases have adopted it in cases where a physician holds himself or herself out as a specialist or where the medical community itself has adopted a national standard for certain types of practice.

The community standard is the rule followed in a majority of jurisdictions. It is likely, however, that with the continued increase in the availability of information and technology and with increasing specialization in medicine, more jurisdictions will adopt the national standard in medical malpractice cases, particularly in cases where the physician holds herself to be a specialist. In determining which standard is applicable, physicians practicing infertility diagnosis and treatment should consider whether they specialize in that type of care, the type of information and technology available, and the extent to which national standards have been established within the medical community. In order to avoid liability, every physician should conform to the requirements of the national standard.

Some physicians practicing artificial insemination have consent forms that include an agreement not to hold the physician liable for any damages. Such provisions may not be enforceable if they are found to be unconscionable or against public policy. Even if such provisions are enforceable, they are only enforceable against the signing parties—parents may not waive an unborn child's right to sue for damages. Perhaps the safest way to avoid liability is to obtain a fully informed consent from the couple.

Informed Consent

Legally valid consent to a medical procedure requires that the consent be voluntarily given by a competent person and the consent be "informed." The consent may be either express or implied from the circumstances surrounding the procedure. If the patient does not authorize the procedure, or if the physician performs a procedure that differs substantially from the procedure authorized, the physician's conduct will be treated as a battery. If the patient consents to the procedure, but the consent is not "informed," the physician will be held liable under a theory of negligence (3). There should be few problems with the voluntariness of the consent or the competence of the patient in the context of infertility diagnosis and treatment because the physician will usually be dealing with adults who come to the physician actively seeking diagnosis and treatment. Most legal cases will deal with whether or not the patient's consent was "informed."

Informed consent is a doctrine defining the information about a medical procedure that a physician must disclose to the patient. There are 2 views regarding the applicable standard for determining whether a physician has disclosed sufficient information. The "professional standard" requires a physician to disclose what other reasonable members of the profession would disclose under similar circumstances. The "objective standard" provides that the physician must disclose all information that a reasonable person would deem "material" to the decision as to whether or not to undergo the procedure.

The professional standard is the one applied by many state courts. Some states have codified this standard. Those favoring the professional standard argue that a lay person is unable to understand adequately complex medical problems and that the physician should decide what information should be disclosed. Those favoring this standard also argue that it is the only standard that permits the physician to make a rational determination as to what disclosures are legally sufficient in any given case.

The objective standard focuses on the patient, rather than on the physician. Courts have adopted a "reasonable person" standard to determine what information is "material" to the patient's decision whether or not to undergo treatment. This standard holds that a physician has a duty to disclose any risk if a reasonable person would consider that risk material to the decision to proceed with the procedure.

Because of the divergence of standards for disclosure among state courts, the physician should determine what standard is applicable in his or her particular state. If the standard in the physician's jurisdiction is uncertain, the safest course would be to adopt the objective standard because it requires a wider range of disclosures than the professional standard. Under either standard, the physician must disclose her diagnosis of the patient's condition or problem, the nature and purpose of the proposed treatment, the probability of success, feasible treatment alternatives, and prognosis if the proposed treatment is not given. By obtaining a patient's informed consent and providing detailed information prior to undertaking any infertility treatment, the physician will not only protect himself or herself from liability on the basis that informed consent was not given, but also will lessen the probability that the patient will bring a suit alleging negligence at a later date.

Artificial Insemination

Legal isssues in artificial insemination are most likely to arise when the sperm is obtained from a donor (AID) or when the sperm is that of the social father (i.e., the husband of a woman artificially inseminated) mixed with that of a donor (AIM). For purposes of this discussion, AID and AIM will be discussed together under the term AID. The issues most likely to arise in AID cases are: (1) the standard of care required, (2) whether informed consent was given, (3) possible contract liability of the doctor or sperm bank providing sperm for the procedure, (4) rights and obligations of the biologic father/donor, social father, and the biologic mother, and (5) the rights of the AID child.

As of October 1979, 19 states have passed laws regulating the practice of artificial insemination (4). These statutes generally serve to establish the legitimacy of the child conceived by AID. Additionally, some of the statutes contain provisions relating to record keeping, screening procedures, husband's consent, and who may perform the procedure. Even in states where AID is regulated by statute, there have been few cases litigated that involve artificial insemination. The cases that have arisen have dealt primarily with the legitimacy of the child and the social father's obligation to support the child (5). Only 1 case has dealt with a physician's liability and informed consent (6). Because of the lack of uniform statutory regulation or litigation establishing a standard of care, the physician should be particularly careful in obtaining a fully informed consent.

MALPRACTICE LIABILITY. There are 3 probable bases upon which an AID recipient or child could bring a malpractice action against the physician. These are negligence in donor selection, failure to maintain adequate records, and lack of informed consent. Of states with statutes regulating AID, some have provisions dealing with these problems. In states with no laws regulating artificial insemination, no uniform standard appears to exist. A survey of physicans performing AID revealed a surprising variability in the screening and record-keeping procedures the physicians employed (7). Until uniform laws regulating AID have been established, the standard of care required will probably remain vague.

DONOR SELECTION. Some states with statutory regulation of AID prescribe the screening tests a physician must perform. The standard of care required in states without regulation is undefined. In determining what screening should be performed, the physician should know the objectives of screening procedures, the availability of the procedures, and whether or not the procedures are commonly used.

The primary objective in screening semen donors is to prevent transmission of infectious or genetic disease to the recipient of the semen or any resulting child. Additional concerns are compatibility of the donor and reciepient's blood group factors, and the possibility of accidental incest between AID children should the physician inseminate a large number of women in the same locality with sperm from a single donor (7). The magnitude of this risk has been estimated (Table 17-7).

Although there is no definitive standard of care required of the physician performing AID, the procedure is analogous to other medical practices. This analogy is helpful in determining what procedures the physician should perform. Recent court decisions have held that genetic counselors may be liable for genetic defects in children whose parents they have counseled. Parents have been allowed to recover for medical expenses and/or emotional pain and suffering.

The position of the physician performing AID is similar to that of the genetic counselor. In both cases, the prospective parents rely on the physician or counselor to detect the possibility of genetic defects before the child is conceived. The parents of the AID child may also rely on the physician to select a donor with physical characteristics closely matching those of the social father. By reason of the genetic counseling cases, the physician performing AID could be held liable if he or she failed to detect a genetic disease in the donor or selected a donor with the wrong physical characteristics.

The situation of the physician performing AID, however, differs from that of the genetic counselor in 3 important respects. First, the genetic counselor deals with 2 known individuals. Physicians performing AID with sperm obtained from a commercial sperm bank will be dealing with only 1 known individual, may or may not have access to the donor's medical records, and will probably have no control over the sperm bank's screening procedures.

Second, the genetic counselor deals with individuals who strongly desire a healthy child and who will have a strong incentive to give any information and submit to any tests required to reach that end. The physician performing AID will be dealing with 3 individuals—the couple and the sperm donor. While the couple desires a healthy child, the sperm donor may be indifferent to the (prospective) child's health. He may not have the time or the desire to answer detailed questions or submit to tests. Even if the donor will answer detailed questions, the physician cannot be sure the donor will recognize genetic disease in his family or that the donor will answer questions honestly. If the donor has a financial incentive to donate sperm, his answers to questions may be less reliable.

Third, the physician, unlike the genetic counselor, may not be trained to perform or interpret screening procedures. While the insemination procedure requires no specialized medical knowledge or technical skill, a general practitioner or even a certified gynecologist performing AID may have little knowledge or training in the increasingly sophisticated technology of human genetics.

The best policy for a physician performing AID is to obtain a fully informed consent from the prospective recipient and her husband.

Record Keeping. Some states have statutes prescribing what records a physician performing AID must keep, under what circumstances the physician may disclose the contents of the records, and to whom the physician may disclose the records. In states with no statutes governing AID, there apparently is a wide disparity in record-keeping procedures. Because of this disparity, it is difficult to define the standard of care required of a physician in keeping records.

The records a physician could reasonably be expected to maintain include records of the consent of the social father, the mother, the physician's statement containing information on the identity, medical background and examination of the donor, records of any tests and their results, date(s) on which the AID procedure was performed, and the names and addresses of the donor and recipient. A physician who obtains sperm from a sperm bank should try to ascertain what record-keeping procedures that sperm bank employs.

The physician who fails to maintain records could be held liable if the AID child later wished to learn something about his or her genetic background. The donor might also wish to inform the AID child of a medical condition that he discovers subsequent to donating sperm. Absence of adequate records precludes this possibility.

A physician could be liable to a donor if she discloses the identity of the donor who wishes to remain anonymous. Physician-patient confidentiality is prescribed by statute in some states. Moreover, the physician who discloses the identity of a donor who has signed a form guaranteeing his anonymity could be liable both for negligence in breaching physician-patient confidentiality and for breach of a contract.

The interests that the social father, recipient, and AID child may have in learning the identity of the biologic father must be carefully balanced against the biologic father's interest in remaining anonymous. In certain situations, such as disclosure of medical records and genetic history of the donor, where the donor's identity need not be disclosed, the interests in obtaining the information may outweigh the privacy interests of the donor. Such information could be provided to the recipient, social father, and AID child after all information identifying the donor has been deleted.

If information contained in records is insufficient, however, the more difficult issue of disclosure of the donor's identity arises. To obviate this, the physician could obtain current medical information about the donor and relay this information to the AID offspring or the parents without disclosing the donor's identity. Alternatively, a court could find that additional information is needed and could appoint a person to locate the donor, obtain the information, and convey the information to the interested parties. In either case, record keeping must be adequate.

Informed Consent. The information the physician must disclose concerning AID may vary because the possible risks of the procedure may depend upon the source of the sperm and the type of procedures used to screen donors. The physician should explain, in as simple terms as possible, the risks and consequences of the particular procedure he or she employs in performing AID. This information should include how donors are selected, what medical history is obtained from them, what tests the donors undergo, what tests (if any) the semen is subjected to, what additional tests could be performed to reduce risks, what risk each test reduces or eliminates, and what risks cannot be eliminated through screening procedures. The physician need not provide the potential recipient with a list of all known genetic diseases that cannot be identified through screening, nor the statistical probability that a donor is a carrier of each. General information on such diseases and whether the donor has them in his family background would be sufficient.

By informing the potential recipient of what tests have been performed and what tests could be performed, the physician will allow the potential recipient to make a decision as to whether to have additional screening done, or whether the decrease in the risks with additional screening are so slight as to be unimportant. In addition, the physician should also advise the potential recipient of any alternative infertility treatments. The recipient's consent to proceed with AID will then be informed.

Although physicians are not expected to know the law, they should also discuss with the potential recipient the difficulties in obtaining future medical information about the donor. This aspect of the discussion might include a description of the record-keeping procedures employed, his or her own policies about disclosing additional information about the donor, and any general legal policies effective in that state governing disclosure of the donor's identity. If the potential recipient is aware of these things prior to undergoing the procedure, she will be less likely to challenge them in the future.

In addition to obtaining the informed consent of the potential recipient and her husband, the physician might also wish to obtain the informed consent of the donor. Here, the information discussed would be legal, rather then medical, in nature. The physician might wish to inform the donor of the fact that he generally will not be able to assert any parental rights over any child conceived with his sperm, and of the possibility that he may be asked to provide additional medical information at a later time.

The physician should obtain consent in writing from both the donor and the recipient. The consent form should include specific information that the physician provided and an acknowledgement that the donor or recipient understands the information. Some states with statutes governing AID also require the consent of a married woman's husband. Even in jurisdictions that do not require it, it would be wise to obtain the husband's consent. The consent forms should be made a part of the physician's records.

FAMILY RIGHTS AND RELATIONSHIPS OF DONOR, RECIPIENT, SOCIAL FATHER, AND AID CHILDREN. Early cases arising from the AID procedure addressed whether AID constituted adultery and whether the AID child was legitimate (5). Some early decisions held that the procedure did constitute adultery and that the AID child was illegitimate, even when the social father had consented to the procedure (8). The trend in recent decisions, however, is to find that AID is not adultery and that the AID child is legitimate (9).

There have been no cases where a recipient has attempted to have the donor accept legal parental responsibilities for an AID child. In one case, however, an AID donor succeeded in securing rights to visit his biologic child (10). That case did not involve the usual anonymous donor/married recipient situation. Rather, it involved a single woman and man who performed the AID procedure themselves. In that case, the court allowed the biologic father visitation rights, and also imposed child-support obligations on him. It is possible that, under certain circumstances, a court would extend this reasoning to impose child-support obligations on a donor.

The problems of legitimacy and child support point to the necessity of having the donor, the recipient, and the recipient's husband sign written agreements outlining what rights they waive or accept.

CRIMINAL LIABILITY. Criminal liability for performance of AID could arise in 1 of 2 ways. In states with statutes governing AID, the statutes may impose criminal sanctions for violations or noncompliance with the statutes. Physicians in states with AID statutes should check the statutes to determine possible criminal sanctions.

There is also a question as to the name of the father the physician must record on the birth certificate of a child conceived by donor insemination. If the physician either performed the AID procedure or is aware that the child is born as a result of AID, he or she may be liable for fraud or falsification of public records if the social father is listed on the birth certificate. While there is no case law regarding this issue, the physician may wish to consult an attorney to determine whether criminal liability is possible.

In Vitro Fertilization

In vitro fertilization (IVF) presents unique legal questions that are difficult to analogize to any other area of the law. In part, these questions arise due to the uncertain legal status of a fertilized ovum. Legislation or a constitutional amendment declaring an embryo to be a "person" from the moment of conception would have a far-reaching impact on the legal obligations and liabilities of a physician performing *in vitro* fertilization. Even without such legislation or a constitutional amendment, a physician performing this procedure may be affected by state laws regarding fetal experimentation.

MALPRACTICE LIABILITY. As with procedures discussed previously, the standard of care required of a physician performing *in vitro* fertilization is impossible to define clearly. The standard of care for a woman undergoing *in vitro* fertilization involves not only the standard care the physician owes to the biologic parents, but also the care the physician owes to the fertilized ovum. Because the procedure is not yet in widespread use, the standard of care required of a physician in performing *in vitro* fertilization will evolve as the procedure becomes more common. In time, legislation and litigation will define what is required of the physician. Most civil litigation will probably focus on the physician's negligence in handling fertilized ova, negligence in failing to detect birth defects in implanted embryos, negligence in performing the laparoscopy and implantation procedures, and failure to obtain informed consent. Additionally, the physician could be held liable under a theory of strict liability.

Negligence in Handling Ova. One court has held that the biologic parents of a fertilized ovum could recover damages from a physician who destroyed the ovum, prior to implantation, without the parent's permission (11). That decision suggests that courts may be willing to hear cases alleging that a physician negligently damaged or destroyed a fertilized ovum.

That case may be distinguishable from usual negligence cases, however, because the physician involved acted intentionally, rather than negligently. The standard applied in determining whether the defendant physician was liable for intentional infliction of emotional distress was whether he "intentionally or recklessly conduct[ed] himself . . . in a manner so shocking and outrageous that it exceed[ed] all bounds of decency . . ." (11). This standard is drastically different from the negligence standard of "reasonable" conduct. Whether a parent of an IVF child could recover damages for negligent handling of a fertilized ovum is very much an open question.

Failure to Detect Birth Defects. Once the physician has successfully performed the IVF procedure, there is a question as to whether he or she has a continuing duty to determine whether or not the IVF child will be born with birth defects. Because of the experimental nature of the procedure, it could be compared to a case where a physician undertakes to give a patient a course of treatment, and then has a duty to the patient to monitor the treatment and the effects until the treatment is completed. If the physician performing IVF has such a duty, he or she should perform all necessary and feasible procedures to ensure the health of the unborn child.

Laparoscopy and Implantation. The laparoscopy procedure is not, in and of itself, experimental. The implantation procedure, while it is only used during IVF, is comparable to other minor surgical procedures. The standard of care required of the physician in performing these procedures would be the standard of care required in the performance of any similar surgical procedure.

Informed Consent. In order to reduce the possibility of having to defend a malpractice action, the physician performing IVF should obtain the patient's fully informed consent to the procedure. The physician should inform the patient of how the procedure is performed, any dangers associated with the laparoscopy and implantation procedures, any increased risks of birth defects, the usual risks of pregnancy, and any measures that will be taken to detect birth defects. Additionally, the physician should inform the patient of procedures for disposal of ova that are fertilized, but not implanted.

Strict Liability. It is possible that a physician could be held strictly liable to a severely defective IVF child. In a strict liability action, the defendant can be held liable for damages even if no moral wrongdoing or departure from a reasonable standard of care is alleged. Strict liability can be imposed when a defendant's actions are unusually dangerous, even when the defendant has taken all possible precautions to assure the actions are safe (12).

Arguably, IVF is an abnormally dangerous activity because of its experimental nature. "The imposition of strict liability would represent a policy judgement that if an experimenter is willing to subject the unborn child to an abnormally dangerous procedure, the experimenter should be willing to share the burden of support if the child is born with severe defects that are attributable to the technique" (12).

Criminal Liability. A physician's potential criminal liability for IVF procedures would be determined by the statutes in his or her particular state. Many states have enacted legislation prohibiting human fetal experimentation. How these statutes will affect the physician performing IVF will depend on the terms of the statute. Of most importance are the statutory definitions of "fetus" and "experimentation." A physician contemplating performing IVF should become acquainted with any state laws that may affect the legality of the procedure. While statutes governing fetal experimentation probably were not intended to cover IVF, some may apply to the IVF procedure by their terms.

In addition to state statutes governing fetal experimentation, proposed federal bills and constitutional amendments would, if passed, raise the possibility of both criminal and civil violations. The relevant provisions of these proposed statutes and amendments provide that a fetus is a "person" entitled to constitutional protections from the moment of conception. If a fertilized ovum is a person for constitutional purposes, a physician could be held liable for murder or federal civil rights violations if he or she destroyed fertilized ova. The extent of a physician's potential liablity under these proposed laws and amendments cannot be determined at this point. This issue would have to be determined by the language of the statutes and amendments, and by litigation in the courts. Currently, the only federal regulation governing *in vitro* fertilization is the requirement that federal funds may not be used for the procedure without prior approval from the Department of Health and Human Services (13).

FUTURE CONCERNS. Developing IVF technology will have a profound effect on family law. In the near future it may be possible to implant a fertilized ovum into the uterus of a woman unrelated to either biologic parent. Such a procedure would combine the legal issues of AID, IVF, and surrogate mother contracts. A full discussion of the issues raised by such a procedure is outside the scope of this chapter. It is most likely, however, that as IVF technology develops further, legislation will be passed to deal with the complex questions raised by new procedures.

Surrogate Mother Agreements

Most legal questions arising from surrogate mother agreements will not directly involve the physician. The major issues likely to arise when a woman contracts with a husband and wife to bear the husband's child will involve the legality and enforceability of any contractual agreements, the necessity for an adoption procedure, and the legitimacy of the child. If a physician is involved in the agreement, he or she may be liable for screening the surrogate for genetic defects, disease, and physiologic suitability. Additionally, there may be questions of legal liability for the physician's role as an intermediary.

MALPRACTICE LIABILITY. When a childless couple who desire to enter into a surrogate mother contract rely on a physician to select a suitable surrogate, the physician has a duty to screen the prospective surrogate for any genetic disease, exposure to any genetically damaging substances, or any infectious disease that may affect the health of the child. Additionally, the physician may be asked to select a surrogate with particular physical characteristics or intellectual capabilities. As in the context of AID, the standard of care required of a physician in screening a prospective surrogate has not yet been defined. The cases involving genetic counselors are analogous, however.

Informed Consent. Since the standard of care required of a physician in screening a prospective surrogate has not been established, he or she should be certain to obtain the fully informed consent of both the husband/donor and his wife, and the prospective surrogate. The nature of the information that must be disclosed would be similar to that given before performing AID. The physician should disclose to the husband/donor and his wife how a surrogate will be selected and what screening procedures will be employed. This could include an explanation of what genetic, infectious, or other diseases will be identified by the screening, what further tests could be performed to identify other risks, and what risks cannot be eliminated by testing. This information will allow the prospective parents to make an informed choice as to what risks they are willing to assume. Additionally, the physician may wish to advise the prospective parents that there may be legal difficulties involved in entering into a surrogate mother contract.

The physician should also obtain the fully informed consent of the surrogate prior to performing artificial insemination. Although the role of the surrogate mother is somewhat analogous to the role of the sperm donor, the surrogate undergoes the pregnancy, with all its inherent risks. The physician should advise the prospective surrogate of the risks of pregnancy and any special risks to her due to her particular physical characteristics. The physician should also advise the prospective surrogate of the potential for legal problems involved in contracts to bear a child.

Record Keeping and Confidentiality. There is no case law involving a physician's duty to keep records of surrogate mothers and parents of children born as a result of surrogate mother contracts; at this time there are no statutes governing such agreements. Since AID is an analogous proecedure, however, the statutes prescribing record-keeping procedures for AID may provide guidelines for what records a physician must keep in surrogate mother agreements.

A physician should maintain records of the contract itself, the identity, medical background, and physical examination of the surrogate and the husband/donor, what screening procedures were employed, dates on which artificial insemination was performed on the surrogate, the social mother's consent to the procedure, and any other information relevant to the procedure. The physician could be held liable if the child or his parents needed information on the surrogate's medical history and/or identity but he or she had failed to keep such records. As in the case of AID, the surrogate might also wish to provide additional information to the child with regard to medical information that she discovers after the birth of the child.

There is some question as to whether a surrogate mother contract could be entered into and still maintain the anonymity of the surrogate. If the surrogate wishes to remain anonymous, the question of whether such an agreement is legally enforceable will only arise if either the surrogate or the social parents breach the contract and the other party attempts to have the contract enforced. Apart from questions of the enforceability of such an agreement, the physician may be liable to the surrogate if he or she has agreed not to disclose the surrogate's identity and subsequently does so. The physician then could be liable both for breach of physician-patient confidentiality and for breach of contract.

When the surrogate wishes to remain anonymous and the child or his parents wish to discover her identity, the competing interests must be balanced. As with AID, the child's or parents' need for medical information from the surrogate may outweigh the surrogate's privacy interests. When the child or her parents wish to obtain information not contained in the physician's records, the invasion of the surrogate's privacy may be more serious. In such a case, however, the surrogate's identity does not necessarily have to be disclosed to the child and his parents. If a court finds that additional information is needed, it could appoint a third party to obtain that information, or the physician could contact the surrogate and obtain the information. The necessity for disclosure of the surrogate's identity and the need to obtain further information from her would be reduced by thorough screening of prospective surrogates, by adequate record keeping by the physician, and by obtaining the fully informed consent of both the prospective parents and the surrogate.

Legal Problems of Surrogate Mother Contracts. Several legal questions arise with surrogate mother contracts: Are the contracts illegal or against public policy? Can specific provisions of the contract be enforced? How are these provisions to be enforced? What is the legal status of a child born as a result of such a contract? and What is the liability of a person who acts as an intermediary in the contract? Some of these questions will arise whether or not the contract specifies compensation of the surrogate; others will arise only in the case of a contract for compensation. Because of the complex legal questions involved in a contract to bear a child, a physician acting as an intermediary and a couple seeking to enter into such a contract may wish to consult an attorney to determine whether such contracts are permitted under state law, and to draw a legally valid and enforceable contract. In the next section we will discuss the major legal issues the physician, the surrogate, and the couple should consider prior to entering into a surrogate mother agreement.

LEGALITY OF SUCH AGREEMENTS. Two problems arise in considering the legality of surrogate mother contracts. First, under some state statutes, the parties to such contracts could be subject to criminal prosecution. Second, even if the parties are not criminally prosecuted, the contracts are not enforceable if such contracts violate state statutory provisions because they call for the performance of an illegal act. There are 2 possible ways such contracts may violate state law: the artificial insemination of the surrogate mother with the husband's sperm may be considered adultery and, if the contract involves payment to the surrogate mother, it may violate criminal statutes prohibiting payment of a parent as an inducement to surrender a child for adoption.

The question of adultery does not present a major problem. Given the widespread acceptance of the practice of artificial insemination, it seems unlikely that any modern court would find that artificial insemination constitutes adultery. Additionally, adultery is no longer a criminal act in many jurisdictions.

A far more serious question involves the legality of agreements to compensate the surrogate mother. In some states it is a criminal offense to pay, or make an offer to pay, a parent to place her child for adoption. In states not having such statutes, such agreements may still be held to violate public policy. In either case, the contract would not be enforceable. In states with such statutes, entering into such a contract could make the parties liable to criminal prosecution.

Although statutes and court decisions involving payment for adoption were intended to curb black market adoptions, at least 1 court has taken the position that such statutes also prohibit surrogate mother contracts that compensate the surrogate. *Doe v. Kelley* involved a couple in which the wife was unable to bear children (14). The Does wished to enter into a surrogate mother contract. Prior to entering into the contract, they filed a complaint in circuit court seeking a declaratory judgment to have the Michigan statutes prohibiting compensation for placing a child for adoption declared unconstitutional and to prevent the state attorney general from prosecuting them for entering into the surrogate mother contract. The court held that the statutes in question were constitutional and that they applied to surrogate mother contracts. Depending upon state statutes and their interpretation, state law may preclude payment to a surrogate mother.

The surrogate mother situation may be distinguished from "black market" adoptions, however, and it is likely that courts will become more flexible in allowing these contracts as such arrangements become more commonplace and accepted. As distinctions between surrogate mother agreements and "black market" adoptions are made, the social evils of the latter will be absent in the former. A major concern of statutes against "black market" adoption is that poor parents or unwed mothers will be forced by financial necessity to give up their children. This does not apply to the surrogate mother situation because the biologic mother never intends to keep the child. The child does not even exist at the time the agreement is entered into.

A second, similar concern is that payment for consenting to adoption "tends to the destruction of one of the finest relations of human life" (15), the relationship between parents and children. The surrogate mother agreement does not constitute bartering away a parent-child relationship, however, because no such relationship exists at the time the contract is made, and, if the provisions of the contract are carried out, no such relationship will form between the surrogate and child. Instead, the contract will allow 2 people, who might otherwise be unable to do so, to benefit from the parent-child relationship.

A third distinction is that the surrogate is paid for her services rather than for the sale of a child. The services of a surrogate are similar to those a sperm donor who generally will be paid for donation of sperm. The child is not yet conceived at the time the contract is made; the surrogate agrees to provide her services in conceiving and bearing the child in return for compensation.

A final distinction is that the parents who will adopt the child are not complete strangers. The child will be adopted by his or her biologic father and his wife. This provides a link of natural affection between the parents and child and promotes the parent-child relationship.

Because of these differences between surrogate mother agreements and the typical "black market adoption" situation, it is likely that courts will become increasingly willing to recognize the legality and validity of such agreements. Even though such agreements may be considered legal, however, there still may be difficult problems involving enforcement of specific provisions of the agreement.

Enforcement of the Surrogate Mother Contract.

ENFORCEMENT AGAINST THE SURROGATE. The provisions that the husband/donor and his wife may seek to enforce against the surrogate will probably involve the agreement to bear the child, to limit her conduct during pregnancy, and to surrender the child for adoption. There are many difficulties in enforcing each of these agreements.

The central provision of the surrogate mother contract will be the agreement to conceive and bear a child. Depending upon the wishes of the husband/donor and his wife, the contract may also include an agreement to abort the child should the results of any prenatal test indicate that the fetus has a genetic defect. It is unlikely that a court would order enforcement of either provision, however, because of the United States Supreme Court decisions regarding abortion.

The Supreme Court has held that the decision whether or not to bear a child is a constitutionally protected liberty (16). Even if the contract states that the surrogate waives this interest, it is unlikely that a court would order her to bear a child or to abort against her wishes. The husband/donor and his wife might have other remedies available to them, however. They could seek return of any compensation or medical expenses already paid by them. Additionally, they could seek compensation for intentional infliction of emotional distress, although it is unlikely that they would prevail on this claim. If the surrogate breached an agreement to abort, they could discontinue payment of medical expenses and refuse to accept the child for adoption.

A surrogate mother contract will probably include a provision calling for the surrogate to restrict her conduct during pregnancy. This provision may also be difficult or impossible to enforce. It is unlikely that a court would order the surrogate to conform her conduct with the contract provisions. Monetary damages would be difficult to prove in many cases. The biologic father would presumably still want the child. The best course of action would probably be to withhold a portion of the monetary compensation.

The compensation might be placed in escrow and paid to the surrogate upon performance of certain contractual provisions. The duties of the surrogate might be divided and a specific amount paid for each. These solutions are not without difficulty, however, and the contracts would have to be carefully drawn to assure their enforceability.

The final responsibility of the surrogate is to surrender the child for adoption. This agreement would be almost impossible to enforce. The initial difficulty in enforcement would involve the legality of the contract as discussed above. If the contract is determined to be illegal or against public policy, it cannot be enforced. Even if it is held to be legal, courts may not be bound by it. The most likely contract remedy would be to rescind and seek to obtain the amount paid in compensation and medical expenses.

If the surrogate's agreement to surrender the child for adoption cannot be enforced through a contract action, it is still possible that the husband/donor and his wife may gain custody through an adoption proceeding brought by the biologic father. The success of such an action would depend largely on state family law and may be affected by some provisions in state legitimacy and artificial insemination statutes.

ENFORCEMENT AGAINST THE BIOLOGIC FATHER. The problem most likely to arise in enforcing the contract against the biologic father would involve enforcement of his agreement to adopt the child. This problem may arise if the child were born with a mental or physical defect. Courts have ordered enforcement of agreements to adopt children; however, those cases involved a situation where children had lived with the families for several years and the adoption agreements were enforced for purposes of inheritance (17). Whether or not a court would extend these decisions to order enforcement of a surrogate mother agreement remains an open question.

Even if the biologic father refused to adopt the child, he may still be liable for support of the child if his paternity could be established. The existence of the agreement itself would provide good evidence of paternity. However, the requirements for establishment of paternity vary, depending upon the jurisdiction. The surrogate mother agreement could include a provision providing for payment of child support and any other costs. If paternity is established, it is likely that the biologic father would be held liable for payment of child support.

STATUS OF THE CHILD. Initially, the status of the child born to a surrogate would depend upon the surrogate marital status. If she were unmarried, the child would be born out of wedlock and would be considered illegitimate. If the biologic father and his wife adopt the child, the child's legitimacy is of no practical legal significance because adopted children generally are treated as the legitimate children of their adoptive parents. If, on the other hand, the biologic father refuses to adopt the child or the surrogate refuses to surrender custody, the child will remain illegitimate. If paternity is established, the child's illegitimacy will generally not affect the biologic father's support obligations. The child's illegitimacy will, however, affect his right to inherit from his biologic father. The extent to which the child's right to inherit would be affected by illegitimacy would depend upon the laws in the jurisdiction.

LIABILITY OF THE INTERMEDIARY. A physician who acts as an intermediary in a surrogate mother agreement may incur legal liability. If the contract is made in a jurisdiction where surrogate mother agreements are held to violate criminal statutes, the physician may be prosecuted as a party to a criminal violation. Other, noncriminal liability would depend upon the terms of the contract and the applicable laws of the state in which the contract was performed.

In some jurisdictions, a physician acting as an intermediary may be deemed a "child placement agency" under state statutory provisions. If the intermediary falls under such state statutory provisions he or she will have to conform to licensing and other provisions contained in the statute.

Depending upon the terms of the contract, the intermediary physician may act as an escrow agent for payment of compensation to the surrogate. If so, the physician will be liable for failure to comply with the terms of the escrow agreement.

If the contract calls for the intermediary physician to assume certain duties, he or she may be liable for negligence in performing those duties, or for breach of contract for failure to perform those duties. The basis for liability would depend upon the terms of the agreement.

Conclusion

Reproductive technology is often fact before society can dictate its will in the form of statutes or court decisions. The keystone to sound medical practice is informed consent, the nature of which depends upon community or national standards of care, and often statutes and court decisions. The legality of many procedures intended to provide a child for the childless varies and the physician performing these would be wise to consult an attorney.

REFERENCES

1. For more detailed discussion of the legal issues discussed in this chapter see general comments in the following references. Artificial human reproduction: legal problems presented by the test tube baby, 28 Emory Law Journal 1045 (1979); Smith, Artificial insemination: disclosure issues, 11 Columbia Human Rights Law Review 87 (1979); Capron, Tort liability in genetic counseling, 79 Columbia Law Review 618 (1979); Black, Legal problems of surrogate motherhood, 16 New England Law Review 373 (1981); Note, Contracts to bear a child, 65 California Law Review 611 (1978); Comment, Surrogate Motherhood in California Legislative Proposals, 18 San Diego Law Review 341 (1981); Annas, Contracts to bear a child, 11 The Hasting Center Report 23 (April 1981); Comment, Surrogate mothers: the legal issues, 7 American Journal of Law and Medicine 323 (1981); Warren, The law of human reproduction: an overview, 3 The Journal of Legal Medicine 1 (1982); Smith, Artificial insemination redivivus: permatuations within a penumbra, 2 The Journal of Legal Medicine 113 (1981).
2. Intentional infliction of mental emotional distress and outrage involve intentional or reckless conduct that is against the accepted standards of conduct, that causes severe emotional distress.
3. In an action for battery the plaintiff need not present expert testimony with regard to the allegedly unauthorized treatment. The plaintiff need only show that the treatment was performed and that it was not authorized. In a negligence action the plaintiff usually must present expert testimony showing that the physician's treatment did not conform to the standards of the medical profession. Additionally, the plaintiff must show that she would not have undergone the procedure had she been fully informed. Some courts have held that a physician who does not fully inform a patient about a proposed treatment may be liable for battery. These courts have held that the physician's failure to fully inform the patient of all material risks negates the patient's consent.
4. Comment, Artificial human reproduction: legal problems presented by the test tube baby, 28 Emory Law Journal 1045, 1046 fn. 10 (1979).
5. Doornbos v. Doornbos, 23 U.S.L.W. 2308 (Superior Court, Cook County, Ill., December 13, 1954); Strand v. Strand, 190 Misc. 786, 78 N.Y.S. 2d 390 (Superior Court 1948); Gurskey v. Gursky, 39 Misc. 2d 1083, 242 N.Y.S. 2d 406 (Superior Court 1963); Anonymous v. Anony-

mous, 41 Misc. 2d 886, 243 N.Y.S. 2d 835 (Superior Court 1964); People v. Sorenson, 68 Cal 2d 280, 436 P.2d 495, 66 Cal. Rptr. 7 (1968).
6. Fitzgerald v. Ruekl, No. 11433 (Nevada 1981).
7. Curie-Cohen M, Luttrell MS, Shapiro S. Current practice of artificial insemination by donor in the United States. N Engl J Med 1979;300:585–590.
8. Doornbos v. Doornbos, 23 U.S.L.W. 2308 (Superior Court, Cook County, Ill., December 13, 1954).
9. People v. Sorenson. Artificial human reproduction: legal problems presented by the test tube baby, 28 Emory Law Journal 1045, 1046 fn. 10 (1979).
10. C.M. v. C.C., 152 N.J. Superior Court 160, 377 A2d 821 (1977).
11. Del Zio v. Vande Wiele, unreported.
12. Cohen. The "Brave New Baby" and the law: fashioning remedies for the victims of in vitro fertilization. Am J Law Med 1978;319.
13. 45 C.F.R. Section 46.204(d) (1979).
14. Reported in the 1980 Report on Human Reproduction and Law II-A-1.
15. Willey v. Lawton, 8 Ill. App. 2d 344, 132 N.E. 2d 34 (1956).
16. Roe v. Wade, 410 U.S. 113 (1973).
17. In re Shirk, 186 Kan 311, 350 P.2d (1960).

Index

Abortion. *See also* Miscarriage
  in ancient civilizations, 2
  clomiphene effect on rate of, 105–106, 107t, 289–290
  ectopic pregnancy and, 168
  from endometriosis, 256, 297
  from gonadotropin-induced cycles, 291, 292t
  habitual, 247–251
    from chronic disease, 249–250, 296
    diagnosis of, 247
    genetic causes of, 250
    from hypothyroidism, 249
    immunologic causes of, 250–251
    from incompetent cervix, 249–250
    from infections, 248
    probability of, 247–248
    from progesterone deficiency, 249
    reproductive performance after, 297–298
    therapy for, 247
    from toxins, 249
    from uterine anomalies and myomas, 250, 295, 296
  after *in vitro* fertilization, 297
  in laws of Hammurabi, 3
  rate of, in normal population, 289
  seminal factors affecting, 297
  tubal, 168, 294, 294t, 295
ACTH, 58–59, 59f
  deficiency of, 66–67
  hypersecretion of, 68–69, 68t, 69f
  in panhypopituitarism, 66, 66f
Acid phosphatase, 85, 87
Acidophils, pituitary, 52
Acromegaly, 51, 69, 70, 180
Acrosin, 164, 186
Acrosome of sperm, 163, 164, 186
Adenohypophysis
  blood supply of, 52, 53f
  cells of, 52
  function of, 51–52
  hormones of, 58–64
    synthesis and release of, 53
  hypothalamic hormones regulating, 33–35
  microanatomy of, 52–53
  origin of, 52
Adenomas
  ACTH-secreting, 68, 69
  growth hormone-secreting, 69, 70
  pituitary, 64, 65, 68

  pregnancy effect on, 293–294, 293t
  prolactin-secreting, 70, 71, 72, 72f, 73, 73f, 74, 74f, 75, 76
Adenosine monophosphate, cyclic
  in acrosome reaction, 186
  in hormone-receptor binding, 55, 55f
  in protein kinase stimulation, 55, 56f
Adenyl cyclase, 55, 61
Adoption of children, 17, 25
  current status of, 331–333
  history of, 329–331
  independent, 334–335
  process of, 333–334
  resources for, 335
Adrenal hyperplasia
  attenuated, 322–323, 323f
  congenital, 316–317
Adrenal insufficiency, 66
Adrenal tumors, 317, 323
Agamede, 4
Age of Enlightenment in history of fertility, 9–11, 10f
Agent Orange, 234, 238
Agonists, 54
Alcohol effects on reproduction, 235
Aldrin, 234
Alkaline phosphatase, 87
Allen, William, 14
5-Alpha reductase, 178–179, 181, 182, 324
17-Alpha-hydroxylase deficiency, 304, 308–309
Ambiguous genitalia. *See* Genital ambiguity
Amenorrhea
  of anorexia nervosa, 41
  athletic, 42, 310, 310t
  diagnosis of, in ancient civilizations, 2
  from growth hormone deficiency, 67
  with hyperprolactinemia, 71
  hypothalamic, 309–311, 310t
  from intrauterine adhesions of, 155
  of Kallmann syndrome, 38
  marijuana-induced, 42
  in panhypopituitarism, 65
  post-pill, 43–44
  primary, 303–324
    adrenal disorders, maternal, 317
    adrenal hyperplasia, attenuated, 322–323, 323f

    adrenal hyperplasia, congenital, 316–317
    adrenal tumors, 317, 323
    17-alpha-hydroxylase deficiency, 308–309
    5-alpha-reductase deficiency, 324
    androgen excess, acquired, 320–324, 324t
    androgen resistance, partial, 319
    androgenic drugs, 318t, 323
    anorchia, congenital, 312
    CNS-hypothalamic-pituitary failure, 314
    causes of, 306–324, 307t
    congenital genital ambiguity, 315–320, 315t, 320t
    Cushing's syndrome, 323
    delayed puberty, 311–312
    drug ingestion, maternal, 317, 318t
    estrous anovulation, chronic, 313
    evaluation of, 305–306, 306f
    general observations on, 303–305, 304t
    gonadal dysgenesis, 306–308, 307f, 308t, 320–321
    hermaphroditism, 319–320, 319f
    hyperthecosis, 322
    hypothalamic amenorrhea, 309–311, 310t
    incomplete puberty, 312–315, 315t
    Leydig cell agenesis, 312
    Müllerian agenesis, 144, 314
    ovarian disorders, maternal, 317
    ovarian failure, 313
    ovarian tumors, virilizing, 322
    pituitary disorders, 311, 311t
    polycystic ovarian disease, 321–322
    pregnancy, 312
    sexual infantilism, 306–312, 312t
    testicular feminization, 314–315, 314f
    testosterone synthesis, deficient, 318–319
    Turner's syndrome, 306–307, 307f, 308t
    vaginal abnormalities, 312–313
  from prolactinoma, 72
  therapy for, 102
  with weight loss, 42

Anaphylaxis from artificial insemination, 284
Ancient civilizations in history of fertility, 2–4, 3f
Androgen-binding protein, 177, 180
Androgens
    acquired excess of, 320–324
        adrenal hyperplasia, attenuated, 322–323, 323f
        adrenal tumors, 323
        5-alpha-reductase deficiency, 324
        amenorrhea from, 320–324, 324t
        from androgenic drugs, 323–324
        Cushing's syndrome, 323
        gonadal dysgenesis, 320–321
        hyperthecosis, 322
        polycystic ovarian disease, 321–322
        virilizing ovarian tumors, 322
    action of, in male reproductive system, 180, 181f
    aromatase effect on, 178
    of athletes, 42
    drugs with side effects of, 317, 318t, 323–324
    for endometriosis, 260–261
    estrogen synthesis from, 61
    in follicular atresia, 90
    insensitivity to, syndrome of, 145–146
    for oligospermia, 193–194
    during ovulation, 91
    resistance to, partial, 190, 192f, 319. *See also* insensitivity to
    in sexual infantilism, 303
    in spermatogenesis, 179
Androstenedione
    of athletes, 42
    estradiol from, 180
    of follicular fluid, 223
    glucocorticoid effect on, 114
    ovarian wedge resection effect on, 115
    synthesis of,
        adrenal cortical, 59
        ^{1}H in, 61
        testicular, 181
Aneuploidy of conceptus, 250
Anorchia, congenital, 312
Anorexia nervosa
    amenorrhea of, 41
    biochemical abnormalities in, 310, 310t
    catecholaminergic activity in CNS with, 41
    diagnosis of, 40, 40f, 41f
    epidemiology of, 40
    estrogen secretion with, 36, 41
    gonadotropin releasing hormone administration with, 36, 41
    signs and symptoms of, 310, 310t
    treatment of, 41–42
Anovulation
    in adolescence, 84
    causes of, 101–102, 102t
    at climacteric, 84
    endocrine evaluation of, 101–102
    with endometriosis, 256, 258
    estrous, chronic, 313
    menstrual cycle length with, 84
    pretreatment assessment of, 101–102
    therapy for, 102
        with bromocriptine, 112–114, 293–294, 293t
        with clomiphene, 102–106, 289–291, 291t
        with gonadotropins, 106–110, 291–293, 292t
    reproductive performance after, 289–294
Antagonists, hormone, 35, 54, 71
Antibiotics
    for cervical factor infertility, 134
    for oligospermia, 194
Antibodies
    antisperm, 129, 130, 136, 194
    in cervical immune response, 130–131
Antiestrogens, 193, 263
Antigens
    seminal plasma, 136
    sperm, 129, 136
Antiprogesterone, 263
Antisperm antibody, 129, 130, 136, 194
Appetite
    in anorexia nervosa, 40
    hypothalamic control of, 31
Aristotle, 4
Aromatase, 178
Artificial insemination
    for azoospermia and oligospermia therapy, 192
    complications of, 284, 284t
    confidentiality of donor in, 24
    counseling on, 277
    donor selection for, 281
    with donor semen, 279–280, 279t
        ethics of, 339–341
        fresh vs frozen, 283
        psychological aspects of, 23–25
        reasons for not starting or stopping, 277, 278t
        results of, 283
    ethical issues of, 284–285
    evaluation of couple for, 280–281
    history of, 12
    with husband's semen, 277–279, 278t, 283
    indications for, 277–280
    instruments for, 282f
    intrauterine, 136, 281
        complications of, 284
    legal issues of, 284–285, 347–350
    psychological aspects of, 23–25, 284–285
    results of, 283, 297
    statistics on, 23
    technique, 281–283
    timing of, 281–283
Asherman syndrome, 154, 155, 155f. *See also* Uterus, synechiae of
Asklepios, 4
Aspiration device for oocyte retrieval, 219, 220, 220f
Athens in history of fertility, 4–5
Azoospermia
    causes of, 188–190, 189f, 191f
    treatment of, 191–192

Basophils, pituitary, 52
Berengarius, 9
Berry, Martin, 12
Beta-lipotropin, 59, 59f
Bioassays, 61
Biopsy
    cervical, 124
    endometrial, 116, 157–158
    testicular, 205, 207
Birth control pills. *See also* Oral contraceptives
    amenorrhea and, 43–44
    hyperestrogenism from, 233
Birth defects
    from clomiphene, 105, 106t, 289, 290
    from diethylstilbestrol, 144
Birth rates in history of fertility, 11–12, 12t
Blood supply
    of adenohypophysis, 52, 53f
    of endometrium, 83
    of male reproductive system, 201, 201f
    of uterus, 83
Bromocriptine, 35, 41, 44
    administration, method of, 112–113
    for anovulation, 112–114, 293–294
    for growth hormone-secreting tumor, 70
    indications for, 102, 112
    for luteal phase dysfunction, 117
    pharmacology of, 112
    for pituitary adenoma therapy, 69
    pregnancy outcomes with, 113, 114
    for prolactinoma, 74, 76
    results of therapy with, 113, 293–294, 293t
    side effects of, 113, 113t
Brown-Sequard, 13

Calcium
    in acrosome reaction, 186
    cAMP dependence on, 55
Calmodulin, 55
Cancer. *See* Tumors
Candida albicans, 128, 134
Carbon monoxide, 235
Casein synthesis, 59
Cervical mucus
    alkaline pH of, 126
    antisperm antibodies in, 131, 296
    clomiphene effect on, 104–105
    composition and structure of, 124–125
    cyclical changes in, during menstrual cycle, 125
    drugs for improvement of quality of, 117
    function of, 125–127
        assessment of, *in vitro*, 133
    leukocytic infiltration of, 123, 128
    plicae palmatae or arbor vitae of, 123
    sperm penetration of, 131, 187–188, 296
        assessment of, *in vitro*, 133
        drugs improving, 134–136
        postcoital test of, 131–133
        problems in, treatment of, 133–137, 134f, 135f
Cervicitis, chronic, 123, 127
Cervix
    abnormalities of, 124
    anatomy of, 123–124
    biopsy of, 124
    cerclage of, 296
    congenitally absent, 124
    embryology of, 123–124
    erosion of, 123, 127
    function of, 125–127
    immune response of, 128–131
    incompetent, 249–250, 296
    infections of, 127–128
    at menarche, 124
    postcoital test and, 131–133
    surgery of, effects of, 124
Chalones, 86
Chlamydia trachomatis, 128, 134, 156, 171
Chlorotrianisene, 103, 103f
Cholesterol, 178, 179
Chorionic gonadotropin, human
    administration, method of, 107
    for azoospermia, 191
    for cervical factor infertility, 134
    complications with use of, 110
    corpus luteum affected by, 94
    for extracorporeal fertilization, 219
    monitoring treatment cycle with, 107
    for oligospermia, 194
    for ovulation induction, 107
    regimens for use of, 108

in spermatogenesis, 179
structural composition of, 61
thyroid hormone receptors and, 64
with varicocelectomy, 204
Christian Church in history of fertility, 6
Chromophobes, pituitary, 52
Cicero, 5
Cimetidine, 236
Circadian rhythms, 31
Clathrins, 55
Clomid. *See* Clomiphene citrate
Clomiphene citrate, 44
    administration, mode of, 103–104, 104f
    antiestrogenic effects of, 104–105
    complications with, 105–106, 106t, 107t
    estrogenic changes with, 104
    with gonadotropins, 110
    for *in vitro* fertilization, 117
    indications for, 102
    for luteal phase dysfunction, 117
    metabolic effects of, 104–105
    mode of action of, 103
    for oligospermia, 193
    pharmacology of, 103, 102f
    results of therapy with, 104, 105t, 105f, 289–291, 291t
Clotting factors, 85, 87
Coitus, 163
Coitus interruptus, 11
Complement, 130
Computed axial tomography
    for growth hormone deficiency diagnosis, 67
    of growth hormone-secreting tumor, 70
    in hypothalamic function testing, 44
    for hypothalamic tumor diagnosis, 43
    for pituitary adenoma diagnosis, 69
    in prolactin-secreting adenoma diagnosis, 72, 73, 74, 74f
Contraceptives, oral, 43–44, 233. *See also* Birth control pills
Corner, George, 14
Corpus luteum, 11, 94
Corticotropin-releasing hormone, 59
Cortisol
    for adrenal hyperplasia, 316, 322–323, 323f
    in anorexia nervosa, 41
    in Cushing's syndrome, 68
    in panhypopituitarism, 66
    synthesis of, adrenal cortical, 59, 309f
Cortisone acetate, 114
Cortrosyn stimulation test, 66, 77
Craniopharyngioma, 43, 44, 72

Cremasteric arteries, 201, 201f
Cryptorchidism, 202
Culpepper, Nicholas, 11
Cumulus oophorus, 163, 164, 186, 222
Cushing's disease or syndrome, 68, 68t, 323
Cyclic AMP. *See* Adenosine monophosphate, cyclic
Cyproheptadine, 69

Danazol therapy for endometriosis, 261–262, 265, 297
DDT, 234, 239
De Graaf, Regner, 10
DeMorsier syndrome, 38
Death rates in history of fertility, 11–12, 12t
Dehydroepiandrosterone sulfate, 59
Denonvilliers' fascia, 199
Desoxycorticosterone, 59
Dexamethasone, 114
Dexamethasone suppression test, 68–69, 77–78
Diabetes insipidus, 32, 44, 65
Dibromochloropropane (DBCP), 232, 253
Diethylstilbestrol, 103, 103f
    cervical abnormalities from, 124, 296
    fallopian tube abnormalities from, 170
    fetal defects from, 144
    uterine abnormalities from, 152–153, 153f, 232f
Digby, Kenelm, 11
Dihydrotestosterone
    function of, in male reproductive system, 177
    in genital ambiguity, 303
    with hirsutism and clitoral enlargement, 314
    receptors for, 180
    from testosterone, 179, 180
    in weight loss, 42
Dioxin, 232, 238
Doisy, Edward, 14
Donor insemination. *See* Artificial insemination, with donor semen
Dopamine, 32, 35
    antagonists of, 35, 71
    GnRH affected by, 177
    monoiodotyrosine effect on, 71
    in prolactin secretion, 35, 59, 70, 71
Douches, 136
Down's syndrome, 298
Doxycycline, 134, 194
Duncan, James Matthew, 13

Ectopic pregnancy, 168–170, 290, 292, 294
Egg. *See* Ovum

Egypt in history of fertility, 2
Ejaculation
  antegrade, 279
  retrograde, 192, 278–279, 279t
Ejaculatory duct, 199, 200, 200f, 205
Embryo
  development of, 164–165
  implantation of, in extracorporeal fertilization, 224
  transfer of, in extracorporeal fertilization, 224–226, 224f
  transport of, to uterus, 164
Embryology
  of cervix, 123–124
  of genital tract, 143–144
  of pituitary gland, 52
Empty sella syndrome, 72, 73
Encephalitis, viral, 43, 43f
Encephalocele, basal, 39–40
Endocervicitis, 128
Endometriosis
  barium enema in diagnosis of, 258
  bleeding from, abnormal, 257
  classification of, 259f, 260
  concomitant disease with, 258
  cytologic smears with, 259
  demography of, 255–256
  diagnosis of, 257–260
  etiology of, 255
  family history of, 257
  histogenesis of, 255
  history and physical examination for, 256–257
  incidence of, 255
  infertility from, 257
  laparoscopy for diagnosis of, 258
  medical therapy for, 260–263
  menopause and, 260
  pain with, 256
  pathophysiology of, 256
  pelvic ultrasound of, 258
  peritoneal lesions and, 259
  pregnancy and, 256, 260, 297
  sites of involvement of, 258
  social history of, 257
  surgical therapy for, 263–265
Endometritis, 155–156
Endometrium
  adhesions of, 154–155, 155f
  basal and functional layers of, 83
  biopsy of, 116, 157–158
  blood supply to, 83
  curettage of, 155
  description of, first, 11
  diseases of, causing infertility, 154–156
  estrogen stimulation of, 87
  in menstrual phase of menstrual cycle, 84–87, 86f, 87ff
  during ovulation, 91
  in proliferative phase of menstrual cycle, 87–91, 88f, 89f, 90f, 91f
  prostaglandin synthesis in, 85
  in secretory phase of menstrual cycle, 92–95, 93f, 95f
Endomitosis, 86
Endorphins, 177
Endosalpinx, 168–169
Environmental agents affecting reproduction, 231–245
  behavioral effects of, 236–237
  carbon monoxide, 235
  cimetidine, 236
  dibromochloropropane (DBCP), 235
  diethylstilbestrol, 231, 232f
  estrogens, 233, 233t
  exposure to, 237–238, 237f, 238f
  fate of, 239–240, 240f
  gossypol, 236
  halogenated polycyclic hydrocarbons, 234
  lead, 233–234
  polycyclic aromatic hydrocarbons, 234–235, 234f
  salicylazosulfapyridine, 235
  screening for, 242
  in spermatogenesis, 235–236, 235t
  spironolactone, 236
  toxicants, mechanism of action of, 240–241, 241t
Epididymal duct, 199
Epididymis
  anatomy of, 199, 200f
  obstruction of, 205, 209, 210f
  sperm storage in, 200
  in vasectomy, 208
  in vasoepididymostomy, 209, 210f, 211f
Epigenesis, 4, 10
Estinyl. See Ethinyl estradiol
Estradiol
  body fat effect on, 36
  endometrial prostaglandins and, 85
  in FSH and LH synthesis and release, 61, 62–63, 63f, 64
  GnRH affected by, 62–63, 63f
  in gonadotropin secretion, 34
  intranasal administration of, 238, 239f
  intravaginal administration of, 237, 238f
  oral ingestion of, 237, 237f
  during ovulation, 91
  in proliferative phase of menstrual cycle, 88
  receptors for, 58
  in secretory phase of menstrual cycle, 94
  testes production of, 179–180
Estradiol dehydrogenase, 94
Estriol
  obesity and, 36
  in endometrial stimulation, 87
Estrogens
  from androgens, 178
  catechol, 36
  cervical effects from, 124, 125, 133
  in follicular phase of ovary, 90
  in hMG therapy, 107, 108t, 109–110
  in proliferative phase of menstrual cycle, 88, 89, 90
  in sexual infantilism, 303
  in uterine leiomyomata etiology, 154
Estrogens, exogenous
  administration of, modes of, 237–238, 237f, 238f, 239f
  for cervical factor infertility, 133–134
  for cervical mucous improvement, 117
  for endometriosis, 261
  for loss of ovarian function, 26–27
  occupational exposure to, 233, 233t
  for ovulation induction, 115
Estrone, 94
Ethics of reproductive intervention, 337–343
  artificial insemination with donor semen, 339–341
  in vitro fertilization, 342–343
  surrogate motherhood, 341–342
  task of, 337–339
Ethinyl estradiol, 133–134
Eunuchoidism, 68
Eustachio, Bartolomeo, 9
Exercise and hypothalamic-pituitary function, 42

Factrel. See Gonadotropin-releasing hormone
Fallopian tubes
  abnormalities of, 165–172
  ampullary-isthmic junction of, 166–167, 166t
  description of, first, 10
  diethylstilbestrol effects on, 170
  in embryo development, 164–165
  in embryo transport, 164
  embryology of, 144
  in endometriosis, 264
  in fertilization, 163–164
  function of, 161–165
  length of, for fertility, 167–168, 167t
  mucus of, 164
  in ovum pickup, 163
  pelvic surgery affecting, 165–166
  pregnancy outcome after operations on, 294–295, 294t
  salpingitis affecting, 170–172
  in sperm capacitation, 163
  in sperm transport, 162–163
  in tubal sterilization, 166–168
  uterotubal junction of, 166t, 167

Fallopius, 10
Fat, body
    in initiation of puberty, 35
    in sex steroid metabolism, 36
Fertility, human
    history of, 1–15
        in Age of Enlightenment, 9–11, 10f
        in ancient riverine civilizations, 2–4, 3f
        in Athens and Rome, 4–6
        birth, death and population growth in, 11–12, 11t, 12t, 13f
        in Ice Age, 1–2, 1f
        in last 250 years, 12–15, 14f, 15f
        in Middle Ages, 6, 7f
        in Renaissance period in England, 6–9, 7f, 8f, 9f, 10f
    infertility. See Infertility
Fertility goddess, 2–3, 3f
Fertilization
    cervix in, 126
    extracorporeal, 215–224
        aspiration device for oocyte retrieval in, 219, 220, 220f
        cleavage following, 224, 224f
        embryo transfer after, 224–226, 225f
        follicular fluid with oocyte retrieval in, 222–223
        granulosa cells with oocyte retrieval in, 222–223, 222f
        historical review of, 215–216
        indications for, 216
        luteal phase after oocyte retrieval in, 227–228
        menstrual cycle and, 217–218, 218f
        oocyte retrieval for, 219–223, 220f, 221f
        oocytes at time of retrieval, 222–223, 222f, 223f
        ovulation induction in, 218–219
        patient selection and preparation for, 216–217
        pregnancies from, 226–227, 226t, 227t, 228–229
        preincubation of oocyte in, 223
        results of, 226–227, 226t, 227t
        sperm penetration for, 223
        in vitro fertilization for, 223–224
    process of, 163
    sperm transport for, 126–127, 162–163
    in vitro, 117
        ethics of, 342–343
        in extracorporeal fertilization, 223–224
        legal issues of, 350–352
Fertilization assay, zona-free hamster, *in vitro*, 187

Fimbria of fallopian tubes, ovum pickup, 163
Fluoxymesterone, 194
Follicle-stimulating hormone
    action of, 61, 61f, 62f
    alpha and beta subunits of, 61, 61f
    in androgen binding protein stimulation, 180
    in azoospermia, 188
    after birth and in childhood, 36
    in corpus luteum formation, 92
    deficiency of, 68
    in estrogen synthesis from androgens, 61
    of follicular fluid, 223
    in follicular phase of ovary, 90
    in gonadotropin secretion regulation, 181–182
    in granulosa cell growth, 61, 62f
    in hyperprolactinemia, 71
    inhibin effect on, 61–62, 61f, 62f, 63
    in Kallmann syndrome, 38
    in oligospermia, 190
    during ovulation, 91
    in primary amenorrhea, 305–306
    in puberty, 36
    in secretory phase of menstrual cycle, 94
    in spermatogenesis, 61, 61f, 179, 185
    structural composition of, 61
    synthesis and release of, 62–64, 62f, 63f, 64f
    synthetic, for ovulation induction, 106–107
    in testicular environment regulation, 178

G-protein, 55
Galactorrhea, 71
Galen, 6, 9
Gallius, 5
Gärtner's duct cysts, 143–144
Gardnerella vaginalis, 128, 134
Gendrin, Augustin, 5
Genetic factors
    in abortion, spontaneous, 250
    in 17-alpha-hydroxylase deficiency, 308, 309
    in anorchia, 312
    in artificial insemination with donor semen, 281
    with delayed puberty, 311
    in endometriosis, 257
    in female pseudohermaphroditism, 316
    in genital ambiguity, 315, 316f
    with gonadotropin therapy, 291
    with hypothalamic dysfunction causing amenorrhea, 309
    in Leydig cell agenesis, 312
    in pituitary dysfunction causing amenorrhea, 311

    in primary amenorrhea, 304–305
    in testicular feminization, 314
    in true hermaphroditism, 319–320, 319f
    in Turner's syndrome, 306, 307, 308
Genital ambiguity, 303, 304
    from adrenal disorders, maternal, 317
    from adrenal hyperplasia, congenital, 316–317
    from adrenal tumor, 317
    amenorrhea with, 315–320
    from androgen resistance, partial, 319
    from drug ingestion, maternal, 317, 318t
    from ovarian disorders, maternal, 317
    from testosterone synthesis, deficient, 318–319
    in true hermaphroditism, 319–320, 319f
Genital tract, female
    duplication of, 144
    embryology of, 143–144
Genital tract, male
    anatomy of, 199–201, 200f, 201f
    arterial supply to, 201, 201f
    embryology of, 143, 144
    nervous system of, 201, 201t
    tubular system of, 199–200, 200f
    venous drainage of, 201
Gestrinone, 263
Gigantism, 69
Glucocorticoids
    administration of, method of, 114–115
    complications with, 115
    for oligospermia, 194
    for ovulation induction, 114
    pharmacology of, 114
    results of therapy with, 115
Gonadal dysgenesis. See also Turner's syndrome
    acquired androgen excess and, 320–321
    mixed, 308
    pure, 307–308
    sexual infantilism and, 306–308, 307f, 308t
Gonadal tumor, dysontogenetic, 304–305
Gonadoblastoma, 321f
Gonadorelin. See Gonadotropin-releasing hormone
Gonadotropin-releasing hormone, 31, 33
    administration of, method of, 111
    for azoospermia, 191
    in FSH and LH synthesis and release, 62–64, 62f, 63f, 64f
    in hyperprolactinemia, 71

Gonadotropin-releasing hormone (*cont.*)
  in hypothalamic function testing, 44
  in Kallmann syndrome, 39
  marijuana effects on, 42
  membrane receptors for, 56
  neurotransmitter effect on, 177
  opioid effect on, 71
  during ovulation, 91
  for ovulation induction, 110
  pharmacology of, 110–111
  in puberty, 36, 38f
  pulse frequency of hypothalamic release of, 177–178
  results of therapy with, 111–112
  side effects and complications with therapeutic use of, 112
  in testicular environment regulation, 177–178, 178f
Gonadotropins
  in anorexia nervosa, 41
  in panhypopituitarism, 65
  pituitary secretion of, 33
  during puberty, 36–37
  testicular regulation of secretion of, 181–182
  with weight loss, 42
Gonadotropins, exogenous. *See also* Chorionic gonadotropin; Menopausal gonadotropin
  administration of, 107
  for cervical factor infertility, 134
  with clomiphene, 110
  complications with therapeutic use of, 109–110
  indications for therapeutic use of, 106
  monitoring of treatment cycle with, 107–108, 108t
  for oligospermia, 194
  pharmacology of, 106–107
  pituitary vs urinary, 106
  regimens for use of, 108
  results of therapy with, 108–109, 109t, 291–293, 292t
Gonorrhea
  cervical infection and, 128
  prevalence of, in nineteenth century, 13
  salpingitis from, 13, 171–172
  treatment of, in ancient civilizations, 2
Gossypol, 236
Graafian follicle, 91–92
Granulocytes, menstrual, 95
Granulosa cells
  in extracorporeal fertilization, 222–223, 222f
  FSH stimulation of, 61, 62f
  luteinization of, 92
  during ovulation, 91
    during proliferative phase of menstrual cycle, 91
Greek customs regarding fertility, ancient, 4
Growth hormone
  deficiency of, 67–68, 67f
  function of, 59, 60
  hypersecretion of, 69–70
  isolation of, 51
  secretion of, factors affecting, 60–61, 60t
Growth hormone releasing factor, 35, 60–61
Guaifenesin, 134
Guanosine 5′-triphosphate, 55
Gynecomastia, 235–236

Hamartomas, 43
Hammurabi, 3
Hand-Schüller-Christian disease, 44, 65
Hartsoeker, Niklaas, 10, 10f
Harvey, William, 9–10
Hellman, Louis M., 14
Heptachlor, 234
Hermaphroditism, 319–320, 319f
Hertwig, Oscar, 12
Hesiod, 5
Hexachlorophene, 234
Hirsutism, 304
Hormones. *See also specific hormone*
  hypothalamic, 32–35
  pituitary, 58–64
    cytoplasmic receptors for, 56–58, 58f
    membrane receptors for, 54–56, 54f, 55f, 56f, 57f
    receptor theory of, 53–54
Hühner, Max, 14
Human chorionic gonadotropin. *See* Chorionic gonadotropin, human
Human menopausal gonadotropin. *See* Menopausal gonadotropin, human
Human placental lactogen, 59
Hunter, William, 12
Hyaluronidase, 164, 186
Hydatidiform mole, 64
Hydrocarbons, halogenated polycyclic, 234
Hydrocarbons, polycyclic aromatic, 234–235, 234f
Hydrosalpinx, 171, 172
2-Hydroxyestradiol, 36
17-Hydroxyprogesterone
  during ovulation, 91
  synthesis of, adrenal cortical, 59, 309f
Hymen, imperforate, 312, 313
Hyperestrogenisms, 233, 233t
Hyperprolactinemia, 70, 70f, 71, 72, 112, 256
Hyperreactio luteinalis, 317
Hyperthecosis, 322
Hypocycloidal polyomography, 72–73, 73f, 74
Hypogonadism, hypogonadotropic, 38, 39, 68, 191–192
Hypospadias, 186
Hypothalamus
  anatomy of, 31, 32f
  development of, 33
  disorders in functioning of, 37–44
    amenorrhea with weight loss, 42
    amenorrhea, athletic, 42
    amenorrhea, marijuana-induced, 42
    amenorrhea, post-pill, 43–44
    amenorrhea, primary, 309–311, 310t
    anorexia nervosa, 40–42, 40f, 41f, 310, 310tt
    in chronic renal failure, 44
    congenital, 38–40
    functional, 40–44
    from neoplasms and inflammatory infiltrates, 44
    precocious puberty, 42–43, 43f
    symptoms of, 37
  function of, 31
  function testing of, 44–45
  in gonadotropin secretion during puberty, 36–37
  historical overview of, 31
  hormones of, 32–35
    dopamine, 35
    gonadotropin releasing hormone, 33–34
    growth hormone releasing factor, 34–35
    oxytocin, 32–33
    posterior pituitary, 32–33
    regulating anterior pituitary function, 33–34
    somatostatin releasing factor, 34–35
    thyrotropin releasing hormone, 33
    vasopressin, 32
  in initiation of puberty, 35–36
  neurons innervating, 31
  physiology of, 35–37
  pituitary relationship to, 31, 32f
  in testicular function regulation, 177, 178f
Hypothyroidism
  abortion from, 249
  of anorexia nervosa, 41
  hyperprolactinemia from, 70
  hypothalamic, 33
  in panhypopituitarism, 65, 66
Hysterectomy
  for endometriosis, 265
  psychological aspects of, 26–27

Hysterosalpingography, 157, 157f
Hysteroscopy, 157–158, 157f

Ice Age in history of fertility, 1–2, 1f
IgA, 130, 131
IgG, 130, 131, 136
IgM, 130, 131
Immune response
 of cervix, 128–131
 systemic vs local, 130, 130f
Immunologic causes of abortion, 250–251
Impotency, sexual, 186
India in history of fertility, 4
Infertility
 denial of, 19
 donor insemination as solution to, 23–25
 emotional support and education in treatment of, 27–28
 environmental factors in, 231–243
  behavioral effects, 236–237
  circumstances of exposure to, 237–238, 237f, 238f
  estrogens, 233, 233t
  fate of, 239–240, 240f
  halogenated polycyclic hydrocarbons, 234
  lead, 233–234
  polycyclic aromatic hydrocarbons, 234–253, 234f
  screening for, 242
  toxicants, mechanism of action of, 240–241, 241t
 feelings of couple faced with, 19–20
 grief with, 20–21
 guilt feelings from, 20
 health professional's role in treatment of, 27–28
 isolation between members of couple due to, 19–20
 as life crisis, 18–19
 management plan for, 27
 "normal," 23
 prediction of, in ancient civilizations, 2
 psychology of, 17–29
 secondary, 25
 statistics on, 17
Infertility, female
 antibody-mediated, 129, 136, 296
 cervical factor, 133–137
 from diethylstilbestrol, 170
 from ectopic pregnancy, 168–170
 from endometrial diseases, 154–156
 with endometriosis, 257
 from endometritis, 155–156
 extracorporeal fertilization for, 216
 from fallopian tube abnormalities, 165–172
 from hysterectomy and premature ovarian failure, 25–27
 from intrauterine adhesions, 154–155
 from miscarriage, 21–22
 from pelvic surgery, 165–166
 from salpingitis, 170–171
 from stillbirth, 22–23
 from tubal sterilization procedures, 166–168
 from uterine abnormalities, 147
  acquired, 152–154
  congenital, 147–151
 from uterotubal junction occlusion, 156
 from vaginal agenesis, 143–147
Infertility, male
 androgen therapy for, 193–194
 antibacterial agents for, 194
 antibody-mediated, 194
 antiestrogens in treatment of, 193
 from azoospermia, 188–190, 189f, 191f
  treatment of, 191–192
 diagnosis of, 189f, 191f, 192f
  cervical mucus penetration test for, in vitro, 187–188
  hamster egg fertilization assay for, in vitro, 187
  history and physical examination for, 186
  hormonal tests for, 188
  laboratory tests for, 186–188
  semen analysis in, 186–187
 environmental factors in, 235–236
 extracorporeal fertilization for, 216
 glucocorticoids for, 194
 gonadotropin therapy for, 194
 medical management of, 191–194
 from oligospermia, 189f, 190, 191f, 192f
  treatment of, 192–194
 statistics on, 199
 surgical management of, 199–213
  for ductal obstruction, 205
  preventive, 201–203
  retroperitoneal, and sympathectomy, 203
  spermatocele creation, 211–212, 211f, 212f
  for varicocele, 203–205
  vasectomy reversal, 208–209, 208f, 209f
  vasoepididymostomy, 209–211, 210f, 211f
  vasography, 205, 207f
Informed consent, 346–374
 for artificial insemination, 349
 for in vitro fertilization, 351
 in surrogate motherhood agreements, 352
Inhibin, 61f, 62, 62f, 63, 63f
 in gonadotropin secretion regulation, 182
 Sertoli cell source of, 177
Insemination, artificial. See Artificial insemination
Insulin tolerance test, 73, 74, 77
Intrauterine device
 ectopic pregnancy from, 168
 for intrauterine adhesions therapy, 155
In vitro fertilization. See Fertilization, in vitro
Islamic society in history of fertility, 6

Jabir, 6
Johnstone, Arthur, 13–14

Kallmann syndrome, 34, 36
 characteristics of, 37–38, 39f
 diagnosis of, 39, 68
 management of, 39
Knaus, H., 14
Knobil, E., 31, 33

Lactation, 59, 60
Lactogen, human placental, 59
Laparoscopy
 for endometriosis diagnosis, 258
 for extracorporeal fertilization, 216, 217, 219–221
Laparotomy, 263
Laurence-Moon-Biedl syndrome, 39
Lead, 233–234
Leeuwenhoek, 10
Legal issues in reproduction, 345–355
 artificial insemination, 347–350
 in vitro fertilization, 350–352
 informed consent, 346–347
 standard of care, 345–346
 surrogate motherhood agreements, 352–356
Leiomyomata, uterine, 154, 250, 258, 295
Leydig cells, 61, 144
 agenesis of, 312
 in azoospermia, 188
 estradiol regulation of function of, 180
 interaction of, with Sertoli cells, 181
 location of, 177
 luteinizing hormone binding to, 178
 testosterone from, 177, 179–180
 with torsion of testes, 203
Light effects on GnRH secretion, 34
Limbic system, 31

Luteinizing hormone
  action of, 61, 61f
  alpha and beta subunits of, 61, 61f
  in artificial insemination timing, 281, 282
  in azoospermia, 188
  after birth and in childhood, 36
  in corpus luteum formation, 92
  deficiency of, 68
  extracorporeal fertilization and, 217, 218f
  of follicular fluid, 223
  in follicular phase of ovary, 90
  gonadotropin releasing hormone effect on, 33–34
  in gonadotropin secretion regulation, 181–182
  in hyperprolactinemia, 71
  in Kallmann syndrome, 38
  in oligospermia, 190
  ontogeny of circadian secretory pattern of, 36, 37f
  during ovulation, 91
  in primary amenorrhea, 305–306
  in puberty, 36
  in secretory phase of menstrual cycle, 94
  structural composition of, 61
  synthesis and release of, 62–64, 62f, 63f, 64f
  synthetic, for ovulation induction, 106–107
  in testicular environment regulation, 178
Luteomas, 317

Maimonides, 6
Malpas, Percy, 247
Malpighi, 11
Malpractice liability
  with artificial insemination, 347
  with *in vitro* fertilization, 350–352
  with surrogate motherhood agreements, 352–355
Malthus, T.R., 12
Mammillary bodies, 31
Marijuana-induced amenorrhea, 42
McCune-Albright syndrome, 43
McIndoe vaginoplasty, 146
Median eminence of hypothalamus, 31
Medroxyprogesterone acetate, 261
Melatonin, 177
Menarche, 83, 124, 303
Menopausal gonadotropin, human. *See also* Gonadotropins, exogenous
  administration of, method of, 107
  for azoospermia, 191
  for cervical mucus quality improvement, 117
  with clomiphene, 110
  complications with use of, 109–110
  for fertilization, extracorporeal, 219
  for fertilization, *in vitro*, 117
Menopausal gonadotropin
  for luteal phase dysfunction, 117
  monitoring treatments cycle with, 107–108, 108t
  for oligospermia, 194
  pharmacology of, 106–107
  regimens for use of, 108
  results of therapy with, 108–109, 109t
Menopause, 260
Menses. *See.* Menstrual cycle
  premature, 313
Menstrual cycle, 83–99
  blood loss with, 84
  cervical mucous changes during, 125
  clinical characteristics of, 83–84
  duration of, 84
  effluvium from, 84–85
  extracorporeal fertilization and, 217–218, 218f
  hematologic disorders affecting, 87
  menstrual phase of, 84–87, 86f, 87f
  onset of, 83
  ovulation, 91–92
  proliferative phase of, 87–91, 88f, 89f, 90f, 91f
  secretory phase of, 92–95, 93f, 95f
  symptoms of, 84
Menstrual granulocytes, 95
Menstruation
  anemia with, 84
  concept of, in ancient Athens and Rome, 4, 5
  retrograde, 312
  spiral arteries in, 85
Mesonephric duct, 143, 144
Mesonephros, 143, 144
Mesopotamia in history of fertility, 2–4, 3f
Mesterolone, 194
Methyltestosterone, 194
Metrial cells, 95
Metroplasty, 147, 148–151, 150f, 151f
Miscarriage. *See also* Abortion
  hospital admission for, 22
  in laws of Hammurabi, 3
  psychological effect of, 21–22
  statistics on, 21
Monoiodotyrosine, 71, 71f
Morgagni, hydatids of, 143
Morris, R.T., 13
Mortality rates in history of fertility, 11–12, 12t

Mucus
  cervical. *See* Cervical mucus
  fallopian tube, 164
Müllerian duct inhibiting factor, 144, 177
Müllerian ducts, 144, 145f
  agenesis of, 144–147, 146f, 304, 314
  anomalies of, affecting uterus, 147–148
Mycoplasma, 128, 134
Myomectomy, 154
Myometrium
  blood supply to, 83
  implantation in, 94
Myxedema, 65. *See also* Hypothyroidism

Neisser, Albert, 13
Neisseria gonorrhoeae, 171
Neoplasms. *See* Tumors
Neurofibromatosis, 43
Neurohypophysis, 32–33
Neurophysin, 32
Noeggerath, Jacob Bruno, 13
Nystatin, 134

Obesity
  estriol excretion with, 36
  hypogonadotropic hypogonadism and, 39
  TEBG levels with, 180
Ogino, K., 14
Olfaction in GnRH function, 34
Oligospermia
  artificial insemination for, 277, 278t
  causes of, 189f, 190, 191f, 192f
  treatment of, 192–194
Opioids, 71
Optic chiasm, 31
Oral contraceptives, 43–44, 233. *See also* Birth control pills
Orchiectomy, 203
Orchiopexy, 202, 203
Osmoregulation
  hypothalamic control of, 31
  with weight loss, 42
Ovarian arteries, 83
Ovaries
  amenorrhea from disorders of, 317
  amenorrhea from premature failure of, 313
  clomiphene effect on, 105
  endocrine function of, discovery of, 13
  in endometriosis, 257, 258, 264
  FSH and LH action in, 61, 61f, 62f
  fetal, 144
  follicular phase of, 90
  granulosa cells of, 61, 62f, 91

hilar cells of, 61, 62f
in hyperreactio luteinalis, 317
luteal phase of, 94, 117
with luteomas, 317
during ovulation, 91–92
during proliferative phase of menstrual cycle, 90–91
psychological effect of loss of function of, 26–27
theca cells of, 61, 62f, 90–91
virilizing tumors of, 322
wedge resection of, 115–116
Ovulation
 basal temperature with, 14, 84
 hypothalamic function during, 91
 induction of, drugs in, 102–115
  bromocriptine, 112–114, 293–294, 293t
  clomiphene citrate, 102–106, 289–291, 291t
  clomiphene-gonadotropin combinations, 110
  estrogen and estrogen/progesterone, 115
  glucocorticoids, 114–115
  gonadotropin releasing hormone, 110–112
  gonadotropins, human, 106–110, 291–293, 292t
 induction of, for extracorporeal fertilization, 218–219
 induction of, ovarian wedge resection for, 115–116
 induction of, patient selection for, 112
 induction of, problems in, 116–117
 ovaries in, 91–92
 pituitary function during, 91–92
 timing of, discovery of, 14
Ovum
 clomiphene effect on, 290
 description of, first, 12
 in extracorporeal fertilization, evaluation of, 222–223, 222f, 223f
  preincubation of, 223
  retrieval of, 219–221, 221f
 in fertilization, 163–164
 life span of, fertilizable, 164
 transfer of, from ovary to oviduct, 163
 vitelline membrane of, 164
 zona pellucida of, 163, 164, 186
Oxytocin, 32, 33

Pampiniform plexus, 201, 203
Panhypopituitarism, 64, 65–66, 65f, 66f
Paramesonephric ducts, 144
Parlodel. *See* Bromocriptine
Parovarian cysts, 143
Pars intermedius, 52

Pelvic inflammatory disease
 ectopic pregnancy and, 168
 etiology of, 171
Pergolide, 76
Pergonal. *See* Menopausal gonadotropin, human
Pesticides, 239, 240
Phenothiazines, 35, 71
Pheromones, 34
Phocomelia, 231
Pituitary gland
 in ACTH deficiency, 66–67
 in ACTH hypersecretion, 68–69, 68t, 69f
 ACTH of, 58–59, 59f
 adenomas of, 64, 65, 68
  ACTH-secreting, 68, 69
  growth hormone-secreting, 69, 70
  prolactin-secreting, 70, 71, 72, 72f, 73, 73f, 74, 74f, 75, 76
 amenorrhea from disorders of, 311, 311t
 anatomy of, 32f, 52–53, 53f
 anterior. *See* Adenohypophysis
 cells of, 52, 54
 deficiency states of, 65–68
 embryology of, 52
 in FSH and LH deficiency, 68
 FSH and LH of, 61–64, 61f, 62f, 63f, 64f
 function testing of, 73–74, 75f
 in growth hormone deficiency, 67–68, 67f
 in growth hormone hypersecretion, 69–70
 growth hormone of, 60–61, 60t
 historical overview of, 51
 hormones regulating function of, 53–54
 hypersecretion states of, 68–76
 hypothalamus relationships to, 31, 32f
 in panhypopituitarism, 65–66, 65f, 66f
 pathology and pathophysiology of, 64–76
 posterior, 32–33
 in prolactin hypersecretion, 70–76, 70f, 71f, 72f, 73f, 74f, 75f
 prolactin of, 59–60, 60t
 in TSH deficiency, 66–67
 TSH of, 64
 in testicular function regulation, 177, 178f
Pituitary gonadotropin, human
 administation of, method of, 107
 complications with use of, 109–110
 monitoring treatment cycle of, 108
 pharmacology of, 106–107

Placenta accreta, 94
Placental chorionic gonadotropin. *See* Chorionic gonadotropin, human
Placental lactogen, human, 59
Polybrominated biphenyls, 239
Polychlorinated biphenyls, 234, 239
Polycystic ovarian disease
 amenorrhea from, 313, 321–322
 drug therapy for, 101, 102, 116–117
 luteomas and, 317
 surgical therapy for, 115
Polyostotic fibrous dysplasia, 43
Population growth rates in history of fertility, 11–12, 11t, 12t, 13f
Postcoital test, 131–133, 133f
Prader-Willi syndrome, 38, 39
Prednisone, 114, 115
Pregnancy
 after age thirty-five, 298, 298t
 from artificial insemination, 283
 after bromocriptine therapy for anovulation, 293–294, 293t
 cardiac output in, 2
 after clomiphene therapy for anovulation, 289–291, 291t
 corpus luteum in, 94
 diagnosis of, Babylonian, 3
 diagnosis of, in ancient civilizations, 2
 ectopic, 168–170, 290, 292, 294
 endometriosis and, 256, 260, 297
 from extracorporeal fertilization, 226–227, 226t, 227t, 228–229
 after gonadotropin therapy for anovulation, 291–293, 292t
 with incomplete puberty, 312
 luteomas in, 317
 after recurrent abortion, 297–298
 with uterine abnormalities, 147–149, 295–296
Pregnenolone, 178, 179–180, 309f
Premarin, 133
Progesterone
 abortion from deficiency of, 249
 cervical effect of, 126, 133
 from corpus luteum, 94
 discovery of, 14
 in FSH and LH synthesis and release, 63, 64, 64f
 of follicular fluid, 223
 GnRH affected by, 62
 in menstrual phase of menstrual cycle, 85
 during ovulation, 91
 for ovulation induction, 115, 116
 receptors for, 58, 58f

Progesterone (cont.)
  in secretory phase of menstrual cycle, 92, 94
  synthesis of, LH in, 61
Progestin
  for endometriosis, 261
  in precocious puberty therapy, 43
  for prolactinoma, 74
Prolactin
  dopamine effect on, 35, 59
  function of, 59
  with growth hormone-secreting tumors, 70
  hypersecretion of, 70–76
  in panhypopituitarism, 65, 65f
  secretion of, 59–60, 60t
  structure of, 59
Prolactin inhibitory factor, 59
Prolactinoma, 70, 71
  diagnosis of, 72–74
  treatment of, 74–76
Prostaglandins
  cAMP activity affected by, 55
  endometrial, 85
  in endometriosis, 256, 259
  in secretory phase of menstrual cycle, 94
Pseudohermaphroditism
  female, 316, 316f
  male, 317, 318, 318f
Puberty
  delayed, 311–312
  gonadotropin secretion during, 36–37
  hypothalamus in initiation of, 35–36
  incomplete, amenorrhea from, 312–320, 320t
    from CNS-hypothalamic-pituitary failure, 314
    from chronic estrous anovulation, 313
    from Müllerian agenesis, 314
    from ovarian failure, 313
    from pregnancy, 312
    from testicular feminization, 314–315, 314f
    from vaginal abnormalities, 312–313
  precocious, 36, 42–43
  restraint of onset of, 36, 38f

Radiation therapy
  of growth hormone-secreting tumor, 70
  for pituitary adenoma treatment, 69
  for prolactinoma, 74, 76
Radioimmunoassays
  bioassays vs, 61
  prolactin, 64, 70
Rathke's pouch, 52
Rathke, M.H., 51

Receptors, hormone
  ACTH, 59
  androgen, 180, 181f
  cytoplasmic, 56–58, 58f
  dihydrotestosterone, 180
  estradiol, 58, 63, 178
  follicle stimulating hormone, 178
  in hypothalamus, 177
  luteinizing hormone, 178
  membrane, 54–56, 54f, 55f, 56f, 57f
  progesterone, 58, 62
  steroid, 58
  testosterone, 180
  theory of, 53–54
  thyroid, 64
Reifenstein syndrome, 190
Relaxin, 85, 95
Renaissance period in history of fertility, 6–9, 7f, 8f, 9f, 10f
Renal failure, chronic, 44
Reproduction
  cervix in, 123–137
  in couples previously infertile, 289–298
    after age thirty-five, 298, 298t
    from anovulation, 289–294
    from cervical factor, 296
    from endometriosis, 297
    from in vitro fertilization, 297
    from male factor, 297
    from recurrent abortion, 297–298
    from tubal disease, 294–295, 294t
    from uterine abnormalities, 295–296
  environmental agents in. See Environmental agents, in reproduction
  ethics of intervention in, 337–343
    with artificial insemination, donor, 339–341
    with in vitro fertilization, 342–343
    with surrogate motherhood, 341–342
    tasks of, 337–339
  fallopian tubes in, 161
  hypothalamic control of, 31
  legal issues in, 345–356
    on artificial insemination, 347–350
    on in vitro fertilization, 350–352
    on informed consent, 346–347
    on standard of care, 345–346
    on surrogate motherhood agreements, 352–356
  uterus in, 143
Resolve, Inc., 18, 28, 29
Rete testis, 199

Rokitansky-Küster-Hauser syndrome, 144
Roman customs regarding fertility, ancient, 5–6
Rubin, Isador, 14
Rufus, 5

Sactosalpinx, 172
Saint Hildegard, 6
Saint Margaret, 8
Salicylazosulfapyridine, 235
Salpingitis
  ectopic pregnancy from, 168
  endometriosis vs, 257–258
  from gonorrhea, 13, 171–172
  infertility from, 171
Salpingoplasty, 172–174, 173t, 174t
Salpingostomy, 172–174, 173t, 174t
Sarcoidosis, 44
Scrotum, 202, 203
Semen analysis, 132, 186–187, 280
Seminal plasma
  antigens of, 136
  sperm capacitation and, 163, 186
Seminal vesicle, 199–200
  absence of, 205, 211
Seminiferous tubules
  anatomy of, 199, 200f
  description of, first, 12
  germ cells of, 179
Serophene. See Clomiphene citrate
Sertoli cells, 61, 144
  5-alpha-reductase activity in, 178
  androgen-binding protein from, 177
  aromatase of, 178
  in azoospermia, 188
  in estradiol synthesis, 180
  follicle stimulating hormone binding to, 178
  inhibin from, 177
  interaction of, with Leydig cells, 181
  location of, 177
  Müllerian inhibiting hormone from, 177
  seminal fluid contribution from, 177
  in spermatogenesis regulation, 177, 179
  with torsion of testes, 203
Sexual development, secondary
  clinical progression of, 37
  hypothalamic control of, 31, 36–37
  with Müllerian agenesis, 145
Sexual impotency, 186
Sexual infantilism
  from 17-alpha-hydroxylase deficiency, 308–309
  amenorrhea with, 303
  from anorchia, congenital, 312
  of anorexia nervosa, 40

of congenital hypothalamic dysfunction, 38, 39
from gonadal dysgenesis, 306–308, 307f
from hypothalamic amenorrhea, 309–311, 310t
from Leydig cell agenesis, 312
from pituitary disorders, 311
puberty delayed and, 311–312
Shortened tube syndrome, 167
Sigmund, Karl, 13
Sims, J. Marion, 12–13
Sims-Hühner test, 131, 162
Smoking, 234
Sodium bicarbonate douches, 136
Somatomedins, 60, 61
 function of, 67
 in growth hormone deficiency, 67, 67f
 with growth hormone-secreting tumors, 70
Somatostatin, 34, 61
Soranus, 5
Spallanzani, Lazzarro, 12
Sperm
 acrosome of, 163, 164, 186
 in azoospermia, 188
 capacitation of, 126, 163, 185–186
 cervical mucous penetration of, 131, 296
  assessment of, *in vitro*, 133
  drugs improving, 134–136
  postcoital test of, 131–133
  problems in, treatment of, 133–137, 134f, 135f
 concentration of, in semen, 187
 description of, first, 10, 10f
 environmental agents affecting, 233, 235–236, 235t
 in extracorporeal fertilization, 223
 in fertilization, 163–164
 graduloma of, 207
 immune response to, 128–131
 life span of, in female genital tract, 164
 morphology of, 187
 motility of, 187, 278
 in oligospermia, 190
 in postcoital tests, 132
 smoking effects on, 234
 storage of, in male genital system, 200
 survival of, in cervical mucus, 126
 transport of, 126–127, 127f, 162–163, 185
Spermatic arteries, 201, 201f
Spermatic vein, 201, 203
Spermatocele, 211–212, 211f, 212f
Spermatogenesis
 androgen binding protein in, 180, 185

in cryptorchidism, 202
duration of, 185
environmental agents inhibiting, 235t, 236
FSH in, 61, 61f, 185
hormonal control of, 179, 185
location for, 199, 200f
Sertoli cells in, 177, 179, 185
Spermatogenic deficiency, mild primary, 192
Spiral arteries, 83, 85, 94
Spironolactone, 236
Sterilization
 from gonorrhea, 13
 tubal, 166–168, 166t, 167t
 vasectomy for, 207–208
Stillbirth, 22–23
Stomodeum, 52
Stuart family, 8, 8f
Sulfamethoxazole, 194
Surgery
 cervical, 124
 for cryptorchidism, 202
 for ectopic pregnancy, 168–169
 for endometriosis, 263–265
 fallopian tube abnormalities from, 165–166
 for growth hormone-secreting tumor excision, 70
 for incompetent cervix, 249–250
 for male infertility prevention, 201–203
 myomectomy, 154
 orchiopexy, 202, 203
 ovarian wedge resection, 115–116
 for ovulation induction, 115–116
 for pituitary adenoma excision, 69
 for prolactinoma therapy, 74, 75–76
 salpingostomy, 172–174, 173t, 174t
 for tubal disease, pregnancy outcome after, 294–295
 for uterine abnormalities, 148–151, 150f, 151f
  pregnancy outcome after, 295, 296
 for vaginal agenesis, 146–147, 147f
Surrogate motherhood, 341–342, 352–356
Sympathectomy, 203

Tamoxifen, 103, 103f, 193
Teslac. *See* Testolactone
Testes
 alcohol ingestion affecting, 235
 anatomy of, 199, 200f
 ancient myths concerning, 4, 5
 arterial supply to, 201, 201f
 biopsy of, 205, 207f

cryptorchid, 202
damage to, penalty for, in laws of Hammurabi, 3
estradiol production by, 179–180
germ cells of, 177
gonadotropin releasing hormone effect on, 177–178, 178f
in hormone production, 179–180
LH action in, 61, 61f
Leydig cells of. *See* Leydig cells
Müllerian duct inhibiting factor of, 144
paracrine control of function of, 180–181
protein synthesis in, 178
out of scrotum, 202
Sertoli cells of. *See* Sertoli cells
steroid sulfates from, 181
steroidogenesis in, 178
testosterone production by, 179–180
torsion of, 202–203, 202f
trauma to, 203
in women, 314
Testolactone, 193
Testosterone
 in androgen insensitivity, 145, 146
 of athletes, 42
 in azoospermia, 188
 cimetidine effect on, 236
 dihydrotestosterone from, 179, 180
 estradiol from, 180
 function of, in male reproductive system, 177
 in genital ambiguity, 303
 glucocorticoid effect on, 114, 115
 in gonadotropin secretion regulation, 182
 with hirsutism and clitoral enlargement, 314
 from Leydig cells, 177
 in male genital formation, 144
 in oligospermia, 190
 ovarian wedge resection effect on, 115
 in primary amenorrhea, 305
 receptors for, 180
 in sexual impotency, 186
 in spermatogenesis, 179, 185
 synthesis of,
  deficient, 318–319
  LH in, 61, 61f
  testicular, 179–180, 181
Testosterone enanthate, 193
Testosterone-estradiol binding globulin, 180
Tetracycline, 134, 194, 226
Thalidomide, 231
Theca cells
 as estradiol source, 90–91
 LH stimulation of, 61, 62f, 90
 during ovulation, 91

Thermoregulation
  hypothalamic control of, 31
  with weight loss, 42
Thyroid stimulating hormone, 33, 44
  action of, 63, 64, 64f
  deficiency of, 66–67
  structural composition of, 61
  synthesis and release of, 64
Thyrotropin releasing hormone, 33, 44
  in infusion tests, 73, 75f, 77
  in prolactin secretion, 59, 70
  in thyroid-stimulating hormone synthesis and release, 64
Thyroxine, 33
  in anorexia nervosa, 41
  cytoplasmic receptors for, 56
  in TEBG synthesis, 180
Tompkins metroplasty, 150–151, 151f, 152f
Toxicants, reproductive, 240–242, 241t
Toxins causing abortion, 249
Trichomonas, 128, 134
Triiodothyronine
  in anorexia nervosa, 41
  in TEBG synthesis, 180
Trophoblast, 168–169
Trotula, 6
Tubal insufflator, 14, 14f
Tuber cinereum of hypothalamus, 31
Tudor family, 7, 7f
Tumors
  adenomas,
    ACTH-secreting, 68, 69
    growth hormone-secreting, 69, 70
    pituitary, 64, 65, 68
      pregnancy effect on, 295, 295t
    prolactin-secreting, 70, 71, 72, 73, 73f, 74, 74f, 75, 76
  adrenal, 317, 323
  craniopharyngiomas, 43, 44, 72
  dysontogenetic gonadal, 304–305

  hypothalamic, 43, 44
  testicular, 203
  uterine leiomyomata, 154
  virilizing ovarian, 322
Tunica albuginea, 199, 201
Tunica vaginalis, 212
Tunica vasculosa, 201
Turner's syndrome, 68, 306–308, 307f, 308f

Urinary tract anomalies, 304
Uterine arteries, 83
Uterus
  abnormal positions of, 154
  abnormalities of,
    abortion from, 250
    acquired, 152–154
    congenital, 144, 147–156, 295–296
  agenesis of, 144, 304
  anatomy of, 83
  bicornuate, 148, 149, 150, 150f, 250
  blood supply of, 83
  clot formation in, 85
  contractions of, in menstrual cycle, 85
  didelphic, 124, 147, 149f
  diethylstilbestrol effects on, 152–153, 153f
  double, 147
  embryology of, 144
  in endometriosis, 257, 258
  function of, 143
  leiomyomata of, 154, 250, 295
  psychological aspects of loss of, 26
  retroflexed, 154
  retroversion of, 154
  rudimentary horns of, 147, 149f
  septate, 148, 149, 150–151, 151f, 152f, 250
  synechiae of, 296
  unicornuate, 147, 149f, 250

Vagina
  agenesis of, 144–147, 146f, 313

  amenorrhea from abnormalities of, 312–313
  with testicular feminization, 314
Vaginitis, 128
Vaginoplasty, 146
Van de Velde, 14
Varicocele, 203–205, 204f, 206f
Varicocelectomy, 204
Vas deferens
  absence of, 205, 211
  anatomy of, 199, 200f
  obstruction of, 205
  sperm storage in, 200
  in vasectomy, 207
  in vasoepididymostomy, 209
  in vasovasostomy, 208
Vasal arteries, 201, 201f
Vasectomy, 207–208
Vasoepididymostomy, 209–211, 210f, 211f
Vasography, 205, 207f
Vasopressin, 32
Vasovasostomy, 208–209, 208f, 209f
Venus of Willendorf, 1, 2f
Vesalius, 9, 10f
Viruses causing abortion, 248
Von Baer, Karl Ernst, 12
Von Kolliker, Albert, 12
Von Willebrand's disease, 87

Weight, body
  amenorrhea with loss of, 42
  in anorexia nervosa, 40, 41
  hypogonadotropic hypogonadism and, 39
  in initiation of puberty, 35
  for menstrual cycle onset, 83
Williams, Whitridge, 13
Wolffian duct, 143, 144, 145f

Yttrium implantation, 69

Zona pellucida of ovum, 163, 164, 186